Novel Anticancer Agents

Strategies for Discovery and Clinical Testing

Novel Anticancer Agents

Strategies for Discovery and Clinical Testing

Editors

Alex A. Adjei
Mayo Clinic and Foundation
Rochester, Minnesota

John K. Buolamwini
College of Pharmacy
University of Tennessee Health Science Center
Memphis, Tennessee

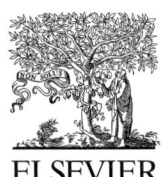

ELSEVIER

AMSTERDAM • BOSTON • HEIDELBERG • LONDON
NEW YORK • OXFORD • PARIS • SAN DIEGO
SAN FRANCISCO • SINGAPORE • SYDNEY • TOKYO
Academic Press is an imprint of Elsevier

Academic Press is an imprint of Elsevier
30 Corporate Drive, Suite 400, Burlington, MA 01803, USA
525 B Street, Suite 1900, San Diego, California 92101-4495, USA
84 Theobald's Road, London WC1X 8RR, UK

This book is printed on acid-free paper.

Library of Congress Cataloging-in-Publication Data
Application submitted

British Library Cataloguing-in-Publication Data
A catalogue record for this book is available from the British Library.

ISBN 13: 978-0-12-088561-9
ISBN 10: 0-12-088561-1

For information on all Elsevier Academic Press publications
visit our Web site at www.books.elsevier.com

Printed in the United States of America

05 06 07 08 09 10   9 8 7 6 5 4 3 2 1

Working together to grow
libraries in developing countries

www.elsevier.com | www.bookaid.org | www.sabre.org

ELSEVIER   BOOK AID
            International   Sabre Foundation

◼ CONTENTS

CONTRIBUTORS XI
PREFACE XV

▮ ▎ STRATEGIES FOR DRUG DISCOVERY

▎ A Survey of Novel Molecular Targets for Anticancer Drug Discovery

JOHN K. BUOLAMWINI

    I. Introduction   1
   II. Overview of Growth Factor Induced Mitogenic Signaling   3
  III. Protein Kinases and Phosphatases   4
  IV. Adapter Proteins   12
   V. GTP-Binding Proteins   12
  VI. Oncogenic Transcription Factors   13
 VII. Apoptosis, Cell Survival, and Life Span Targets   15
VIII. Angiogenesis and Metastasis Molecular Factors   17
  IX. Protein Degradation and Chaperoning Targets   19
   X. Chromatin Remodeling Factors   19
  XI. Conclusion   20
     References   20

v

2 Microarrays: Small Spots Produce Major Advances in Pharmacogenomics

M. NEES, W. KUSNEZOW, AND C. D. WOODWORTH

I. Introduction to Microarrays 38
II. Advantages of DNA Microarrays 44
III. Major DNA Array Formats: Something for Everyone 45
IV. What is the Best Way to Interface with Microarrays? 52
V. Microarrays and Pharmacogenomics: Revolutionizing Discovery of New Drugs and Gene Function 55
VI. What Can Go Wrong in cDNA Microarray Experimentation? 65
VII. Array-Based Proteomics: How to Investigate Protein Complexity 68
VIII. Emerging Microarray Technologies for High-Throughput Proteome Investigation: A Technical Overview 68
IX. Current and Future Applications of Protein Arrays in Drug Discovery 71
X. How to Deal with all that Data 73
XI. The Future is Only Going to Get Better 74
References 76

3 Strategies to Target Chemotherapeutics to Tumors

CHARLES F. ALBRIGHT AND PEARL S. HUANG

I. Background and Rationale 83
II. Antibody-Directed Enzyme Prodrug Technique 84
III. Passive Tumor Targeting 84
IV. Targeting by Binding to Tumor Cell Surface Molecules 85
V. Enzyme-Activated Targeting 85
VI. Summary and Future Directions 90
References 90

4 QSAR and Pharmacophore Mapping Strategies in Novel Anticancer Drug Discovery

JAMES J. KAMINSKI

I. Introduction 93
II. Pharmacophore Definition 94
III. Pharmacophore Validation 99
IV. Conclusions 104
References 104

5 Applications of Nuclear Magnetic Resonance and Mass Spectrometry to Anticancer Drug Discovery

ROBERT POWERS AND MARSHALL M. SIEGEL

I. Introduction 107
II. NMR in Anticancer Drug Discovery 109
III. Mass Spectrometry in Anticancer Drug Discovery 140

IV. MS/NMR Screening Assay 162
V. Conclusions 172
Acknowledgements 172
References 173

6 Antisense Strategies for the Development of Novel Cancer Therapeutics

RUIWEN ZHANG AND HUI WANG

I. Introduction 191
II. Design and Evaluation of Antisence Oligonucleotides 193
III. Conclusion 202
Acknowledgements 203
References 203

7 Antibodies and Vaccines as Novel Cancer Therapeutics

SVETOMIR N. MARKOVIC AND ESTEBAN CELIS

I. Introduction 207
II. Anti-Tumor Antibodies 207
III. Cancer Vaccines 212
IV. Conclusion 218
References 219

8 Inhibitors of Apoptosis as Targets for Cancer Therapy

M. SAEED SHEIKH AND YING HUANG

I. The Inhibitors of Apoptosis 223
II. Concluding Remarks 229
References 230

9 Preclinical Testing and Validation of Novel Anticancer Agents

LLOYD R. KELLAND

I. Introduction 233
II. Target Validation 234
III. A Generic Cascade for Anticancer Drug Discovery 235
IV. High-Throughput Cell-Free Screens for Activity Against the Target 237
V. *In Vitro* Cell Line Models 238
VI. *In Vivo* Testing of Novel Compounds 240
VII. Cassette-Dosing 240
VIII. Pharmaceutical Considerations 241
IX. High-Throughput *In Vivo* Anti-Tumor Testing: The Hollow Fiber Assay 241
X. Human Tumor Xenografts 242
XI. Orthotopic, Transgenic, and Other Animal Models 243

XII. Pharmacodynamics   244
XIII. Summary   245
    Acknowledgements   245
    References   245

▌▌ METHODS FOR CLINICAL TESTING OF NOVEL AGENTS

10 Surrogate End Points and Biomarkers for Early Trials of Novel Anticancer Agents

ALEX A. ADJEI

   I. Introduction   249
  II. What are Targeted Agents?   250
 III. Surrogate Markers or Biomarkers?   250
 IV. Biomarkers as Indicators of Drug Effect *In Vivo*   252
  V. Biomarkers as Predictive Factors   252
 VI. Biomarkers as Prognostic Factors   253
VII. Technical Issues in the Evaluation of Drug Effects *In Vivo*   254
VIII. Lessons for the Future   261
    Acknowledgements   261
    References   261

11 Regulatory Considerations in Clinical Trials of Novel Anticancer Drugs

GRANT WILLIAMS AND RICHARD PAZDUR

  I. Introduction   263
 II. Overview of Cancer Drug Regulation   264
III. Regulatory Considerations in Early Cancer Drug Development   267
IV. Regulatory Considerations in Late Drug Development   271
 V. Conclusion   283
    Acknowledgements   283
    References   283

12 Improving the Efficacy and Safety of Anticancer Agents—The Role of Pharmacogenetics

MARGARET-MARY AMEYAW AND HOWARD L. MCLEOD

  I. Introduction   286
 II. Thiopurine Methyltransferase   286
III. DPD   288
IV. Thymidylate Synthase   289
 V. ABC Family of Drug Transporters   291

VI. UDP-Glucuronosyltransferase IAI Pharmacogenetics and Irinotecan   292
VII. MTHFR Reductase Pharmacogenetics   293
VIII. Cytochrome P4503A Pharmacogenetics   293
IX. Conclusion   293
Acknowledgements   294
References   294

13 Imaging of Pharmacodynamic End Points in Clinical Trials

ERIC O. ABOAGYE, A. R. PADHANI, AND PATRICIA M. PRICE

I. Introduction   300
II. PET   300
III. Evaluation of Cancer Therapeutics with PET   302
IV. MRI Assessment of Microvessel Function   311
V. Conclusions   328
References   328

14 Devising Proof-of-Concept Strategies in Oncology Clinical Trials

PAUL S. WISSEL

I. Introduction   337
II. Proof-of-Concept   338
III. Elements of "The Concept"   339
IV. Application of Surrogate End Points in Proof-of-Concept Decision Making   343
V. Selected Statistical Considerations in Proof-of-Concept Studies   349
VI. Pharmacodynamic Proof-of-Concept End Points   352
VII. Pharmacokinetic Proof-of-Concept End Points   356
VIII. Proceeding From Proof-of-Concept Directly to Phase III   359
IX. Guidelines and Summary   360
Acknowledgements   361
References   361

15 Clinical Trial Designs for Cytostatic Agents and Agents Directed at Novel Molecular Targets

EDWARD L. KORN, LARRY V. RUBINSTEIN, SALLY A. HUNSBERGER, JAMES M. PLUDA, ELIZABETH EISENHAUER, AND SUSAN G. ARBUCK

I. Introduction   366
II. Phase I Dose-Finding Trials   366
III. Preliminary Efficacy Trials   372
IV. Definitive Randomized Efficacy Trials   376
V. Conclusions   377
References   377

16 Cancer Gene Therapy Clinical Trials: From the Bench to the Clinic

EVANTHIA GALANIS

   I. Regulatory Requirements and Good Manufacturing Practices for Gene Transfer Products 381
  II. Preclinical Development of Gene Therapy Vectors/Toxicology Testing 382
  III. Federal and Institutional Approval Processes for Clinical Gene Therapy Trials 383
  IV. Gene Therapy Clinical Trial Design 384
  V. Correlative End Points 386
    References 389

17 Molecular Targets for Radiosensitization

ROGER OVE AND JAMES A. BONNER

   I. Introduction 391
  II. Growth Factor Receptors 394
  III. Ras 399
  IV. Modulation of p53 401
  V. DNA Damage Recognition and Repair 402
  VI. Other Promising Approaches 405
  VII. Conclusions 407
  VIII. Addendum 407
    Addendum References 409
    References 409

18 Patient Accrual to Clinical Trials

SUSAN QUELLA

   I. Introduction 415
  II. Setting Up the Environment 415
    References 425

Index 427

CONTRIBUTORS

Numbers in parentheses indicate the pages on which the authors' contributions begin.

Eric O. Aboagye (299) PET Oncology Group, Department of Cancer Medicine, Imperial College School of Medicine, London, United Kingdom

Alex A. Adjei (249) Mayo Clinic and Foundation, Rochester, Minnesota

Charles F. Albright (83) Dupont Pharmaceuticals, Department of Cancer Research, Glenolden, Pennsylvania

Margaret-Mary Ameyaw (285) Departments of Medicine, Molecular Biology and Pharmacology, and Genetics, Washington University School of Medicine, The Siteman Cancer Center, St. Louis, Missouri

Susan G. Arbuck (365) Aventis Pharmaceuticals, Bridgewater, New Jersey; Current affiliation: Schering Plough Research Institute, Kenilworth, New Jersey

James A. Bonner (391) Department of Radiation Oncology, University of Alabama at Birmingham, Birmingham, Alabama

John K. Buolamwini (1) Department of Pharmaceutical Sciences, College of Pharmacy, University of Tennessee Health Science Center, Memphis, Tennessee

Esteban Celis (207) Mayo Clinic, Department of Immunology, Rochester, Minnesota

Elizabeth Eisenhauer (365) National Cancer Institute of Canada, Clinical Trials Group, Kingston, Ontario, Canada

Evanthia Galanis (379) Division of Medical Oncology, Mayo Clinic and Foundation, Rochester, Minnesota

Pearl S. Huang (83) Dupont Pharmaceuticals, Department of Cancer Research, Glenolden, Pennsylvania

Ying Huang (223) Department of Pharmacology, SUNY Upstate Medical University, Syracuse, New York

Sally A Hunsberger (365) Biometric Research Branch, National Cancer Institute, Bethesda, Maryland

James J. Kaminski (Deceased) (93) Schering-Plough Research Institute, Kenilworth, New Jersey

Lloyd R. Kelland (233) St. George's Hospital Medical School, London, United Kingdom

Edward L. Korn (365) Biometric Research Branch, National Cancer Institute, Bethesda, Maryland

W. Kusnezow (37) Division of Functional Genome Analysis, German Cancer Research Center, Heidelberg, Germany

Svetomir N. Markovic (207) Mayo Clinic, Department of Hematology, Rochester, Minnesota

Howard L. Mcleod (285) Departments of Medicine, Molecular Biology and Pharmacology, and Genetics, Washington University School of Medicine, The Siteman Cancer Center, St. Louis, Missouri

M. Nees (37) Division of Molecular Diagnostics and Therapy, Department of Surgery, University of Heidelberg Germany

Roger Ove (391) Department of Radiation Oncology, University of Alabama at Birmingham, Birmingham, Alabama

A.R. Padhani (299) Paul Strickland Scanner Centre, Mount Vernon Hospital, Middlesex, United Kingdom

Richard Pazdur (263) Division of Oncology Drug Products, Center for Drug Evaluation and Research, Food and Drug Administration, Rockville, Maryland

James M. Pluda (365) Investigational Drug Branch, Cancer Therapy Evaluation Program, National Cancer Institute, Bethesda, Maryland

Robert Powers (107) Department of Chemistry, University of Nebraska Lincoln, Lincoln, Nebraska

Patricia M. Price (299) PET Oncology Group, Department of Cancer Medicine, Imperial College School of Medicine, London, United Kingdom

Susan Quella (413) Mayo Clinic, Mayo Alliance for Clinical Trials (Mayo ACT), Rochester, Minnesota

Larry V. Rubinstein (365) Biometric Research Branch, National Cancer Institute, Bethesda, Maryland

M. Saeed Sheikh (223) Department of Pharmacology, SUNY Upstate Medical University, Syracuse, New York

Marshall M. Siegel (107) Discovery Analytical Chemistry, Wyeth Research, Pearl River, New York

Hui Wang (191) Department of Pharmacology and Toxicology, Cancer Pharmacology Laboratory, Comprehensive Cancer Center, and Gene Therapy Center, University of Alabama at Birmingham, Birmingham, Alabama

Grant Williams (263) Division of Oncology Drug Products, Center for Drug Evaluation and Research, Food and Drug Administration, Rockville, Maryland

Paul S. Wissel (337) Group Director, Clinical Development, GlaxoSmith Kline, Collegeville, Pennsylvania and Adjunct Associate Professor, University of Pennsylvania, Philadelphia, Pennsylvania

C. D. Woodworth (37) Department of Biology, Clarkson University, Potsdam, New York

Ruiwen Zhang (191) Department of Pharmacology and Toxicology, Cancer Pharmacology Laboratory, Comprehensive Cancer Center, and Gene Therapy Center, University of Alabama at Birmingham, Birmingham, Alabama

PREFACE

These are exciting times for the discovery and development of anticancer drugs. Through unprecedented advances in molecular biology and genetics, a myriad of drug targets have been identified in cancer cells. Likewise, advances in combinatorial chemistry, high through-put screening, computational and chemical synthesis have provided hundreds of agents in the clinic and many more in preclinical testing, that attack and inhibit these numerous targets, in an effort to improve the outcomes of patients with malignant neoplasms. While there have been exciting successes with imatinib mesylate and bevacizumab, there have been multiple failures. The current challenge for physicians and scientists involved in research and therapy of cancer is to devise robust methods for identifying and credentialing valid cancer targets, followed by hypothesis-driven rational development strategies that aim at selecting patients who are most likely to respond to particular therapies and to reduce toxicity of therapy. This book brings together basic and clinical scientists who discuss approaches to address the challenges outlined above. The first part provides a survey of validated and emerging novel molecular targets for drug development, and addresses methods of identifying and testing agents pre-clinically. The second part focuses on the challenges facing clinicians in performing rational, hypothesis-driven clinical trials and provides suggestions to overcoming a number of scientific and practical problems. This book should be useful to scientists and clinicians involved in drug development and novel therapeutics in academia, government,t and industry. The editors wish to thank all contributors for their patience during the long and arduous journey that brought this project to fruition.

Alex A. Adjei, M.D., Ph.D.
Rochester, MN
John K. Buolamwini, Ph.D.
Memphis, TN
November 2005

I

STRATEGIES FOR DRUG DISCOVERY

1

A SURVEY OF NOVEL MOLECULAR TARGETS FOR ANTICANCER DRUG DISCOVERY

JOHN K. BUOLAMWINI

Department of Pharmaceutical Sciences
College of Pharmacy
University of Tennessee Health Science Center, Memphis, Tennesse

I. INTRODUCTION
II. OVERVIEW OF GROWTH FACTOR INDUCED MITOGENIC SIGNALING
III. PROTEIN KINASES AND PHOSPHATASES
IV. ADAPTER PROTEINS
V. GTP-BINDING PROTEINS
VI. ONCOGENIC TRANSCRIPTION FACTORS
VII. APOPTOSIS, CELL SURVIVAL, AND LIFE SPAN TARGETS
VIII. ANGIOGENESIS AND METASTASIS MOLECULAR FACTORS
IX. PROTEIN DEGRADATION AND CHAPERONING TARGETS\
X. CHROMATIN REMODELING FACTORS
XI. CONCLUSION

I. INTRODUCTION

Advances in cancer biology over the last decade and a half have uncovered numerous genetic and epigenetic alterations that induce and/or promote oncogenesis and cancer progression by activating oncogenes and/or inactivating tumor supressor genes [1–4]. The completion human genome sequence project [5], and the enormous progress made on the human cancer genome anatomy project [6], have laid solid foundations for the application of tools from the burgeoning fields of genomics (i.e., DNA microarrays, siRNA), proteomics, and bioinformatics for the rapid identification and validation of novel cancer molecular targets [7]. It is now possible to go from gene to target in a short span of time, as shown recently by the use of bioinformatics tools in mining the expressed sequence tags (ESTs) in the human cancer genome anatomy database to identify and validate a novel potential solid tumor therapeutic target, the SIM2-s gene [8]. These targets are providing unprecedented opportunities for developing new cancer therapies that have less-severe side effects than current cytotoxic drugs [9]. Concurrently, innovative drug discovery technologies comprising computer-, crystallography-, and NMR-aided drug design [10–12], as well as combinatorial chemistry and high throughput screening [13, 14] have combined to create fertile grounds for exploiting the targets for novel anticancer drug discovery. At the clinical development level, new trial design approaches will foster the rapid translation of the new agents into effective molecularly targeted cancer therapeutics.

Already, the paradigm of molecularly targeted cancer therapeutics has taken hold in the new millennium, starting with the introduction of Herceptin (trastuzumab) for the treatment of metastatic breast cancer patients whose tumors overexpress the receptor tyrosine kinase oncoprotein HER-2/neu (erbB-2) [15]. Validation of the more widely applicable small molecule drug approach for molecularly targeted cancer therapy was provided by the introduction of Gleevec in 2001. Gleevec (STI571, imatinib) is targeted at the Bcr-Abl tyrosine kinase for the treatment of chronic myelogenous leukemia (CML) [16]. Another small molecule novel cancer drug targeting a receptor tyrosine kinase is Iressa (ZD1389, gefitinib), which was introduced in the United States last year (May, 2003) for treating refractory lung cancer [17]. Iressa inhibits the kinase activity the epidermal growth factor receptor (EGFR), a member of the erbB tyrosine kinase family to which HER-2 also belongs. These successes have served to establish protein tyrosine kinases as a novel class of "druggable" targets for cancer as well as other diseases. In addition to kinases, many other potential cancer therapeutic targets in deregulated or dysregulated molecular pathways of cancer cells have been identified for cancer drug development; and many more will be discovered.

This chapter provides a general survey of validated and emerging novel molecular targets for cancer drug discovery and development, with a focus on those explored for the discovery of molecularly targeted cancer therapeutics. Due to the extensive breadth of coverage and space limitations, details relating to individual molecular targets are limited mainly to those most relevant to drug discovery. Also, it should be noted that not every potential novel target has been considered, but most functional categories are represented.

After an introductory overview of growth factor mitogenic signaling, novel molecular targets are discussed in functional context in the following classes: (1) protein kinases and phosphatases; (2) adaptor proteins; (3) GTP-binding proteins; (4) oncogenic transcription factors; (5) apoptosis, cell survival, and lifespan targets; (6) angiogenesis and metastasis factors; (7) protein degradation and chaperoning targets; and (8) chromatin remodeling factors. Strategies that have been used to develop novel cancer therapies against the novel targets include small molecule and peptide drug development [18, 19], antibody therapeutics [20], antisense therapeutics [21], and gene therapy [23, 23]. It is hoped that the comprehensive and global treatment of novel anticancer cancer targets included in this chapter will further stimulate interest in their exploitation for more effective cancer therapies devoid of the severe toxicities associated with most current cancer drugs.

II. OVERVIEW OF GROWTH FACTOR INDUCED MITOGENIC SIGNALING

The targeting of oncogenic protein tyrosine kinase signal transduction pathways in cancer cells ushered in the molecularly targeted approach to therapeutics [24, 25]. These enzymes are involved in the initiation and relaying of growth and proliferation signals. A general illustration of the relaying of growth factor induced mitogenic signals is given in see Figure 1.1. The signaling cascade is initiated by the growth factors binding to their cognate receptor tyrosine kinases (RTKs) at the extracellular domain. This binding causes receptor dimerization, which induces phosphorylation of the receptors in the intracellular domain. This leads to the recruitment of downstream members particularly adaptor proteins like Grb2, which bind through SH2 domains at phosphorylated sites on the RTK. Grb2 is in turn activated and binds to the guanine nucleotide exchange factor, the sos (son of sevenless), causing its translocation to the cell membrane where it rendevous with the GTP-binding protein Ras. This causes Ras to undergo a critical molecular switch that releases a bound GDP from Ras replaced by GTP instead, which results in the activation of Ras. Ras is a signaling hub that has several other upstream regulators, and downstream effectors [26–29]. In the most studied Ras, signaling cascade, activated Ras binds to raf-1 kinase, which it activates to start a mitogen-activated protein (MAP) serine/threonine kinase cascade. Activated raf-1 phosphorylates the kinase MEK, which in turn phosphorylates the last member in the cascade, extracellular regulated kinase (ERK). Phosphorylated ERK then translocates to the cell nucleus to propagate the mitogenic signal by phosphorylating transcription factors that cause the expression of cell division cycle genes [30–32].

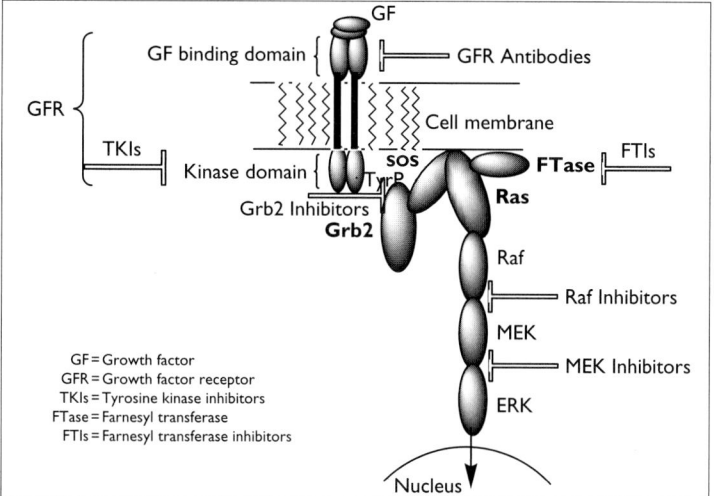

FIGURE 1.1 A simplified outline mitogenic growth factor signaling pathway prior to cell division. Points of potential attack by therapeutic agents are indicated.

The overexpression and/or activating mutations of growth factors and their receptors, as well as other tyrosine kinases and factors in mitogenic signal transduction pathways, have been implicated in many of the major human cancers including breast, ovarian, and non-small cell lung and brain cancers [30, 33], and are pursued intensely as novel molecularly targeted cancer therapy [9, 34–43]. These and other emerging novel cancer molecular targets are discussed in the following sections.

III. PROTEIN KINASES AND PHOSPHATASES

Protein and/or lipid kinases (enzymes that transfer the γ-phosphate group from ATP to OH groups of amino acids in proteins or lipid molecules like phosphatidyl inositols) modulate the cellular functions of numerous other proteins and play critical roles in signal transduction pathways of cell growth, proliferation, differentiation, and survival. Phosphatases are proteins that catalyze the removal of phosphate groups from these phosphorylated species and are important in these signaling pathways as well. It is estimated that of the approximately 32,000 human genes identified in the human genome sequence about 20% code for signal transduction-related proteins, including over 520 known protein kinases and 130 protein phosphatases [44]. They are, as a group, some of the most prone cellular constituents to oncogenic change [44]. In fact, their aberrant expression and/or activation, which results in perturbation of signaling [44], have been observed in various human cancers and other proliferative diseases [37, 45]. Protein kinases are generally divided into two classes: tyrosine kinases and serine/threonine kinases. Tyrosine kinases have been identified as front-end or upstream players in mitogenic signal transduction pathways encompassing both receptor and cytosolic (non-receptor) tyrosine types. Serine/threonine kinases, on the other hand, are more downstream in proliferative signaling and involved in the likes of the MAP kinase signaling cascades as well as cell cycle progression and cell survival pathways.

A. Tyrosine Kinases

The major receptor and cytosolic (non-receptor) tyrosine kinases that have been identified as novel cancer targets will be discussed here as well as strategies taken to develop cancer therapeutics targeting them [37, 46].

1. The HER/ErbB Receptor Tyrosine Kinase Family

The HER/ErbB receptor tyrosine kinase family comprises the EGFR (erbB1, HER-1), HER-2/neu (erbB2), HER-3 (erbB3), and HER-4 (erbB4) receptor tyrosine kinases [32, 47–50]. These RTKs form homo- or heterodimers upon binding with their specific growth factors (ligands), with the exception of HER-2 for which no specific ligand has been identified. Consequently, HER-2 depends on heterodimerization with the other family members to be activated under normal conditions [50]. The erbB receptors and their role in cancer progression have been reviewed recently [51]. EGFR and HER-2 have emerged as probably the most viable novel cancer molecular targets in this family. However, there is much cooperativity among members, even though they have their distinctive substrates and activating triggers. For example, EGFR is activated by either overexpression or mutation whereas HER-2 appears to be activated only by overexpression resulting from gene amplification. ErbB receptor overexpression or activating mutation is frequently encountered in breast, ovarian, and non-small cell lung cancers [30, 33, 46, 48]. It has recently been demonstrated that ErbB3/HER-3 is an essential partner in transformation by HER-2, coupling its effects to the phosphatidylinositol 3-kinase/protein kinase B pathway in breast cancer cells [51]. Therefore HER-2 signaling through a mitogen-activated protein kinase (MAPK) arm alone is not sufficient for transformation. Interestingly. HER3 is said to have a nonfunctional kinase domain.

Antibody anticancer therapeutics based on EGFR or HER-2 have been developed [34, 52, 53]. Cetuximab (erbitux, IMC-C225) is a monoclonal antibody targeted to EGFR that is in advanced clinical trials for cancer therapy [52]. In the case of HER-2, monoclonal antibody drug, trastzumamab (Herceptin, Genentech, South San Francisco, CA) is already in the clinic for treating metastatic breast cancers that overexpress HER-2 [54]. Small molecule anticancer drug discovery approaches based on EGFR and/or c-erbB-2 tyrosine are being pursued extensively. Success has been forthcoming with agents that inhibit their kinase activity in competition against ATP in the catalytic site [34, 36, 38, 42, 55]. The availability of the X-ray crystal structures of the catalytic domains of several RTKs alone or in complex with substrates or inhibitors [56], which includes the recent structures of EGFR [57], is facilitating selective kinase inhibitor design. The most successful compounds are the anilinoquinazolines and analogs. A major attractive feature about these agents is that not only are they not as toxic as current cytotoxic chemotherapy drugs, but they can be administered orally. In this regard, the quinazoline ZD1839 (Iressa, gefitinib) has been approved in the United States for the treatment of refractory lung cancer [34]. Other EGFR-targeted small molecules in clinical development include OSI-774 (erlotinib/Tarceva), PD-153053, PD-168393, and CI-1033 [58, 59]. No small molecule drugs against HER-2 have been approved yet, but there are some in the cancer drug development pipelines. Interestingly, HER-2 has been shown to be a client of the heat shock protein Hsp90, which is important for the function of several oncogenic kinases including bcr-able and src kinases. Actively pursued inhibitors of Hsp90, like the geldanamycin analogs, would be indirect inhibitors of HER-2 function as well [60, 61]. Antisense therapy against these RTKs is being explored [62, 63].

2. Other Receptor Tyrosine Kinase Cancer Molecular Targets

In addition to the HER or erbB family of oncogenic RTKs, several other RTKs constitute potential novel molecular targets for cancer drug discovery such as the platelet-derived growth factor receptor (PDGFR). Its signaling is known to control cell proliferation and tumor angiogenesis and to maintain cell survival [64]. Gliomas are particularly noted for deregulated PDGFR signaling [33]. Small molecule selective inhibitors of PDGFR have been identified, which include 2-phenylaminopyrimidines such as STI571 (Gleevec or imatinid) [40]. This is also currently used to treat CML. It has been reported recently that mutations involving the fusion of the Fip1-like 1 (FIP1L1) gene to the PDGFR-alpha (PDGFRalpha;) gene produces a constitutively activated tyrosine kinase, FIP1L1-PDGFRalpha, that is the molecular target of imatinib in hypereosinophilic syndrome [65]. 3-Arylsubstituted quinoxalines and quinolines are also among PDGFR kinase inhibitors [40]. Leflunomide (SU101) is an effective inhibitor of PDGFβ-promoted glioma tumor growth *in vivo* [66]. Interestingly the small molecule agent SCH 13929 interacts with, and competitively inhibits the binding of PDGF to its receptors, thus inhibiting its functions both *in vitro* and *in vivo* [67].

The vascular endothelial growth factor receptors, VEGFR-1 (flt-1), VEGFR-2, and VEGFR-3, as well as basic fibroblast growth factor receptor (bFGFR) are RTKs implicated in tumor angiogenesis through induction of the proliferation of endothelial cells [68–71]. Small molecular and antibody approaches have identified effective inhibitors of these targets that are being developed for clinical use. The compounds include SU5416, a VEGFR-2 (flk-1)-selective kinase inhibitor in advanced clinical development [72]. PTK787 is a new potent kinase inhibitor of both VEGFR-1 and VEGFR-2 receptors, with IC_{50} values of 0.077 and 0.037 μM, respectively [73]. Interestingly in the case of the VEGF/VEGFR system targeting the growth factors themselves with antibodies have also been productive to the extent that bevacizumab (Avastin), a humanized antibody targeted to circulating VEGF, has been useful as an antiangiogenic agent for the treatment of metastatic colorectal cancer [74]. PD145709 and SU5402 are selective bFGFR receptor kinase inhibitors [75, 76]. In addition to its angiogenesis promotion function, bFGFR has been implicated in the induction of the MDM2 protein through a p53-independent mechanism resulting in cell survival and drug resistance [77].

Another potential novel cancer molecular target in the RTK genre is c-kit, which has been shown to be mutated and constitutively active in certain human gastrointestinal stromal cancers [78]. c-Kit has also been shown to be overexpressed in about 75% of small cell lung cancers (SCLC), and is being pursued for drug development in this regard [79]. Interestingly, STI571 (imitinib) again inhibits its kinase activity and is being tested.

The c-Met receptor tyrosine kinase and its ligand, hepatocyte growth factor (HGF), constitute another receptor tyrosine kinase system implicated in the development and progression of several human cancers that might be a target for cancer therapy. Recently, a small molecule selective ATP-competitive inhibitor of c-Met kinase activity, PHA-665752, inhibited HGF-stimulated and constitutive c-Met phosphorylation, as well as HGF and c-Met-driven cell proliferation, survival, and invasion [80]. This compound was also shown to suppress gastric tumor growth in a xenograft model.

The IGF-I receptor tyrosine kinase (IGF-IR) is also an important player in oncogenesis. In addition to its own transforming effects, it is also required for transformation by other oncogenes, including src, Ras, PDGFR, and EGFR in some cell systems [81]. It has been shown to enhance invasion and induce resistance to apoptosis in colon cancer cells through the Akt/Bcl-xL pathway [82]. High levels of circulating IGF-I, a ligand of IGF-IR have been associated with increased risk for development of breast cancer in premeno-pausal women [83]. IGF-IR would appear to be a potential novel molecular target for cancer therapy, although it is less vigorously pursued than other RTKs like HER-2 and EGFR. A potential problem is that inhibitors of IGF-IR would also inhibit insulin receptor function. Several small molecule inhibitors of IGF-IR have been reported including the tyrphostins such as AG1024 and AG1034 and heterarylurea compounds. Interestingly, AG1024 was shown to overcome the resistance of human primary glioblastoma cells to anti-EGR therapy, which was thought to be mediated by IGF-IR signaling through PI3-kinase/Akt [84]. The availability of several high-resolution X-ray crystal structures of catalytic domain of IGF-IR in activated forms and in complex with substrates [85, 86] should facilitate structure-based discovery of selective small molecule inhibitors.

Another potential cancer molecular target is FLT3, receptor tyrosine kinase involved in hematopoiesis. It is the most frequently mutated gene in acute myelogenous leukemia (AML) and is associated with poor prognosis; it may be a therapeutic target for patients with this disease as well [87]. It has been identified as an oncogene and a therapeutic target for a mixed lineage leukemia — rearranged acute lymphoblastic leukemia (MLL). The Flt3 inhibitor PKC412 has been shown to inhibit the proliferation of Ba/F3 cells dependent upon its activation [88]. The therapeutic efficacy of CT53518, a piperazinyl quinazoline inhibitor of FLT3, has been demonstrated in both in a nude mouse model and in a murine bone marrow transplant model of FLT3-ITD-induced disease [89].

The RTKs EPH-A2/ECK and EPH-B3 are overexpressed in over 90% of melanoma cell lines and might constitute drug development targets for melanoma [90]. Ret is a RTK that is required for development of the kidneys and enteric system and for neuronal differentiation and survival. In response to ligand, Ret is activated by heterodimer formation with one of four struc-turally related glycosylphosphatidylinositol (GPI)-linked cell-surface receptors, GFR-α1–4 [44]. Somatic rearrangements that result in fusions between the N terminus of various proteins and the TK domain of Ret can lead to constitu-tive dimerization of the fusion proteins, and result in papillary thyroid carcino-mas (PTCs). Activating mutations in Ret cause multiple endocrine neoplasia 2A (MEN2A), MEN2B, and familial medullary thyroid carcinoma. Targeting Ret activity in these neoplasias might constitute a viable therapeutic approach, which has yet to be explored.

3. Non-Receptor/Cytosolic Tyrosine Kinases

In addition to the receptor tyrosine kinases, non-receptor or cytosolic tyrosine kinases are also involved in mitogenic signaling transduction. The src gene product pp60^{src} is an important oncogenic non-receptor protein tyrosine kinase, which is important for signaling from many RTKs and has been associated with several cancer types [91], such as colon [33] and pan-creatic [92]. In addition to other kinase activation mechanisms available to src, including dephosphorylation by several protein tyrosine phos-phatases, RTKs can also activate src by providing phosphorylated tyrosine SH2 domain docking sites [44]. This makes src an important downstream signaling target utilized by several oncogenic RTKs to augment their transformation capacity. Another major known oncogenic member of the src family is the lck gene product p56[lck] [93], which is deregulated in T-cell lymphomas and as such is a potential therapeutic target for these malignancies [94]. Lck transduces signals important for the development of alphabeta and gammadelta T cells [95].

The bcr-abl gene product p210[bcr-abl] is deregulated in most chronic myelogenous leukemias [33]. 2-Substituted aminopyrido[2,3-d]pyrimidinones [96] have been found to have selective inhibitory activity against pp60[src]. Other small molecule pp60[src]-specific inhibitors include 5,10-dihydropyrimidino[4,5-b] quinolin-4[1H]-ones and 3-[N-phenyl]carboxamide-2-iminochromene derivatives [40]. The 3-[N-phenyl]carboxamide-2-iminochromene derivatives also inhibit the kinase activity p56[lck]. X-ray crystal structure-based design of novel small molecule inhibitors has also been undertaken [97]. The 2-phenylaminopyrimidine derivative, CGP 57148 [STI571, Gleevec], is a potent inhibitor of the bcr-abl gene product p210[bcr-abl] tyrosine kinase *in vitro* and *in vivo* [98] and has recently been approved for the treatment of CML [16]. This drug, as mentioned in the previous section, also inhibits c-kit tyrosine kinase [78, 99], as well as PDGFR kinase [40]. Key small molecule inhibitors have also been identified for p56[lck], including dihydroxystyrene salicylic acid, a dihydroxyisoquinoline derivative and a pyrazolo[3,4-d]pyrimidine derivative [40].

B. Serine/Threonine Kinases

1. Cytoplasmic Serine/Threonine Kinases

Several cytoplasmic oncogenic serine/threonine kinases have also been identified, such as some members of the protein kinase C (PKC) family, protein kinase A (PKA), protein kinase B (PKB; Akt), and the MAP kinases. They are also being investigated as novel targets for cancer therapy.

2. PKC, PKA, and PKB

Efforts are underway to develop specific inhibitors targeting the serine/ threonine kinases designated PKC, PKA, and PKB, commonly referred to as Akt as novel anticancer drugs. PKC isozymes, some of which are calcium-dependent [100], participate in cell growth regulation and tumor promotion, and are the prime molecular targets of tumor promoting phorbol esters [101–103]. Most are activated by the endogenous molecule, diacylglycerol [104]. There is cross-talk between PKC and the Ras-Raf-MEK-ERK signaling pathway [28]. PKC overexpression has been observed in estrogen receptor negative breast cancer, thyroid cancer, gliomas, and melanoma [105]. PKC overexpression has also been implicated in tumor angiogenesis [105]. These observations have focused attention on this family for novel anticancer drug development [105–111]. The PKCα isoform has been shown to be overexpressed in multidrug resistant cancers [105, 107, 112, 113]. The antiproliferative effect of PKC inhibitors has been shown to be cell context dependent [107]. Several nonspecific PKC inhibitors have been discovered and these include 7-hydroxystaurosporin (UCN-01), a Chk1 inhibitor [114], and safingol

[106, 107, 109, 115]. CGP 53506 is said to be selective against PKCα and it has been shown to inhibit tumor growth [116]. The X-ray crystal structure of PKC δ in complex with a phorbol ester is used in structure-based design for the discovery of novel PKC modulators [117–119]. The attractive feature about PKC inhibitors is their ability to induce apoptosis independent of p53 functional status. However, enthusiasm dampened when it was discovered that most of the inhibitors inhibited other cellular proteins. A case in point was the finding that UCN-01 was a potent inhibitor of Chk1 kinase [114]. The lack of specificity of current PKC modulators makes it questionable whether their effects are really due to modulation of PKC, as many also inhibit other serine/threonine kinases, especially cyclin-dependent kinases. Altered protein kinase C-α (PKC-α) expression has been implicated in tumor promotion and carcinogenesis. Antisense approaches to the inhibition of PKCα have advanced into clinical trials [120], particularly the ISIS agent LY900003 (ISIS 3521, afinitak). This agent has shown good clinical activity especially in combination with chemotherapy [120]. Protein kinase Cζ has been shown to regulate p70 S6 kinase in conjunction with phosphoinositide 3-kinase [121].

Cyclic AMP-dependent protein kinase (PKA), has also been the target of novel anticancer drug discovery. In this regard, a cyclic AMP analog, 8-chloro-cyclic AMP targeted at PKA has been shown to inhibit tumor growth [122]. Antisense oligonucleotides have also been designed against this target and are being evaluated in preclinical models [123].

PKB isoforms, also known as Akts, have been shown to be key participants in cell survival pathways via the PI-3 kinase signaling pathways [124, 125] in several cancers such as breast, prostate, colon, and brain [44]. Akts bind to membrane phosphatidylinositide 3-phosphates, and are subsequently activated through phosphorylation by phosphatidylinositol-dependent kinases [126–128]. Akt phosphorylates GSK-3β, the anti-apoptotic protein BAD, the forkhead transcription factors, and other targets [129, 130]. Akt also signals through transcription factors such as NF-κB to promote cell survival [131]. It has been shown that Akt also has metastatic promoting capacity [132].

It is worth noting that PI-3 kinase is different from the other kinases discussed in this chapter, in that it phosphorylates membrane phosphoinositide lipids at the 3-position hydroxyl group. PI-3 kinase is negatively regulated by the tumor-suppressor gene PTEN (phosphatase and tensin homolog detected in chromosome 10) [133, 134]. PI-3 kinase activation promotes cell cycle entry by inducing cyclin D synthesis, and also controls cell growth (increase in mass) by regulating the activities of the mammalian target of rapamycin (mTOR) and p70 S6K [135]. mTOR as a downstream effector PI-3K/Akt signaling pathway that mediates cell survival and proliferation, is an attractive target for anticancer drug development [136–138]. The flavonoid derivative, LY294002 is an ATP-binding site competitive, reversible potent inhibitor of the PI-3K [139]. By targeting mTOR, the immunosuppressant and antiproliferative agent rapamycin and its analogs CCI-779, RAD 001, and AP23573 inhibit signals required for cell cycle progression, cell growth, and proliferation, and are now pursued as clinical agents [136].

3. MAP Kinases

The classical MAP kinase cascade downstream from Ras [1, 140–143] harbors two important protooncogenic proteins that are explored as potential novel anticancer drug targets: Raf-1 and MEK [144–146]. Activated Ras binds and activates MEK, which in turn phosphorylates and activates the MAP kinase ERK. This causes ERK to translocate into the cell nucleus to induce the transcription of genes required for cell division. In addition to mitogenic signaling, Raf-1 also participates in anti-apoptotic signaling through both MEK-dependent and -independent mechanisms. MEK-dependent Raf anti-apoptotic effects involve ERK activation, which promotes Rsk1 phosphorylation and inactivation of the pro-apoptotic protein BAD [147] and/or activation of the cell survival transcription factor CREB [148]. MEK-independent cell survival signaling by raf is thought to involve its targeting to mitochondria and possible interaction with the Bcl-2 family of proteins [149–151].

In addition to kinase-dependent cell survival effects, raf-1 also promotes cell survival in a kinase-independent mechanism by antagonizing the apoptosis signal-regulating kinase 1 (ASK-1) protein through protein-protein interaction [152]. Antisense oligonucleotides against raf-1 mRNA have been developed and are tested in the clinic as molecular cancer therapeutics [21, 153]. Small molecule approaches to Raf-1 kinase inhibition are also being pursued. Thus, BAY-43–9006 is in clinical trails [146]. Selective small molecule inhibitors of MEK have also been discovered: PD 98059, which inhibits cell growth and reversed Ras transformation [154], and CI-1040, which suppresses colon tumor growth *in vivo* [146].

4. Oncogenic Cell Cycle Serine/Threonine Kinases

When activated MAP kinases translocate to the cell nucleus they initiate transcription programs that induce the expression of genes to begin the cell division cycle process. Serine/threonine kinases, termed cyclin-dependent kinases (CDKs), function in complexes with their activating cyclins (regulatory units) to drive progression through the different phases of the cell division cycle [155–157]. CDKs are kept under control by nuclear proteins termed cyclin-dependent kinase inhibitors (CKIs) and exemplified by p21, p27, p57, and p16 [158–162]. G1 cyclins and their CDK complexes phosphorylate the retinoblastoma (Rb) tumor-suppressor protein and related proteins, as well as the E2F transcription factor family [163–165]. CDKs have emerged as potential targets for novel anticancer drug discovery [166–170], with several small molecule ATP-site competitive CDK inhibitor drugs under development [101, 157, 171]. Important CDK inhibitors in this regard are flavopiridol, olumoucine, and its analog roscovitine. Flavopiridol is quite non-selective, inhibiting CDK1, CDK2, CDK4, CDK6, and CDK9 [169]. This CDK inhibition has been shown to result in cell cycle arrest in G1, independent of functional status of p53 or Rb [172], as well as cell cycle arrest at G2. The latter is attributed to the inhibition of the kinase activity of cyclin B-CDK1. Flavopiridol is being studied in clinical trials [105, 173]. The ability of CDK inhibitors to induce apoptosis independent of p53 status has been an attractive property of the group. This has been attributed to the ability of CDK inhibitors to perturb the function of CDK-cyclin complexes like CDK9/cyclin T, which is not involved with the progression of the cell cycle, but participates in regulating RNA polymerase [174]. The anti-HIV activity of flavopiridol is thought to be derived from the inhibition of RNA polymerase [175], which is an emerging potential target for anti-HIV drug development.

The purine-derivative CDK inhibitors olumoucine and analog roscovitine are more selective than flavopiridol and are also under clinical study [176]. Other significant CDK inhibitors are the purvalanols [177], the paulones [178], indigoids [179], and aminothiazoles [180]. Recent evidence seems to suggest that the cell cycle can proceed in the absence of CDK2 and cyclin E [181]. This may have to be taken into consideration by drug discovery projects based on this system.

The oncogenic serine/threonine kinases polo-like kinase [182] and aurora-2 kinase [183] are also emerging as attractive potential cancer targets in the cell cycle progression machinery. These have been shown to the aberrantly expressed predominantly in non-small cell lung cancer and colorectal cancers, respectively. The potential of aurora-2 as a novel cancer target has been reviewed recently [184]. A derivative of the natural product shikonin, beta-hydroxyisovalerylshikonin, it has recently been reported to induce apoptosis in human leukemia K562 cells by inhibiting polo-like kinase 1 [185]. This agent is said to be a substrate competitive inhibitor of protein kinases [186]. No small molecule inhibitors have been reported for aurora kinase; However, this situation may soon change with the publication of X-ray crystal structures of Aurora-2 kinase [187, 188].

Chk1 is also a serine/threonine kinase that is an important mediator of cell cycle arrest in G2 following DNA damage, and has a potential role in cancer therapeutics [134]. The ability of 7-hydroxystaurosporine (UCN-01) to abrogate the G2 checkpoint is attributed to inhibition of Chk1 kinase activity [189]. High-resolution X-ray crystal structures of human Chk1 kinase domain in complex with staurosporine, UCN-01, or the related compound SB-218078 have been reported [190], and should serve as templates for structure-based design of small molecule inhibitors. Drugs that target Chk1 and Chk2 have the potential to improve the efficacy of DNA-damaging agents in cancer patients [191].

C. Protein Phosphatases

Unlike the protein kinases, aberrant protein phosphatase activity has not been shown to be extensively involved in malignancies. Nevertheless, a few oncogenic protein phosphatases have been identified such as those in the Cdc25 family that are oncogenic [192]. These dual specific phosphatases are involved primarily in cell cycle progression. There are three in the family; namely Cdc25A, Cdc25B, and Cdc25C [192]. The oncogenic members of the family of three (A, B, and C) isoforms are Cdc25A and B. Overexpression of Cdc25B has been demonstrated in 32% of human primary breast cancers [192]. Widespread overexpression of Cdc25A and Cdc25B has been documented in many human cancers, including breast, colon, gastric, head-and-neck and non-small-cell lung cancers, esophageal squamous-cell carcinoma, colorectal carcinoma, non-Hodgkin's lymphoma, and neuroblastoma [193].

Overexpression of Cdc25A is associated with poor survival in breast cancer patients [193]. Combinatorial libraries have been synthesized and screened for Cdc25 inhibitors, which resulted in the discovery of potent inhibitors like SC-$\alpha\alpha\delta$9, which suppress tumor growth [193, 194]. Novel arylating K vitamin analogs have also been shown to inhibit Cdc25A [195].

IV. ADAPTER PROTEINS

As illustrated in Figure 1, adaptor proteins like the Grb2 bind to tyrosine kinases and provide docking sites to recruit downstream targets for signal propagation. Inhibiting them will provide a means for simultaneously block-ing mitogenic signals deriving from both receptor and non-receptor tyrosine kinases [196, 197]. Grb2 has emerged as one of the important potential can-cer molecular targets in this category [198]. There are two types of domains on the Grb2 protein, which it uses to perform its adapter function: SH2 (src homology 2) and SH3 (src homology 3) [199]. The SH2 domain is used to bind to phosphotyrosine. The Grb2 SH2 domain has been successfully tar-geted by peptides and small molecule inhibitors [196]. A cyclic tetrapeptide has recently been reported that binds the GrB2 SH2 domain with picomolar level affinity, and is able to block Grb2-Her-2 association as well as inhibit the mitogenic effects of HER-2 [200].

V. GTP-BINDING PROTEINS

Ras, a 21-kDa GTP-binding protein is the flagship member of this class of novel anticancer molecular targets. Ras is a critical signal-relaying hub in cell proliferation and differentiation and survival [201]. Three members, K-Ras, H-Ras, and N-Ras, have been identified in humans [202, 203]. Ras oncogenic mutations are found in 30% of human cancers, and are particularly prevalent in pancreatic cancer (90%), colorectal cancer (50%), lung cancer (40%), and myeloid leukemias (30%) [204]. Currently there are no agents that can disrupt either Ras-sos or Ras-raf interactions. The availability of the X-ray crystal structure of the Ras-sos complex [205] may allow attempts at structure-based design of Ras-sos interaction inhibitors. However, this will be a difficult task as the binding interface is large and is not a preferred scenario for small molecule inhibitor design. The Ras-related GTP-binding proteins Rac and Rho have also been proposed as potential drug discovery targets [206]. These proteins are key players in cytoskeletal reorganizations. Rho suppresses p21 to allow Ras to drive cells into S phase [29]. The Rho family GTPases Rac1 and Cdc42 have also been shown to regulate p70S6K [207]. Recently it has also been demonstrated that RhoB is critical for vascular development in terms of sprout morphology and colocalizes with Akt to promote cell survival in sprouting endothelial cells of newly forming vessels [208]. This has uncov-ered a link between RhoB and the Akt survival-signaling pathway. It appears that RhoB association with Akt allows its nuclear localization. This suggests that RhoB is a potential angiogenic cancer molecular target.

Anticancer drug discovery targeting oncogenic Ras has focused on antisense oligonucleotides [21] and small molecule inhibitors of Ras farnesyl transfeRase [209, 210]. Most of the successful antisense therapeutics are those that target mutant H-Ras mRNA, which have shown efficacy in preclinical models and are currently being evaluated in clinical trials with some clinical activity being reported [21, 211, 212]. Ras farnesylation is required to anchor newly translated Ras protein to the cell membrane before it can perform its signal transduction functions [213, 214]. This is accomplished by Ras farnesyl transfeRase (FTase). Ras farnesylation involves the transfers of a farnesyl moiety from farnesyl pyrophosphate to the cysteine in the CAAX amino acid sequence at the C terminus of Ras (where C is cystein, A is any aliphatic amino acid, and X is any amino acid) [209, 215]. Many FTase-selective inhibitors have been discovered for targeting the Ras for cancer chemotherapy [215–217]. SCH66336 and R115777 are two orally active Ras FTase inhibitors in clinical trials for several cancers [210, 218]. In view of the high frequency of Ras mutations in pancreatic cancer, Ras-directed agents might provide effective therapies for this cancer, which has been very difficult treat. Advanced clinical trials of SCH66336 and R115777 in pancreatic cancer are under way [219].

VI. ONCOGENIC TRANSCRIPTION FACTORS

Several oncogenic transcription factors have been identified including myc, ets, fos, jun, NF-κB, and myb. These play important roles in proliferation, differentiation, and/or cell survival pathways [1, 220, 221]. Myc, which was one of the first oncogenic transcription factors identified, was shown to cooperate with Cyclin D1 in promoting malignancy of B-cell lymphoma [222, 223]. Myc cooperation with the anti-apoptotic protein Bcl-2 in oncogenic transformation has also been shown [224]. Further, myc has also been shown to activate telomerase in human mammary epithelial cells and normal human diploid fibroblasts [225]. C-Myc overexpression has been associated with the etiology of many major types of human neoplasia including Burkitt's lymphoma, colorectal cancer, breast cancer, prostate cancer, and melanoma [226]. The related N-myc and L-myc oncogenes are potential molecular targets in neuroblastoma and small cell lung cancer, respectively. Inhibiting c-myc expression can induce differentiation and reverse transformation [227]. Antisense and antigene approaches to c-myc-targeted cancer therapy are being pursued [21]. In addition, G-quadruplex oligonucleotides are also being explored based on studies of the c-myc promoter region [226]. Small molecule specific inhibitors of myc oncogenes are not yet available. It has recently been shown in osteosarcoma cells that a sustained loss of c-myc function and reversal of neoplastic phenotype occur even by a brief period of inactivation [228]. Phosphorodiamidate morpholino oligomer (PMO) antisense oligonucleotides have been successfully used to inhibit of c-myc expression. One such oligomer, AVI-4126, has demonstrated efficacy in a PC-3 androgen-independent human prostate cancer xenograft mouse model, which has been shown to be suitable for human clinical trials [229].

NF-κB (nuclear factor-κB) is another transcription factor that is emerging as a potential anticancer drug target [230, 231]. NF-κB has been implicated in both carcinogenesis and tumor progression, playing a role in proliferation and cell survival. In the inactivated form, NF-κB resides in the cytoplasm as a heterodimeric protein composed of different combinations of members of the Rel family of transcription factors, which are bound to inhibitory proteins, the IκBs [232, 233]. The IκB keeps NF-κB from entering the cell nucleus, thereby inactivating it. The NF-κB family is involved mainly in stress-induced, immune, and inflammatory responses. The phosphorylation of IκB by IκB kinases, IKKα or IKKβ, causes its 26S proteasome-assisted degradation and the release of NF-κB, which then translocates into the nucleus to effect the transcription of target genes [234]. The anticancer activity of the proteasome inhibitor PS-341 (a newly introduced novel molecularly targeted anticancer drug is said to involve inhibition of the degradation of IκB, thereby inhibiting the transcriptional activity of NF-κB) [235]. Inhibitors of IKK activity that prevent IκB phosphorylation like PS-1145, also inhibit NF-κB activation [236]. PI-3 kinase/Akt signaling has been shown to cause phosphorylation and activation of IKKs, and thus participate in NF-κB transcriptional activation, albeit in cell-type-dependent fashion based on the cellular level of the IKKα isoforms [237]. NF-κB has been shown to be involved in apoptosis and cell survival signaling in a cell-context-dependent manner [238, 239] and to be important in oncogenesis and cancer progression [240].

Recently, the transcription factor hypoxia-inducible factor 1 (HIF-1) has also been shown to be important in cancer progression and angiogenesis. Its overexpression has been correlated with treatment failure and mortality in brain, breast, cervical, esophageal, oropharyngeal, and ovarian cancers [241]. Tumor-suppressor proteins such as VHL, PTEN, and p53 have all been reported to inhibit HIF-1α function, but in different ways. The VHL tumor-suppressor gene is a ubiquitously expressed cellular regulator of HIF-1α half-life. VHL is an E3 ligase that binds HIF-1α, and targets it for ubiquitin-mediated degradation. Tumor cells that have decreased VHL expression have increased concentrations of HIF-1α, as well as of HIF-1α target gene products, under aerobic conditions. A luciferase reporter based cell screen has been used to discover inhibitors of HIF-1α as reported in a recent study [242]. Among these inhibitors were analogs of the topoisomeRase I inhibitor anticancer agent camptothecin. HIF-1α has been touted as an attractive molecular target for cancer drug development, as was demonstrated by the inhibition of colon tumor xenograft growth by disruption of the interaction between HIF-1α and the coactivator p300/CREB [243]. The potential of HIF-1α as a general therapeutic target has been reviewed, and cancer stands out as a major disease area that could benefit from selective HIF-1α inhibitors [244].

The peroxisome proliferator-activated receptors (PPARs) are nuclear hormone receptors that mediate the transcriptional effects of peroxisome proliferators. These are ligand-activated transcription factors and have been implicated in various diseases including cancer [245]. PPARs heterodimerize with another nuclear hormone receptor, retinoid X receptor, and exert their effects via regulation of gene transcription upon binding of the ligand. Three isotypes are known: α, γ, and δ. At present PPARγ ligands are used in the treatment of type 2 diabetes exemplified by the thiazolidinedione like troglitazone. PPARγ activity has been shown to control the cell cycle and induce cell differentiation and apoptosis, and agonists of this nuclear receptor are potential cancer therapeutic agents [246]. These agonists were shown to inhibit cell proliferation and induce apoptosis in human melanoma cells [247]. It has also been reported that genetic disruption of PPARδ decreases the tumorigenicity of human colon cancer cells [248]. These examples indicate the attempts at exploration of PPARs as novel targets for cancer therapeutics.

The transcription factor Gli is activated by a sonic hedgehog signaling pathway, and its abnormal activation has been implicated in familial and sporadic cancers, which include basal cell carcinomas, medulloblastomas, and rhabdomyosarcoma, especially medulloblastoma [249–252]. Small molecule inhibitors of smoothened, a key molecular target in the pathway, may be developed as treatment for medulloblastoma. Examples of such compounds are cyclopamine [253] and Cur41414 [254, 255].

VII. APOPTOSIS, CELL SURVIVAL, AND LIFE SPAN TARGETS

Apoptosis (i.e., programmed cell death) is an evolutionary conserved cellular suicide program with defined biochemical and morphologic characteristics [256]. Apoptosis is essential for maintaining cell number balance in developing organisms as well as the homeostasis of adult tissues. In addition, apoptosis is used by cellular surveillance mechanisms to eliminate cells carrying deleterious mutations, fatal abnormalities, or infectious agents. Cancer is characterized by clonal expansion of abnormal cells that resist the apoptotic machinery that should have caused their elimination [257]. Methods to induce apoptosis are sought in current cancer therapeutics [258].

The p53 tumor suppressor gene is a key inducer of apoptosis in the intrinsic pathway, and has been dubbed the "guardian of the genome" [259]. Research on p53 arguably dominated cancer research in the early 1990s, which resulted in p53 named as molecule of the year in *Science* magazine in 1993 [260]. p53 functions mainly as a transcription factor, which causes cell cycle arrest or apoptosis in response to DNA damage [189, 261]. p53 is also involved in DNA repair as well as other functions [262]. The cell cycle arrest function of p53 is achieved primarily through the transcriptional induction of the cyclin-dependent kinase inhibitor p21 and/or GADD45 gene product [263], while its apoptosis induction function stems mainly from transcriptional induction of the Bax gene product [264]. Transcription-independent mechanisms of apoptosis induction by p53 have also been documented [262, 265, 266]. Mutations in the p53 gene occur in more than 50% of human cancers [267] with loss of function [268, 269], which leads to aggressiveness and drug resistance in many cancers [270, 271]. Many genotoxic anticancer agents elicit cytotoxicity by inducing apoptosis in the context of functional (wild-type) p53 [268, 269, 272].

A variety of novel anticancer therapeutic approaches have been taken to manipulate p53 pathways [267, 273]. These include gene therapy, exploitation of lack of p53 function for selective oncolytic viral therapy, pharmacological restoration of function to mutant p53 through conformational changes, and inhibition of p53 binding to Mdm2.

The overexpression of the Mdm2 gene product [274] suppresses normal p53 function [275, 276]. The Mdm2 protein is transcriptionally induced by p53 in a negative feedback control loop [277–279]. The mechanism by which Mdm2 suppresses p53 function involves abrogation of transactivation function as well as ubiquitin E3 ligase activity, which promotes p53 degradation. This suppression of p53 by Mdm2 is an attractive potential intervention target for anticancer drug action. Mdm2 overexpression, which may result from gene amplification, increased transcription, or enhanced translation [280, 281] has been shown to occur in many human tumors such as sarcomas; brain tumors; and breast, ovarian, cervical, lung, and colon cancers as well as pediatric solid tumors [274, 280]. This makes Mdm2 a potential novel anticancer molecular target [282, 283]. Peptides, small molecules, and antibodies that bind to Mdm2 protein, as well as anti-Mdm2 antisense oligonucleotides that inhibit Mdm2 expression [282–290] are in development as potential anticancer therapies. These agents could be developed as cancer treatments in their own right or be combined with other cancer therapeutic regimens to enhance apoptosis (see Chapter 6).

The Bcl-2 protein is an anti-apoptotic member of a large family of apoptosis-regulating proteins comprising both anti- and pro-apoptotic members that are differentially regulated, but share sequence-homology domains. Pro- and anti-apoptotic family members heterodimerize to modulate one another's function [291]. Overexpression of the anti-apoptotic proteins Bcl-2 and Bcl-xL has been observed in various tumors, and this is thought to cause anti-cancer drug resistance by inhibiting cytochrome *c* release from mitochondrial and activation of caspase-3 [292]. Bcl-2, the first member of the group, was originally identified at the chromosomal breakpoint of t-bearing [14, 18] B-cell lymphomas [293] and has been more widely explored as an anticancer drug target [294]. As mentioned above, Bcl-2 cooperates with myc to cause oncogenic transformation [224]. Bcl-2 overexpression is especially prevalent in B-cell lymphomas [295]. Other cancers such as prostate, breast, colorectal, small cell lung, and non-small cell lung cancers have also been shown to over-express Bcl-2 [296].

Bcl-xL is also a potential novel anticancer molecular target [296]. Peptidyl blockers of the dimerization of the Bcl-2 family have been designed [297], and small molecule Bcl-2 inhibitors obtained by structure-based design have been reported [298, 299]. An antisense oligonucleotide against Bcl-2 (G3139, oblimersen, Genanse) is currently undergoing clinical trial for cancer therapy [300]. An antisense oligonucleotide, 4259, targeting Bcl-xL has been shown to induce apoptosis in a variety of human breast cancer cell lines [301]. The interesting concept of using a bi-specific antisense oligonucleotide inhibiting both Bcl-2 and Bcl-xL expression has also been applied to induce apoptosis in tumor cells [302]. Small molecule inhibitors of Bcl-xL have also been identified [303, 304]. One concern while attempting to use Bcl-2 inhibitors in cancer therapy may be their adverse effects in patients with ischemic cardiac disease, where the anti-apoptotic effects of Bcl-2 are beneficial [296].

Another important emerging anti-apoptosis molecular target is survivin [305]. Survivin is a recently described member of the inhibitor-of-apoptosis

(IAP) family [306] of proteins, which also has spindle checkpoint control functions in the cell cycle [307–309]. Survivin is expressed in the most common human cancers but not in normal adult tissues [305, 310]. About 85% of non-small cell lung cancer tumors were shown to overexpress survivin mRNA [311]. The overexpression of survivin mutants has been shown to inhibit melanoma tumor growth *in vivo* [312] as well as induce tumor apoptosis and suppress tumor angiogenesis [313]. The widespread expression of survivin in cancer and its relative absence in normal cells have made it an attractive target for cancer diagnosis and immunotherapeutics [314]. XIAP (X-linked IAP), a highly effective member of the anti-apoptotic protein family [315] has also been shown to be widely overexpressed in many types of cancer [316], and is another potential a novel target for inducing apoptosis in cancer therapy.

The protein chaperone, Hsp70, is also been shown to be an anti-apoptotic factor [317–319]. Hsp70 blocks the assembly of a multi-protein complex termed the apoptosome. This is essential for activating the cascade of cysteine-aspartyl proteases (caspases), which are "the executioners" in the apoptotic programs. The overexpression of Hsp70 in transfected cells protects against stress-induced apoptosis [319]. This implies that Hsp70 might provide an apoptosis-inducing therapeutic target in cancers that have a dependence on it for survival. The expression of antisense DNA of Hsp70 was used in glioblastoma and breast and colon cancer in a xenograft model [320].

The enzyme telomeRase is a ribonucleoprotein DNA polymeRase that lengthens telomeres, which are specialized nucleotide sequences at the ends of chromosomes consisting of long tandem repeats of the sequence TTAGGG [321]. This function promotes the prolongation of the proliferation life span in cells [322, 323]. TelomeRase maintains telomere length by using its integral RNA template to add the TTAGGG tracks to telomeres. TelomeRase is induced in actively dividing cells and cancer cells, but not in other normal cells [322, 324]. TelomeRase activity has been shown to be elevated in 86% of cancers studied [325], and may serve as a candidate molecular target for selective cancer chemotherapy [325–328]. Quite a number of telomeRase inhibitors have been identified including porphyrins, anthraquinones, and 7-deaza-nucleotide analogs [325, 329, 330]. The use of telomeRase inhibitors in cancer therapy will have to contend with toxicity problems that might arise due to the requirement of telomeRase activity in renewable tissues such as the liver [324].

VIII. ANGIOGENESIS AND METASTASIS MOLECULAR FACTORS

For incipient cancers to establish and metastasize, they need nutrient supplies, which they obtain by developing blood vessels to tap into the host blood supply [68, 69]. This process of developing new blood vessels is termed angiogenesis. Tumor angiogenesis is critical for cancer progression and metastasis [331–333]. VEGFR and bFGFR are RTKs discussed earlier as promoting tumor angiogenesis. These induce endothelial cell growth and proliferation. In addition to these, several non-tyrosine kinase tumor angiogenesis factors have been identified, and will be the focus in this section [334]. An important angiogenic factor in this regard is angiogenin, which is a polypeptide that can induce or suppress angiogenesis [335]. The peptidyl compounds angiostatin and endostatin antagonize the angiogenic actions of angiogenin, and were shown to be highly effective in elimination of tumors in mice, which led to human clinical trials of these agents [336]. Structure-activity relationships among endostatin analogs are being studied to discover more potent peptides [337, 338]. Thalidomide and the fumagilin AG-1470, are also prominent antiangiogenic agents, albeit with mechanisms of action that are still unclear [70]. The thalidomide analog, S-3-[3-aminophthalimido]-glutarimide (S-3APG) has been shown to inhibit angiogenesis and growth in mouse models of B-cell malignancies [339]. Indirect induction of angiogenesis has also been demonstrated, with HIF-1 signaling as one example of such a mechanism [241]. The use of natural products as antiangiogenic agents has been reviewed recently [340], which showed an increasing repertoire of potential antiangiogenic therapeutics. It has recently been reported that Ras induces the sequential activation of PI-3 kinase, Rho, and ROCK, which leads to activation of myc through phosphorylation. This action enables it to repress the expression of the antiangiogenic factor thrombospondin-1 to promote tumor angiogenesis [341].

Matrix metalloproteinases (MMPs) are a large family of zinc-binding proteins that degrade extracellular matrix and allow cancer invasion [342, 343]. MMPs can be classified into five categories based on substrate preference: (1) type 1 collagenases, comprising MMP-1, MMP-8, and MMP-13; (2) type IV collagenases, MMP-2 and MMP-9; (3) stromelysins, MMP-3, MMP-7, MMP-10, and MMP-11; (4) elastases, MMP-12; and (5) membrane-type matrix metalloproteases, MT-MMPs [344]. They generated a lot of interest initially as molecular targets for controlling cancer metastasis [345], and many small molecule inhibitors have been discovered with varying selectivities against the different MMPs. Several MMP inhibitors were tested and advanced into clinical trials. These include marimastat, prinomastat (AG3340), and BAY 12–9566 [343, 346], but the results of those trials were disappointing [347]. Although more understanding of the role of MMPs in tumor invasion is still evolving [224], better inhibitors and better clinical trials designs may help to attain the potential of MMP inhibitors as anti-metastatic agents [343].

The serine protease formed urokinase (uPA) has been shown to be involved in tumor metastasis and angiogenesis [344, 348]. The uPA/uPAR have been shown to cooperate with MMPs in tumor cell intravasation [349]. These observations as well as others have attracted attention to the uPA/uPAR system for developing molecularly targeted anticancer drugs [350]. The potential role of urokinase receptor antagonists in metastatic disease has been summarized [348]. Amiloride analogs that inhibit uPA have shown anti-tumor invasion properties *in vivo* [70].

The cell adhesion class of extracellular matrix interacting molecules (CAMs), which mediate cell-matrix and cell-cell interactions, have roles in cancer invasion and organ-specific metastasis [351, 352] and also constitute potential cancer molecular targets [353]. The largest group of CAMs are the integrins, which are transmembrane heterodimeric proteins comprising α- and β-subunits. They function as receptors for matrix proteins such as fibronectin, vitronectin, laminin, and collagen [354]. Cadherins, selectins, mucins, hyaluronan (CD44); the MHC antigens, CD2, CD4, and CD8; and other Igs such as ICAM-1, ICAM-2, VCAM-1, CEA, C-CAMs, and DCC [351, 353], as well as gangliosides [355]. Synthetic peptides designed to antagonize adhesion which incorporate an RGD [Arg-Gly-Asp] motif, have been shown to prevent metastasis [70, 351, 353].

IX. PROTEIN DEGRADATION AND CHAPERONING TARGETS

Inhibition of the 26S proteasome has been shown to be a promising new approach to cancer therapy. In this regard, bortezomib (Velcade, PS-341), a dipeptide boronic acid analog proteasome inhibitor, is currently available for the treatment of relapsed and refractory multiple myeloma. Further trials are underway to assess its efficacy against a range of other cancers [356]. The strategy of proteasome inhibition using bortezomib has been shown to combat cancer resistance to radiation and chemotherapy attributable to induction of NF-κB [236, 357].

Heat shock protein 90 (Hsp90) is a molecular chaperone that plays a key role in the conformational maturation of oncogenic signaling proteins including HER-2/ErbB2, Akt, Raf-1, Bcr-Abl, cyclin D1, met, and mutant p53 [358]. Hsp90 inhibitors bind to Hsp90, abrogating its ATPase activity and inducing the proteasomal degradation of Hsp90 client proteins. Geldanamycin analog ansamycins were the first Hsp90 inhibitors discovered. The geldanmycin analog, 17-allylamino, 17-demethoxygeldanamycin (17AAG) has emerged as the clinical development candidate among these. Its performance in clinical trials has been good thus far [359, 360]. Further tests are warranted to move it into advanced clinical trials. In the meantime, efforts to discover new Hsp90 inhibitors are underway [361, 362].

It has been shown that the selective killing of cancer cells by the 17AAG is the result of the higher affinity (100-fold) conformation of the activated Hsp90 found in tumor cells compared to normal cells. Tumor Hsp90 is present entirely in multi-chaperone complexes with high ATPase activity, whereas Hsp90 from normal tissues is in a latent, uncomplexed state [363]. This provides a novel mechanism for achieving selective cancer cell killing, as well as less toxic cancer chemotherapy. The promise of targeting of Hsp90 as a cancer therapeutic target was made evident in a recent special issue of the journal, *Current Cancer Drug Targets* [364].

X. CHROMATIN REMODELING FACTORS

Chromatin structure is an important factor in gene expression. Among the proteins involved in chromatin remodeling, histone deacetylases (HDACs) are the most studied and targeted with regard to the development of novel cancer therapeutics [365]. HDACs function in opposition to histone acetylases (HATs) by deacetylating lysine residues on histone tails that HATs have acetylated that have been shown to be deregulated in cancer. Development of HDAC inhibitors for cancer therapy is an active area of research [365, 366–368]. Trichostatin A (TSA) and suberoylanilide hydroxamic acid (SAHA) are much-studied small molecules that inhibit HDAC by binding to its catalytic site [369]. Hydroxamic acid based HDAC inhibitors like SAHA have entered clinical trials and have shown good tolerability [367].

XI CONCLUSION

We are in an era of great opportunities and hope for tackling the formidable problem of cancer chemotherapy. The plethora of potential novel anticancer targets surveyed in this chapter attest to this. Harnessing these targets will improve the chances of effectively treating many cancers that are currently intractable. Proof of principle has already been demonstrated for these novel anticancer targets, and success has been achieved in developing small molecule and antibody therapeutics against several oncogenic tyrosine kinase novel targets for use in cancer patients. There are still challenges in developing effective and selective cancer therapies in terms of the selection of the right targets for drug development, for the treatment of the appropriate cancers, and for the selection of the appropriate patient population end points for clinical testing of novel therapies, as well as how to tailor treatments to individual patients' tumor target profiles. Genomics and proteomics hold promise for addressing some of these problems. Overall, the field is fertile and the stage is set for many new breakthroughs in the war against cancer. For the most part, the tools needed are already in place. It is now time to harness innovative drug discovery and development and translational strategies to achieve the goal of developing novel clinically effective cancer treatments without severe toxicities.

REFERENCES

1. Hunter T. Oncoprotein networks. *Cell* 1997; 88:573–582.
2. Weinberg RA. Tumor suppressor genes. *Science* 1991; 254:1138–1146.
3. Hanahan D, Weinberg A. The hallmarks of cancer. *Cell* 2000; 100:57–70.
4. Workman P. The potential for molecular oncology to define new drug targets. In *New Molecular Targets for Cancer Chemotherapy* (Kerr DJ and Workman P, eds.), CRC Press, Boca Raton FL, 1994; pp.1–44.
5. Venter JC, Adams MD, Myers EW, Li PW, Mural RJ, Sutton GG, Smith HO, Yandell M, Evans CA, Holt RA et al. The sequence of the human genome. *Science* 2001; 291:1304–1351.
6. http://cgap.nci.nih.gov/
7. Lindsey MA. Target discovery. *Nat. Rev. Drug Discov.* 2003; 2:831–838.
8. DeYoung MP, Tress M, Narayanan R. Identification of Down's syndrome critical locus gene SIM2-s as a drug therapy target for solid tumors. *Proc. Natl. Acad. Sci. U. S. A.* 2003; 100:4760–4765.
9. Buolamwini JK, Assefa H. Overview of Novel Anticancer Drug Targets In *Novel Anticancer Drug Protocols* (Buolamwini JK and Adjei AA, eds.), Humana Press, Totowa NJ, 2003; pp. 3–28.
10. Neamati N, Barchi JJ Jr. New paradigms in drug design and discovery. *Curr. Top. Med. Chem.* 2002; 2:211–227.
11. Blundell TL. Structure-based drug design. *Nature* 1996; 384(Suppl. 6604):23–26.

12. Pellecchia M, Sem DS, Wüthrich K. NMR in drug discovery. *Nat. Rev. Drug Discov.* 2002; 1:211–219.
13. Geysen HM, Schoenen F, Wagner D, Wagner R. Combinatorial compound libraries for drug discovery: An ongoing challenge. *Nat. Rev. Drug Discov.* 2003; 2:222–230.
14. Bajorath J. Integration of virtual and high-throughput screening. *Nat. Rev. Drug Discov.* 2002; 1:882–894.
15. Shak S. Overview of the tRastuzumab [Herceptin] anti-HER2 monoclonal antibody clinical programme in HER-2 overexpressing metastatic breast cancer. Herceptin Multinational Investigator Study Group. *Semin. Oncol.* 1999; 26:71–77.
16. Druker BJ. STI571 [Gleevec™] as a paradigm for cancer therapy. *Trends Mol. Med.* 2002; 8(Issue 4 Suppl.):S14–S18.
17. Wakeling AE, Guy SP, Woodburn JR, Ashton SE, Curry BJ, Barker AJ, Gibson KH. ZD1839 (Iressa): An orally active inhibitor of epidermal growth factor signaling with potential for cancer therapy. *Cancer Res.* 2002; 62:5749–54.
18. Seymore L. Novel anti-cancer agents in development: Exciting prospects and new challenges. *Cancer Treat. Rev.* 1999; 25:301–312.
19. Buolamwini JK. Novel molecular targets for cancer drug discovery. In *The Molecular Basis of Human Cancer* (Coleman WB and Tsongalis GJ, eds.), Humana Press, Totowa NJ, 2002; pp. 521–540.
20. Jurcic JG, Scheinberg DA, Houghton AN. Monoclonal antibody therapy of cancer. *Cancer Chemother. Biol. Response Modif.* 1997; 17:195–216.
21. Wang H, Prasad G, Buolamwini JK, Zhang R. Antisense anticancer oligonucleotide therapeutics. *Curr. Cancer Drug Tar.* 2001; 1:177–196.
22. Chong C, Vile R. Gene therapy for cancer. *Drugs Future* 1997; 22:857–874.
23. Gomez-Navarro J, Bilbao G, Curiel DT. Gene therapy in the treatment of human cancer. In *The Molecular Basis of Human Cancer* (Coleman WB and Tsongalis GJ, eds.), Humana Press, Totowa NJ, 2002; pp. 541–565.
24. Sausville EA, Longo DL. Growth factors and growth factor inhibitors. In *Cancer Therapeutics: Experimental and Clinical Agents* (Teicher B, ed.), Humana Press, Totowa NJ, 1994; pp. 337–370.
25. Adjei AA. Signal transduction pathway targets for anticancer drug discovery. *Curr. Pharm. Design* 2000; 6:361–378.
26. Gishizky ML. Tyrosine kinase induced mitogenesis. Breaking the link with cancer. *Annu. Rep. Med. Chem.* 1995; 30:247–253.
27. Katz ME, McCormick F. Signal transduction from multiple Ras effectors. *Curr. Opin. Genet. Dev.* 1997; 7, 75–79.
28. Marais R, Light Y, Mason C, Paterson H, Olson MF, Marshall CJ. Requirement of Ras-GTP-Raf complexes for activation of Raf-1 by protein kinase C. *Science* 1998; 280:109–112.
29. Olson MF, Paterson HF, Marshall CJ. Signals from Ras and Rho GTPases interact to regulate expression of p21$^{Waf1/Cip1}$. *Nature* 1998; 394:295–299.
30. Ullrich A, Schlessinger J. Signal transduction by receptors with tyrosine kinase activity. *Cell* 1991; 61:203–212.
31. Schlessinger J, Ullrich A. Growth factor signaling by receptor tyrosine kinases. *Neuron* 1992; 9:383–391.
32. Fantl WJ, Johnson DE, Williams LT. Signalling by receptor tyrosine kinases. *Annu. Rev. Biochem.* 1993; 62:453–481.
33. Kolibaba KS, Druker BJ. Protein tyrosine kinases and cancer. *Biochim. Biophys. Acta* 1997; 1333:F217–F248.
34. de Bono JS, Rowinsky EK. The ErbB receptor family: a therapeutic target for cancer. *Trends Mol. Med.* 2002; 8(Issue 4 Suppl.):S19–S26.
35. Lofts FJ, Gullick WJ. Growth factor receptors as targets. In *New Molecular Targets for Cancer Chemotherapy* (Kerr DJ and Workman P, eds.), CRC Press, Boca Raton FL, 1994; pp. 45–66.
36. Levitzki A. Protein tyrosine kinase inhibitors. In *New Molecular Targets for Cancer Chemotherapy* (Kerr DJ. and Workman P, eds.), CRC Press, Boca Raton FL, 1994; pp. 67–79.
37. Levitzki A, Gazit A. Tyrosine kinase inhibition: an approach to drug development. *Science* 1995; 267, 1782–1788.

38. Burke TR. Protein tyrosine kinase inhibitors. *Drugs Future* 1992; 17:119–131.

39. Zwick E, Bange J, Ullrich A. Receptor tyrosine kinases as targets for anticancer drugs. *Trends Mol. Med.* 2002; 8:17–23.

40. Fry DW. Recent advances in tyrosine kinases inhibitors. *Annu. Rep. Med. Chem.* 1996; 31:151–160.

41. Traxler P, Lydon N. Recent advances in protein tyrosine kinase inhibitors. *Drugs Future* 1995; 20:1261–1274.

42. Traxler P, Furet P, Met H, Buchdunger E, Meyer T, Lydon N. Design and synthesis of novel tyrosine kinase inhibitors using a pharmacophore model of the ATP-binding site of the EGF-R. *J. Pharm. Belg.* 1997; 52:88–96.

43. Fry DW, Kraker AJ, Connors RC, Elliot WL, Nelson JM, Showalter HDH, Leopold WR. Strategies for the discovery of novel tyrosine kinase inhibitors with anticancer activity. *Anticancer Drug Design* 1994; 9:331–351.

44. Blume-Jensen P, Hunter T. Oncogenic kinase signalling. *Nature* 2001; 411:355–356.

45. Cohen P. The development and therapeutic potential of protein kinase inhibitors. *Curr. Opin. Chem. Biol.* 1999; 3:459–465.

46. Vlahovic G, Crawford J. Activation of tyrosine kinases in cancer. *Oncologist* 2003; 8:531–538.

47. Klapper LN, Kirschbaum MH, Sela M, Yarden Y. Biochemical and clinical implications of the ErbB/HER signaling network of growth factor receptors. *Adv. Cancer Res.* 2000; 77:25–79.

48. Aaronson SA. Growth factors and cancer. *Science* 1991; 254:1146–1152.

49. Tzahar E, Yarden Y. The ErbB-2/HER2 oncogenic receptor of adenocarcinomas: From orphanhood to multiple stromal ligands. *Biochim. Biophys. Acta* 1998; 1377:M25-M37.

50. Yarden Y, Sliwkowski MX. Untangling the ErbB signalling network. *Nat. Rev. Mol. Cell Biol.* 2001; 2:127–137.

51. Holbro T, Civenni G, Hynes NE. The ErbB receptors and their role in cancer progression. *Exp. Cell Res.* 2003; 284:99–110.

52. Baselga J. The EGFR as a target for anticancer therapy: focus on Cetuximab. *Eur. J. Cancer* 2001; 37:S16–S22.

53. Grunwald V, Hidalgo M. Developing inhibitors of the epidermal growth factor receptor for cancer treatment. *J. Natl. Cancer Inst.* 2003; 95:851–67.

54. Slamon DJ, Leyland-Jones B, Shak S, Fuchs H, Paton V, Bajamonde A, Fleming T, Eiermann W, Wolter J, Pegram M, Baselga J, Norton L. Use of chemotherapy plus a monoclonal antibody against HER2 for metastatic breast cancer that overexpresses HER2. *N. Engl. J. Med.* 2001; 344:783–792.

55. Yaish P, Gazit A, Gilom C, Levitzki A. Blocking of EGF-dependent cell proliferation by EGF receptor kinase inhibitors. *Science* 1988; 242:933–935.

56. Hubbard SR, Jeffrey HT. Protein tyrosine kinase structure and function. *Annu. Rev. Biochem.* 2000; 69:373–398.

57. Stamos J, Sliwkowski MX, Eigenbrot C. Structure of the epidermal growth factor receptor kinase domain alone and in complex with a 4-anilinoquinazoline inhibitor. *J. Biol. Chem.* 2002; 277:46265–46272.

58. Khalil MY, Grandis JR, Shin DM. Targeting epidermal growth factor receptor: Novel therapeutics in the management of cancer. *Expert Rev. Anticancer Ther.* 2003; 3:367–380.

59. Ciardiello F, Tortora G. A novel approach in the treatment of cancer: Targeting the epidermal growth factor receptor. *Clin. Cancer Res.* 2001; 7:2958–2970.

60. Miller P, DiOrio C, Moyer M, Schnur RC, Bruskin A, Cullen W, Moyer JD. Depletion of the erbB-2 gene product p185 by the benzoquinone ansamycins. *Cancer Res.* 1994; 54:2724–2730.

61. Neckers L. Hsp90 inhibitors as novel cancer chemotherapeutic agents. *Trends Mol. Med.* 2002; 8(Issue 4 Suppl.):S55–S61.

62. Witters L, Kumar R, Mandal M, Bennett CF, Miraglia L, Lipton A. Antisense oligonucleotides to the epidermal growth factor receptor. *Breast Cancer Res. Tr.* 1999; 53:41–50.

63. Roh H, Pippin JA, Green DW, Boswell CB, Hirose CT, Mokadam N, Drebin JA. HER2/neu antisense targeting of human breast carcinoma. *Oncogene* 2000; 19:6138–6143.

64. Heldin C-H, Ostman A, Ronnstrand L. Signal transduction via platelet-derived growth factor receptors. *Biochim. Biophys. Acta* 1998; 1378:F79–F113.

65. Cools J, DeAngelo DJ, Gotlib J et al. A tyrosine kinase created by fusion of the PDGFRA and FIP1L1 genes as a therapeutic target of imatinib in idiopathic hypereosinophilic syndrome. *N. Engl. J. Med.* 2003; 348:1201–1214.

66. Shawver LK, Schwartz DP, Mann E et al. Inhibition of platelet-derived growth factor-mediated signal transduction and tumor growth by N-[4-[trifluoromethyl]phenyl]-5-methylisoxazole-4-carboxamide. *Clin. Cancer Res.* 1997; 3:1167–1177.

67. Mullins DE, Hamud F, Reim R, Davis HR. Inhibition of PDGF receptor binding and PDGF-stimulated biological activity in vitro and of intimal lesion formation in vivo by 2-bromomethyl-5-chlorobenzene sulfonylphthalimide. *Arterioscler. Thromb.* 1994; 14:1047–1055.

68. Hanahan D. Signaling vascular morphogenesis and maintenance. *Science* 1997; 277:48–50.

69. Risau W. Mechanisms of angiogenesis. *Nature* 1997; 386:671–674.

70. Powell D, Skotnicki J, Upeslacis J. Angiogenesis inhibitors. *Annu. Rep. Med. Chem.* 1997; 32:161–170.

71. Kubo H, Fujiwara T, Jussila L, Hashi H, Ogawa M, Shimizu K, Awane M, Sakai Y, Takabayashi A, Alitalo K, Yamaoka Y, Nishikawa SI. Involvement of vascular endothelial growth factor receptor-3 in maintenance of integrity of endothelial cell lining during tumor angiogenesis. *Blood* 2000; 96:546–553.

72. Fong TA, Shawver LK, Sun L et al. SU5416 is a potent and selective inhibitor of the vascular endothelial growth factor receptor (Flk-1/KDR) that inhibits tyrosine kinase catalysis, tumor vascularization, and growth of multiple tumor types. *Cancer Res.* 1999; 59:99–106.

73. Zhu Z, Bohlen P, Witte L. Clinical development of angiogenesis inhibitors to vascular endothelial growth factor and its receptors as cancer therapeutics. *Curr. Cancer Drug Tar.* 2002; 2:135–156.

74. O'Neil BH, Goldberg RM. Novel chemotherapeutic and targeted agents in metastatic colorectal cancer: The time has arrived. *Expert Opin. Inv. Drugs* 2003; 12:1939–1949.

75. Fry DW, Nelson JM. Inhibition of fibroblast growth factor-mediated tyrosine phosphorylation and protein synthesis by PD 145709, a member of the 2-thioindole class of tyrosine kinase inhibitors. *Anticancer Drug Design* 1995; 10:604–622.

76. Mohammadi M, McMahon G, Sun L, Tang C, Hirth P, Yeh BK, Hubbard SR, Schlessinger J. Structures of the tyrosine kinase domain of fibroblast growth factor receptor in complex with inhibitors. *Science* 1997; 276:955–960.

77. Shaulian E, Resnitzky D, Shifman O, Blandino G, Amsterdam A, Yayon A, Oren M. Induction of Mdm2 and enhancement of cell survival by bFGF. *Oncogene* 1997; 15:2717–2725.

78. Hirota S, Isozaki K, Moriyama Y et al. Gain-of-function mutations of c-kit in human gastrointestinal stromal tumors. *Science* 1998; 279:577–580.

79. O'Dwyer ME, Druker BJ. The role of the tyrosine kinase inhibitor STI571 in the treatment of cancer. *Curr. Cancer Drug Tar.* 2001; 1:49–57.

80. Christensen JG, Schreck R, Burrows J et al. A selective small molecule inhibitor of c-Met kinase inhibits c-Met-dependent phenotypes in vitro and exhibits cytoreductive antitumor activity in vivo. *Cancer Res.* 2003; 63:7345–7355.

81. Wang Y, Sun Y. Insulin-like growth factor receptor-1 as an anti-cancer target: Blocking transformation and inducing apoptosis. *Curr. Cancer Drug Tar.* 2002; 2:191–207.

82. Sekharam M, Zhao H, Sun M, Fang Q, Zhang Q, Yuan Z, Dan HC, Boulware D, Cheng JQ, Coppola D. Insulin-like growth factor 1 receptor enhances invasion and induces resistance to apoptosis of colon cancer cells through the Akt/Bcl-xL pathway. *Cancer Res.* 2003; 63:7708–7716

83. Hankinson SE, Willett WC, Colditz GA, Hunter DJ, Michaud DS, Deroo B, Rosner B, Speizer FE, Pollak M. Circulating concentrations of insulin-like growth factor-I and risk of breast cancer. *Lancet* 1998; 351:1393–1396.

84. Chakravarti A, Loeffler JS, Dyson NJ. Insulin-like growth factor receptor I mediates resistance to anti-epidermal growth factor receptor therapy in primary human glioblastoma cells through continued activation of phosphoinositide 3-kinase signaling. *Cancer Res.* 2002; 62:200–207.

85. Favelyukis S, Till JH, Hubbard SR, Miller WT. Structure and autoregulation of the insulin-like growth factor 1 receptor kinase. *Nat. Struct. Biol.* 2001; 8:1058–1063.

86. Pautsch A, Zoephel A, Ahorn H, Spevak W, Hauptmann R, Nar H. Crystal structure of bisphosphorylated IGF-1 receptor kinase. Insight into domain movements upon kinase activation. *Structure* 2001; 9:955–965.

87. Gilliland DG, Griffin JD. Role of FLT3 in leukemia. *Curr. Opin. Hematol.* 2002; 9:274–281.

88. Armstrong SA, Kung AL, Mabon ME et al. Inhibition of FLT3 in MLL. Validation of a therapeutic target identified by gene expression based classification. *Cancer Cell* 2003; 3:173–183.

89. Kelly LM, Yu JC, Boulton CL et al. CT53518, a novel selective FLT3 antagonist for the treatment of acute myelogenous leukemia (AML). *Cancer Cell* 2002; 1:421–432.

90. Easty DJ, Bennett DC. Protein tyrosine kinases in malignant melanoma. *Melanoma Res.* 2000; 10:401–411.

91. Bjorge JD, Jakymiw A, Fujita DJ. Selected glimpses into the activation and function of src kinase. *Oncogene* 2000; 19:5620–5635.

92. Lutz MP, Eber IBS, Flossmann-Kast BBM, Vogelmann R, Luhrs H, Friess H, Buchler MW, Adler G. Overexpression and activation of the tyrosine kinase Src in human pancreatic carcinoma. *Biochem. Biophys. Res. Commun.* 1998; 243:503–508.

93. Bolen JB, Veillet AA. Function for the lck proto-oncogene. *Trends Biochem. Sci.* 1989; 14:404–407.

94. Cheung RK, Dosch HM. The tyrosine kinase lck is critically involved in the growth transformation of human B lymphocytes. *J. Biol. Chem.* 1991; 266:8667–8670.

95. Zamoyska R, Basson A, Filby A, Legname G, Lovatt M, Seddon B. The influence of the src-family kinases, Lck and Fyn, on T cell differentiation, survival and activation. *Immunol. Rev.* 2003; 191:107–118.

96. Klutchko SR, Hamby J, Boschelli DH et al. 2-Substituted aminopyrido[2,3-d]pyrimidin-7[8H]-ones. Structure-activity relationships against selected tyrosine kinases and in vitro and in vivo anticancer activity. *J. Med Chem.* 1998; 41:3276–3292.

97. Lunney EA, Para KS, Rubin JR, Humblet C, Fergus JH, Marks JS, Sawyer TK. Structure-based design of a novel series of ligands that bind to the pp60^{src} SH2 domain. *J. Am. Chem. Soc.* 1997; 119:12471–12476.

98. Buchdunger E, Zimmerman J, Mett H, Meyer T, Muller M, Druker BJ, Lydon BN. Inhibition of the Abl protein-tyrosine kinase in vitro and in vivo by a 2-phenylaminopyrimidine derivative. *Cancer Res.* 1996; 56:100–104.

99. Heinrich MC, Griffith DJ, Druker BJ, Wait CK, Ott KA, Zigler AJ. Inhibition of c-kit receptor tyrosine kinase activity by STI 571, a selective tyrosine kinase inhibitor. *Blood* 2000; 96:925–932.

100. Dekker LV, Parker PJ. Protein kinase C. A question of specificity. *Trends Biochem. Sci.* 1994; 19:73–77.

101. Lee JC, Adams JL. Inhibitors of serine/threonine kinases. *Curr. Opin. Biotechnol.* 1995; 6:657–661.

102. Castagna M, Takai Y, Kaibuchi K, Sano K, Kikkawa U, Nishizuka Y. Direct activation of calcium-activated phospholipid-dependent protein kinase by tumor-promoting phorbol esters. *J. Biol. Chem.* 1982; 257:7847–7851.

103. Niedel JE, Kuhn LJ, Vandenbank GR. Phorbol diester receptor copurifies with protein kinase C. *Proc. Natl. Acad. Sci. U. S. A.* 1983; 80:36–40.

104. Exton JH. Cell signalling through guanine-nucleotide-binding regulatory proteins [G proteins] and phospholipases. *Eur. J. Biochem.* 1997; 243:10–20.

105. Capronigro F, French RC, Kaye SB. Protein kinase C: A worthwhile target for anticancer drugs? *Anticancer Drugs* 1997; 8:26–33.

106. Grescher A, Dale IL. Protein kinase C — a novel target for rational anticancer drug design? *Anticancer Drug Design* 1989; 4, 93–105.

107. Basu A. The potential of protein kinase C as a target for anticancer treatment. *Pharmacol. Ther.* 1993; 59:257–280.

108. Philip PA, Harris AL. Potential for protein kinase C inhibitors in cancer therapy. *Cancer Treat. Res.* 1995; 178:3–27.

109. Schwartz GK. Protein kinase C inhibitors as inducers of apoptosis for cancer treatment. *Expert Opin. Inv. Drugs* 1996; 5:1601–1615.

110. Goekjian PG, Jirousek MR. Protein kinase C inhibitors as novel anticancer drugs. *Expert Opin. Inv. Drugs* 2001; 10:2117–2140.

111. Hofmann J. Modulation of protein kinase C in antitumor treatment. *Rev. Physiol. Biochem. Pharmacol.* 2002; 142, 1–96.

112. Blobe GC, Sachs CW, Khan WA, Fabbro D, Stabel S, Wetsel WC, Obeid LM, Fine RL, Hannun YA. Selective regulation of expression of protein kinase C (PKC) isozymes in multidrug-resistant MCF-7 cells. Functional significance of enhanced expression of PKCα. *J. Biol. Chem.* 1993; 268:658–664.

113. Gill PK, Gescher A, Gant TW. Regulation of MDR1 promoter activity in human breast carcinoma cells by protein kinase C isozymes alpha and theta. *Eur. J. Biochem.* 2001; 268:4151–4157.

114. Graves PR, Yu L, Schwarz JK, Gales J, Sausville EA, O'Connor PM, Piwnica-Worms H. The Chk1 protein kinase and the Cdc25C regulatory pathways are targets of the anticancer agent UCN-01. *J. Biol. Chem.* 2000; 275:5600–5605.

115. Harris, Hill CH, Lewis EJ, Nixon JS, Wilkinson SE. Protein kinase C inhibitors. *Drugs Future* 1993; 18:727–735.

116. Zimmermann J, Caravatti G, Mett H, Meyer T, Muller M, Lydon NB, Fabbro D. Phenylamino-pyrimidine (PAP) derivatives: a new class of potent and selective inhibitors of protein kinase C (PKC). *Arch. Pharm.* 1996; 329:371–376.

117. Wang S, Milne GWA, Nicklaus MC, Marquez VE, Lee J, Blumberg PM. Protein kinase C. Modeling of the binding site and prediction of binding constants. *J. Med. Chem.* 1994; 37:1326–1338.

118. Wang S, Zaharevitz DW, Sharma R, Marquez VE, Milne GWA, Lewin NE, Du L, Lee J, Blumberg PM. Discovery of novel, structurally diverse protein kinase C agonists through computer 3D-database pharmacophore search. Molecular modeling studies. *J. Med. Chem.* 1994; 37:4479–4489.

119. Qiao L, Wang S, George C, Lewin LE, Blumberg PM, Kozikowski AP. Structure-based design of a new class of protein kinase C modulators. *J. Am. Chem. Soc.* 1998; 120:6629–6630.

120. Tortora G, Ciardiello F. Antisense strategies targeting protein kinase C: Preclinical and clinical development. *Semin. Oncol.* 2003; 30(4 Suppl. 10):26–31.

121. Romanelli A, Martin KA, Toker A, Blenis J. p70 S6 Kinase is regulated by protein kinase Cα and participates in a phosphoinositide 3-kinase-regulated signalling complex. *Mol. Cell Biol.* 1999; 19:2921–2928.

122. Ramage AD, Langdon SP, Ritchie AA, Urns DJ, Miller WR. Growth inhibition by 8-chloro-cyclic AMP of human HT29 colorectal and ZR-75–1 breast carcinoma xenografts is associated with selective modulation of protein kinase A isoenzymes. *Eur. J. Cancer* 1995; 31A:969–973.

123. Cho YS, Cho-Chung YS. Antisense protein kinase A RIalpha acts synergistically with hydroxycamptothecin to inhibit growth and induce apoptosis in human cancer cells: molecular basis for combinatorial therapy. *Clin. Cancer Res.* 2003; 9:1171–1178.

124. Toker A. Protein kinases as mediators of phosphoinositide 3-kinase signaling. *Mol. Pharmacol.* 2000; 57:652–658.

125. Vivanco I, Sawyers CL. The phosphatidylinositol 3-kinase/AKT pathway in human cancer. *Nat. Rev. Cancer* 2002; 2:489–501.

126. Alessi DR, Andjelkovic M, Caudwell B, Cron P, Morrice N, Cohen P, Hemmings BA. Mechanism of activation of protein kinase B by insulin and IGF-1. *EMBO J.* 1996; 15:6541–6551.

127. Toker A, Cantley LC. Signalling through the lipid products of phosphoinositide-3OH kinase. *Nature* 1997; 387:673–676.

128. Franke TF, Kaplan DR, Cantley LC, Toker A. Direct regulation of the Akt protooncogene product by phosphatidylinositol-3,4-bisphosphate. *Science* 1997; 275:665–668.

129. Datta SR, Dudek H, Tao X, Masters S, Fu H, Gotoh Y, Greenberg ME. Akt phosphorylation of BAD couples survival signals to the cell-intrinsic death machinery. *Cell* 1997; 91:231–241.

130. Brunet A, Bonni A, Zigmond MJ, Lin MZ, Juo P, Hu LS, Anderson MJ, Arden KC, Blenis J, Greenberg ME. Akt promotes cell survival by phosphorylating and inhibiting a Forkhead transcription factor. *Cell* 1999; 96:857–868.

131. Ozes ON, Mayo LD, Guston JA, Pfeffer SR, Pfeffer LM, Donner DB. NF-kappa B activation by tumor necrosis factor requires the Akt serine-threonine kinase. *Nature* 1999; 401:82–85.

132. Nakanishi K, Sakamoto M, Yasuda J, Takamura M, Fujita N, Tsuruo T, Todo S, Hirohashi S. Critical involvement of the phosphatidylinositol 3-kinase/Akt pathway in anchorage independent growth and hematogeneous intrahepatic metastasis of liver cancer. *Cancer Res.* 2002; 62:2971–2975.

133. Leslie LR, Downes PC. PTEN: the down side of PI 3-kinase signalling. *Cell. Signal.* 2002; 14:285–295.

134. Zhong H, Chiles K, Feldser D, Laughner E, Hanrahan C, Georgescu MM, Simons JW, Semenza GL. Modulation of hypoxia-inducible factor 1-alpha expression by the epidermal growth factor/phosphoinositide-3 kinase/PTEN/AKT/FRAP pathway in human prostate cancer cells: Implications for tumor angiogenesis and therapeutics. *Cancer Res.* 2000; 60:1541–1545.

135. Alvarez B, Garrido E, Garcia-Sanz JA, Carrera AC. Phosphoinositide 3-kinase activation regulates cell division time by coordinated control of cell mass and cell cycle progression rate. *J. Biol. Chem.* 2003; 278:26466–26473.

136. Hidalgo M, Rowinsky EK. The rapamycin-sensitive signal transduction pathway as a target for cancer therapy. *Oncogene* 2000; 19:6680–6686.

137. Sawyers CL. Will mTOR inhibitors make it as cancer drugs? *Cancer Cell* 2003; 4:343–348.

139. Hu L, Zaloudek C, Mills GB, Gray J, Jaffe RB. In vivo and in vitro ovarian carcinoma growth inhibition by a phosphatidylinositol 3-kinase inhibitor (LY294002). *Clin. Cancer Res.* 2000; 6:880–886.

140. Stein B, Anderson D. The MAP kinase family: new "MAPs" for signal transduction pathways targets. *Annu. Rep. Med. Chem.* 1996; 31:289–298.

141. Lewis TS, Shapiro PS, Ahn NG. Signal transduction through MAP kinase cascades. *Adv. Cancer Res.* 1998; 74:49–139.

142. Cobb MH. MAP kinase pathways. *Prog. Biophys. Mol. Biol.* 1999; 71:479–500.

143. Kolch W. Meaningful relationships: The regulation of the Ras/Raf/MEK/ERK pathway by protein interactions. *Biochem. J.* 2000; 351:289–305.

144. Kumar CC, Madison V. Drugs targeted against protein kinases. *Expert Opin. Emerging Drugs* 2001; 6:308–315.

145. Herrera R, Sebolt-Leopold JS. Unraveling the complexities of the Raf/MAP kinase pathway for pharmacological intervention. *Trends Mol. Med.* 2002; 8(4):S27–S31.

146. Sebolt-Leopold JS, Dudley DT et al. Blockade of the MAP kinase pathway suppresses growth of colon tumors in vivo. *Nat. Med.* 1999; 5:810–816.

147. Shimamura A, Ballif BA, Richards SA, Blenis J. Rsk1 mediates a MEK-MAP kinase cell survival signal. *Curr. Biol.* 2000; 10:127–135.

148. Bonni A, Brunet A, West AE, Datta SR, Takasu MA, Greenberg ME. Cell survival promoted by the Ras-MAPK signalling pathway by transcription-dependent and -independent mechanisms. *Science* 1999; 286:1358–1362.

149. Wang HG, Miyashita T, Takayama S et al. Apoptosis regulation by interaction of Bcl-2 protein and Raf-1 kinase. *Oncogene* 1994; 9, 2751–2756.

150. Pardo OE, Arcaro A, Salerno G, Raguz S, Downward J, Seckl MJ. Fibroblast and growth factor-2 induces translational regulation of Bcl-X$_L$ and Bcl-2 via a MEK-dependent pathway. Correlation with resistance to etoposide-induced apoptosis. *J. Biol. Chem.* 2002; 277:12040–12046.

151. Zhong J, Troppmai J, Rapp UR. Independent control of cell survival by Raf-1 and Bcl-2 at the mitochondria. *Oncogene* 2001; 20:4807–4816.

152. Chen J, Fujii K, Zhang L, Roberts T, Fu H. Raf-1 promotes cell survival by antagonizing signal-regulating kinase 1 through a MEK-ERK independent mechanism. *Proc. Natl. Acad. Sci. U. S. A.* 2001; 98, 7783–7788.

153. Monia BP. First- and second-generation antisense inhibitors targeted to human c-raf kinase: in vitro and in vivo studies. *Anticancer Drug Design* 1997; 12:327–339.

154. Dudley DT, Pang L, Decker SJ, Bridges AJ, Saltiel AR. A synthetic inhibitor of the mitogen-activated protein kinase cascade. *Proc. Natl. Acad. Sci. U. S. A.* 1995; 92:7686–7689.

155. Draetta G. Cell cycle control in eukaryotes: Molecular mechanisms of cdc2 activation. *Trends Biol. Sci.* 1990; 15:378–383.

156. Sherr CJ. Mammalian G1 cyclins. *Cell* 1993; 73:1059–1065.

157. Coleman KG, Lyssikatos JP, Yang BV. Chemical inhibitors of cyclin-dependent kinases. *Annu. Rep. Med. Chem.* 1997; 32:171–179.

158. Hunter T, Pines J. Cyclins and cancer II: Cyclin D and CDK inhibitors come of age. *Cell* 1994; 79:573–582.

159. Morgan DO. Principles of CDK regulation. *Nature* 1995; 374:131–134.

160. Lee MH, Renisdottir I, Massague J. Cloning of p57KIP2, a cyclin-dependent kinase inhibitor with unique domain structure and tissue distribution. *Gene Dev.* 1995; 9:639–649.

161. Sherr CJ, Roberts JM. CDK inhibitors, positive and negative regulators of G1-phase progression. *Gene Dev.* 1999; 13:1505–1512.

162. Ortega S, Malumbres M, Barbacid M. Cyclin-dependent kinases, INK4 inhibitors and cancer. *Biochim. Biophys. Acta* 2002; 1602:73–87.

163. Lees EM, Harlow E. Cancer and the cell cycle. In *Cell Cycle Control* (Hutchison C and Glover DM, eds.), IRL Press, New York, 1995; pp. 228–263.

164. Weinberg RA. The retinoblastoma protein and cell cycle control. *Cell* 1995; 81, 323–330.

165. Draetta G, Pagano M. Cell cycle control and cancer. *Annu. Rep. Med. Chem.* 1996; 31:241–248.

166. Imoto M. Molecular target therapy of cancer: a. cell cycle. *Kagaku Ryo Ryoiki* 1998; 14, 13–19.

167. Buolamwini JK. Cell cycle molecular targets in novel anticancer drug discovery. *Curr. Pharm. Design* 2000; 6, 379–392.

168. Buolamwini JK. Cell cycle molecular targets and drug discovery. In *Cell Cycle Checkpoints and Cancer* (Blagosklonny MV, ed.), Landes Bioscience, Georgetown TX, 2001; pp. 235–246.

169. Sausville EA. Complexities in the development of cyclin-dependent kinase inhibitor drugs. *Trends Mol. Med.* 2002; 8(Issue 4 Suppl.):S32–S37.

170. Hardcastle IR, Golding BT, Griffin RJ. Designing inhibitors of cyclin-dependent kinases. *Annu. Rev. Pharmacol. Toxicol.* 2002; 42:325–348.

171. Meijer L. Chemical inhibitors of cyclin dependent kinases. *Trends Cell Biol.* 1996; 6:393–397.

172. Carlson BA, Dubay MM, Sausville EA, Brizuella L, Worland PJ. Flavopiridol induces G1 arrest with inhibition of cyclin-dependent kinase (CDK) 2 and CDK4 in human breast carcinoma cells. *Cancer Res.* 1996; 56:2973–2978.

173. Christain MC, Puda JM, Ho PTC, Arbuck SG, Murgo AJ, Sausville EA. Promising new agents under development by the division of cancer treatment, diagnosis, and centers of the national cancer institute. *Semin. Oncol.* 1997; 24:219–140.

174. Chao S-H, Price DH. Flavopiridol inactivates P-TEFb and blocks most RNA polymeRase II transcription in vivo. *J. Biol. Chem.* 2001; 276:31793–31799.

175. Wang D, de la Fuente C, Deng L, Wang L, Zilberman I, Eadie C, Healey M, Stein D, Denny T. Harrison LE, Meijer L, Kashanchi F. Inhibition of human immunodeficiency virus type-1 transcription by chemical cyclin-dependent kinase inhibitors. *J. Virol.* 2001; 75:7266–7279.

176. Iseki H, Ko TC, Xue XY, Seapan A, Hellmich MR, Townsend CW. Cyclin-dependent kinase inhibitors block proliferation of human gastric cancer cells. *Surgery* 1997; 122:187–194.

177. Gray NS, Wodika L, Thunnissen A-M et al. Exploiting chemical libraries, structure, and genomics in the search for kinase inhibitors. *Science* 1998; 281:533–538.

178. Sauseville EA, Zaharevitz D, Gussio R et al. Cyclin-dependent kinases: Initial approaches to exploit a novel therapeutic target. *Pharmacol. Ther.* 1999; 82:285–292.

179. Hoessel R, Leclerc S, Endicott JA et al. Indirubin, the active constituent of a Chinese antileukemia medicine, inhibits cyclin-dependent kinases. *Nat. Cell Biol.* 1999; 1:60–67.

180. Toogood P. Cyclin-dependent kinase inhibitors for treating cancer. *Med. Res. Rev.* 2001; 21:487–498.

181. Tetsu O, McCormick F. Proliferation of cancer cells despite CDK2 inhibition. *Cancer Cell* 2003; 3:233–245.

182. Wolf G, Elez R, Doermer A, Holtrich U, Ackermann H, Stutte HJ, Altmannsberger HM, Rubsamen-Waigmann H, Strebhardt K. Prognostic significance of polo-like kinase [PLK] expression in non-small cell lung cancer. *Oncogene* 1997; 14:543–549.

183. Bischoff JR, Anderson L, Zhu Y et al. A homologue of *Drosophila aurora* kinase is oncogenic and amplified in human colorectal cancers. *EMBO J.* 1998; 17:3052–3065.

184. Warner SL, Bearss DJ, Han H, Von Hoff DD. Targeting Aurora-2 kinase in cancer. *Mol. Cancer Ther.* 2003; 2:589–595.

185. Masuda Y, Nishida A, Hori K, Hirabayashi T, Kajimoto S, Nakajo S, Kondo T, Asaka M, Nakaya K. Beta-hydroxyisovalerylshikonin induces apoptosis in human leukemia cells by inhibiting the activity of a polo-like kinase 1 (PLK1). *Oncogene* 2003; 22:1012–1023.

186. Nakaya K, Miyasaka T. A shikonin derivative, beta-hydroxyisovalerylshikonin, is an ATP-non-competitive inhibitor of protein tyrosine kinases. *Anticancer Drugs* 2003; 14:683–693.

187. Coll JT, Renwick SB, Swenson L, Weber P, Lippke JA, Austen DA. Crystal structure of aurora-2, an oncogenic serine/threonine kinase. *J. Biol. Chem.* 2002; 277:42419–42422.

188. Nowakowski J, Cronin CN, McRee DE, Knuth MW, Nelson CG, Pavletich NP, Rogers J, Sang BC, Scheibe DN, Swanson RV, Thompson DA. Structures of the cancer-related Aurora-A, FAK, and EphA2 protein kinases from nanovolume crystallography. *Structure* 2002; 10:1659–1667.

189. Bates S, Vousden KH. p53 in signaling checkpoint arrest or apoptosis. *Curr. Opin. Genet. Dev.* 1996; 6:12–19.

190. Zhao B, Bower MJ, McDevitt PJ, Zhao H, Davis ST, Johanson KO, Green SM, Concha NO, Zhou BB. Structural basis for Chk1 inhibition by UCN-01. *J. Biol. Chem.* 2002; 277: 46609–46615.

191. Zhou BB, Sausville EA. Drug discovery targeting Chk1 and Chk2 kinases. *Prog. Cell Cycle Res.* 2003; 5:413–421.

192. Galaktionov K, Lee AK, Eckstein J, Draetta G, Meckler J, Loda M, Beach D. CDC25 phosphatases as potential human oncogenes. *Science* 1995; 269:1575–1577.

193. Lyon MA, Ducruet AP, Wipf P, Lazo JS. Dual-specificity phosphatases as targets for antineoplastic agents. *Nat. Rev. Drug Discov.* 2002; 1:961–976.

194. Ducruet AP, Rice RL, Tamura K, Yokokawa F, Yokokawa S, Wipf P, Lazo JS. Identification of new Cdc25 dual specificity phosphatase inhibitors in a targeted small molecule array. *Bioorg. Med. Chem.* 2000; 8:1451–1466.

195. Wang Z, Southwick EC, Wang M, Kar S, Rosi KS, Wilcox CS, Lazo JS, Carr BI. Involvement of Cdc25A phosphatase in Hep3B hepatoma cell growth inhibition induced by novel K vitamin analogs. *Cancer Res.* 2001; 61:7211–7216.

196. Botfield MC, Green J. SH2 and SH3 domains: choreographers of multiple signaling pathways. *Annu. Rep. Med. Chem.* 1995; 30:227–237.

197. Gishizky ML. Tyrosine kinase induced mitogenesis. Breaking the link with cancer. *Annu. Rep. Med. Chem.* 1995; 30:247–253.

198. Lowenstein EJ, Daly RJ, Batzer AG, Li W, Margolis B, Lammers R, Ullrich A, Skolnic EY, Bar-Sagi D, Schlessinger J. The SH2 and SH3 domain-containing protein GRB2 links receptor tyrosine kinases to Ras signaling. *Cell* 1992; 70:431–442.

199. Mayer BJ, Gupta R. Functions of SH2 and SH3 domains. *Curr. Top. Microb. Immunol.* 1998; 228:1–22.

200. Shi ZD, Lee K, Liu H, Zhang M, Roberts LR, Worthy KM, Fivash MJ, Fisher RJ, Yang D, Burke TR Jr. A novel macrocyclic tetrapeptide mimetic that exhibits low-picomolar Grb2 SH2 domain-binding affinity. *Biochem. Biophys. Res. Commun.* 2003; 310:378–383.

201. Bourne HR, Sanders DA, McCormic F. The GTPase superfamily: A conserved switch for diverse cell functions. *Nature* 1990; 348:125–132.

202. Mulcahy LS, Smith MR, Stacey D. Requirement for Ras proto-oncogene function during serum-stimulated growth in NIT 3T3 cells. *Nature* 1985; 313:241–243.

203. Barbacid M. Ras genes. *Annu. Rev. Biochem.* 1987; 56:779–827.

204. Bos JL. Ras oncogenes in human cancer: A review. *Cancer Res.* 1989; 49:4682–4689.

205. Boriack-Sjodin PA, Margait SM, Bar-Sagi D, Kuriyan J. The structural basis of the activation of Ras by Sos. *Nature* 1998; 394, 337–343.

206. Symons M. The Rac and Rho pathway as a source of drug targets for Ras-mediated malignancies. *Curr. Opin. Biotechnol.* 1995; 6:668–674.

207. Chou MM, Blenis J. The 70kD S6 kinase complexes with and is activated by the Rho family G proteins Cdc42 and Rac1. *Cell* 1996; 85:573–583.

208. Adini I, Rabinovitz I, Sun JF, Prendergast GC, Benjamin LE. RhoB controls Akt trafficking and stage-specific survival of endothelial cells during vascular development. *Gene Dev.* 2003; 17:2721–2732.

209. Sebolt-Leopold JS. A case for Ras targeted agents as antineoplastics. In *Cancer Therapeutics: Experimental and Clinical Agents* (Teicher, B., ed.), Humana Press, Totowa NJ, 1994; pp. 395–415.

210. Herrera R, Sebolt-Leopold JS. Unraveling the complexities of the Raf/MAP kinase pathway for pharmacological intervention. *Trends Mol. Med.* 2002; 8(Issue 4 Suppl.): S27–S31.

211. Adjei AA, Dy GK, Erlichman C, Reid JM, Sloan JA, Pitot HC, Alberts SR, Goldberg RM, Hanson LJ, Atherton PJ, Watanabe T, Geary RS, Holmlund J, Dorr FA. A phase I trial of ISIS 2503, an antisense inhibitor of H-Ras, in combination with gemcitabine in patients with advanced cancer. *Clin. Cancer Res.* 2003; 9:115–123.

212. Cunningham CC, Holmlund JT, Geary RS, Kwoh TJ, Dorr A, Johnston JF, Monia B, Nemunaitis J. A Phase I trial of H-Ras antisense oligonucleotide ISIS 2503 administered as a continuous intravenous infusion in patients with advanced carcinoma. *Cancer* 2001; 92:1265–1271.

213. Jackson JH, Cochrane CG, Bourne JR, Solski PA, Buss JE, Der CJ. Farnesol modification of Kirsten-Ras Exon 4B protein is essential for transformation. *Proc. Natl. Acad. Sci. U. S. A.* 1990; 87:3042–3046.

214. Kato K, Cox AD, Hisaka MM, Graham SM, Buss JE, Der CJ. Isoprenoid addition to Ras protein is the critical modification for its membrane association and transformation activity. *Proc. Natl. Acad. Sci. U. S. A.* 1992; 89:6403–6407.

215. Cox AD, Der CJ. Farnesyl transfeRase inhibitors and cancer treatment: Targeting simply Ras? *Biochim. Biophys. Acta* 1997; 1333:F51–F71.

216. Bolton GL, Sebolt-Leopold JS, Hodges JC. Ras oncogene directed approaches in cancer chemotherapy. *Annu. Rep. Med. Chem.* 1994; 29:165–174.

217. Leonard DM. Ras farnesyltransfeRase: A new therapeutic target. *J. Med. Chem.* 1997; 40:2971–2990.

218. Zujewski J. 1998; NCI Cancernet Web site. http://cancernet.nci.gov/cgi-bin/cancer-phy.

219. Dempke WC. FarnesyltransfeRase inhibitors — a novel approach in the treatment of advanced pancreatic carcinomas. *Anticancer Res.* 2003; 23:813–818.

220. Latchman DS. Transcription-factor mutations in disease. *N. Engl. J. Med.* 1996; 334:28–33.

221. Papavassiliou AG. Transcription factor-based drug design in anticancer drug development. *Mol. Med.* 1997; 3:99–810.

222. Lovec H, Grzeschiczek A, Kowalski M-B, Moroy T. Cyclin D1/bcl-1 cooperates with myc genes in the generation of B-Cell lymphoma in transgenic mice. *EMBO J.* 1994; 13:3487–3495.

223. Bodrug SE, Warner BJ, Bath ML, Linderman DJ, Harris AW, Adams JM. Cyclin D1 transgene impedes lymphocyte maturation and collaborates in lymphomagenesis with the myc gene. *EMBO J.* 1994; 13:2124–2130.

224. Gauwerky CE, Haluska FG, Tsujimoto Y, Nowell PC, Croce CM. Evolution of B-Cell malignancy: pre-B-cell leukemia resulting from MYC activation in a B-cell neoplasm with a rearranged Bcl2 gene. *Proc. Natl. Acad. Sci. U. S. A.* 1988; 85:8548–8552.

225. Wang J, Xie L, Y, Allan S, Beach D, Hannon GJ. Myc activates telomeRase. *Gene Dev.* 1998; 12:1769–1774.

226. Hermeking H. The MYC oncogene as a cancer drug target. *Curr. Cancer Drug Tar.* 2003; 3:163–675.

227. Wickstrom EL, Bacon TA, Gonzalez A, Freeman DL, Lyman GH, Wickstrom E. Human promyelocytic leukemia HL-60 cell proliferation and c-myc protein expression are inhibited by an antisense pentadecadeoxynucleotide targeted against c-myc mRNA. *Proc Natl. Acad. Sci. U. S. A.* 1988; 85:1028–1032.

228. Jain M, Arvanitis C, Chu K, Dewey W, Leonhardt E, Trinh M, Sundberg CD, Bishop JM, Felsher DW. Sustained loss of a neoplastic phenotype by brief inactivation of MYC. *Science* 2002; 297:102–104.

229. Iversen PL, Arora V, Acker AJ, Mason DH, Devi GR. Efficacy of antisense morpholino oligomer targeted to c-myc in prostate cancer xenograft murine model and a Phase I safety study in humans. *Clin. Cancer Res.* 2003; 9:2510–2519.

230. Hideshima T, Chauhan D, Richardson P, Mitsiades C, Mitsiades N, Hayashi T, Munshi N, Dang L, Castro A, Palombella V, Adams J, Anderson KC. NF-kappa B as a therapeutic target in multiple myeloma. *J. Biol. Chem.* 2002; 277:16639–16647.

231. Haefner B. NF-kB: Arresting a major culprit in cancer. *Drug Discov. Today* 2002; 7:653–663.

232. Baldwin AS Jr. The NF-kappa B and I kappa B proteins: New discoveries and insights. *Annu. Rev. Immunol.* 1996; 14:649–683.

233. Mercurio F, Manning AM. Multiple signals converging on NF-kappaB. *Curr. Opin. Cell Biol.* 1999; 11:226–232.

234. Mercurio F, Zhu H, Murray BW, Shevchenko A, Bennett BL, Li J, Young DB, Barbosa M, Mann M, Manning A, Rao A. IKK-1 and IKK-2: Cytokine-activated IkappaB kinases essential for NF-kappaB activation. *Science* 1997; 278:860–866.

235. Zandi E, Karin M. Bridging the gap: Composition, regulation, and physiological function of the IκB kinase complex. *Mol. Cell Biol.* 1999; 19:4547–4551.

236. Cusack JC, Liu R, Houston M et al. Enhanced chemosensitivity to CPT-11 with proteasome inhibitor PS-341: implications for systemic nuclear factor-kB inhibition. *Cancer Res.* 2001; 61:3535–3540.

237. Gustin JA, Ozes ON, Akca H, Pincheira R, Mayo L, Li Q, Rivera GJ, Korgaonkar CK, Donner DB. Cell type specific expression of the IkB kinases determines the significance of PI 3-kinase/Akt signaling to NF-kB activation. *J. Biol. Chem.* Oct 2003; 10.1074/jbc. M306976200.

238. Wang CY, May MW, Komeluk RG, Goeddel DV, Baldwin AS Jr. NF-KB antiapoptosis: Induction of TRAF1 and TRAF2 and C-IAP1 and C-IAP2 to suppress caspase 8 activation. *Science* 1998; 28:1680–1683.

239. Ryan KM, Ernsi ME, Rice NR, Vousden KH. Role of NF-kB in p53-mediated programmed cell death. *Nature* 1999; 404:892–896.

240. Baldwin AS. Control of oncogenesis and cancer therapy resistance by the transcription factor NF-κB. *J. Clin. Invest.* 2001; 107:241–246.

241. Semenza GL. HIF-1 and tumor progression: pathophysiology and therapeutics. *Trends Mol. Med.* 2002; 8(Issue 4 Suppl.):S62–S67.

242. Rapisarda A, Uranchimeg B, Scudiero DA, Selby M, Sausville EA, Shoemaker RH, Melillo G. Identification of small molecule inhibitors of hypoxia-inducible factor 1 transcriptional activation pathway. *Cancer Res.* 2002; 62:4316–4324.

243. Kung AL, Wang S, Klco JM, Kaelin WG, Livingston DM. Suppression of tumor growth through disruption of hypoxia-inducible transcription. *Nat. Med.* 2000; 6:1335–1340.

244. Giaccia A, Siim BG, Johnson RS. HIF-1 as a target for drug development. *Nat. Rev. Drug Discov.* 2002; 2:803–811.

245. Kersten S, Desvergne B, Wahli W. Roles of PPARs in health and disease *Nature* 2000; 405:421–424.

246. Panigrahy D, Shen LQ, Kieran MW, Kaipainen A. Therapeutic potential of thiazolidinediones as anticancer agents. *Expert Opin. Inv. Drugs* 2003; 12:1925–1937.

247. Placha W, Gil D, Dembinska-Kiec A, Laidler P. The effect of PPARgamma ligands on the proliferation and apoptosis of human melanoma cells. *Melanoma Res.* 2003; 13:447–456.

248. Park BH, Vogelstein B, Kinzler KW. Genetic disruption of PPARdelta decreases the tumorigenicity of human colon cancer cells. *Proc. Natl. Acad. Sci. U. S. A.* 2001; 98:2598–2603.

249. Oro AE, Higgins KM, Hu Z, Bonifas JM, Epstein EH, Scot MP. Basal cell carcinomas in mice overexpressing sonic hedgehog. *Science* 1997; 276:817–821.

250. Stecca B, Altaba AR. The therapeutic potential of modulators of the Hedgehog-Gli signaling pathway. *J. Biol.* 2002; 1:9.1–9.4.

251. Taipale J, Beachy PA. The Hedgehog and wnt signalling pathways in cancer. *Nature* 2001; 411:349–354.

252. Taylor MD, Liu L, Raffel C et al. Mutations in *SUFU* predispose to medulloblastoma. *Nat. Genet.* 2002; 31:306–310.

253. Taipale J, Chen JK, Cooper MK, Wang B, Mann RK, Melinkovic L, Scott MP, Beachy PA. Effects of oncogenic mutations in Smoothened and Patched can be reversed by cyclopamine. *Nature* 2000; 406:1005–1009.

254. Frank-Kamenetsky M, Zhang XM, Bottega S, Guicherit O, Wichterle H, Dudet H, Bumcrot D, Wang FY, Jones S, Shulok J, Rubin LL, Porter JA. Small molecule modulators of hedgehog signaling: Identification and characterization of smoothened agonists and antagonists. *J. Biol.* 2002; 1:10.

255. Chen JK, Taipale J, Young KE, Maiti T, Beachy PA. Small molecule modulation of Smoothened activity. *Proc. Natl. Acad. Sci. U. S. A.* 2002; 99, 14071–14076.

256. Hengartner MO. The biochemistry of apoptosis. *Nature* 2000; 407:770–776.

257. Reed JC. Dysregulation of apoptosis in cancer. *J. Clin. Oncol.* 1999; 17:2941–2953.

258. Sellers WR, Fisher DE. Apoptosis and cancer drug targeting. *Clin. Invest.* 1999; 104:1655–1661.

259. Lane DP. p53 guardian of the genome. *Nature* 1992; 358, 15–16.

260. Culotta E, Koshland DE. Molecule of the year: p53 sweeps cancer research. *Science* 1993; 262, 1958–1961.

261. Levine AJ. p53 the cellular gate keeper for growth and division. *Cell* 1997; 88:323–331.

262. Harris CC. Structure and function of the p53 tumor suppressor gene: Clues for rational cancer therapeutic strategies. *J. Natl. Cancer Inst.* 1996; 88:1442–1455.

263. Kastan MB, Zhan Q, El-Deiry WS, Carrier F, Jacks T, Walsh WV, Plunkett BS, Vogelstein B, Fornace AJ Jr. A mammalian cell cycle checkpoint pathway utilizing p53 and GADD45 is defective in ataxia-telangiectasia. *Cell* 1992; 71:587–597.

264. Miyashita T, Reed JC. Tumor suppressor p53 is a direct transcriptional activator of the bax gene. *Cell* 1995; 80:293–299.

265. White E. Life, death and the pursuit of apoptosis. *Gene Dev.* 1996; 10:1–15.

266. Caelles C, Helmberg A, Karin M. p53-dependent apoptosis in the absence of transcriptional activation of p53-targeted genes. *Nature* 1994; 370:220–223.

267. Lane DP, Lain S. Therapeutic exploitation of the p53 pathway. *Trends Mol. Med.* 2002; 8[4], S38–S42.

268. Lowe SW, Ruley HE, Jacks T, Housman DE. p53-dependent apoptosis modulates the cytotoxicity of anticancer agents. *Cell* 1993; 74:957–967.

269. Kerr DJ, Workman P, eds. *New Molecular Targets for Cancer Chemotherapy*, CRC Press, Boca Raton, FL 1994.

270. Buttitta F, Marchetti A, Gadducci A, Pellegrini S, Morganti M, Carnicelli V, Cosio S, Gagetti O, Genazzani AR, Bevilacqua G. p53 alterations are predictive of chemoresistance and aggressiveness in ovarian carcinomas: A molecular and immunohistochemical study. *Br. J. Cancer* 1997; 75:230–235.

271. Aas T, Borressen A-L, Geisler S, Smith-Sorensen B, Johnse H, Varhau JE, Akslen LA, Lonning PE. Specific p53 mutations are associated with de novo resistance to doxorubicin in breast cancer patients. *Nat. Med.* 1996; 2:811–814.

272. Herr I, Debatin K-M. Cellular stress response and apoptosis in cancer therapy. *Blood* 2001; 98:2603–2614.

273. upp TR, Lane DP, Ball KL. Strategies for manipulating the p53 pathway in the treatment of human cancer. *Biochem. J.* 2000; 352:1–17.

274. Liner JD, Kinzler KW, Meltzer PS, George PL, Vogelstein B. Amplification of a gene encoding a p53-associated protein in human sarcomas. *Nature* 1992; 358:80–83.

275. Inlay CA. The mdm-2 oncogene can overcome wild-type p53 suppression of transformed cell growth. *Mol. Cell Biol.* 1993; 13:301–306.

276. Midgley CA, Lane DP. p53 protein stability in tumor cells is not determined by mutation but is dependent on mdm2 binding. *Oncogene* 1997; 15:1179–1189.

277. Thut CJ, Goodrich JA, Tjian R. Repression of p53-mediated transcription by MDM2: A dual mechanism. *Gene Dev.* 1997; 11:1974–1986.

278. Barak Y, Juven T, Haffner R, Oren M. mdm-2 Expression is induced by wild-type p53 activity. *EMBO J.* 1993; 12:461–468.

279. Chen J, Lin J, Levine AJ. Regulation of transcription function of the p53 tumor suppressor by the mdm-2 oncogene. *Mol. Med.* 1995; 1:142–152.

280. Momand J, Jung D, Wilczynski S, Niland J. The MDM2 gene amplification database. *Nucleic Acids Res.* 1998; 26:3453–3459.

281. Landers JE, Cassel SL, George DL. Translational enhancement of Mdm2 oncogene expression in human tumor cells containing a stabilized wild-type p53 protein. *Cancer Res.* 1997; 57, 3562–3568.

282. Wang H, Oliver P, Zeng X, Le LP, Chen J, Chen L, Zhou W, Agrawal S, Zhang R. MDM2 oncogene as a target for cancer therapy: An antisense approach. *Int. J. Oncol.* 1999; 15, 653–660.

283. Zhang R, Wang H. MDM2 oncogene as a novel target for human cancer therapy. *Curr. Pharm. Design* 2000; 6:393–416.

284. Bottger A, Bottger V, Garcia-Echeverria C, Chene P, Hochkeppel H-K, Sampson W, Ang K, Howard SF, Picksley SM, Lane DP. Molecular characterization of the mdm2-p53 interactions. *Mol. Biol.* 1997; 9:744–756.

285. Bottger V, Bottger A, Howard SF, Picksley SM, Chene P, Garcia-Echeverria C, Hochkeppel H-K, Lane DP. Identification of novel mdm2 binding peptides by phage display. *Oncogene* 1996; 13:2141–2147.

286. Garcia-Echeverria C, Chene P, Blommers MJJ, Furet P. Discovery of potent antagonists of the interaction between human double minute 2 and tumor suppressor p53. *J. Med. Chem.* 2000; 43:3205–3208.

287. Arriola EL, Lopez AR, Chresta CM. Differential regulation of p21/waf-1/cip-1 and mdm2 by etoposide: etoposide inhibits the p53-mdm2 autoregulatory feedback loop. *Oncogene* 1999; 18:1081–1091.

288. Stoll R, Renner C, Hansen S et al. Chalcone derivatives antagonize interactions between the human oncoprotein mdm2 and p53. *Biochemistry* 2001; 40:336–344.

289. Chen L, Agrawal S, Zhou W, Zhang R, Chen Z. Synergistic activation of p53 by inhibition of mdm2 expression and DNA damage *Proc. Natl. Acad. Sci. U. S. A.* 1998; 95:195–200.

290. Chen L, Lu W, Agrawal S, Zhou W, Zhang R, Chen J. Ubiquitous induction of p53 in tumor cells by antisense inhibition of mdm2 expression. *Mol. Med.* 1999; 5:21–34.

291. Chao DT, Korsmeyer SJ. BCL-2 family: Regulators of cell death. *Annu. Rev. Immunol.* 1998; 16:395–419.

292. Kojima H, Endo K, Moriyama H, Tanaka Y, Alnemri ES, Slapak CA, Teicher B, Kufe D, Datta R. Abrogation of mitochondrial cytochrome c release and caspase-3 activation in acquired multidrug resistance. *J. Biol. Chem.* 1998; 273:16647–16650.

293. Tsujimoto Y, Gorham J, Cossman J, Jaffe E, Croce CM. The t[14;18] chromosome translocations involved in B-cell neoplasms result from mistakes in VDJ joining. *Science* 1985; 229:1390–1393.

294. Bissonnette R, Echeverri F, Mahboubi A, Green DR. Apoptotic cell death induced by c-myc is inhibited by bcl-2. *Nature* 1992; 359:552–554.

295. Korsmeyer SJ. Bcl-2 initiates a new category of oncogenes: Regulators of cell death. *Blood* 1992; 80:879–886.

296. Oltersdorf T, Fritz LC. The bcl-2 family: targets for the regulation of apoptosis. *Annu. Rep. Med. Chem.* 1998; 33:253–262.

297. Diaz J-L, Oltersdorf T, Horne W, McConnell M, Wilson G, Weeks S, Garcia T, Fritz LC. A common binding site mediates heterodimerization and homodimerization of bcl-2 family members. *J. Biol. Chem.* 1997; 272:11350–11355.

298. Enyedy IJ, Ling Y, Nacro K, Tomita Y, Wu X, Cao Y, Guo R, Li B, Zhu X, Huang Y, Long YQ, Roller PP, Yang D, Wang S. Discovery of small-molecule inhibitors of Bcl-2 through structure-based computer screening. *J. Med. Chem.* 2001; 44:4313–4324.

299. Wang JL, Liu D, Zhang ZJ, Shan S, Han X, Srinivasula SM, Croce CM, Alnemri ES, Huang Z. Structure-based discovery of an organic compound that binds Bcl-2 protein and induces apoptosis of tumor cells. *Proc. Natl. Acad. Sci. U. S. A.* 2000; 97:7124–7129.

300. Nahta R, Esteva FJ. Bcl-2 antisense oligonucleotides: A potential novel strategy for the treatment of breast cancer. *Semin. Oncol.* 2003; 30:143–149.

301. Simoes-Wust AP, Olie RA, Gautschi O, Leech SH, Haner R, Hall J, Fabbro D, Stahel RA, Zangemeister-Wittke U. Bcl-xl antisense treatment induces apoptosis in breast carcinoma cells. *Int. J. Cancer* 2000; 87:582–590.

302. Zangemeister-Wittke U, Leech SH, Olie RA, Simoes-Wust AP, Gautschi O, Luedke GH, Natt F, Haner R, Martin P, Hall J, Nalin CM, Stahel RA. A novel bispecific antisense oligonucleotide inhibiting both bcl-2 and bcl-xL expression efficiently induces apoptosis in tumor cells. *Clin. Cancer Res.* 2000; 6:2547–2555.

303. Degterev A, Lugovskoy A, Cardone M, Mulley B, Wagner G, Mitchison T, Yuan J. Identification of small-molecule inhibitors of interaction between the BH3 domain and Bcl-XL. *Nat. Cell Biol.* 2001; 3:173–182.

304. Wang S, Yang D, Lippman ME. Targeting Bcl-2 and Bcl-XL with nonpeptidic small-molecule antagonists. *Semin. Oncol.* 2003; 30(5 Suppl. 16):133–142.

305. Ambrosini G, Adida C, Altieri DC. A novel anti-apoptosis gene, survivin, expressed in cancer and lymphoma. *Nat. Med.* 1997; 3:917–921.

306. Deveraux QL, Reed JC. IAP family proteins — suppressors of apoptosis. *Gene Dev.* 1999; 13:239–252.

307. Li F, Ambrosini G, Chu EY, Plescia J, Tognin S, Marchisio PC and Altieri DC. Control of apoptosis and mitotic spindle checkpoint by survivin. *Nature* 1998; 396:580–584.

308. Altieri DC. Survivin, versatile modulation of cell division and apoptosis in cancer. *Oncogene* 2003; 22:8581–8589.

309. Altieri DC. Survivin and apoptosis control. *Adv. Cancer Res.* 2003; 88:31–52.

310. Ambrosini G, Adida C, Sirugo G, Altieri DC. Induction of apoptosis and inhibition of cell proliferation by survivin gene targeting. *J. Biol. Chem.* 1998; 273:11177–11182.

311. Monzo M, Rosell R, Felip E, Astudillo J, Sanchez JJ, Maestre J, Martin C, Font A, Barnadas A, Abad A. A novel anti-apoptosis gene: Re-expression of surviving messenger RNA as a prognosis marker in non-small cell lung cancers. *J. Clin. Oncol.* 1999; 17:2100–2104.

312. Grossman D, Kim PJ, Schechner JS, Altieri DC. Inhibition of melanoma tumor growth in vivo by survivin targeting. *Proc. Natl. Acad. Sci. U. S. A.* 2001; 98:635–640.

313. Blanc-Brude OP, Mesri M, Wall NR, Plescia J, Dohi T, Altieri DC. Therapeutic targeting of the survivin pathway in cancer: Initiation of mitochondrial apoptosis and suppression of tumor-associated angiogenesis. *Clin. Cancer Res.* 2003; 9:2683–2692.

314. O'Driscoll L, Linehan R, Clynes M. Survivin: Role in normal cells and in pathological conditions. *Curr. Cancer Drug Tar.* 2003; 3:131–152.

315. Deveraux QL, Takahashi R, Salvesen GS, Reed JC. X-linked lAP is a direct inhibitor of cell-death proteases. *Nature* 1997; 388:300–304.

316. LaCasse EC, Baird S, Komeluk RG, MacKenzie AE. The inhibitors of apoptosis [IAPs] and their emerging role in cancer. *Oncogene* 1998; 17:3247–3259.

317. Beere HM, Wolf BB, Cain K, Mosser DD, Mahboubi A, Kuwana T, Tailor P, Morimoto RI, Cohen GM, Green DR. Heat-shock protein 70 inhibits apoptosis by preventing recruitment of procaspase-9 to the Apaf-1 apoptosome. *Nat. Cell Biol.* 2000; 2:469–475.

318. Saleh A, Srinivasula SM, Balkir L, Robbins PD, Alnemri ES. Negative regulation of the Apaf-1 apoptosome by Hsp70. *Nat. Cell Biol.* 2000; 2:476–483.

319. Nylandsted J, Rohde M, Brand K, Bastholm L, Elling F, Jaattela M. Selective depletion of heat shock protein 70 [Hsp70] activates a tumor-specific death program that is independent of caspases and bypasses Bcl-2. *Proc. Natl. Acad. Sci. U. S. A.* 2000; 97:7871–7876.

320. Nylandsted J, Wick W, Hirt UA, Brand K, Rohde M, Leist M, Weller M, Jaattela M. Eradication of glioblastoma, and breast and colon carcinoma xenografts by Hsp70 depletion. *Cancer Res.* 2002; 62:7139–7142.

321. Blackburn EH. TelomeRases. *Annu. Rev. Biochem.* 1992; 61:113–129.

322. Kim NW, Piatyszek MA, Prowse KR, Harley CB, West MD, Ho PLC, Coviello GM, Wright WE, Weinrich SL, Shay JW. Specific association of human telomeRase activity with immortal cells and cancer. *Science* 1994; 266:2011–2015.

323. Mergny JL, Riou JF, Mailliet P, Teulade-Fichou MP, Gilson E. Natural and pharmacological regulation of telomeRase. *Nucleic Acids Res.* 2002; 30:839–865.

324. Burger AM, Bibby MC, Double JA. TelomeRase activity in normal and malignant mammalian tissues: Feasibility of telomeRase as a target for cancer chemotherapy. *Br. J. Cancer* 1997; 75:516–522.

325. Sharma S, Raymond E, Soda H, Von Hoff DD. TelomeRase and telomere inhibitors in preclinical development. *Expert Opin. Inv. Drugs* 1997; 6:1179–1185.

326. Hamilton SE, Corey DR. TelomeRase: anti-cancer target or just a fascinating enzyme? *Chem. Biol.* 1996; 3:863–867.

327. Parkinson EK. Do telomeRase antagonists represent a novel anti-cancer strategy? *Br. J. Cancer* 1996; 73:1–4.

328. Stewart SA, Hahn WC. Prospects for anti-neoplastic therapies based on telomere biology. *Curr. Cancer Drug Tar.* 2002; 2:1–17.

329. Aszalos A, Eckhardt S. Molecular events as targets of anticancer drug therapy. *Pathol. Oncol. Res.* 1997; 3:147–158.

330. Perry PJ, Gowan SM, Reszka AP, Polucci P, Jenkins TC, Kelland LR, Niedle S. 1,4- and 2,6-disubstituted amidoanthracene-9,10-dione derivatives as inhibitors of human telomeRase. *J. Med. Chem.* 1998; 41:3253–3260.

331. Folkman J. Angiogenesis in cancer, vascular rheumatoid and other diseases. *Nat. Med.* 1995; 1, 27–31.

332. Folkman J. Clinical applications of research on angiogenesis. *N. Engl. J. Med.* 1995; 333:1757–1763.

333. Folkman J. Fighting cancer by attacking its blood supply. *Sci. Am.* 1996; 275:150–154.

334. Gourley M, Williamson JS. Angiogenesis: New targets for the development of anticancer chemotherapies. *Curr. Pharm. Design* 2000; 6:417–439.

335. Folkman J, Klagsbrun M. Angiogenic factors. *Science* 1987; 235:442–447.

336. Nelson NJ. News item: inhibitors of angiogenesis enter phase III testing. *J. Natl. Cancer Inst.* 1998; 90:960–963.

337. Chillemi F, Francescato P, Ragg E, Cattaneo MG, Pola S, Vicentini L. Studies on the structure-activity relationship of endostatin: Synthesis of human endostatin peptides exhibiting potent antiangiogenic activities. *J. Med. Chem.* 2003; 46:4165–4172.

338. Cattaneo MG, Pola S, Francescato P, Chillemi F, Vicentini LM. Human endostatin-derived synthetic peptides possess potent antiangiogenic properties in vitro and in vivo. *Exp. Cell Res.* 2003; 283:230–236.

339. Lentzsch S, Rogers MS, LeBlanc R, Birsner AE, Shah JH, Treston AM, Anderson KC, D'Amato RJ. S-3-Amino-phthalimido-glutarimide inhibits angiogenesis and growth of B-cell neoplasias in mice. *Cancer Res.* 2002; 62:2300–2305.

340. Singh RP, Agarwal R. Tumor angiogenesis: a potential target in cancer control by phyto-chemicals. *Curr. Cancer Drug Tar.* 2003; 3:205–217.

341. Watnick RS, Cheng YN, Rangarajan A, Ince TA, Weinberg RA. Ras modulates Myc activity to repress thrombospondin-1 expression and increase tumor angiogenesis. *Cancer Cell* 2003; 3:219–231.

342. Mazzieri R, Masiero L, Zanetta L, Monea S, Onisto M, Garbisa S, Mignatti P. Control of type IV collagenase activity by components of the urokinase-plasminsystem: A regulatory mechanism with cell-bound reactants. *EMBO J.* 1997; 16, 2319–2332.

343. Vihinen P, Kahari V-M. Matrix metalloproteinases in cancer: Prognostic markers and thera-peutic targets. *Int. J. Cancer* 2002; 99:157–166.

344. Rabbani SA. Metalloproteases and urokinase in angiogenesis and tumor progression. *In Vivo* 1998; 12:135–142.

345. Foda HD, Zucker S. Matrix metalloproteinases in cancer invasion, metastasis and angio-genesis. *Drug Discov. Today.* 2001; 6:478–482.

346. Zucker S, Cao J, Chen WT. Critical appraisal of the use of matrix metalloproteinase inhibitors in cancer treatment. *Oncogene* 2000; 19:6642–6650.

347. Coussens LM, Fingleton B, Matrisian LM. Matrix metalloproteinase inhibitors and cancer: Trials and tribulations. *Science* 2002; 295:2387–2392.

348. Weidle UH, Konig B. Urokinase receptor antagonists: Novel agents for the treatment of cancer. *Expert Opin. Inv. Drugs* 1998; 7:391–404.

349. Kim J, Wu W, Kovalski K, Ossowski L. Requirement of specific proteases in cancer cell intravasation as revealed by a novel semi-quantitative PCR-based assay. *Cell* 1998; 94:335–362.

350. Edwards DR, Murphy G. Proteases — invasion and more. *Nature* 1998; 394:527–528.

351. Huang Y-W, Baluna R, Vitetta ES. Adhesion molecules as targets for cancer therapy. *Histol. Histopathol.* 1997; 12:467–477.

352. Shaw LM, Rabinovitz I, Wang HH-F, Toker A, Mercurio AM. Activation of phosphoinosi-tol 3-OH kinase by the α6β4 integrin promotes carcinoma invasion. *Cell* 1997; 91:949–960.

353. El-Hariry I, Pignatelli M. Adhesion molecules: Opportunities for modulation and a paradigm for novel therapeutic approaches in cancer. *Expert Opin. Inv. Drugs* 1997; 6:1465–1478.

354. Engleman VW, Kellogg MS, Rogers TE. Cell adhesion integrins as pharmaceutical targets. *Annu. Rep. Med. Chem.* 1996; 31:191–200.

355. Fish RG. Role of gangliosides in tumor progression: a molecular target for cancer therapy? *Med. Hypotheses* 1996; 46:140–144.

356. Adams J. Potential for proteasome inhibition in the treatment of cancer. *Drug Discov. Today* 2003; 8:307–315.

357. Ma MH, Yang HH, Parker K, Manyak S, Friedman JM, Altamirano C, Wu ZQ, Borad MJ, Frantzen M, Roussos E, Neeser J, Mikail A, Adams J, Sjak-Shie N, Vescio RA, Berenson JR. The proteasome inhibitor PS-341 markedly enhances sensitivity of multiple myeloma tumor cells to chemotherapeutic agents. *Clin. Cancer Res.* 2003; 9:1136–1144.

358. Workman P. Overview: Translating Hsp90 biology into Hsp90 drugs. *Curr. Cancer Drug Tar.* 2003; 3:297–300.

359. Sausville EA, Tomaszewski JE, Ivy P. Clinical development of 17-allylamino, 17-demethoxygeldanamycin. *Curr. Cancer Drug Tar*. 2003; 3:377–383.

360. Banerji U, Judson I, Workman P. The clinical applications of heat shock protein inhibitors in cancer — present and future. *Curr. Cancer Drug Tar*. 2003; 3:385–390.

361. Chiosis G, Lucas B, Huezo H, Solit D, Basso A, Rosen N. Development of purine-scaffold small molecule inhibitors of Hsp90. *Curr. Cancer Drug Tar*. 2003; 3:371–376.

362. Soga S, Shiotsu Y, Akinaga S, Sharma SV. Development of radicicol analogues. *Curr. Cancer Drug Tar*. 2003; 3:359–369.

363. Kamal A, Thao L, Sensintaffar J, Zhang L, Boehm MF, Fritz LC, Burrows FJ. A high-affinity conformation of Hsp90 confers tumour selectivity on Hsp90 inhibitors. *Nature* 2003; 425:407–410.

364. Workman P, ed., *Curr. Cancer Drug Tar*. 2003; 3, Issue4

365. Johnstone RW. Histone-deacetylase inhibitors: Novel drugs for the treatment of cancer. *Nat. Rev. Drug Discov*. 2002; 1:287–299.

366. Gabrielli BG, Johnstone RW, Saunders NA. Identifying molecular targets mediating the anticancer activity of histone deacetylase inhibitors: A work in progress. *Curr. Cancer Drug Tar*. 2002; 2:337–353.

367. Kelly WK, O'Connor OA, Marks PA. Histone deacetylase inhibitors: From target to clinical trials. *Expert Opin. Inv. Drugs* 2002; 11:1695–1713.

368. Chen JS, Faller DV, Spanjaard RA. Short-chain fatty acid inhibitors of histone deacetylases: Promising anticancer therapeutics? *Curr. Cancer Drug Tar*. 2003; 3:219–236.

369. Finnin et al. Structures of a histone deacetylase homologue bound to the TSA and SAHA inhibitors. Nature 1999; 401:188–193.

2

MICROARRAYS: SMALL SPOTS PRODUCE MAJOR ADVANCES IN PHARMACOGENOMICS

M. NEES

Division of Molecular Diagnostics and Therapy
Department of Surgery
University of Heidelberg, Germany

W. KUSNEZOW

Division of Functional Genome Analysis
German Cancer Research Center
Heidelberg, Germany

C. D. WOODWORTH

Department of Biology
Clarkson University
Potsdam, New York

   I. INTRODUCTION TO MICROARRAYS
  II. ADVANTAGES OF DNA MICROARRAYS
 III. MAJOR DNA ARRAY FORMATS: SOMETHING FOR EVERYONE
 IV. WHAT IS THE BEST WAY TO INTERFACE WITH MICROARRAYS?
  V. MICROARRAYS AND PHARMACOGENOMICS: REVOLUTIONIZING DISCOVERY OF NEW DRUGS AND GENE FUNCTION
 VI. WHAT CAN GO WRONG IN cDNA MICROARRAY EXPERIMENTATION
VII. ARRAY-BASED PROTEOMICS: HOW TO INVESTIGATE PROTEIN COMPLEXITY
VIII. EMERGING MICROARRAY TECHNOLOGIES FOR HIGH-THROUGHPUT PROTEOME INVESTIGATION: A TECHNICAL OVERVIEW
 IX. CURRENT AND FUTURE APPLICATIONS OF PROTEIN ARRAYS IN DRUG DISCOVERY
  X. HOW TO DEAL WITH ALL THAT DATA
 XI. THE FUTURE IS ONLY GOING TO GET BETTER

The advent of microarray technology has led to fundamental improvements in the way that researchers address biomedical questions. DNA microarrays provide extensive information on gene function and interaction by simultaneously measuring the expression of thousands of RNAs or proteins. Microarray technology has many applications for clinical and basic research. These include identification of novel drug targets and marker genes for disease progression, improving clinical diagnosis, discovering mechanisms of drug action, and providing information on drug efficacy and toxicity. Great advancements have occurred in array technology within the last two years. In this chapter basic aspects of DNA and protein microarrays and their applications for pharmacogenomics are discussed. Specifically, microarray instrumentation and experimentation are described and each of the major array formats including oligonucleotides arrays, spotted arrays, and macroarrays are presented. The advantages, disadvantages, and options for using each array format are also discussed. Important factors in the design and analysis of microarray experiments are reviewed. The most recent developments in microarray technology, which include peptide and antibody arrays, are presented. Most important, provide examples of new applications of microarrays are provided with a focus on cancer research and drug discovery.

I. INTRODUCTION TO MICROARRAYS

Within the last few years the genomes of more than 40 organisms have been completely sequenced and a rough map of the human genome has been completed [1, 2]. Biomedical research has been revolutionized through the knowledge of these sequences. The next important goal will be to understand the function of these newly identified genes and how normal function is altered in human disease [3, 4]. The science of genomics examines how individual genes operate in the context of a complex organism [5, 6]. Pharmacogenomics focuses on identification of new drug targets and prediction of drug activity [7, 8]. Oncogenomics is the use of genomic approaches to study cancer biology. A diversity of novel techniques has emerged recently to study differential gene expression, and one of the most promising is microarrays [9]. Microarrays are composed of many thousands of oligonucleotides or cDNAs that have been deposited on a small substrate. Nucleic acids are labeled with radioactivity, biotin, or a fluorescent tag and then hybridized to DNA sequences immobilized on the substrate. Differences in hybridization are detected using autoradiography, laser scanning, light emission by charge coupled device cameras, or most recently, by electronic semiconductor chips (Nanogen Inc., San Diego, CA). Microarrays are commonly used to analyze a wide variety of questions involving differential mRNA gene expression, genomic alterations [10], mutations in DNA, or single nucleotide polymorphisms (SNPs). They are also appropriate for DNA sequencing. For instance, HySeq Inc. (Sunnyvale, CA) markets the "HyChip" technology, which can analyze up to 5000 bases in a single experiment. Spotted peptides or antibodies have been developed to study protein expression on a global scale [11–13] and will be discussed in detail. Tissue microarrays are currently revolutionizing clinical diagnostics. Small arrays of paraffin-embedded tissue fragments represent a powerful tool with which to localize gene expression within normal or diseased clinical samples [14–16]. Recently, arrays of living cells were pioneered by Cellomics, Inc., (Pittsburgh, PA). Chemical arrays with spotted ligands and other small synthetic molecules have been introduced most recently by Graffinity (Heidelberg, Germany), and Caliper Instruments has developed a similar system (LibraryCard Reagent Array). Chemical arrays are an important novel tool to define and quantify biochemical interactions between drugs or ligands and biological macromolecules. These systems will be extremely important for pharmaceutical companies that screen thousands of chemical compounds for drug evaluation. All of these high-throughput microtechnologies allow one to locate and quantitatively assess the level of multiple DNAs, mRNAs, proteins, or biochemical interactions in a complex sample.

Microarray technology continues to evolve rapidly. A critical factor for the breakthrough of cDNA array or gene chip technology during the 1990s was the availability of cDNA clones from public repositories such as the IMAGE consortium. The expressed sequence tag (EST) sequencing projects and the construction of comprehensive genomic databases such as GenBank and UniGene were a prerequisite for the success of microarrays. Recently, the availability of complete sequence data from humans and other organisms has hastened developments in array technology. Although arrays were constructed to analyze thousands of genes several years ago, now all genes encoded by an organism can be analyzed simultaneously in one array experiment. Full-genome studies were initially performed for yeast [17], which has a total of 6307 open reading frames. Other organisms followed, which included a number of important human pathogens. The complete catalogue of genes and messenger RNAs revealed by the human genome project now requires careful experimental annotation and validation on a genomic scale [1, 2]. Oligonucleotide arrays that contain all currently known or deduced human exons have been developed [18]. Shoemaker et al. [18] used "exon" and "tiling" arrays fabricated by ink-jet oligonucleotide synthesis to validate and refine computational gene predictions and identify co-expressed genes. This array-based method will help to provide an accurate count of human genes and allow detection of alternative mRNA splice variants. Although complete genome data are not yet available for the mouse, Riken (Japan) has made public 18,000 full-length mouse cDNA clones. This large collection has been used to produce cDNA microarrays for gene expression profiling in diverse mouse tissues [19]. Similar large, comprehensive mouse arrays have been used to monitor global gene expression patterns in various tissues and cell types and during mammalian development (particularly at an early stage) [20].

A large number of algorithms and software packages have been developed to organize the vast amount of data generated by microarrays (reviewed in references 21–23). Hundreds of companies market arrays, array services, analysis software, or detection devices for arrays. An information-intensive Web page maintained by Shi (www.gene-chips.com) provides an excellent overview of currently available techniques and possibilities. In summary, microarrays are an extremely powerful new tool for discovery of how genes function, how they interact with other genes, and how altered gene function contributes to human disease. The objectives of this chapter are to describe new developments in microarray technology and to emphasize their potential for pharmacogenomics, cancer research, and discovery of gene function. For this purpose, the focus is mainly on expression arrays, but this chapter also discusses protein, peptide, and other non-DNA arrays. The latter represents the next generation of high-throughput tools for analysis of gene expression and will become increasingly important with the growing interest in proteomics in the post-genomic era. Microarray-related online resources mentioned in this chapter are listed in Tables 1 and 2. Table 1 lists a number of non-commercial Web sites related to microarray production, analysis, gene expression databases, functional genomics, and bioinformatics. Web sites from commercial suppliers of microarrays and related techniques are listed in Table 2.

TABLE 2.1 Selection of Non-Commercial Web Sites Related to Microarray Production, Analysis, Gene Expression Databases, Functional Genomics and Bioinformatics

Organization or database	Contents	Web site L
Arabidopsis Functional Genomics Consortium AFGC	Microarray technologies and their applications in plant biology	http://afgc.stanford.edu/
Array Express	Microarray database at EBI (European Bioinformatics Institute, Hinxton, UK)	http://www.ebi.ac.uk/arrayexpress
Association of Biomolecular Resource Facilities ABRF	ABRF's Microarray Research Group (MARG)	http://www.abrf.org/ABRF/ ResearchCommittees/MARG/marg.html
CGAP (Cancer Genome Anatomy Project) at NCBI	Resources and databases on cancer specific gene expression	http://www.ncbi.nlm.nih.gov/CGAP/
Chemical Industry Institute of Toxicology (CIIT)	Information on toxicogenomics and microarrays	http://www.ciit.org/TOXICOGENOMICS/ homepage.html
CSNDB	Cell signaling networks database	http://geo.nihs.go.jp/csndb/
DbEST	Sequence data and other information on single pass cDNA sequences	http://www.ncbi.nlm.nih.gov/web/genbank
Eisen Lab	Mike Eisen's software resources	http://rana.lbl.gov/
ENTREZ	PubMed/Medline, protein and nucleotide database	http://www.ncbi.nlm.nih.gov/Entrez
EPD	Eukaryotic promoter database	http://www.epd.isb-sib.ch/
EuroBioChips	Information on microarray and microfluidic technologies	http://www.eurobiochips.com/index2.html
Genbank at NCBI	Genetic sequence database of publicly available sequences	http://www.ncbi.nlm.nih.gov/web/genbank
GeneCards at Weitzmann Institute	Database at Weitzmann Institute of Science, Israel	http://bioinformatics.weizmann.ac.il/cards http://genome.www.stanford.edu/genecards
GeneX	Repository of gene expression data	http://www.ncgr.org/genex/
GGEG Global Gene Expression Group	SAGE-related information and databases at MD Anderson Cancer Center	http://sciencepark.mdanderson.org/ggeg/ default.html
Harvard University, Lipper Center for Computational Genomics	Computational Genomics, software development	http://arep.med.harvard.edu/

(*Continues*)

TABLE 2.1 (*Continued*)

Organization or database	Contents	Web site L
IMAGE consortium	The world largest public collection of genes and clones	http://image.llnl.gov/
ISYS	Bioinformatics software tools and databases	http://www.ncgr.org/isys/
GEML	Gene Expression Markup Language	http://www.GEML.org
Gene-Chips	Excellent list of web links on microarray technology	http://www.gene-chips.com/
LLMPP	Lymphoma/Leukemia Molecular Profiling Project Gateway (Dr. Lou Staudt)	http://LLMPP.NCI.NIH.GOV/
MatInspector	Library of transcription factor binding sites plus search tools	http://genomatix.gsf.de/products/ matinspector.html
McDermott Center for Human Growth and Development	Identification of gene networks	http://innovation.swmed.edu/
MedMiner	Genomics and Bioinformatics Group at NCI (J. Weinstein)	http://discover.nci.nih.gov/
MGD	Genetics of laboratory mice (Jackson Lab)	http://www.informatics.jax.org
MIPS	Munich Information Center for Protein Sequences and full length cDNAs	http://www.mips.biochem.mpg.de/ proj/human/
National Cancer Institute, NCI	NCI Microarray project at the Advanced Technology Center ATC, NCI	http://nciarray.nci.nih.gov
Lab-on-a-chip	Overview of "lab-on-a-chip" microarrays systems	http://www.lab-on-a-chip.com/
LocusLink at NCBI	Human Genome Database	http://www.ncbi.nlm.nih.gov/ genome/guide/human/
MGED	Microarray gene expression database group	http://www.mged.org/Annotations-wg/ index.html)
National Human Genome Research Institute NHGRI	Microarray projects at the NHGRI	http://www.nhgri.nih.gov/DIR/LCG/ 15K/HTML/
National Institute of Environmental Health Science	Microarray projects at the NIEHS	http://dir.niehs.nih.gov/microarray/
Nature Genome Gateway	Nature magazine's genome pages	http://www.nature.com/genomics/
Nylon Microarrays Site	Information on how to produce and hybridize macroarrays	http://tagc.univ-mrs.fr/microarrays/
Oak Ridge National Laboratory	Information on the Human Genome Project	http://www.ornl.gov
PathDB	Research tools for functional genomics	http://www.ncgr.org/pathdb/
PGA (Program for Genomic Application)	Genomics and proteomics of cell injury and inflammation	http://pga.swmed.edu/deliverables.htm

(*Continues*)

TABLE 2.1 (*Continued*)

Organization or database	Contents	Web site L
Plant Array Website	Resources for plant DNA microarrays	http://www.ensam.inra.fr/biochimie/plant_arrays/index.html
Protocols Online Web Site	Online resource for microarray protocols	http://www.protocolonline.net/molbio/DNA/dna_microarray.htm
PubGene	Online literature data mining tools	http://www.pubgene.org/
RIKEN	Gene banks for mouse and other organisms	http://www.rtc.riken.go.jp/
Rockefeller Institute, New York, NY	List of academic microarray facilities	http://linkage.rockefeller.edu/wli/microarray/core.html
Rockefeller Institute, New York	*Xenopus* microarray project	http://arrays.rockefeller.edu/xenopus/
SageNet	Serial analysis of gene expression	http://www.sagenet.org/SAGEData/sagedata.htm
Sanger Center, Cambridge, UK	*Saccharomyces pombe* (fission yeast) functional genomics	http://www.sanger.ac.uk/PostGenomics/S_pombe/
Science Magazine	Functional genomics resources	http://www.sciencemag.org/feature/plus/sfg
Source	Stanford Online Universal Resource for cDNA Clones & ESTs	http://genome-www4.stanford.edu/cgi-bin/SMD/source/sourceSearch
Stanford University Microarray Database SMD	Microarray database	http://genome-www4.stanford.edu/MicroArray/SMD/
Stanford University Microarray Links	Microarray protocols, software, and tools	http://genome.www4.stanford.edu/MicroArray/SMD/restech.html
Stanford University, Patrick O.Brown's Web site	Microarray resources, databases,	http://cmgm.stanford.edu/pbrown/
SWISS-PROT	Protein database	http://expasy.ch/sprot
Systems Biology, Dr. Leroy Hood	Software for microarray analysis, Institute for Systems Biology	http://www.systemsbiology.org/
The Genome Database	Human genome database	http://gdbwww.gdb.org/
TIGR	Microbial genome databases	http://www.tigr.org/tdb/mdb/mdbcomplete.html
Transfac	Transcription Factor Database	http://transfac.gbf.de
U. S. Environmental Protection Agency Microarray Consortium	Forum for collaboration in development and application of microarray technology	http://www.epa.gov/nheerl/epamac/
UniGene at NCBI	mRNA database	http://www.ncbi.nlm.nih.gov/Unigene
University of Ontario Cancer Institute (OCI)	Information on microarray projects at OCI	http://www.oci.utoronto.ca/services/microarray/
Whitehead Institute for Biomedical Research/ MIT Center for Genome Research	Information on map and sequence software and microarray projects at the MIT Genome Center (E. Lander)	http://www.genome.wi.mit.edu/

TABLE 2.2 Selection of Commercial Suppliers of Microarray-Related Technologies

Company name	Products and services	Web site URL
Affymetrix	Oligonucleotide arrays	http://www.affymetrix.com/
Agilent Technologies	Custom microarrays, scanners	http://www.agilent.com
AlphaGene	DNA microarrays and libraries	http://www.alphagene.com/
AmershamPharmacia	Microarray supplies, dyes, spotters,	http://www.apbiotech.com/
Applied Biosystems	Gene analysis, informatics	http://www.applera.com/
Axon Instruments	Microarray scanners	http://www.axon.com/
Beecher Instruments	Tissue microarrays	http://www.beecherinstruments.com/
Biacore	Microarrays, informatics	http://www.biacore.com/
BioDiscovery	Image analysis software	http://www.biodiscovery.com/
BioForce Laboratory	Nanoscale microarrays	http://www.bioforcelab.com/
BioMerieux	Microarrays, informatics	http://www.biomerieux.com/
BioRobotics	Microarray production	http://www.biorobotics.com/
Capital Biochip	Microarrays	http://www.capitalbiochip.com
Cartesian Technologies	Microarray spotters	http://www.cartesiantech.com/
Celera Genomics	Bioinformatics	http://www.celera.com/
Cellomics	Cell-based arrays	http://www.cellomics.com/
Ciphergen Biosystems	Protein chips (SELDI)	http://www.ciphergen.com/
Clontech Laboratories BD	Atlas microarrays	http://www.clontech.com/
Compugen	DNA microarrays, informatics	http://www.compugen.com/
Corning	Microarrays, glass slides	http://www.cmt.corning.com/
Cruachem	Custom microarrays	http://www.cruachem.co.uk
CuraGen	Bioinformatics	http://www.curagen.com/
Display Systems	Microarrays, informatics	http://www.displaysystems.com/
EuroGenTech	Microarray spotters, microarrays	http://www.eurogentec.com/
Ferrarius Biotechnology	Lab-on-a-chip system	http://www.febit.com/
Gene Logic	Informatics	http://www.genelogic.com/
Gene Machines	Arrayers	http://www.genemachines.com/
GeneScan	Microarrays	http://www.genescan.com/
Genetix	Robotics, microarray supplies	http://www.genetix.co.uk
Genisphere 3DNA	Oligodendromeric detection	http://www.genisphere.com/
Genomatix	Bioinformatics and sequence analysis	http://genomatix.gsf.de/free_services/
Genometrix	DNA microarrays	http://www.genometrix.com/
Genomic Solutions	Arrayers	http://www.genomicsolutions.com/
GENPAK	Arrayers	http://www.genpakdna.com/
GENSET	Microarray services	http://www.genxy.com/
Graffinity AG	Chemical Arrays	http://www.graffinity.com
Hitachi	Microarrays	http://www.hitachi.co.jp
Hypromatix	Antibody arrays	http://www.hypromatrix.com/
HySeq Inc.	DNA Sequencing by hybridization	http://www.hyseq.com/
Illumina	Bead-based microarrays	http://www.illumina.com/
Incyte Genomics	Microarray services, informatics	http://www.incyte.com/
Intelligent Bio-Instruments	Microarraying robots	http://www.intelligentbio.com/
Interactiva	Oligonucleotide microarrays	http://www.interactiva.com/
LION bioscience	Informatics	http://www.lionbioscience.com/
Lynx	Bead-based microarrays	http://www.lynxgen.com/
Mergen	DNA microarrays	http://www.mergen-ltd.com/
Motorola Biochip Systems	Gel-pad microarrays	http://www.motorola.com/ biochipsystems
Motorola Clinical Micro Sensors	Electronic DNA biochips	http://www.microsensor.com/
MWG Biotech	Scanners, robots	http://www.mwgbiotech.com/

(Continues)

TABLE 2.2 (*Continued*)

Company name	Products and services	Web site URL
Nanogen Inc.	Electronic detection of DNA on chips	http://www.nanogen.com
NEN Life Science (PE)	Microarrays, Tyramid	http://www.NEN.com/
NimbleGen	High-density microarrays	http://www.nimblegen.com/
Operon	Oligonucleotide microarrays	http://www.operon.com/
Origene Technologies	DNA microarrays	http://www.origene.com/
Packard BioScience	Robotics, Imaging systems, microarrays	http://www.packardbioscience.com/
Perkin Elmer Life Science	Microarrays	http://www.perkinelmer.com/
Phylos	Protein microarrays	http://www.phylos.com/
Radius Biosciences	Microarray services	http://www.ultranet.com/~radius
Research Genetics	Macroarrays, microarrays	http://www.resgen.com/
Rosetta Inpharmatics	Informatics	http://www.rii.com/
Sequenom	Microarray analysis, informatics	http://www.sequenom.com/
Soma-Logic	Protein chips	http://www.somalogic.com/
Spotfire	Informatics	http://www.spotfire.com/
Stratagene	Microarrays	http://www.stratagene.com/
SuperBioChips	Tissue microarrays	http://www.tissue-array.com/
Takara Shuzo Co Ltd.	Microarray supplies	http://www.takara.co.jp
Telechem International	Microarray and spotting supplies	http://arrayit.com/
Virtek Vision	Microarray scanners	http://www.virtek.com/
Vysis	Microarrays, microarray scanners	http://www.vysis.com/
Xanthon	Microarray detection and analysis	http://www.xanthoninc.com/
Xenometrix	Cell-based microarrays	http://www.xeno.com/
Zyomyx	Protein biochips	http://www.zyomyx.com/

II. ADVANTAGES OF DNA MICROARRAYS

A large number of molecular techniques have been used to assess differential gene expression. Many of these are termed open systems because they require no specific sequence information to generate a gene expression profile (they are open to discovery of new genes). Several important examples include serial analysis of gene expression (SAGE), differential display (DD), representational difference analysis (RDA), and subtractive suppression techniques (SSH). It is also possible to subtract large cDNA libraries by electronic subtraction (digital differential display; DDD). While open systems clearly have advantages for gene discovery, they are usually labor intensive, have a high rate of false positive results (in particular DD), and are difficult and tedious to perform. Furthermore, most of these methods are biased toward detection of highly expressed genes. For SAGE, hundreds of thousands of small gene tags (10 to 13 mers) must be sequenced and analyzed, yet expression data for many low abundance RNAs may not reach a sufficiently high level for statistical significance. In contrast, microarrays are considered closed systems because sequence knowledge of genes or ESTs is provided prior to construction (arrays are closed to discovery of new genes). Considering the high representation of the estimated 34,000 human genes by EST clusters (e.g., in the UniGene and Incyte LifeSeq human databases) and the completion of the first draft of the human genomic sequence [1, 2], the use of closed systems no longer appears to be a major disadvantage. The same is true for the 40 or more other organisms whose genomes have been sequenced. It is unclear what percentage of human genes is not represented in public or private cDNA and EST databases (LifeSeq, UniGene, GenBank, embl, etc.). The analysis of the first draft of the human genome provides all the necessary data and is publicly available. Online genome resources are also available for many other organisms including the mouse, rat, zebrafish, *Drosophilia melanogaster*, *Caenorhabditis elegans*, and *Saccharomyces cerevisiae* and many pathogenic microorganisms at *Nature* magazine's genome gateway. Known genes and ESTs can be mapped and annotated, and the function of novel genes can be predicted from the genomic sequence, even if no representative cDNA fragment has been cloned. The human genome is about to become a closed system, with all the necessary sequence information provided. Microarrays are already taking advantage of fully sequenced genomes [18]. The major advantages of microarrays are that they are high-throughput, versatile, and fast. Arrays are also relatively easy to use and manufacture, and they can be reasonably cheap (after an initial investment in equipment necessary to produce, hybridize, and/or scan arrays). Anyone can design or purchase (see below) their own custom arrays, regardless of their specific interest.

III. MAJOR DNA ARRAY FORMATS: SOMETHING FOR EVERYONE

Several major microarray formats have been used in the past, and new and increasingly sensitive formats are constantly being developed. For decades, genes, clones, or DNA fragments have been spotted onto nylon membranes in an arrayed fashion [24]. However, the breakthrough for cDNA expression microarrays occurred with the use of DNA molecules (primarily oligonucleotides and PCR products) immobilized or synthesized on glass surfaces. Although these modern arrays have been available for only about 5 years, they have become powerful and popular tools.

A. Nylon Filter Arrays

DNA spotted on nylon or nitrocellulose filters represents the oldest array format. This was the forerunner of modern cDNA filter arrays and has been produced and hybridized for decades. In particular, routine hybridization of filter arrays containing thousands of genomic clones has been used extensively in genomic mapping projects to construct large contigs and to help assemble bacterial and microbial genomes. However, these supports were not called arrays but simply filters. Simple dot or slot blot hybridizations, performed in virtually any molecular biology lab, can actually be considered small-scale filter array hybridizations. However, these experiments usually have a low complexity (i.e., the number of genes spotted ranges from dozens to no more than a few hundred). Many research projects using DD, SSH, or representational difference analysis (RDA) still utilize self-made dot blot filters as a rapid prescreening method for the evaluation and confirmation of differential gene expression. The average spot size in modern filter arrays has a diameter of 0.5–1 mm. This is considerably larger compared to oligonucleotide chips or glass-based expression arrays, which have spot sizes that range between 20 and 200 μm.

Nylon membranes are usually hybridized with radioactively labeled nucleic acids (^{33}P, ^{35}S, or ^{33}P). Although non-isotopic detection of array hybridization is generally possible, it is considerably less sensitive and can result in severe background problems. For these reasons, non-isotopic detection is rarely used for nylon filters.

Despite larger spot formats, filter arrays can still accommodate very large numbers of cDNA fragments/clones. Up to 50,000 clones have been arranged on a single filter set (UniGene set filters I and II from the Resource Center for Genome Research at Berlin, Germany). A number of different filter arrays with >9000 human genes are marketed by Research Genetics. Clontech markets the Atlas Array System, which was among the first filter array products that together with Research Genetics arrays were commercially available at a reasonable price. The first generation of these filters contained only 588 human, rat, or murine genes spotted in duplicate, but they were used by many laboratories. Smaller sets with genes involved in apoptosis or cell proliferation were also available dating back to 1997. Clontech now sells a full palette of different arrays on nylon, glass, and even plastic supports. It also markets the software necessary for data extraction. Proper filter array analysis is performed with the use of a phosphor imager or related technology (Molecular Dynamics, Fuji) and appropriate software for data analysis is mandatory.

A number of software packages are available, but data extraction can be tedious, especially using larger arrays. The alignment of thousands of spots with a grid that is necessary for data management can take hours with very large arrays. Poor hybridization quality and low signal intensities can make perfect spot alignment impossible. Another major disadvantage of filter arrays is that they do not offer the possibility of dual or competitive hybridizations on one array. Data analysis and comparison of several filter hybridizations must take into account the local heterogeneity of hybridization, considerable background, and other artifacts like uneven hybridization that are mainly due to the large format. However, a clear advantage of filter arrays is that they are easily produced in house, and they can be stripped and reused several times. Glass-based microarrays are usually used only once. In comparison to the equipment necessary for production of arrays on glass slides, spotters for medium size nylon membranes (macroarray spotters) are relatively cheap. Furthermore, expensive array scanners that detect fluorescent signals are not necessary, and the required supplies (autoradiographic materials or a phosphor imager plus a few cassettes) can be found in most molecular biology laboratories.

B. High-Density Oligonucleotide Chips

One of the most successful formats is synthetic oligonucleotide microarrays. These high-density arrays are constructed on glass or silicon wafers by a process of miniaturized photolithography [25–27], which was adapted from semiconductor technology. The process synthesizes thousands of different oligonucleotides directly on the glass or sometimes a silicon substrate (chip). Many chips can be produced in parallel. After completion, the wafer is cut into individual slides, and these are enclosed in plastic devices that facilitate automated hybridization. For these chips, a specialized hybridization device is mandatory. This powerful method was pioneered by Affymetrix in the mid-1990s. One major advantage of this array format is that genes can be arrayed at extremely high density (currently >400,000 features/1.28 × 1.28 cm array). Each feature has a diameter the size of about 20μm. On Affymetrix arrays, each gene is represented by 20 different oligonucleotides from different regions of the gene (perfect match oligos; PM). Affymetrix arrays also include oligonucleotides with a single base exchange in the middle (mismatch oligos; MM), which prevents specific hybridization and, therefore, minimizes the number of false positives. Signal intensities derived from the MM oligos are subtracted from those derived from the PM oligo set. The result indicates the expression level of a particular gene, and if a gene is considered as present or absent in a particular sample. The large probe volume (>200 μl) and the constant mixing of the sample throughout the hybridization process in the proprietary fluidics station help to minimize artifacts that are frequently observed in other array systems (e.g., local depletion of probe leading to low individual signal strength on large arrays). Arrays for a number of different organisms are available, including humans, mouse, rat, *Arabidopsis*, *Drosophila*, *S. cerevisiae*, and *Escherichia coli*. Affymetrix also offers specialized chips such as those for detection of p53 mutations in human cancer or SNPs. For the human genome, several arrays that cover the named human genes as well as unnamed ESTs are available. The full set of human genes offered by Affymetrix comprises 5 chips with 12,000 genes/oligo sets each.

Analysis of Affymetrix expression data is performed with the proprietary Jaguar software package. Other programs are also available (ArraySuite). Spots are located by an automatic grid algorithm, but can also be manually defined by the user. This can help to reduce the impact of hybridization artifacts. The program also automatically performs data normalizations using either the sum of all data points (global normalization) or selected controls, which can be defined by the user. Furthermore, statistical measurements can be performed that allow interpretation of individual spot intensities. Links to spot content information are provided. However, the sequence information for the oligos used for detection is not provided. Occasionally, errors have been detected in oligonucleotide sequences and are replaced in subsequent versions of these chips. In-depth analyses of individual chips can eliminate potential artifacts, which include identification of cross hybridizing probes and image processing errors [28]. Affymetrix also maintains a central Laboratory Information Management System (LIMS) that offers tools for data mining and interaction with other users of their GeneChip systems.

Although Affymetrix chips have been used with considerable success in profiling gene expression, they also have disadvantages. Individual chips are still relatively expensive and cannot be reused. RNA labeling by biotin incorporation prior to hybridization can be tedious and time-consuming. It also requires considerable amounts of RNA. Parallel hybridizations of two samples cannot be performed, and data analysis is totally dependent on the

Affymetrix software packages and workstations. The system including the hybridization station, the chip reader plus computer workstation, and software is expensive and smaller labs cannot easily afford this technology. The proprietary kits for mRNA labeling can also contribute to render this technology cost-intensive. For that reason, larger institutions usually buy one system for a central chip analysis facility.

Another disadvantage of oligonucleotide chips is that they cannot be readily constructed in most research laboratories. However, this fact can also be considered an advantage. Because only a few different Affymetrix chip designs are sold worldwide, results from different labs can easily be compared. Reproducibility and a standardized chip design will be critical for novel initiatives that intend to generate and collect information on gene expression on a wide variety of human diseases and cancers. For instance, the International Genomics Consortium (IGC), funded and headed by the National Human Genome Research Institute (NHGRI), has considered using Affymetrix oligonucleotide arrays to generate standardized and comparable data that will eventually be stored in one database that would be publicly accessible to academic researchers.

Affymetrix now offers custom-designed oligonucleotide arrays using a specialized spotting technology that is more versatile. However, in the near future, the "lab-on-a-chip" approach could allow the massive parallel design of up to 40,000 different oligonucleotides on a single glass array directly by the user (e.g., FeBiT or Ferrarius Biotechnology, Mannheim, Germany; Caliper Instruments, Mountain View, CA; Agilent, etc.). Comprehensive information on this issue is available at www.lab-on-a-chip.com. In FeBiT's lab-on-a-chip approach, chip synthesis, hybridization, and data analysis are consecutively performed by the same machine. A considerable disadvantage of this system is that only one chip at a time can be synthesized by photolithography and hybridized, and of course, these systems will be expensive. However, chips can be reused, and the master files for production of novel chips can be used many times. Master files can also be easily modified so that new genes can be added or others omitted.

A similar novel development in photolithographic chip production is the use of virtual masks that replace the photolithographic masks used by Affymetrix. A set of lasers and an array of micromirrors is used to design a custom oligo microarray overnight. The method, Maskless Array Synthesizer (MAS), was pioneered at the University of Michigan, and is now developed at NimbleGene Systems (Madison, WI).

C. Spotted Arrays

The third major microarray format consists of PCR products, plasmids, and more recently, oligonucleotides that are spotted onto pretreated glass microscope slides. The DNA on these arrays can be bound covalently or electrostatically to the glass surface. A decisive factor for the success of spotted arrays was the simultaneous development of quantitative fluorescent labeling methods that enable the user to detect two or more labeled RNA samples in parallel on one array. This beautiful concept clearly facilitates data analysis and evaluation of differential gene expression. The ratios of differential expression obtained by this method can usually be confirmed by other techniques (RT-PCR, Northern hybridization). RNA labeling is comparably fast and easy to perform using dyes and labeling protocols that have been adapted for this purpose. The first glass arrays and detection methods were developed in the laboratory of Patrick O. Brown in the mid-1990s [29–32]. DNA fragments were and still are primarily generated by PCR amplification of cloned cDNA inserts in bacterial vectors. Printing or spotting of DNA is accomplished using special print heads, pins, and robotic devices (spotter or arrayer) to deposit small droplets (100–300 nl) of DNA solutions, which generate spots with diameters between 50 and 300 μ. Spot size largely depends on the pins used and can be controlled by the user. However, spot sizes deposited by this method can vary considerably. Affymetrix developed a "pin and ring" technology that guarantees defined and even spot sizes and DNA deposition. In this method, a stamp rather than a metal pin is used to print DNA solutions on glass surfaces. Alternatively, a number of different ink-jet techniques have been developed. These are usually combined with oligonucleotide synthesizers [33, 34]. Packard Biosystems (Meridan, CT) developed a piezoelectronic dispensing technology to print exactly defined volumes of DNA solutions that generate spots with minimal size variations. Printing occurs "on demand," controlled by an electronic signal. This non-contact printing process (Packards BioChip Arrayer) is expected to be used for protein chips as well.

Different strategies for immobilization of DNA on glass surfaces have been used, but a common and inexpensive method is to coat ordinary microscope slides with poly-L-lysine. This is performed easily in any lab. Alternatively, one can purchase glass slides precoated with a number of different chemical substances. Samples of RNA or DNA from the experimental and control groups can be labeled with different fluorophores and co-hybridized on the array. The most widely used dyes are Cy3 and Cy5 (CyDye; Amersham Pharmacia Biotech). ALEXA dyes (Molecular Probes Inc.) are available in a wide range of different excitation and emission wavelengths. They provide robust fluorescence signals and are easy to use. ALEXA dyes are usually indirectly coupled to cDNA or protein molecules. Other dyes including BODIPY dyes, fluorescein isothiocyanate (FITC), or rhodamine are used less frequently. Regardless of which dye is used, the false color images generated by array scanners are usually defined as red and green. Genes that are not differentially expressed in both samples appear yellow due to the combination of similar intensities in both red and green channels (provided the channel intensities have been normalized). Predominantly red or green colors indicate higher intensity in one channel compared to the other, and therefore, differential expression of the gene printed on that spot.

Fluorescent signals are detected using specialized array scanners that contain at least two lasers with different wavelengths (Axon Instruments; Packard BioSystems, Molecular Dynamics) and a set of appropriate photomultiplier tubes (PMT) to detect the signal. A single image file is generated for each channel. Array analysis software packages (GenePix, ScanAlyze, ScanArray, ArrayVision, LifeExpress, etc.) use the single-channel input files to generate dual false color images by a simple overlay technique that combines data from both fluorescence channels. In a second critical step, intensity data are processed, normalized, and compared. Different methods and strategies for data collection, normalization, and computational analysis of microarray data have been recently reviewed by Quackenbush [21]. For analysis, researchers frequently transfer array data directly to a central array database (Oracle or Web-based databases) and perform normalization, quality control, background determination, multiple array comparison, and statistical evaluation with the help of proprietary or in-house designed software. A good example is the National Cancer Institute (NCI) Array Web site. A similar site including databases and other resources was developed by the NHGRI. Array data can also be mined with commercial software packages including Spotfire, GeneSpring, Mineset, and SAS.

D. Spotted Oligonucleotide Arrays

Within the last year, the use of arrays containing spotted oligonucleotides constantly grew. Usually, single-stranded oligonucleotides between 25 and 80 bases long are used. In comparison to PCR products, oligonucleotides offer easier optimization of hybridization kinetics and guarantee standardized DNA concentrations for spotting, which results in defined amounts of DNA immobilized per spot. Proper selection of oligonucleotide also helps to minimize the number of cross-hybridizing probes on the chip. Several companies already offer oligonucleotide arrays spotted on glass (Affymetrix, Operon, etc.). The first full genome chip for yeast using spotted oligonucleotides has been produced and was marketed by Operon. The first complete genome chips for humans using spotted oligonucleotides were recently introduced by Rosetta Inpharmatics, Inc. (Kirkland, WA) [18]. Rosetta's FlexJet technology allows the production of arrays of tens of thousands of oligonucleotides synthesized *in situ* by an ink-jet printing method (adapted from Hewlett-Packard), employing standard phosphoramidite chemistry [33]. In general, 60–70 mer oligonucleotides are sufficient to reliably detect transcript ratios at one copy per cell in complex biological samples. Results using a single, carefully selected oligonucleotide per gene correlate closely with those obtained using cDNA arrays. Most of the genes for which measurements differ are members of gene families that show alternative mRNA processing. These splice variants can only be distinguished and analyzed by oligonucleotides [18]. The ink-jet technology has also been modified by Agilent, Inc. (Palo Alto, CA) to produce high-density arrays that contain up to 14,000 cDNAs/array. The advantages of these systems are uniform spot sizes and the extremely rapid production of arrays. In parallel, Agilent also developed a lab-on-a-chip system that uses Rosetta's FlexJet technology to synthesize and print up to 8500 different oligonucleotides *in situ*. A number of commercial suppliers offer bulk oligonucleotide production at reasonable prices for custom array design or software to design and optimize oligonucleotides in the lab. Oligonucleotide arrays will become increasingly important with decreasing production costs for bulk orders of small-scale oligonucleotide synthesis.

The use of oligonucleotide arrays also means that the tedious process of choosing, ordering, growing, freezing and amplifying thousands of bacterial clones with cDNA inserts will become obsolete. For many labs, this might be sufficient encouragement to join the growing list of universities or industries that have developed their own core array production facilities. The falling prices for custom oligonucleotide synthesis are also an invitation to settle on oligonucleotide chips rather than spotted Patent Cooperative Treaty (PCT) products.

E. Novel DNA Array Technologies

A number of novel technologies have been introduced in the past months that increase array sensitivity and sample throughput. For instance, 3D microarrays have been developed at the Argonne National Laboratory in collaboration with the Russian Engelhardt Institute of Molecular Biology. Thousands of microscopic 3D gel pads are affixed to glass slides. Each pad contains a defined cDNA sequence and allows thousands of simultaneous biological reactions on the chip. This approach might be interesting as a sensitive and cost-effective alternative to other biochips in clinical research. Similar gel-pad arrays are also developed at Motorola BioChip Systems (Northbrook, IL). A completely different 3D approach was developed by Illumina, Inc. (San Diego, CA). For this technology, thousands of individual microscopic glass fibers are chemically etched to create microscopic wells at the end of each fiber. These fibers are combined with beads that, in a separate process, can be coated with specific sensor molecules such as DNA fragments or peptides. Fibers loaded with beads can then be arranged to match the layout of 96-, 384-, and 1536-well microplates. Many of these fiber-optic bundles can then be combined to create larger structures. Up to 3 million individual assays can be performed in parallel in a single experiment. This technology has been primarily developed for high-throughput genotyping, but can also be used for expression profiling. One major advantage of the Illuminas design is the extreme flexibility in terms of the nature of immobilized molecules as well as the possibilities of user-defined variations from experiment to experiment. Corning, Inc. (Corning, NY) developed another 3D array system that consists of a honeycomb-like glass substrate that offers thousands of individual, microscopic reaction cells. These cone-shaped structures serve as reservoirs that hold increased amounts of cDNA sequences or other molecules. This design helps to increase the sensitivity of detection in hybridization experiments. Corning also developed a printing technology that allows the simultaneous stamping of 10,000 individual elements in about 1 minute. Basically, each pin used for printing delivers its contents to just one opposing channel or reservoir on the glass slide. This method minimizes cross contamination that can occur with ordinary arrayers.

IV. WHAT IS THE BEST WAY TO INTERFACE WITH MICROARRAYS?

The decision to use microarrays should be considered thoroughly. There are many different levels at which a lab can use gene chips. These range from outsourcing (the possibility with the least direct handling) to establishment of a core facility for microarray production and analysis.

A. Mining The Existing Information

Considering the increasing availability of published data on global gene expression profiling, it might be advantageous to mine existing data rather than undertake new microarray experiments. There were 27 publications on microarrays in 1999, and in 2000 the number swelled to 97. In 2002, there was a dramatic increase to 1900. Recently published studies using microarrays have cataloged lists of hundreds of genes that are differentially expressed as a result of drug treatment or human disease [35–40]. This trend will certainly continue in the future.

These large gene or clone lists can be downloaded from supplementary Web pages that contain the original "raw" data sets. For example, vast data sets of genes that are expressed in different human tissues and human diseases (mostly cancer) can be downloaded from the SAGE databases at NCBI or the Cancer Genome Anatomy Project (CGAP). No laboratory can evaluate all interesting candidate genes that have been identified in these studies. Therefore, after comprehensive expression profiling (even if done by others), it is necessary to return to the traditional one gene–one paper strategy and carefully identify biological functions of novel candidate genes. This is particularly important if one considers that the vast majority of the 12,000 named human genes are described in only one publication and most of these contain little or no information on biological function. The remaining two-thirds of human genes are not named and await future characterization.

These thoughts are not intended to discourage use of arrays. They are just a reminder that microarray experiments are not appropriate for the detailed biological and biochemical characterization of novel genes. The important but difficult task of gene characterization will continue for many years after completion of the human genome sequence.

B. Commercial Array Hybridization Services

Often, outsourcing of microarray experiments to commercial service labs is the best, fastest, and cheapest alternative. Incyte Pharmaceuticals, Inc. has offered custom array hybridization for a number of years. All that is necessary is to provide two or more RNA samples to Incyte, and a few weeks later a list of genes that are up- or downregulated is returned. This approach can be fast and successful, yet still affordable [41]. This is extremely important because it allows the devotion of time and resources to confirming differential gene expression and assigning biological meaning to specific candidate genes. This process can be far more time-consuming than the initial identification of candidate genes.

C. Commercial or Self-Made Microarrays

For laboratories that are interested in hands-on array work, plenty of commercial alternatives are available. However, with constantly increasing numbers of new commercial suppliers offering a wide range of different array formats or custom arrays, it is necessary to do a thorough cost/time analysis. It is also worthwhile to develop some practical experience with filter or glass array hybridization before deciding which system to use for expression profiling. If a large number of chips are necessary, in-house production will definitely help to reduce costs — even if the necessary equipment for start up is expensive. Frequent use of commercial arrays is costly. For experiments that do not need to be repeated many times, the use of commercially available chips (or even an array service) might be a wise decision. However, a problem can arise with specimens or cells that are characterized by significant biological diversity (like human tissues or tumor biopsies). In these cases, it is necessary to repeat hybridizations many times to get an idea which natural fluctuations in gene expression can occur. For this reason, a cheap source of microarrays is advisable, which makes these experiments affordable.

D. In-House Production of Microarrays

Large customized microarrays in various formats (filter- or glass-based) can be synthesized in many research labs. An ordinary glass microscope slide (25 × 75 mm) easily accommodates up to 23,000 spots. It is possible to print all of the genes in the human genome on just two slides and even have space for controls and duplicate spots. Although a few labs might be interested in producing complete genomic chips, most will definitely focus on smaller arrays; for example, for specific pathways (apoptosis or cell cycle related genes). In-house production of microarrays is an interesting opportunity to speed up throughput of hybridization experiments that otherwise would have to be performed the traditional way. For academic institutions, the cost-saving possibility of ordering hundreds or thousands of clones royalty free from the IMAGE consortium (or related organizations) might be an important issue. One has to be aware that the purchase of chemicals and equipment necessary for generating thousands of PCR products from these clones (PCR machines in 96- or 384-well format, plus considerable amounts of Taq DNA polymerase), printing on glass slides (arrayers), and feature detection (scanners) require sufficient funding and wide utilization to be cost-effective. Central core facilities that serve the special needs of a number of research labs within an institution are the best way to deal with this situation. The Rockefeller Institute maintains a list of such academic facilities.

When it comes to gathering specific information on a limited number of individual target genes or defined cell signaling pathways, a small gene array designed in house can be far more flexible and cheaper compared to commercial arrays with scores of clones or oligonucleotides. Thousands of arrays can be produced once the DNA has been generated that is used for spotting. This approach is appropriate for academic institutions or companies that are involved in drug design targeted to a limited set of genes, such as the family of tyrosine kinases or phosphatases [42, 43]. A full set of all known members of a certain gene family can be arrayed or spotted and used to screen for effects of hundreds of different drugs in dozens of different cell lines or tissues [44]. Similar experiments have been performed using peptide chips that contained a number of recombinant kinases. Kinetics of phosphorylation reactions could be measured and quantified directly on the chip [45, 46]. This approach is also useful for the generation of tissue-specific arrays or arrays of genes from defined chromosomal regions [47] or diseased tissues [48, 49]. To generate microarrays in the lab, there exists only one limiting factor: exact sequence information and/or a large number of cDNA clones must be available. Labs that perform open techniques to identify differential gene expression (DD, RDA, SSH, SAGE) might also be interested in small custom arrays, because cDNA libraries and other collections of clones from past experiments can be easily printed on identical chips and used to confirm differential expression in the original cells or tissues of interest [50]. This approach offers very high throughput compared to the more conventional evaluation methods including dot blot or Northern hybridization.

Despite these obvious advantages of self-made arrays, there are also a number of disadvantages. There are many opportunities for human error and technical problems in microarray production. For instance, errors exist in the clone collections used for the generation of DNA fragments. In part, mislabeling and inappropriate handling of clones by lab personnel can lead to such problems. Clones can also be contaminated by other clones. Bacteria can easily contaminate other wells in the 96- or 384-well plates that are commonly used for storage, growth, and transfer of clones. In PCR amplification that is used to generate the DNA fragments that are used for spotting, contamination can also be an issue.

Between 1 and 5% of all bacterial clones even in well-maintained clone sets are estimated not to contain the sequence they are supposed to contain. These rates can go up to 40% in other libraries. Very high error rates have been found in clone sets from some commercial suppliers (e.g., Research Genetics). For this reason, it is advisable to purchase sequence-verified clone sets, which are available from a number of companies and non-commercial suppliers (e.g., Incyte, Lion Bioscience, etc.). Alternatively, a lab might be interested in sending out its own clone set for sequencing. It might be worthwhile to pay for sequence information in order to avoid the risk of wasting precious time with results that cannot be confirmed. Even with sequence-verified clone sets, handling errors cannot be excluded. With every freezing and thawing cycle, the risk of bacterial cross contamination increases. Therefore, it is necessary to confirm cDNA results by other techniques, e.g., conventional or real-time RT-PCR, *in situ* hybridization, fluorescence *in situ* hybridization (FISH), or Northern blot analysis.

An expensive, but increasingly interesting alternative to bacterial clones is the use of oligonucleotides for spotting. It would be extremely useful to make databases publicly available that contain sequence information for suitable 60–80 mer oligonucleotides for all human genes, which can be used for array production. To date, no such database exists. The >2 million oligos designed by Rosetta Inpharmatics would be an extremely valuable and time-saving resource for academic researchers. However, a number of computer programs have been developed that can be used to define optimal oligonucleotides. Some of these are shareware available at no charge.

V. MICROARRAYS AND PHARMACOGENOMICS: REVOLUTIONIZING DISCOVERY OF NEW DRUGS AND GENE FUNCTION

Progress in sequencing of the human genome has made the full set of genetic information available for pharmacogenomics. This sequence data will be invaluable for development of novel drugs for treatment of human disease. There are at least three major applications for microarrays in pharmacogenomics. First, microarray experiments aid in discovery of new drug targets. They simultaneously compare expression of thousands of genes in normal versus pathologic tissue. Genes that are uniquely expressed in disease and are potential targets for drug development can be identified. These same genes are, in principle, also interesting as potential early detection markers for diagnostic purposes. Secondly, arrays are used to clarify molecular mechanisms of drug action and to predict drug efficacy and toxicity. By monitoring differential gene expression in response to drug treatment, arrays identify clusters of genes that define specific signal pathways. Finally, arrays are used to catalog genetic polymorphisms in a population. As information accumulates to link specific polymorphisms with differences in drug responsiveness, it may become possible to customize treatment of individual patients.

A. Discovery of Drug Targets

Knowledge about where and when a specific gene is expressed can provide clues regarding its importance in pathogenesis. Such information can implicate a specific gene as a potential target for drug therapy. For example, microarrays have been used to compare gene expression profiles in osteosarcomas with low versus high metastatic potential [51]. These studies identified 53 RNAs that were differentially expressed. One of the genes that was upregulated in metastatic cells encoded ezrin, a potential target that regulates motility, invasion, and adherence of cancer cells. Although altered expression can link a gene to a specific disease, it does not definitively implicate the gene as an etiologic factor. Many co-regulated genes are altered as a consequence rather than as a cause of disease. Targeting drugs to these genes may reduce symptoms, but they may not interfere with the underlying cause of disease. Potentially important drug targets can be validated using animal models (reviewed in reference 52). For example, it is possible to systematically compare gene expression profiles in normal mice versus those that over express a specific transgene, or mice that have a targeted gene disruption. In this regard, expression profiling has been used to identify genes with altered expression in mice deficient in high-density lipoprotein [53].

Several of these genes regulated steroid metabolism and oxidative processes. The impact of genomic methylation on gene expression has been studied using fibroblasts from DNA methyltransferase defective mice [54]. Using mouse cell lines and an *in vivo* mouse model for cancer progression and metastasis, a strong correlation was shown between genes activated by NF-κB and those that were overexpressed in metastasis [55]. Another example is the analysis of the time course of inflammation-related gene expression in the mouse urogenital tract [56]. Similar approaches can be performed using yeast [57]. Yeast mutants that are defective in calcineurin, immunophilins, or other genes were treated with the immunosuppressants cyclosporin A or FK506. In these studies, the presence or absence of a drug-induced pattern of altered gene expression could establish whether the mutant gene was required to generate the drug signature.

Another application of microarrays is that they allow one to profile expression of a specific gene in many different tissues, which may be important for selection of drug targets. Highly tissue-specific expression of a potential target is attractive because it would minimize the potential for side effects in other tissues. For example, Miki et al. [19] analyzed tissue-specific mRNA gene expression in 49 different mouse tissues, and they were able to define sets of genes that ubiquitously expressed in many organs as well as genes that are uniquely expressed in a particular tissue. A novel use of microarrays involves gene transfection by culturing cells directly on an array chip [58]. Cells growing on a spot of DNA take up and express the respective gene. The transfected clones are then examined for biological changes in response to each of the arrayed DNAs. Arrays using living cells are also being developed by Cellomics, Inc. (Pittsburgh, PA). Cellomics' CellChip system consists of a micropatterned chemical array to which cells are attached, and a reaction chamber that contains a fluid delivery system for delivering drugs and other reagents directly to the cells.

B. Mechanism of Drug Action

Gene expression microarrays are potentially useful for investigating the mechanism of drug action and for predicting toxicity. Gray and co-workers have used microarrays to screen for targets of different protein kinase inhibitors in yeast [44]. In these studies, most genes that were downregulated by different inhibitors were involved in cell cycle progression. However, each specific inhibitor also induced distinct changes in RNA profiles, which suggested different modes of action. In another study, microarray analysis was performed on yeast after treatment with the alkylating agent methyl methanosulfonate [59, 60]. Then 400 of the 6200 genes analyzed were up- or downregulated. When 50 were selected for validation by Northern blot analysis, 48 could be confirmed. Although some of these RNAs were known to be induced by DNA damage, many additional genes were perturbed, which suggested alternate pathways that the cell might use to cope with genetic damage. Cho et al. [61] examined effects of UV irradiation and alkylating agents on global gene expression in human fibroblasts. Not surprisingly, many DNA damage-inducible genes correlate with cell cycle regulatory genes that control progression from G2 to M phase. This approach also identified a number of genes that had not previously been associated with cell cycle progression or arrest, which included a large set of genes involved in extracellular matrix formation and turnover. A recent study combined cancer research, cancer prevention, and pharmacogenomics. Mariadason et al. [36] examined the effects of the chemopreventive drugs curcumin, trichostatin A, sulindac, and butyrate on gene expression of colorectal cancer cell lines. For each drug, unique expression profiles were identified, which suggested overlapping but different mechanisms of action. Human cell lines have been used as model systems to examine drug action in the NCI60 project. In one study, the gene expression patterns of 60 cell lines derived from different classes of human tumors were generated, compared, and used for cluster analysis to identify tissue-specific expression patterns [62]. These cell lines were also used in the National Cancer Institute's screen for anticancer drugs [63, 64]. Since 1990, the National Cancer Institute has screened more than 60,000 compounds against a panel of 60 human cancer cell lines that were derived from different tumor types. Detailed information on mechanisms of drug action, toxicity, and drug resistance can be retrieved from the NCI60 database [65].

cDNA microarrays also have the potential to aid in screening drug candidates for toxicity (reviewed in reference 66). Testing large numbers of drug candidates requires a high throughput method that is fast, accurate, and uses minimal amounts of drug. Arrays can identify genes that are up- or downregulated in response to chemotherapeutic treatment, and some of these genes may serve as surrogate markers for toxicity. When used as a prescreen, microarrays can rapidly identify toxic drug candidates and suggest others that are more likely to have low toxicity when tested in animal models. An interesting example for this approach is the identification of genes induced or repressed by different classes of human interferons (IFN) [35]. IFNs alpha and beta induce a very different pattern of altered gene expression compared to IFN gamma, and high doses of IFN can have increased toxicity. These findings provide insight into the basic mechanisms of IFN action and ultimately may contribute to better therapeutic uses for IFNs.

C. Pharmacogenetics

Significant differences exist in both the toxicity of drugs and in their efficacy among individuals. Pharmacogenetics refers to identification of genomic sequence alterations that can modify and/or potentially predict the individual's response to a drug. Most genes that are involved in drug metabolism are subject to common genetic polymorphisms that might contribute to individual variability in drug response. Genetic polymorphisms also influence drug uptake and activity (reviewed in reference 8). SNPs involve one base pair change and are the most common sequence variation with a frequency estimated at 1/1000 bases. To date, about 2.4 million SNP have been identified. Microarrays have the potential to identify SNPs or alterations in gene copy number that are associated with disease. Brown and co-workers have used microarrays to develop a sensitive comparative genomic hybridization method and have used this technique to compare variation in copy number of breast cancer cell lines and tumors [67]. This approach provides a gene by gene measure of copy number, thus achieving a dramatic increase in resolution compared to chromosome-based comparative genomic hybridization methods.

Microarrays are also useful for identifying SNPs that might be associated with drug susceptibility. Array technology might allow physicians to identify a subset of patients who are most likely to have an adverse response to a drug due to an inherited gene polymorphism, such as a drug metabolizing enzyme. By profiling variations in the sequence of an individual's DNA, it might be possible to predict the patient's response to specific treatments [67]. Microarrays might also be used to screen microorganisms for mutations that confer drug resistance. In this regard, oligonucleotide arrays detected mutant alleles of the *Mycobacterium tuberculosis rpoB* gene that mediate resistance to rifampin [68]. Thus, microarrays have the potential to influence diagnosis of drug-resistant strains and subsequent treatment.

D. Disease Classification and Cancer Research

Microarrays have been extensively used to classify diverse types of human disease and in particular human cancers based on their pattern of differential gene expression [40, 69, 70]. Each disease and cancer type or subtype is associated with its own unique pattern of mRNA gene expression. By comparing these distinct patterns, detailed information can be extracted that is useful for understanding and refining molecular diagnosis and therapy. A growing number of publications describe expression profiling of a variety of human cancers. However, thousands of experiments will be needed to analyze, define, and monitor disease-specific expression patterns of these tumor types with sufficient accuracy. For this purpose, the IGC, funded and headed by the NHGRI in Bethesda, Maryland, plans on organizing a large-scale project intended to gather information on gene expression in a wide variety of human diseases and cancers. The IGC seeks to collect microarray data from more than 10,000 tumor samples of different tumor locations that are collected in a number of cancer centers worldwide. These data will be stored in one database that would be publicly accessible to academic researchers.

This project is called EXpression Project for Oncology (expO). It seeks to increase the amount of information on gene expression available to the public as well as improve the benefits and reduce the risk of using genetic information from patients. One mandatory issue will be the use of standardized expression arrays that can be easily compared. Currently, oncologists use many different array types and technologies that are difficult to compare. Furthermore, anonymized, but detailed and comprehensive patient data and clinical records would also be linked to the expression data. Clinical researchers would be able to use these data sets for development of novel diagnostic assays, to improve monitoring of disease progression and relapse, and eventually for drug development.

In any case, a large-scale project as described above would partially duplicate efforts that are already published or in progress. The following section is intended to summarize some examples for interesting projects and experimental data on cancer gene expression that have been recently made available.

1. Leukemia and Lymphoma

Golub et al., have shown that expression profiling is a sophisticated method for pathological diagnosis [69]. They used oligonucleotide array data to classify human leukemias as either acute myeloid (AML) or acute lymphocytic (ALL) without previous knowledge of the pathologic diagnosis. Furthermore, tumors that had previously been misinterpreted as ALL or AML could be identified and correctly classified. The ability to distinguish subtle differences between apparently similar tumors also has the potential to lead to improved therapy.

Microarrays have been used to identify two distinct forms of diffuse B-cell lymphoma based on tumor expression profiles [70]. One profile contained genes expressed at an early stage of B-cell differentiation and was associated with increased survival. The second profile was associated with poor prognosis and included a different set of genes associated with B-cell activation. Thus, microarrays identified two previously undefined, yet clinically different types of cancer, each associated with a different prognosis. A recent study used protein (antibody) arrays for immunophenotyping different classes of normal peripheral blood lymphocytes and a number of different leukemic cells [12]. Cells were directly bound to an array containing antibodies against 50 of the 247 currently known cluster of differentiation antigens (CDs). Patterns of immobilized cells corresponded well with clinical classifications such as chronic lymphocytic leukemia, hairy cell leukemia, mantle cell lymphoma, AML, and ALL.

2. Colorectal Cancer

Expression profiling has been applied by several groups to define different classes, stages, and grades of colorectal cancer [37–39]. Alon et al. [37] and Nottermann et al. [39] used oligonucleotide arrays to analyze global gene expression in normal, preneoplastic adenomas, and malignant colorectal cancer. Kitahara et al. [38] combined laser capture microdissection, linear mRNA amplification, and hybridization of glass-based cDNA microarrays. Array data were confirmed by standard RT-PCR methods. Another Japanese group designed a moderate-sized, colon-specific cDNA expression microarray to confirm differential expression of a large number of candidates that were defined by other methods, which included SAGE, mRNA differential display, and electronic subtraction of cDNA libraries [48]. Interestingly, only a minor fraction of genes identified by these different groups are overlapping. One possible explanation for this observation might be the different composition of the microarrays that were used for expression analysis. Additionally, the biological heterogeneity of the patient samples in combination with different methods of RNA extraction and other technical variations might also account for the striking differences. A larger number of samples and patients needs to be analyzed to show which genes are most consistently overexpressed or repressed in malignant tissue.

A number of groups use a strategy that combines identification of novel candidate genes by microarray hybridization with detailed biological characterization of one or a few of these. For instance, Scherl-Mostageer et al. [71] identified a novel tumor associated gene by a combination of representational difference analysis and cDNA arrays. The novel gene CDCP1 (cub domain containing protein) represents a transmembrane domain protein with unknown functions that is localized on chromosome 3p21-p23. A different approach was chosen by Lin et al. [72]. A cell culture model system was used to identify genes that are regulated by the beta catenin/T-cell factor pathway. Mutation of the tumor suppressor gene APC (adenomatous polyposis coli) is a common and early event in colorectal carcinogenesis, which leads to constitutive activation of the beta catenin/T-cell factor pathway in preneoplastic and tumor cells. The novel gene AF17 was identified as one of more than 80 genes that respond to this critical signal transduction pathway. Others include well-known genes like IGF2 (insulin like growth factor 2) and cytokeratin K5. Both are overexpressed in many colorectal cancers.

Another important gene that negatively regulates cell growth and promotes differentiation in intestinal epithelial cells is the nuclear hormone peroxisome proliferator-activated receptor gamma (PPAR γ). Gupta et al. [73] identified genes that are induced or repressed by PPAR γ. To induce or inhibit PPAR γ function, highly specific PPAR γ agonists and one inhibitor were used, and RNA expression patterns were analyzed by oligonucleotide array hybridization. The PPAR γ target genes identified included several growth inhibitory and regulatory factors and proteins that regulate cell adhesion and aggregation.

Several studies analyzed expression patterns that correlated with inflammatory bowel diseases (ulcerative colitis and Crohn's disease), and identified a large number of genes that associate with disease progression or genetic susceptibility of affected patients [74, 75]. Interestingly, the two different colorectal inflammatory diseases displayed overlapping, but also markedly different expression patterns.

3. Esophageal Cancer

Genes upregulated in malignant esophageal cancer tissue were identified by Kan et al. [76]. Interestingly, cell lines derived from esophageal tumor specimens differed markedly from cancer tissues. This is probably due to complex biological interactions between tumor cells, inflammatory reaction, and the tumor stroma, which cannot be analyzed using tumor cell lines. The effect of different chemotherapeutic drugs on gene expression patterns of esophageal tumors was investigated by Kihara et al. [77]. Cancer tissues from patients that were treated with the commonly used chemotherapeutic drugs 5-fluorouracil or cisplatin were analyzed using fluorescence-based cDNA microarrays, and statistical approaches were used to characterize genes that correlated with clinical data. A total of 52 genes were identified that showed some correlation with differential sensitivity to drug treatment, prognosis, and survival of patients.

4. Bladder Cancer

Very detailed and comprehensive data on gene expression patterns in superficial and invasive bladder cancer have been published by Thykjaer et al. [40] Different expression patterns are characteristic for superficial and invasive cancers, and also correlate with different grades of bladder cancers (grades I–IV). Furthermore, expression patterns showed several functionally related clusters that include genes promoting cell cycle progression, growth factors, cell adhesion and extracellular matrix molecules, and genes that play a role in inflammation.

5. Prostate Cancer

Important gene expression data have been recently generated for prostate cancer and premalignant prostate neoplasias. Dhanasekaran et al. [79] analyzed more than 50 normal and neoplastic prostate samples, which included benign prostatic hyperplasia and invasive prostate cancer by cDNA microarrays. Expression patterns of two strong candidate marker genes, pim-1 and the protease hepsin, were analyzed using tissue microarrays. The combination of two related high-throughput techniques is a powerful approach to identify, confirm, and consolidate data that are important for diagnostic early detection and potentially treatment. Very similar data have also been published by Luo et al. [78]. This work identified more than 200 genes that showed statistically relevant differences in gene expression between normal tissue, preneoplastic hyperplasia, and prostate cancer. Interestingly, this group also identified the serine protease hepsin as a major candidate gene overexpressed in neoplastic prostatic tissues. Bull et al. [49] used a specialized, prostate-specific cDNA microarray to analyze gene expression patterns in prostate cancers and prostate cell lines.

6. Breast Cancer

Tumor gene expression profiles and genes differentially expressed in human breast cancer were first described by Perou et al. [80, 81]. Functionally related genes were usually found within identical clusters. Distinct clusters of genes were identified that share functions in cell adhesion, immunological responses (e.g., interferon-induced genes), cell cycle response, and differentiation. The association between estrogen receptor (ER) status of breast cancer tissues and gene expression patterns was analyzed by Gruvberger et al. [82]. Tumors could be successfully classified as ER+ or ER−, according to expression patterns. Microarray expression data from a total number of 100 genes was sufficient to clearly identify each tumor class. However, most of the genes used for discrimination between as ER+ or ER− status were not directly induced by estrogen or ER. Therefore, ER+ and ER− tumors display very different gene expression profiles that are not exclusively based on the direct effects of estrogen and estrogen receptor signaling. By microarray hybridization, Houghton et al. [83] identified a collection of potential candidate tumor antigens that were subsequently used for detection of circulating tumor cells in patients with known metastatic disease. This approach is promising to identify novel markers that can be successfully applied for detection of minimal residual disease and monitoring of patients at risk of relapse.

7. Ovarian Cancer

A number of genes upregulated in ovarian cancer were identified by Tapper et al. [84]. These significant changes not only correlated with tumor malignancy and progression, but also with differentiation of the tumors.

8. Hepatocellular Carcinoma

Okabe et al. [85] analyzed global gene expression patterns in hepatocellular carcinoma (HCC). The expression patterns of hepatitis B and C virus associated HCC differed markedly from those associated with hepatitis C virus. In both, mitosis-promoting genes were upregulated. Similar to findings in other tumor types, there were a number of genes that associated with different histological types and invasive properties. Similar, partially overlapping data were generated by Tackels-Horne et al. [86] using Affymetrix GeneChips. A total of 800 genes were overexpressed in tumor tissues, and 400 were more strongly expressed in normal liver tissue. However, the authors did verify differential gene expression by RT/PCR or Northern blot hybridization. The role of hypoxia and the importance of hypoxia-related signal transduction pathways in HCC was investigated by Scandurro et al. [87]. This group identified upregulation of integrin-linked kinase (ILK) and glycogen synthase kinase 3 (GSK-3 beta) in response to low oxygen levels. Both GSK-3 beta and ILK play a role in activation of major signaling pathways, which include protein kinase B (AKT), and the Wnt signaling pathway. GSK-3 beta also plays an important role in colorectal cancer [72]. Genes induced by hepatocyte growth factor (HGF, or scatter factor) in hepatocellular cells were identified by microarray analysis by Medico et al. [88]. Overexpression of HGF and oncogenic activation of the HGF receptor c-MET is involved in hepatocellular carcinogenesis and progression. The secreted phosphoprotein osteopontin was identified as a major target of gene activation by HGF. The growth promoting function of osteopontin on liver cells could be impaired by specific antibodies against this protein.

9. Melanoma

mRNA gene expression patterns of malignant melanoma were mathematically analyzed by Bittner et al. [88a]. Groups of genes were identified that clearly distinguish highly aggressive melanoma from other, less malignant types. This analysis revealed new, previously unknown subtypes of cutaneous melanoma that are defined by typical phenotypic characteristics. Distinct melanoma subtypes might respond differently to treatment or could have different, more or less aggressive metastatic properties.

A small number of tumors of other localizations have also been analyzed by microarray hybridization, which include pituitary adenomas [89] and mesotheliomas [90]. More publications of this kind will certainly be published in the near future.

An important issue that has not been appropriately addressed thus far is the effect of ischemia on gene expression of normal and malignant biopsies that have been removed during surgery. Huang et al. used medium-sized microarrays to investigate the kinetics of altered gene expression at time points up to 1 h after surgery, and found a number of gene groups that are induced by ischemia showing different kinetics [91].

E. Pathogenic Mechanisms

cDNA microarrays have the potential for identifying important molecular changes that contribute to pathogenesis. Using this methodology, groups of genes may be identified as associated with a characteristic disease. Clustering of these genes can subsequently identify specific signal transduction pathways or related functional changes. In this way, arrays provide insight into the molecular alterations that cause or accompany pathogenesis. For example, microarrays and cluster analysis have identified groups of genes that are expressed differentially in normal breast or colon tissue relative to their malignant counterparts [37, 39, 81]. To directly address the etiologic importance of a specific RNA, it can be inhibited or overexpressed in cells and the resulting gene expression profiles can be compared. For example, microarrays have been used to search for RNAs whose levels are altered in response to inducible expression of the Wilms tumor suppressor protein (WT). These experiments identified amphiregulin, an epidermal growth-factor-like molecule, as an important target of the tumor suppressor WT [92]. In another study, mouse keratinocytes that contained a targeted disruption of the epidermal growth factor receptor gene failed to progress to papillomas or carcinomas after xenografting to nude mice. Microarray analysis determined that among others, the cyclin-dependent kinase inhibitor p27 and insulin-like growth factor binding protein 2 were upregulated specifically in the knock-out cells [93].

Microarrays have also been used to study the pathogenesis of infectious diseases (reviewed in reference 94). Many microbial genomes have been completely sequenced and sequence information to generate comprehensive microbial arrays is available.

Microbial or viral arrays have the potential to identify genes associated with important properties such as virulence or latency (as an example, see reference 95). Microarrays of host genes have led to an increased understanding of microbial pathogenesis. For example, infection of macrophages with either *Salmonella typhimurium* or purified lipopolysaccharide (LPS) results in expression of the same subset of cytokine genes [96]. This indicates that LPS is important for stimulating the early response of macrophages to bacterial infection. In other studies, expression of human papillomavirus type 16 E6 and E7 proteins activated expression of NF-κB regulated genes, diminished expression of many IFN-regulated genes [97], and inhibited genes induced by transforming growth factor β2 [98]. These experiments demonstrate that microarrays are useful for dissecting cytokine-mediated signal pathways that are altered in response to microbes.

F. Discovery of Gene Function

The overall pattern of gene expression can suggest clues to the function of newly identified genes. Genes that are expressed similarly (increase or decrease due to a common circumstance) are likely to be functionally related. Gene expression patterns can be compared by clustering software (self-organizing map, hierarchical clustering, K-means clustering, and principle component analysis algorithms) that sort gene expression data by similarity. A prerequisite for clustering is a data set that consists of a preferably large number of array experiments using either different conditions (increasing drug concentrations or increasing incubation times) or multiple experiments with biological material from different sources (different patients). Genes that show similar expression patterns are placed close to each other in groups or "clusters" [99]. A recent review describes many of these "higher level" gene expression analysis tools in detail [21]. Using clustering algorithms, co-expressed genes can be identified, and the function of previously unidentified or unknown genes may be inferred. For example, Cho et al. examined genome-wide expression during progression of the cell cycle in *S. cerevesiae* [61, 100]. Over 6% of genes were cell cycle dependent. Of these, 60% were known to vary during the cell cycle. The remaining 40% were newly described. Many of these genes have human homologs suggesting similar functions in humans. Similar sets of genes can be identified in almost all large-scale microarray experiments. Usually, the potential importance of a cluster is defined by a subset of genes with well-established biological functions. Other genes that show similar expression patterns might have related functions, or at least related regulatory mechanisms. Hughes et al. described a method for gene discovery via a compendium of expression profiles [101]. They constructed a reference database of expression profiles corresponding to 300 diverse mutations and chemical treatments in *S. cerevisiae*, and showed that the cellular pathways affected can be determined by pattern matching, even among very subtle profiles.

Miki et al. [19] characterized gene expression patterns in 49 adult and embryonic mouse tissues by using cDNA microarrays that contain 18,816 full-length mouse cDNAs. Cluster analysis was used to define unique or overlapping sets of genes that are characteristically expressed in diverse mouse tissues. Furthermore, cluster analysis revealed that genes coding for known enzymes in 78 different metabolic pathways usually showed strong coordination of expression within the pathways among very different tissues. Unknown genes can be grouped into such functional or metabolic classes by similarity of their gene expression patterns with those of genes with known enzymatic function.

Despite the advantages in identification of co-expressed genes that might implicate similar functions, microarrays are often of less help in actually confirming the molecular function of novel genes. For example, IFN-induced genes represent a large cluster of coordinately expressed genes that can be identified in many different experiments [35, 97]. These genes usually respond to pro-inflammatory stimuli, cell differentiation, and stress, and are also differentially expressed in a large number of human tumors. Analysis of promoter elements within these genes reveals a common sequence, the IFN specific response element. This group contains nameless ESTs as well as some well-defined genes with known function, such as the 2'-5' oligoadenylate synthetases. The cluster also contains a number of IFN-inducible transmembrane proteins, but little is known about their function. Thus, microarray experiments provide important initial data concerning regulation of mRNA transcription, but they can not replace thorough biochemical investigations of gene function.

G. Gene Regulation

Gene expression patterns can provide information regarding transcriptional regulation by identifying common *cis*-acting regulatory elements within the co-expressed genes. Identification of common *cis* elements within the promoters of co-expressed genes might imply regulation by similar combinations of transcription factors. Transcription factor databases (Transfac, EPD) offer tools to explore promoter structure and also possible complex interactions between different transcription factors that are critical for regulation of mRNA gene expression. With the sequencing of the human genome, promoter sequences for most human genes have become available. Therefore, a promising approach is to combine gene expression profiling by microarrays with large-scale promoter analysis to identify common patterns that might explain coordinate mRNA expression at a molecular level (compare Genomatix, Inc.). Expression data generated from yeast have also been used to pioneer this novel area of genomic research. Statistical algorithms of whole genome RNA data have identified transcriptional regulatory networks in yeast without any prior knowledge of their structure [102]. Microarray analysis during yeast sporulation identified at least seven distinct temporal patterns of gene expression. Consensus sequences that are either known or proposed to be involved in temporal regulation could be identified solely from analysis of sequences of coordinately expressed genes [103].

VI. WHAT CAN GO WRONG IN cDNA MICROARRAY EXPERIMENTATION?

Many factors influence the design and results of microarray experiments, and several important parameters are described below. Technical aspects of microarray experimentation have been reviewed recently [104–106].

A. Sensitivity of Detection

A high level of sensitivity is important for comparison of genes that regulate biological processes. While some RNAs are expressed at high levels (housekeeping genes, structural proteins, or proteins associated with terminal differentiation), many important regulatory genes (transcription factors) normally function at low levels of expression. The sensitivity of detection is influenced by the strength of specific hybridization and the level of nonspecific background. It is also defined by the choice of DNA elements immobilized on the chip or filter surface. Therefore, elimination of DNA sequences that produce hybridization artifacts is a critical issue for chip design.

The use of well-designed oligonucleotides instead of PCR products generated from cDNA clones can strongly reduce the risk of cross-hybridizing probes and other artifacts [33, 34]. Inadequate sensitivity or high/inconsistent background hybridization can also result in an increased rate of false positive or false negative results. This can become a critical issue for macroarrays spotted on nylon membranes. Nylon filters generally tend to generate more background compared to glass microarrays. However, in fluorescent microarray experiments, inappropriate drying of hybridized glass arrays and other technical issues can also lead to severe background problems. In theses cases, affected areas have to be excluded (flagged) from analysis. The inclusion of many different samples or experimental groups in array studies can help to minimize this potential problem. Generally, false negative and positive results can become less deleterious if the experimental objective is to cluster large groups of genes in order to identify regulatory pathways. False positive or negative results are critical to consider if the sample size is limited or if the objective is to identify specific drug targets.

For fluorescent array hybridizations using direct label incorporation, at least 25–30 µg of total RNA or 0.5–1 µg of poly(A) mRNA are necessary. With large amounts of starting material available (e.g., using RNA from cell culture experiments), this is usually not a limiting issue. However, a problem arises with the use of very small amounts of RNA as starting material, for example, from laser capture microdissection [38, 107], embryonic tissues [20], or small organisms like *Drosophila*. In such cases, amplification of either the RNA or the hybridization signal is critical. A number of systems have been developed for signal amplification. The Tyramide system introduced by NEN (Micromax cDNA arrays) uses an antibody-mediated signal amplification method adapted from immunohistochemistry. With the Tyramide system, array hybridizations can be performed with as little as 2–5 µg of total RNA as starting material. Genisphere (Genisphere 3DNA Inc., NJ) markets an oligodendromeric fluorescent signal amplification system [108] that allows array hybridization with as little as 0.5µg of total RNA as starting material. Radioactive hybridization methods can also be considered as an alternative to fluorescent labeling of cDNA if limited sample material is available. Even for large filter hybridizations, 5–10 µg of total RNA are usually sufficient. As an alternative, RNA can be amplified using a T7-directed linear amplification protocol [38, 109]. This technique has been pioneered by Eberwine and colleagues [110, 111]. Amplification of as little as 2 ng total RNA is possible without generation of major qualitative and quantitative differences in representation of individual mRNAs [112]. The reliability of the RNA amplification can be tested by co-hybridizing amplified and nonamplified RNA samples. Other, nonlinear amplification protocols have been described (Clontech's SMART-PCR). All of these methods are potentially prone to artifacts that must be carefully detected and eliminated. Time will show which approach proves to be the most reliable.

B. Choice of Controls

Changes in mRNA expression must be compared to a standard. Without proper normalization of array experiments, it is difficult to extract reliable expression data or ratios of differential expression. Housekeeping genes are often used for this purpose because it is assumed that they are not significantly altered under most experimental conditions. However, this assumption may be incorrect. Some individual housekeeping genes do vary in expression during different experimental treatments, thus, a large number of housekeeping genes must be analyzed in any one experiment for standardization. For example, expression of beta actin differs by as much as 36-fold between different tumor samples, and marked differences have also been observed for glyceraldehyde phosphate dehydrogenase. Both genes have been used for decades to normalize mRNA gene expression data. A large number of potentially useful housekeeping genes have been identified and cataloged by Affymetrix [113]. Many of these genes are expressed in different cell types and levels of expression are similar. A second method for determining the baseline level of gene expression is to spike the probe with a known amount of labeled cDNA that hybridizes to the array. This provides an internal standard for comparison. A third useful control is to use nonspecific DNA (plasmid vectors, fragments from unrelated organisms like *Arabidopsis* or Lambda phages, or poly(A) sequences) spotted on the array. Ideally, the sample should not interact with these targets. One or all of these methods are helpful in determining whether changes in gene expression are significant. Another important control for reproducibility consists of flipping the two dyes that are used for cDNA labeling. This procedure is useful for identifying artifacts due to incomplete sample labeling.

C. Validation of Results

Confirmation of array results by independent methods such as semiquantitative RT-PCR, Northern blotting, RNase protection, Western blotting, or ELISA is important. In recent years, quantitative real-time RT-PCR has become available (TaqMan, LightCycler, iCycler). These rapid high-throughput methods allow quantitative PCR in a 96-well format and significantly speed up the validation process. RNA *in situ* hybridization is also useful for localization of expressed genes to a specific cell type within the tissue. However, detection sensitivity is frequently limiting. Recently, tissue arrays have emerged as a high-throughput approach to validate specific genes previously identified by DNA microarrays (references 14, 15 and reviewed in references 114–116). As many as ~1000 tissue samples from paraffin blocks can be deposited on a glass slide and simultaneously analyzed for expression of either RNA or protein. The diameter of these tissue samples ranges from 0.5 and 1.2 mm. Larger spots can simplify analysis.

Tissue arrays are an excellent method for extending and confirming microarray results. Tissue arrays have also been used to identify genes that are differentially expressed in hormone-sensitive and resistant forms of prostate cancer. In these experiments, arrays of tumor samples confirmed that the insulin-like growth factor binding protein 2 was overexpressed in 100% of hormone refractory clinical tumors [117]. Tissue microarrays can be produced in any lab that has access to paraffin-embedded tissue sections. Several companies offer arraying services. Other companies offer complete tissue arrays, already mounted on glass slides, for several human tumor localizations. The problem with these commercially available arrays is that clinical patient data for the samples mounted are usually lacking (see below). Therefore, the most important step in good tissue microarray design is careful histological examination of samples by a trained pathologist. Tissue array data with properly assigned clinical follow-up data is extremely useful, whereas specimens of unclear origin are useless. In a typical tissue microarray project, sample requisition can take up to 1 year prior to chip production.

VII. ARRAY-BASED PROTEOMICS: HOW TO INVESTIGATE PROTEIN COMPLEXITY

Although gene expression is regulated primarily at the level of transcription, many posttranscriptional mechanisms significantly influence this process. A logical question is: "Why not focus on protein rather than DNA?" In the following section, this issue will be discussed in depth.

According to a recent report by the Bioinsights consulting group, the international market for protein chips and high-throughput protein analysis will grow from $45 million in 2000 to an estimated $500 million in 2006. In comparison, the cDNA microarray market is expected to reach approximately $1.2 billion in 2006. (www.smalltimes.com/document.cfm?section-1d= 514document-1d=2831). This demand will occur in part from the inability to reliably identify drug targets simply by knowledge of genomic sequences or RNA expression profiling.

Thus far, there have been limited studies that investigate the correlation between protein and mRNA expression. One interesting study investigated this relationship in *S. cerevisiae*. Protein expression levels differed significantly from mRNA levels for many genes. The expected correlation value for all 6000 yeast proteins was less than 0.4 [118]. No comparable data are yet available for higher organisms. It is also clear that changes in protein level do not necessarily reflect changes in protein activity [119]. Moreover, changes in protein activity do not necessarily correlate with changes in specific biological responses within the cell [120]. Thus, a very important issue for protein activity that may not apply for mRNA is the localization of a particular protein within different cellular compartments. A number of posttranslational modifications (phosphorylation, acetylation, cleavage of signal peptides, glycosylation, and myristylation) contribute to the complexity and perplexity in the proteome. Additionally, alternative splicing at the mRNA level further complicates the situation. Consequently, the complexity in the human proteome is expected to range from 100,000 to 1 million different protein molecules [120, 121], in striking contrast to the 34,000 to 46,000 genes [1, 2]. There is growing evidence that drugs perturb cellular processes that are regulated by multiple genes, transcripts, and proteins [119]. Therefore, there is an enormous need for large-scale methodologies in proteomics research. One should also be aware that no known function exists for >75% of human genes [122].

VIII. EMERGING MICROARRAY TECHNOLOGIES FOR HIGH-THROUGHPUT PROTEOME INVESTIGATION: A TECHNICAL OVERVIEW

The generation of protein arrays is far more expensive and laborious compared to cDNA expression arrays, which have become a routine method in many laboratories. The following problems have to be resolved. First, there is no method for protein amplification such as PCR. Second, proteins are chemically more complex and heterogeneous in comparison to mRNAs and DNA. It will be difficult to define general protein detection and immobilization strategies that do not discriminate between specific types of proteins [123]. Third, in contrast to DNA, proteins easily lose biochemical activity due to denaturation, dehydration, or oxidation. For many proteins, narrow ranges of pH or salt concentrations are critical for enzymatic performance. Fourth, the detection of proteins by antibody–antigen interactions is characterized by a broad range of specificity and affinity. These binding affinities are generally weaker than DNA-DNA or DNA-RNA interactions [124].

A variety of novel experimental methods and different platforms for protein and peptide arrays have been described, most of them in the last year. Emili et al. [124] proposed to classify protein arrays into nonliving and living arrays. The first group consists of a grid of proteins, peptides, or antibodies that offer the possibility of high-throughput quantitation of proteins in complex biological solutions and the screening of discrete biochemical activities. In contrast, living arrays are constructed from cells growing on a grid in an arrayed order. They provide an experimental tool to investigate biochemical and biophysical reactions in the context of a living cell. In the following section, different protein array technologies are subdivided as living and nonliving arrays.

A. Nonliving Arrays

Nonliving arrays have been used for ELISA for decades [125]. Mendoza et al. [126] created multiple small antibody arrays consisting of 8 different antibodies in the format of 96-well plates. Standard ELISA technique and a scanning CCD detector were used to image the arrayed antigens. This strategy allowed parallel incubation and multiplex analysis of up to 96 different samples at once. For the purpose of screening a human fetal brain cDNA expression library, Büssow et al. [127] developed a membrane-based antigen array from a set of 37,830 *E. coli* that express His-tagged fusion proteins. These were probed with antibodies using standard ELISA techniques and analyzed with CCD cameras. The same group also used special transfer stamps that deposit minute drops (5 nl) of purified protein onto small rectangular (25 × 75 mm) PVDF membranes at a density of 300 samples/cm² [11]. Whole expression libraries of arrayed proteins can be screened in a single experiment [128, 129].

de Wildt et al. [130] used the reverse approach by spotting an antibody array with 18,342 immobilized bacterial clones, each one expressing a different single chain recombinant antibody. This technique was developed for identification of recombinant antibodies that bind with high affinity to selected antigens. It also allows for the determination of the strength of individual antigen binding and level of expression for each antibody clone. These antibody selection filters are useful as a novel antibody selection technique and present an alternative to phage display. Filter membranes can also be applied to screen for different biochemical activities on a large scale. Ge [131] used low-density protein arrays that contained 48 highly purified proteins primarily involved in transcription [131]. These arrays were used to study specific interaction of proteins with radioactive-labeled DNA, RNA, ligands, and other small chemicals. More important, these protein filters could be reused by stripping. Filter membranes remain the most applicable platform for protein arrays because of superior protein binding capacity. However, the limiting factors for filter protein arrays are the low resolution and considerable background problems. Furthermore, it will be difficult to construct high-density protein arrays that are comparable to large cDNA microarrays (density 1000–3000 spots/cm^2). Hence, it is difficult to use this technology for applications with limiting sample quantities such as protein expression profiling of tumor biopsies.

B. Glass-Based Protein Arrays

A protein array fabrication strategy using glass surfaces was described by MacBeath and Schreiber [132]. Proteins and antibodies were spotted on a glass surface coated with a cross-linking reagent that reacts with primary amines. Standard robotic instrumentation adapted from cDNA array production was used for spotting. This strategy was used to screen protein-protein or protein-ligand interactions and for identification of specific substrates for several protein kinases. A single spot of the FKBP12-rapamycin binding protein (FRB) could be identified within an array of 10,000 spots containing other proteins. Other modified surfaces such as aldehyde activated, poly-L-lysine, nitrocellulose, or nickel-coated glass slides (for His-tag containing proteins) were also evaluated for the production of protein microarrays [12, 13, 133–136].

Striking differences in specificity of antigen and antibody interactions on glass-based arrays were demonstrated by Haab et al. [135]. Of 115 antibody/antigen pairs, only 50% of the antigens and 20% of the arrayed antibodies provided specific and accurate measurements. In contrast, several antibody/antigen interactions could be detected in concentrations as low as 1 ng/ml. Protein mixtures were labeled with the standard dyes Cy5 and Cy3, which are also used in many cDNA array experiments. This technique allows simultaneous comparison of two biological samples and detection with a standard microarray laser scanner. Thus, the glass slide format allows the design of true high-density protein arrays that are comparable to cDNA microarrays and also compatible with standard microarray instrumentation (robotic spotters, imaging laser scanners, microarray software). A major disadvantage of arraying proteins on glass slides is the risk of protein denaturation due to solvent evaporation.

An alternative glass-slide-based strategy was developed in a joint program between the Argonne National Laboratory and the Engelhardt Institute of Molecular Biology, Russian Academy of Sciences, Moscow [137, 138]. Three-dimensional arrays are produced by immobilization of proteins in tiny gel packets that are dotted across a glass surface. Because of the three-dimensional structure, this approach allows immunoassays, antigen detection, and detection of enzymatic activity with a high efficiency of protein immobilization [139]. This technique uses a homogenous aqueous environment that reduces drying and excludes protein denaturation. Another nanowell technology was applied by Zhu et al. [45, 46] to analyze practically all known yeast protein kinases. Substrates as well as protein kinases were bound to the chip surface using epoxysilane, which reacts with amino groups of proteins. This technology allows the creation of a microenvironment for proteins and is applicable for solution-based assays.

C. Living Arrays

There are only a limited number of reports on biochemical assays carried out on arrayed living cells. The first living arrays were developed by Uetz et al. [140] to study yeast two-hybrid interactions. More than 6000 yeast colonies that expressed different Gal4-fusion proteins were arrayed on a solid medium and used for library screening. Ross-MacDonald et al. [141, 142] characterized 8000 yeast strains from the same genetic background that were mutagenized using yeast transposons. Mutant phenotypes were observed after growth of the arrayed yeast colonies on 21×21 cm agar plates under 20 different growth conditions. Living protein array for mammalian cells were produced by Ziauddin et al. [58]. Human embryonic kidney cells (HEK 293) were cultured on glass slides that were spotted with plasmid DNA (expression vectors), which contained a number of different cDNA inserts. Cells growing on particular spots take up plasmid DNA and express the recombinant protein of interest. Each DNA spot had a diameter of 120–150 μm in diameter and was colonized by a of cluster of 30–80 cells. Using classical detection techniques such as autoradiography, fluorescence, and *in situ* immunofluorescence, the authors were able to identify expression of various proteins involved in tyrosine kinase signaling, apoptosis, and cell adhesion. Additionally, the subcellular localization for many proteins could be determined. Most interestingly, effects of recombinant protein expression on cell phenotype could be addressed using this technology.

IX. CURRENT AND FUTURE APPLICATIONS OF PROTEIN ARRAYS IN DRUG DISCOVERY

Because levels of mRNA and protein do not necessarily correlate in many regulatory processes involving posttranscriptional alterations, it is important to investigate the relevance of a specific protein or groups of proteins in disease. However, there have been few studies to date that describe the application of protein arrays in clinical investigation. Joos et al. [13] used high-density antigen microarrays to detect autoantibodies in the sera of patients suffering from different autoimmune diseases. Huang et al. [143, 144] used low-density antibody arrays on filter membranes to detect cytokines in patient sera. The same arrays were used to analyze conditioned media derived from human glioblastoma U251 cell cultures stimulated with rTNFα. Both approaches used ELISA for protein detection. Compared to standard ELISA, these protein microarrays are considerably more sensitive. The method developed by Joos et al. [13] was one of the most sensitive glass slide-based protein microarray techniques yet developed. This type of antibody microarray could also be used for diagnostic and prognostic studies of disease. To characterize expression of surface CD antigens on leukocytes and leukemia cells, an antibody microarray was developed by Belov et al. [12]. A suspension of unlabeled leukocytes isolated from peripheral blood of patients with chronic lymphocytic leukemia, hairy cell leukemia, mantle cell lymphoma, AML, and T-cell acute lymphoblastic leukemia was applied to an array that contained 60 anti-CD antibodies. The resulting dot patterns were highly characteristic for each hematologic malignancy. This type of antibody array allows rapid and sensitive immunophenotyping that could be performed in a clinical setting. The intact cells that bound to the array could be further characterized using fluorescent labeled antibodies. Protein microarray techniques that catalog differences in protein expression in various tissues, in different diseases, or as a consequence of drug treatment are a powerful tool for drug discovery. However, these arrays do not elucidate functional characteristics of the proteins.

A. Functional Characterization of Proteins

Many known proteins as well as other hypothetical or predicted proteins have not been functionally characterized. To date, most comprehensive studies of protein function and interaction were carried out with the yeast *S. cerevisiae*, whose genome was sequenced in 1997. Nevertheless, a significant portion of the 6300 open reading frames encode proteins with undiscovered biological function [46]. Presumably, it will be possible to use similar techniques to prepare protein arrays for large-scale protein analysis in humans and higher eukaryotes. An example of successful application of protein arrays in biochemical research is the investigation of protein kinase functions. It is estimated that 2–3% of the eukaryotic genomes encode protein kinases or phosphorylases that regulate phosphorylation of up to 25% of cellular proteins. These proteins are involved in nearly every major regulatory process [145]. Human diseases including cancer, atherosclerosis and immune dysfunctions usually involve mutation, overexpression, or malfunction of at least one protein kinases [146, 147]. Zhu et al. [45] evaluated nearly all known yeast protein kinase (119 of 122) for their affinity to 17 different potential substrates as well as autophosphorylation using a protein microarray. Not surprisingly, the authors found that most protein kinases prefer specific substrates. They also identified a large number of tyrosine kinases in yeast. Previously, only seven yeast tyrosine kinases were known. This is the first genome-wide attempt to analyze a specific protein function using protein chip technology.

Most proteins perform their function as multiple protein complexes. Thus, it is mandatory to analyze protein-protein interactions in order to understand cellular processes. Living protein arrays with nearly all predicted open reading frames (ORFs) of *S. cerevisiae* were used by Uetz et al. [140] to study protein-protein interactions in yeast (see above). Using the two-hybrid system, 192 proteins were screened for putative interaction partners and a total of 281 specific protein-protein interactions were identified. These studies identified a complex network of known and functionally uncharacterized proteins that are involved in functions such as the cell cycle, meiotic recombination, and RNA splicing. Zhu et al. [136] constructed a yeast proteome microarray on nickel-coated glass slides that included approximately 80% of all yeast proteins. Yeast cDNAs were cloned and expressed as fusion proteins with glutathione-S-transferase and a His$_6$ tag. The microarrays were probed with biotinylated proteins and lipids that were subsequently detected using fluorescent labeled streptavidin. The authors identified 39 calmodulin-binding proteins, 33 of which were novel. A total of 150 proteins were shown to bind to various phospholipids. The function of 52 proteins within this group had been completely unknown. Additionally, some proteins that are involved in glucose metabolism were identified as high-affinity binding partners for phospholipids. This led to speculation that phospholipids could regulate some aspects of glucose metabolism and that some steps of glucose metabolism might occur on membrane surfaces.

B. Mass Spectrometry Based Protein Chip Technologies

Ciphergen's proprietary reverse-phase ProteinChip uses a number of different surfaces immobilized on small aluminum chips. These absorb proteins by a variety of noncovalent interactions [148]. Therefore, the complexity of proteins in biological samples can be significantly reduced. These chip surfaces probe for hydrophobic, electrostatic (anion and cation exchange surfaces), or metal affinity binding of proteins. In a second step, proteins bound to the surface are analyzed by surface-enhanced laser desorption mass spectrometry (SELDI), and protein profiles are generated that can be directly compared. The resolution of this mass spectrometry-based system is immense, and small changes in protein mass due to glycosylation or phosphorylation can be exactly identified. The SELDI protein chip technology can measure molecular masses with a deviation of less than 0.2%. The system can detect a few femtomoles of protein, and estimate the amount of hundreds of proteins and peptides simultaneously. The system offers a useful and rapid alternative to two-dimensional gel electrophoresis. However, the initial investment cost is high. The major disadvantage (as with 2D gels) is that interesting peaks cannot easily be identified.

SELDI is currently the most commonly used chip-based technology for protein profiling. In one recent publication [149], patient-matched normal, premalignant, malignant, and metastatic cell populations were microdissected from human esophageal, prostate, breast, ovary, colon, and hepatic tissue sections. Reproducible protein profiles could be obtained from as few as 25 cells in less than 5 minutes after microdissection. The authors have shown reproducible downregulation of a 28-kDa protein in most of the cancer specimens.

X. HOW TO DEAL WITH ALL THAT DATA

A major future goal is to develop centralized databases for public distribution of cDNA and eventually peptide array results [22, 23]. However, the lack of standard array formats and analysis protocols until recently interfered with the development of a universal resource. Many different types of arrays exist, and analysis of signal intensity is performed using different algorithms. These factors complicate comparison of data generated in different laboratories. For these reasons, the Microarray Gene Expression Database Group (MGED) is interested in establishing international standards. MGED would like to define minimal requirements of information necessary to describe a microarray experiment. The definitions used to annotate and define microarray experiments including quality control and repeats of identical experiments have recently been made public. The MGED group and others are also interested in establishing an international language format for description of microarray data. Rosetta Inpharmatics, Inc. recently initiated the development of a gene expression markup language (GEML) that is intended to facilitate the exchange of gene expression data between different laboratories or even between different expression profiling technologies (e.g., SAGE and microarrays). For this purpose, the GEML Conductor program was developed, which allows researchers to visualize and exchange expression data. GEML Conductor is available free (see Table 2.1 for Web site). Exchange of microarray data also indicates that microarray databases can be used to store expression data from many different laboratories using different experiments, organisms, or cell types. A number of public microarray databases have been established to date. These include the Stanford Microarray Database at Stanford University, the ArrayExpress Database at European Bioinformatics Institute (EBI) and the Gene Expression Omnibus GEO at NCI to name a few. A number of additional databases are listed in Table 2.1.

An important point for analysis and interpretation of microarray data is screening of the literature to identify common features in co-expressed genes. Many of the genes on an array have unknown function or have been described by just one or two publications in PubMed. However, a vast amount of published information is available on other genes. To screen this huge data source within a reasonable time, a number of data mining tools have been developed. All of these tools are Web based. Medminer filters, extracts, and organizes relevant sentences in the literature based on a gene, gene-to-gene, or gene-drug query. This tool combines the GeneCards and PubMed search engines with user input and automated server-side scripts in an integrated text filtering system [150]. Another important database for identification of co expressed genes and cellular signaling pathways is PubGene [151]. This program basically represents a database that was created by the automated analysis of titles and abstracts in over 10 million MEDLINE records. PubGene contains literature links and cross references for 13,712 named human genes (June 2001). The associations between genes have been annotated by linking genes to terms from the medical subject heading (MeSH) index and terms from the gene ontology database.

XI. THE FUTURE IS ONLY GOING TO GET BETTER

What was an unusual and difficult technology in the past is rapidly becoming the norm. The emphasis has progressed from the design or improvement of array technology to practical applications including pharmacogenomics. Arrays may develop in several stages. These include large chips that contain tens of thousands of genes that can be used to examine global gene expression, often at reasonable cost. With the growing market for arrays, prices will fall and access to this technology will become available for smaller labs. However, smaller specialty arrays will also become popular for focusing on specific signal pathways or diseases.

As more and more investigators utilize microarrays, and novel companies decide to produce microarrays or related products, new technology will improve their sensitivity and reproducibility. In a few years, microarray technology might be used as a standardized and inexpensive routine lab procedure, comparable to automated DNA sequencing today. An important area in the future will be data handling and analyses. It will be useful to develop databases that accommodate results from different labs using dissimilar techniques. It would be desirable to make at least some of these databases publicly available with unlimited access for institutional and academic researchers. It will also be important to develop improved tools for analysis of complex comparisons such as correlation of expression patterns with genomic localization or promoter analysis. Novel programs that mine transcriptional regulatory sequences from clustered gene groups might provide insight into important mechanisms of transcriptional regulation by *cis* elements.

The emerging technology of high-density protein, peptide, and antibody arrays might eventually allow routine analysis of major subsets of the human proteome. It is conceivable that 5000 to 10,000 cellular proteins could be analyzed in a single experiment. Currently, protein microarray techniques are at an early stage of development. Numerous technical difficulties still have to be solved to establish protein arrays as a reliable tool in proteomics. Future versions of antibody microarrays for protein expression profiling must be able to detect proteins with very high sensitivity and specificity in complex biological samples. However, many monoclonal antibodies will not be suitable for this purpose. Hence, the production of highly specific antibodies with minimal cross reactivity for a large number of human proteins represents the most critical bottleneck for future array development. The production of high-quality monoclonal antibodies will be an extremely important issue. One possible alternative platform for future protein arrays could be based on phage display libraries, which can generate very high-affinity recombinant antibodies. The large-scale biochemical analysis by means of antibody arrays would also be greatly expedited by the possibility of low cost, large-scale expression and purification of recombinant proteins and antigens. With the currently available technology, these goals are unachievable, but efforts are under way to develop appropriate purification processes. These include:

- the Structure Factory in Germany (http://www.psf-ag.com/company.htm)
- the Harvard Institute for Proteomics (www.hip.harvard.edu/)
- the RIKEN Genomic Sciences Center in Japan (www.gsc.riken.go.jp/)
- several collaborative Structural Genomics Centers soon to be funded by the NIH (www.nigms.nih.gov/funding/psi.html)

Membrane-bound proteins account for an estimated 20–40% of all cellular proteins. Biochemical analysis of membrane-associated proteins will be a difficult task because these proteins usually require a lipid bilayer for optimal activity and stability [152]. However, analysis of membrane-associated proteins by arrays is an extremely promising task and would be rewarding for virtually all fields of life science, including pharmacogenomics and drug development. Membrane proteins make up a large portion of known drug targets for substances that are currently used as drugs. Methods are already established that circumvent some of the technological problems imparted by the special properties of membrane proteins [153].

In a number of years, it is likely that individuals will be assessed at birth for genetic polymorphisms that might allow prediction of disease later in life. In particular, these would be SNPs. This SNP mapping could also be performed by genomic microarray hybridization (SNP-Chips). Currently, arrays for SNP detection are at a comparably early stage of development. However, huge databases that contain data for millions of SNPs are set up at several, predominantly commercial genome centers (e.g., Celera). Genomic array results could serve as a map that would suggest appropriate alterations in lifestyle to prevent disease and focusing medical testing on patients with a high risk for a specific disease. It is possible that Web-based databases that contain all patients SNPs or other genetic polymorphisms will be developed, and these will be used to customize each individual's diagnosis and treatment. Although accumulation of patient databases would be useful for prevention and treatment of human disease, there is clearly a great potential for abuse and loss of privacy.

REFERENCES

1. Lander ES, Linton LM, Birren B et al. Initial sequencing and analysis of the human genome. *Nature* 2001; 409:860–921.
2. Venter JC, Adams MD, Myers EW et al. The sequence of the human genome. *Science* 2001; 291:1304–1351.
3. Brown PO, Hartwell L. Genomics and human disease — variations on variation. *Nat. Genet.* 1998; 18:91–93.
4. Brown PO, Botstein D. Exploring the new world of the genome with DNA microarrays. *Nat. Genet.* 1999; 21:33–37.
5. Collins, FS. Contemplating the end of the beginning. *Genome Res.* 2001; 11:641–643.
6. Collins FS, Mansoura MK. The human genome project. *Cancer* 2001; 91:221–225.
7. Collins FS. Genetics: An explosion of knowledge is transforming clinical practice. *Geriatrics* 1999; 54:41–47.
8. Evans WE, Relling MV. Pharmacogenomics: Translating functional genomics into rational therapeutics. *Science* 1999; 286:487–491.
9. Jain KK. Applications of biochip and microarray systems in pharmacogenomics. *Pharmacogenomics* 2000; 1:289–307.
10. Lichter P, Joos S, Bentz M, Lampel S. Comparative genomic hybridization: Uses and limitations. *Semin. Hematol.* 2000; 37:348–357.
11. Lueking A, Horn M, Eickhoff H, Bussow K, Lehrach H, Walter G. Protein microarrays for gene expression and antibody screening. *Anal. Biochem.* 1999; 270:103–111.
12. Belov L, de LV, dos Remedios CG, Mulligan SP, Christopherson RI. Immunophenotyping of leukemias using a cluster of differentiation antibody microarray. *Cancer Res.* 2001; 61:4483–4489.
13. Joos TO, Schrenk M, Hopfl P et al. A microarray enzyme-linked immunosorbent assay for autoimmune diagnostics. *Electrophoresis* 2000; 21:2641–2650.
14. Kononen J, Bubendorf L, Kallioniemi A et al. Tissue microarrays for high-throughput molecular profiling of tumor specimens. *Nat. Med.* 1998; 4:844–847.
15. Nocito A, Bubendorf L, Maria TE et al. Microarrays of bladder cancer tissue are highly representative of proliferation index and histological grade. *J. Pathol.* 2001; 194:349–357.
16. Schraml P, Kononen J, Bubendorf L et al. Tissue microarrays for gene amplification surveys in many different tumor types. *Clin. Cancer Res.* 1999; 5:1966–1975.
17. DeRisi JL, Iyer VR, Brown PO. Exploring the metabolic and genetic control of gene expression on a genomic scale. *Science* 1997; 278:680–686.
18. Shoemaker DD, Schadt EE, Armour CD et al. Experimental annotation of the human genome using microarray technology. *Nature* 2001; 409:922–927.

19. Miki R, Kadota K, Bono H et al. Delineating developmental and metabolic pathways *in vivo* by expression profiling using the RIKEN set of 18,816 full-length enriched mouse cDNA arrays. *Proc. Natl. Acad. Sci. U. S. A.* 2001; 98:2199–2204.

20. Tanaka TS, Jaradat SA, Lim MK et al. Genome-wide expression profiling of mid-gestation placenta and embryo using a 15,000 mouse developmental cDNA microarray. *Proc. Natl. Acad. Sci. U. S. A.* 2000; 97:9127–9132.

21. Quackenbush J. Computational genetics computational analysis of microarray data. *Nat. Rev. Genet.* 2001; 2:418–427.

22. Brazma A, Vilo J. Gene expression data analysis. *FEBS Lett.* 2000; 480:17–24.

23. Brazma A, Robinson A, Cameron G, Ashburner M. One-stop shop for microarray data. *Nature* 2000; 403:699–700.

24. Augenlicht LH, Wahrman MZ, Halsey H, Anderson L, Taylor J, Lipkin M. Expression of cloned sequences in biopsies of human colonic tissue and in colonic carcinoma cells induced to differentiate *in vitro*. *Cancer Res.* 1987; 47:6017–6021.

25. Lockhart DJ, Dong H, Byrne MC et al. Expression monitoring by hybridization to high-density oligonucleotide arrays. *Nat. Biotechnol.* 1996; 14:1675–1680.

26. Lipshutz RJ, Fodor SP, Gingeras TR, Lockhart DJ. High density synthetic oligonucleotide arrays. *Nat. Genet.* 1999; 21:20–24.

27. Lipshutz RJ. Applications of high-density oligonucleotide arrays. *Novartis Found. Symp.* 2000; 229:84–90.

28. Li C, Wong WH. Model-based analysis of oligonucleotide arrays: Expression index computation and outlier detection. *Proc. Natl. Acad. Sci. U. S. A.* 2001; 98:31–36.

29. Schena M, Shalon D, Davis RW, Brown PO. Quantitative monitoring of gene expression patterns with a complementary DNA microarray. *Science* 1995; 270:467–470.

30. DeRisi J, Penland L, Brown PO et al. Use of a cDNA microarray to analyse gene expression patterns in human cancer. *Nat. Genet.* 1996; 14:457–460.

31. Schena M, Shalon D, Heller R, Chai A, Brown PO, Davis RW. Parallel human genome analysis: microarray-based expression monitoring of 1000 genes. *Proc. Natl. Acad. Sci. U. S. A.* 1996; 93:10614–10619.

32. Shalon D, Smith SJ, Brown PO. A DNA microarray system for analyzing complex DNA samples using two-color fluorescent probe hybridization. *Genome Res.* 1996; 6:639–645.

33. Hughes TR, Mao M, Jones AR. Expression profiling using microarrays fabricated by an ink-jet oligonucleotide synthesizer. *Nat. Biotechnol.* 2001; 19:342–347.

34. Hughes TR, Shoemaker DD. DNA microarrays for expression profiling. *Curr. Opin. Chem. Biol.* 2001; 5:21–25.

35. Der SD, Zhou A, Williams BR, Silverman RH. Identification of genes differentially regulated by interferon alpha, beta, or gamma using oligonucleotide arrays. *Proc. Natl. Acad. Sci. U. S. A.* 1998; 95:15623–15628.

36. Mariadason JM, Corner GA, Augenlicht LH. Genetic reprogramming in pathways of colonic cell maturation induced by short chain fatty acids: Comparison with trichostatin A, sulindac, and curcumin and implications for chemoprevention of colon cancer. *Cancer Res.* 2000; 60:4561–4572.

37. Alon U, Barkai N, Notterman DA et al. Broad patterns of gene expression revealed by clustering analysis of tumor and normal colon tissues probed by oligonucleotide arrays. *Proc. Natl. Acad. Sci. U. S. A.* 1999; 96:6745–6750.

38. Kitahara O, Furukawa Y, Tanaka T et al. Alterations of gene expression during colorectal carcinogenesis revealed by cDNA microarrays after laser-capture microdissection of tumor tissues and normal epithelia. *Cancer Res.* 2001; 61:3544–3549.

39. Notterman DA, Alon U, Sierk AJ, Levine AJ. Transcriptional gene expression profiles of colorectal adenoma, adenocarcinoma, and normal tissue examined by oligonucleotide arrays. *Cancer Res.* 2001; 61:3124–3130.

40. Thykjaer T, Workman C, Kruhoffer M et al. Identification of gene expression patterns in superficial and invasive human bladder cancer. *Cancer Res.* 2001; 61:2492–2499.

41. Chang YE, Laimins LA. Microarray analysis identifies interferon-inducible genes and Stat-1 as major transcriptional targets of human papillomavirus type 31. *J. Virol.* 2000; 74:4174–4182.

42. Fambrough D, McClure K, Kazlauskas A, Lander ES. Diverse signaling pathways activated by growth factor receptors induce broadly overlapping, rather than independent, sets of genes. *Cell* 1999; 97:727–741.

43. Sweeney C, Fambrough D, Huard C et al. Growth factor-specific signaling pathway stimulation and gene expression mediated by ErbB receptors. *J. Biol. Chem.* 2001; 276:22685–22698.

44. Gray NS, Wodicka L, Thunnissen AM et al. Exploiting chemical libraries, structure, and genomics in the search for kinase inhibitors. *Science* 1998; 281:533–538.

45. Zhu H, Klemic JF, Chang S et al. Analysis of yeast protein kinases using protein chips. *Nat. Genet.* 2000; 26:283–289.

46. Zhu H, Snyder M. Protein arrays and microarrays. *Curr. Opin. Chem. Biol.* 2001; 5:40–545.

47. Sudbrak R, Wieczorek G, Nuber UA et al. X chromosome-specific cDNA arrays: Identification of genes that escape from X-inactivation and other applications. *Hum. Mol. Genet.* 2001; 10:77–83.

48. Takemasa I, Higuchi H, Yamamoto H et al. Construction of preferential cDNA microarray specialized for human colorectal carcinoma: Molecular sketch of colorectal cancer. *Biochem. Biophys. Res. Commun.* 2001; 285:1244–1249.

49. Bull JH, Ellison G, Patel A et al. Identification of potential diagnostic markers of prostate cancer and prostatic intraepithelial neoplasia using cDNA microarray. *Br. J. Cancer* 2001; 84:1512–1519.

50. Martin KJ, Graner E, Li Y et al. High-sensitivity array analysis of gene expression for the early detection of disseminated breast tumor cells in peripheral blood. *Proc. Natl. Acad. Sci. U. S. A.* 2001; 98:2646–2651.

51. Khanna C, Khan J, Nguyen P et al. Metastasis-associated differences in gene expression in a murine model of osteosarcoma. *Cancer Res.* 2001; 61:3750–3759.

52. Kimura S, Gonzalez FJ. Applications of genetically manipulated mice in pharmacogenetics and pharmacogenomics. *Pharmacology* 2000; 61:147–153.

53. Callow MJ, Dudoit S, Gong EL, Speed TP, Rubin EM. Microarray expression profiling identifies genes with altered expression in HDL-deficient mice. *Genome Res.* 2000; 10:2022–2029.

54. Jackson-Grusby L, Beard C, Possemato R et al. Loss of genomic methylation causes p53-dependent apoptosis and epigenetic deregulation. *Nat. Genet.* 2001; 27:31–39.

55. Dong G, Loukinova E, Chen Z et al. Molecular profiling of transformed and metastatic murine squamous carcinoma cells by differential display and cDNA microarray reveals altered expression of multiple genes related to growth, apoptosis, angiogenesis, and the NF-κB signal pathway. *Cancer Res.* 2001; 61:4797–4808.

56. Saban MR, Hellmich H, Nguyen NB, Winston J, Hammond TG, Saban R. Time course of LPS-induced gene expression in a mouse model of genitourinary inflammation. *Physiol. Genomics* 2001; 5:147–160.

57. Marton MJ, DeRisi JL, Bennett HA et al. Drug target validation and identification of secondary drug target effects using DNA microarrays. *Nat. Med.* 1998; 4:1293–1301.

58. Ziauddin J, Sabatini DM. Microarrays of cells expressing defined cDNAs. *Nature* 2001; 411:107–110.

59. Jelinsky SA, Estep P, Church GM, Samson LD. Regulatory networks revealed by transcriptional profiling of damaged *Saccharomyces cerevisiae* cells: Rpn4 links base excision repair with proteasomes. *Mol. Cell. Biol.* 620: 8157–8167.

60. Jelinsky SA, Samson LD. Global response of *Saccharomyces cerevisiae* to an alkylating agent. *Proc. Natl. Acad. Sci. U. S. A.* 1999; 96:1486–1491.

61. Cho RJ, Huang M, Campbell MJ et al Transcriptional regulation and function during the human cell cycle. *Nat. Genet.* 2001; 27:48–54.

62. Ross DT, Scherf U, Eisen MB et al. Systematic variation in gene expression patterns in human cancer cell lines. *Nat. Genet.* 2000; 24:227–235.

63. Weinstein JN, Myers TG, O'Connor PM et al. An information-intensive approach to the molecular pharmacology of cancer. *Science* 1997; 275:343–349.

64. Weinstein JN, Buolamwini JK. Molecular targets in cancer drug discovery: Cell-based profiling. *Curr. Pharm. Des.* 2000; 6:473–483.

65. Scherf U, Ross DT, Waltham M et al. A gene expression database for the molecular pharmacology of cancer. *Nat. Genet.* 2000; 24:236–244.

66. Rininger JA, DiPippo VA, Gould-Rothberg BE. Differential gene expression technologies for identifying surrogate markers of drug efficacy and toxicity. *Drug Discov. Today* 2000; 5:560–568.

67. Pollack JR, Perou CM, Alizadeh AA et al. Genome-wide analysis of DNA copy-number changes using cDNA microarrays. *Nat. Genet.* 1999; 23:41–46.

68. Troesch A, Nguyen H, Miyada CG et al. Mycobacterium species identification and rifampin resistance testing with high-density DNA probe arrays. *J. Clin. Microbiol.* 1999; 37, 49–55.

69. Golub TR, Slonim DK, Tamayo P et al. Molecular classification of cancer: Class discovery and class prediction by gene expression monitoring. *Science* 1999; 286:531–537.

70. Alizadeh AA, Eisen MB, Davis RE et al. Distinct types of diffuse large B-cell lymphoma identified by gene expression profiling. *Nature* 2000; 403:503–511.

71. Scherl-Mostageer M, Sommergruber W, Abseher R, Hauptmann R, Ambros P, Schweifer N. Identification of a novel gene, CDCP1, overexpressed in human colorectal cancer. *Oncogene* 2001; 20:4402–4408.

72. Lin YM, Ono K, Satoh S et al. Identification of AF17 as a downstream gene of the beta-catenin/T-cell factor pathway and its involvement in colorectal carcinogenesis. *Cancer Res.* 2001; 61:6345–6349.

73. Gupta RA, Brockman JA, Sarraf P, Willson TM, DuBois RN. Target genes of peroxisome proliferator-activated receptor {gamma} in colorectal cancer cells. *J. Biol. Chem.* 2001; 276:29681–29687.

74. Lawrance IC, Fiocchi C, Chakravarti S. Ulcerative colitis and Crohn's disease: Distinctive gene expression profiles and novel susceptibility candidate genes. *Hum. Mol. Genet.* 2001; 10:445–456.

75. Dieckgraefe BK, Stenson WF, Korzenik JR, Swanson PE, Harrington CA. Analysis of mucosal gene expression in inflammatory bowel disease by parallel oligonucleotide arrays. *Physiol. Genomics* 2000; 4:1–11.

76. Kan T, Shimada Y, Sato F et al: Gene expression profiling in human esophageal cancers using cDNA microarray. *Biochem. Biophys. Res. Commun.* 2001; 286:792–801.

77. Kihara C, Tsunoda T, Tanaka T et al. Prediction of sensitivity of esophageal tumors to adjuvant chemotherapy by cDNA microarray analysis of gene-expression profiles. *Cancer Res.* 2001; 61:6474–6479.

78. Luo J, Duggan DJ, Chen Y et al. Human prostate cancer and benign prostatic hyperplasia: Molecular dissection by gene expression profiling. *Cancer Res.* 2001; 61:4683–4688

79. Dhanasekaran SM, Barrette TR, Ghosh D et al. Delineation of prognostic biomarkers in prostate cancer. *Nature* 2001; 412:822–826.

80. Perou CM, Jeffrey SS, van de RM et al. Distinctive gene expression patterns in human mammary epithelial cells and breast cancers. *Proc. Natl. Acad. Sci. U. S. A.* 1999; 96:9212–9217.

81. Perou CM, Sorlie T, Eisen MB et al. Molecular portraits of human breast tumours. *Nature* 2000; 406:747–752.

82. Gruvberger S, Ringner M, Chen Y et al. Estrogen receptor status in breast cancer is associated with remarkably distinct gene expression patterns. *Cancer Res.* 2001; 61:5979–5984.

83. Houghton RL, Dillon DC, Molesh DA et al. Transcriptional complementarity in breast cancer: Application to detection of circulating tumor cells. *Mol. Diagn.* 2001; 6:79–91.

84. Tapper J, Kettunen E, El Rifai W, Seppala M, Andersson LC, Knuutila S. Changes in gene expression during progression of ovarian carcinoma. *Cancer Genet. Cytogenet.* 2001; 128:1–6.

85. Okabe H, Satoh S, Kato T et al. Genome-wide analysis of gene expression in human hepatocellular carcinomas using cDNA microarray: Identification of genes involved in viral carcinogenesis and tumor progression. *Cancer Res.* 2001; 61:2129–2137.

86. Tackels-Horne D, Goodman MD, Williams AJ et al. Identification of differentially expressed genes in hepatocellular carcinoma and metastatic liver tumors by oligonucleotide expression profiling. *Cancer* 2001; 92:395–405.

87. Scandurro AB, Weldon CW, Figueroa YG, Alam J, Beckman BS. Gene microarray analysis reveals a novel hypoxia signal transduction pathway in human hepatocellular carcinoma cells. *Int. J. Oncol.* 2001; 19:129–135.

88. Medico E, Gentile A, Lo CC et al. Osteopontin is an autocrine mediator of hepatocyte growth factor- induced invasive growth. *Cancer Res.* 2001; 61:5861–5868.

88a. Bittner M, Meltzer P, Chen Y et al. Molecular classification of cutaneous malignant melanoma by gene expression profiling. *Nature* 2000; 406:536–540.

89. Evans CO, Young AN, Brown MR et al. Novel patterns of gene expression in pituitary adenomas identified by complementary deoxyribonucleic acid microarrays and quantitative reverse transcription-polymerase chain reaction. *J. Clin. Endocrinol. Metab.* 2001; 86:3097–3107.

90. Kettunen E, Nissen AM, Ollikainen T et al. Gene expression profiling of malignant mesothelioma cell lines: cDNA array study. *Int. J. Cancer* 2001; 91:492–496.

91. Huang J, Qi R, Quackenbush J, Dauway E, Lazaridis E, Yeatman T. Effects of ischemia on gene expression. *J. Surg. Res.* 2001; 99:222–227.

92. Lee SB, Huang K, Palmer R et al. The Wilms tumor suppressor WT1 encodes a transcriptional activator of amphiregulin. *Cell* 1999; 98:663–673.

93. Woodworth CD, Gaiotti D, Michael E, Hansen L, Nees M. Targeted disruption of the epidermal growth factor receptor inhibits development of papillomas and carcinomas from human papillomavirus-immortalized keratinocytes. *Cancer Res.* 2000; 60:4397–4402.

94. Cummings CA, Relman DA. Using DNA microarrays to study host-microbe interactions. *Emerg. Infect. Dis.* 2000; 6:513–525.

95. Zhu H, Cong JP, Mamtora G, Gingeras T, Shenk T. Cellular gene expression altered by human cytomegalovirus: global monitoring with oligonucleotide arrays. *Proc. Natl. Acad. Sci. U. S. A.* 1998; 95:14470–14475.

96. Rosenberger CM, Scott MG, Gold MR, Hancock RE, Finlay BB. *Salmonella typhimurium* infection and lipopolysaccharide stimulation induce similar changes in macrophage gene expression. *J. Immunol.* 2000; 164:5894–5904.

97. Nees M, Geoghegan JM, Hyman T, Frank S, Miller L, Woodworth CD. Papillomavirus type 16 oncogenes downregulate expression of interferon-responsive genes and upregulate proliferation-associated and NF-κB-responsive genes in cervical keratinocytes. *J. Virol.* 2001; 75:4283–4296.

98. Nees M, Geoghegan JM, Munson P, Prabhu V, Liu Y, Androphy E, Woodworth CD. Human papillomavirus type 16 E6 and E7 proteins inhibit differentiation-dependent expression of transforming growth factor-beta2 in cervical keratinocytes. *Cancer Res.* 2000; 60:4289–4298.

99. Eisen MB, Spellman PT, Brown PO, Botstein D. Cluster analysis and display of genome-wide expression patterns. *Proc. Natl. Acad. Sci. U. S. A.* 1998; 95:4863–14868.

100. Cho RJ, Campbell MJ, Winzeler EA et al. A genome-wide transcriptional analysis of the mitotic cell cycle. *Mol. Cell* 1998; 2:65–73.

101. Hughes TR, Marton MJ, Jones AR et al. Functional discovery via a compendium of expression profiles. *Cell* 2000; 102:109–126.

102. Tavazoie S, Hughes JD, Campbell MJ, Cho RJ, Church GM. Systematic determination of genetic network architecture. *Nat. Genet.* 1999; 22:281–285.

103. Chu S, DeRisi J, Eisen M et al. The transcriptional program of sporulation in budding yeast. *Science* 1998; 282:699–705.

104. Hegde P, Qi R, Abernathy K et al. A concise guide to cDNA microarray analysis. *Biotechniques* 2000; 29:548–554, 556.

105. Wildsmith SE, Elcock FJ. Microarrays under the microscope. *Mol. Pathol.* 2001; 54:8–16.

106. Wildsmith SE, Archer GE, Winkley AJ, Lane PW, Bugelski PJ. Maximization of signal derived from cDNA microarrays. *Biotechniques* 2001; 30:202–206, 208.

107. Emmert-Buck MR, Bonner RF, Smith PD et al. Laser capture microdissection. *Science* 1996; 274:998–1001.

108. Stears RL, Getts RC, Gullans SR. A novel, sensitive detection system for high-density microarrays using dendrimer technology. *Physiol. Genomics* 2000; 3:93–99.

109. Wang E, Miller LD, Ohnmacht GA, Liu ET, Marincola FM. High-fidelity mRNA amplification for gene profiling. *Nat. Biotechnol.* 2000; 18:457–459.

110. Van Gelder RN, von Zastrow ME, Yool A, Dement WC, Barchas JD, Eberwine JH. Amplified RNA synthesized from limited quantities of heterogeneous cDNA. *Proc. Natl. Acad. Sci. U. S. A.* 1990; 87:1663–1667.

111. Eberwine J, Spencer C, Miyashiro K, Mackler S, Finnell R. Complementary DNA synthesis *in situ*: methods and applications. *Methods Enzymol.* 1992; 216:80–100.

112. Baugh LR, Hill AA, Brown EL, Hunter CP. Quantitative analysis of mRNA amplification by *in vitro* transcription. *Nucleic Acids Res.* 2001; 29, E29.

113. Warrington JA, Nair A, Mahadevappa M, Tsyganskaya M. Comparison of human adult and fetal expression and identification of 535 housekeeping/maintenance genes. *Physiol. Genomics* 2000; 2:143–147.

114. Moch H, Kononen T, Kallioniemi OP, Sauter G. Tissue microarrays: what will they bring to molecular and anatomic pathology? *Adv. Anat. Pathol.* 2001; 8:14–20.

115. Moch H, Schraml P, Bubendorf L et al. High-throughput tissue microarray analysis to evaluate genes uncovered by cDNA microarray screening in renal cell carcinoma. *Am. J. Pathol.* 1999; 154:981–986.

116. Horvath L, Henshall S. The application of tissue microarrays to cancer research. *Pathology* 2001; 33:125–129.

117. Bubendorf L, Kolmer M, Kononen J et al. Hormone therapy failure in human prostate cancer: analysis by complementary DNA and tissue microarrays. *J. Natl. Cancer Inst.* 1999; 91:1758–1764.

118. Gygi SP, Rochon Y, Franza BR, Aebersold R. Correlation between protein and mRNA abundance in yeast. *Mol. Cell Biol.* 1999; 19:1720–1730.

119. Miklos GL, Maleszka R. Protein functions and biological contexts. *Proteomics* 2001; 1:169–178.

120. Bailey JE. Lessons from metabolic engineering for functional genomics and drug discovery. *Nat. Biotechnol.* 1999; 17:616–618.

121. Cahill DJ. Protein and antibody arrays and their medical applications. *J. Immunol. Methods* 2001; 250:81–91.

122. Harry JL, Wilkins MR, Herbert BR, Packer NH, Gooley AA, Williams KL. Proteomics: Capacity versus utility. *Electrophoresis* 2000; 21:1071–1081.

123. Irving RA, Hudson PJ. Proteins emerge from disarray. *Nat. Biotechnol.* 2000; 18:932–933.

124. Emili AQ, Cagney G. Large-scale functional analysis using peptide or protein arrays. *Nat. Biotechnol.* 2000; 18:393–397.

125. Walter G, Bussow K, Cahill D, Lueking A, Lehrach H. Protein arrays for gene expression and molecular interaction screening. *Curr. Opin. Microbiol.* 2000; 3:298–302.

126. Mendoza LG, McQuary P, Mongan A, Gangadharan R, Brignac S, Eggers M. High-throughput microarray-based enzyme-linked immunosorbent assay (ELISA). *Biotechniques* 1999; 27:778–776, 788.

127. Bussow K, Cahill D, Nietfeld W, Bancroft D, Scherzinger E, Lehrach H, Walter G. A method for global protein expression and antibody screening on high-density filters of an arrayed cDNA library. *Nucleic Acids Res.* 1998; 26:5007–5008.

128. Holt LJ, Bussow K, Walter G, Tomlinson IM. By-passing selection: Direct screening for antibody-antigen interactions using protein arrays. *Nucleic Acids Res.* 2000; 28:E72.

129. Holt LJ, Enever C, de Wildt RM, Tomlinson IM. The use of recombinant antibodies in proteomics. *Curr. Opin. Biotechnol.* 2000; 11:445–449.

130. de Wildt RM, Mundy CR, Gorick BD, Tomlinson IM. Antibody arrays for high-throughput screening of antibody-antigen interactions. *Nat. Biotechnol.* 2000; 18:989–994.

131. Ge H. UPA, a universal protein array system for quantitative detection of protein-protein, protein-DNA, protein-RNA and protein-ligand interactions. *Nucleic Acids Res.* 2000; 28:E3.

132. MacBeath G, Schreiber SL. Printing proteins as microarrays for high-throughput function determination. *Science* 2000; 289:1760–1763.

133. Stillman BA, Tonkinson JL. Expression microarray hybridization kinetics depend on length of the immobilized DNA but are independent of immobilization substrate. *Anal. Biochem.* 2001; 295:149–157.

134. Stillman BA, Tonkinson JL. FAST slides: A novel surface for microarrays. *Biotechniques* 2000; 29:630–635.

135. Haab BB, Dunham MJ, Brown PO. Protein microarrays for highly parallel detection and quantitation of specific proteins and antibodies in complex solutions. *Genome Biol.* 2001; 2(2); Research 0004.

136. Zhu H, Bilgin M, Bangham R et al. Global analysis of protein activities using proteome chips. *Science* 2001; 293:2101–2105.

137. Vasiliskov VA, Prokopenko DV, Mirzabekov AD. Parallel multiplex thermodynamic analysis of coaxial base stacking in DNA duplexes by oligodeoxyribonucleotide microchips. *Nucleic Acids Res.* 2001; 29:2303–2313.

138. Guschin D, Yershov G, Zaslavsky A et al. Manual manufacturing of oligonucleotide, DNA, and protein microchips. *Anal. Biochem.* 1997; 250:203–211.

139. Arenkov P, Kukhtin A, Gemmell A, Voloshchuk S, Chupeeva V, Mirzabekov A. Protein microchips: use for immunoassay and enzymatic reactions. *Anal. Biochem.* 2000; 278: 123–131.

140. Uetz P, Giot L, Cagney G et al. A comprehensive analysis of protein-protein interactions in *Saccharomyces cerevisiae*. *Nature* 2000; 403:623–627.

141. Ross-MacDonald P, Coelho PS, Roemer T et al. Large-scale analysis of the yeast genome by transposon tagging and gene disruption. *Nature* 1999; 402:413–418.

142. Ross-MacDonald P, Sheehan A, Friddle C, Roeder GS, Snyder M. Transposon mutagenesis for the analysis of protein production, function, and localization. *Methods Enzymol.* 1999; 303:512–532.

143. Huang RP, Huang R, Fan Y, Lin Y. Simultaneous detection of multiple cytokines from conditioned media and patient's sera by an antibody-based protein array system. *Anal. Biochem.* 2001; 294:55–62.

144. Huang RP. Simultaneous detection of multiple proteins with an array-based enzyme-linked immunosorbent assay (ELISA) and enhanced chemiluminescence (ECL). *Clin. Chem. Lab. Med.* 2001; 39:209–214.

145. Williams DM, Cole PA. Kinase chips hit the proteomics era. *Trends Biochem. Sci.* 2001; 26:271–273.

146. Hunter T. Signaling — 2000 and beyond. *Cell* 2000; 100:113–127.

147. Stern DF. Phosphoproteomics. *Exp. Mol. Pathol.* 2001; 70:327–331.

148. Paweletz CP, Charboneau L, Bichsel VE et al. Reverse phase protein microarrays which capture disease progression show activation of pro-survival pathways at the cancer invasion front. *Oncogene* 2001; 20:1981–1989.

149. Paweletz CP, Liotta LA, Petricoin EF III. New technologies for biomarker analysis of prostate cancer progression: Laser capture microdissection and tissue proteomics. *Urology* 2001; 57:160–163.

150. Tanabe L, Scherf U, Smith LH, Lee JK, Hunter L, Weinstein JN. MedMiner: An Internet text-mining tool for biomedical information, with application to gene expression profiling. *Biotechniques* 1999; 27:1210–1217.

151. Jenssen TK, Laegreid A, Komorowski J, Hovig E. A literature network of human genes for high-throughput analysis of gene expression. *Nat. Genet.* 2001; 28:21–28.

152. Stevens TJ, Arkin IT. Do more complex organisms have a greater proportion of membrane proteins in their genomes? *Proteins* 2000; 39:417–420.

153. Bieri C, Ernst OP, Heyse S, Hofmann KP, Vogel H. Micropatterned immobilization of a G protein-coupled receptor and direct detection of G protein activation. *Nat. Biotechnol.* 1999; 17:1105–1108.

3

STRATEGIES TO TARGET CHEMOTHERAPEUTICS TO TUMORS

CHARLES F. ALBRIGHT

PEARL S. HUANG

Dupont Pharmaceuticals
Department of Cancer Research
Glenolden, Pennsylvania

I. BACKGROUND AND RATIONALE
II. ANTIBODY-DIRECTED ENZYME PRODRUG TECHNIQUE
III. PASSIVE TUMOR TARGETING
IV. TARGETING BY BINDING TO TUMOR CELL SURFACE MOLECULES
V. ENZYME-ACTIVATED TARGETING
VI. SUMMARY AND FUTURE DIRECTIONS

I. BACKGROUND AND RATIONALE

Most tumors are treated with cytotoxic chemotherapeutics that were discovered over 20 years ago using cell-based screening methods. While these agents are widely used, only a small subset of cancers, including Hodgkin's lymphoma, testicular cancer, acute lymphoid leukemia, and non-Hodgkin's leukemia, are routinely cured using these agents (reviewed in reference 1). More modern efforts to improve cancer treatment involve identification of rational biochemical targets and design of anticancer agents that appropriately affect these targets. Although significant effort continues in this area, this approach has yielded only a few successful drugs, e.g., STI571, an inhibitor of the bcr-abl kinase [2]. This experience has motivated renewed efforts to selectively deliver chemotherapeutics to tumors based on the hypothesis that increased chemotherapeutic levels in tumors will improve cancer treatment. Although this hypothesis logically follows from our current understanding of chemotherapy, targeted chemotherapeutics are needed to test this hypothesis for cancers that are rarely cured by chemotherapy because current chemotherapeutics are already administered at their maximally tolerated doses (MTD). Targeted chemotherapies employ prodrug strategies designed to selectively deposit the active metabolite in tumor tissue. For these approaches to increase the therapeutic index of the active metabolite, the prodrug must be selectively activated in the tumor and the active metabolite must remain in the tumor for a reasonable time relative to the time it takes for the drug to trigger cell death. If the active metabolite diffuses out of the tumor before it can trigger cell death, then selective delivery of the metabolite to the tumor will not significantly improve the therapeutic index. For this reason, targeted chemotherapeutics have used doxorubicin because it binds tightly to DNA. Other agents that bind tightly to intracellular components, such as DNA or microtubules, may benefit from tumor targeting. In contrast, enzyme inhibitors that bind weakly to their respective enzymes are unlikely to benefit from chemotherapeutic targeting approaches.

II. ANTIBODY-DIRECTED ENZYME PRODRUG TECHNIQUE

Early efforts to target chemotherapeutics to tumors used antibody-directed enzyme prodrug technique (ADEPT) (reviewed in reference 3). In this approach, a prodrug-activating enzyme is first administered in the form of a tumor-specific antibody/enzyme conjugate. At a subsequent time, a chemotherapeutic prodrug that can be activated by the targeted enzyme is systemically administered. The time between enzyme and prodrug administration is critical because the antibody-conjugate is present at substantial levels in non-tumor tissue at short times and dissociates or becomes metabolized at longer times. The potential antigenicity of the antibody-enzyme conjugate, the specificity of the antibody for tumor cells, and problems in distributing macromolecules throughout tumors are additional complexities with the ADEPT approach. These significant technical hurdles have prevented its clinical use.

III. PASSIVE TUMOR TARGETING

The endothelial cells in many tumor vessels are poorly organized thereby leading to abnormal openings between the circulatory system and tumors. This leaky tumor vasculature combined with poor lymphatic drainage leads to a preferential accumulation of large macromolecules in tumors, an effect often referred to as enhanced permeability and retention (reviewed in reference 4). Liposome-encapsulated and polymer-linked chemotherapeutics exploit this passive targeting to preferentially deliver cytotoxic compounds to tumors. Once in the tumor, cytotoxic agents most likely diffuse out of liposomes, whereas polymer-conjugated cytotoxics require endocytosis and subsequent release of the active metabolite in lysosomes. Although early preclinical data suggested liposomal doxorubicin (liposomal Dox) was superior to free Dox (reviewed in reference 5), subsequent preclinical data found that liposomal Dox was similar to free Dox [6]. In clinical trials, liposomal Dox is more effective and less toxic than standard therapy for Kaposi's sarcoma [7, 8], but the efficacy of liposomal Dox for other tumors is unclear because phase II trials for ovarian cancer report conflicting results (reviewed in reference 9). While liposomal Dox was effective at reducing doxorubicin-induced cardiotoxicity, new dose-limiting toxicities, including stomatitis, were induced by liposomal preparations. To further improve liposomal delivery, liposomes coated with antitumor antibodies, or immunoliposomes, were developed by several groups. Liposomes coated with anti-HER2 antibodies showed improved efficacy in preclinical models (reviewed in reference 10). Interestingly, these improvements resulted from increased internalization of liposomes in cancer cells, not from increased targeting of liposomes to tumors. Clinical studies to test anti-HER2 immunoliposomes are in progress.

IV. TARGETING BY BINDING TO TUMOR CELL SURFACE MOLECULES

Several conjugates have been made that target cytotoxics to tumors by coupling them to molecules that bind cell surface receptors, such as bombesin, luteinizing hormone-release hormone, somatostatin, and folate, or antigens, such as Lewis Y, that are overexpressed on tumors [11, 12]. Following binding of the chemotherapeutic conjugate to the tumor cell surface, the conjugate is internalized and the chemotherapeutic is released in lysosomes due to the decreased pH or enzymatic activities. Impressive preclinical results were obtained with some of these conjugates, including a doxorubicin conjugated to the BR96 antibody and a myatansinoid conjugate to the C242 antibody [13, 14]. In contrast to these impressive preclinical findings, BR96-doxorubicin was less effective than doxorubicin at inhibiting the growth of metastatic breast carcinomas in a phase II clinical trial [15]. The BR96-doxorubicin dose was limited by gastrointestinal toxicity that probably resulted from the expression of Lewis Y antigen in the gastric mucosa and small intestine. These toxicities were not observed in mice because mice do not express Lewis Y antigen. The results with BR96-doxorubicin suggest that targeting using tumor cell surface proteins will require tumor-specific molecules, not just tumor-enriched molecules.

V. ENZYME-ACTIVATED TARGETING

The therapeutic strategies discussed thus far rely primarily on cell surface binding and biophysical properties of tumors to direct cytotoxics to the tumor. An alternative strategy is to design chemotherapeutic prodrugs that are activated by proteases or other enzymes that are elevated in tumors. Because these compounds are typically peptide-chemotherapeutic conjugates that are activated outside tumor cells, this approach does not face the challenge of distributing high-molecular mass agents uniformly to tumors or the limitations of endocytosis. These conjugates must, however, have sufficient tumor specificity.

A. Leu-Doxorubicin

N-l-leucyl-doxorubicin (Leu-Dox), contains a leucine residue conjugated to the primary amine of doxorubicin (Figure 3.1). Leucine derivatives of anthracyclines were developed based on the hypothesis that elevated aminopeptidase and

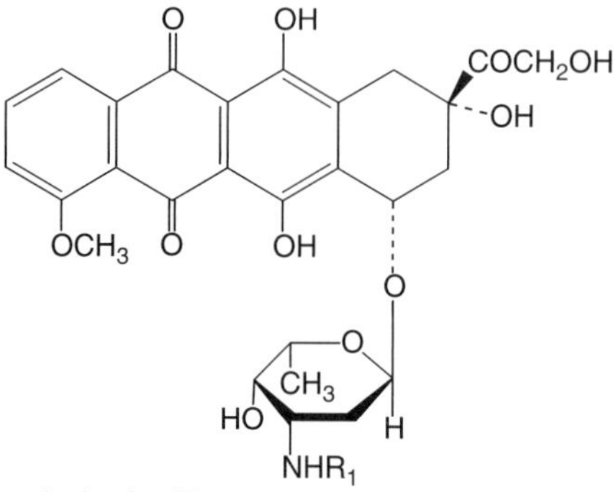

Compound	Activating Enzyme	R1
Doxorubicin		hydrogen
Leu-Dox	unknown	L
HMR 1826	Glucuronidase	4-β-glucuronyl-nitroZ
L-377,202	Prostate-specific antigen	glutaryl-Hyp-A-S-Chg-Q-S-L
Super-Leu-Dox	unknown	βA-L-A-L
	Plasmin	dV-L-K
	Fibroblast activation protein α	Z-P-A-G-P
	Cathepsin B	Ac-F-K-PABC

FIGURE 3.1 Summary of enzyme-activated doxorubicin conjugates. Conjugates replace the hydrogen in doxorubicin at R1 with the indicated R1 structures. Peptides are conjugated at their C terminus. Amino acids are abbreviated using the single letter code. Other abbreviations: nitroZ (3-nitrobenzyloxycarbonyl), Hyp (trans-4-hydroxyproline), Chg (cyclohexylglycine), βA (beta alanine), dV (d-isomer valine), Z (benzyloxycarbonyl), Ac (acetyl), and PABC (p-aminobenzyl carbonyl).

lysosomal protease activity in tumors would preferentially activate Leu-Dox in tumors [16, 17]. Consistent with this hypothesis, studies in several xenograft models showed that Leu-Dox (28 mg/kg) was slightly more effective at reducing tumor growth than Dox (8 mg/kg) when both compounds were administered at their MTD [18–20]. The magnitude of these improvements, however, was modest. For instance, Dox and Leu-Dox inhibited tumor growth by an average of 59 and 77%, respectively, in three ovarian cancer xenografts [18]. Furthermore, a pharmacokinetic analysis showed that Leu-Dox did not significantly change the ratio of Dox in tumor and heart, relative to Dox [21].

B. Glucuronidase-Activated Doxorubicin

Glucuronide-doxorubicin, such as HMR 1826, was originally developed for use with antibody-linked enzyme delivery to tumors (Figure 3.1). To circumvent the problems with this approach, the ability of tumors to directly activate HMR 1826 was tested. Initial preclinical studies were encouraging in that HMR 1826 caused tumor-selective deposition of Dox in a human tumor xenograft and a perfused lung model [22, 23]. In both cases, HMR 1826 appeared to increase to tumor-selective deposition of doxorubicin at least 10-fold. In the perfused lung model, Dox deposition from HMR 1826 depended upon glucuronidase activity since d-saccharolactone, a glucoruonidase inhibitor, reduced Dox deposition. The major extracellular source of glucuronidase in these tumors derived from infiltrating monocytes/granulocytes, which were primarily localized to necrotic regions of the tumor. Initial studies suggested that this increased Dox deposition led to an improved therapeutic index. In particular, 400 mg/kg HMR 1826 was more effective than 4.5 mg/kg doxorubicin in reducing the growth of several tumor xenografts. A subsequent study, however, questions the improved therapeutic index of HMR 1826 since HMR 1826 only showed statistically significant improvement in one of seven xenograft models [6]. The major difference between these studies was that the second study used HMR 1826 and doxorubicin at 200 and 7 mg/kg, respectively. Hence, the improved efficacy of HMR 1826 in the first study may have resulted from the failure to compare the cytotoxics administered at their MTD. Taken together, these studies suggest that although HMR 1826 led to an improved deposition of doxorubicin in tumor tissue, only a modest improvement in tumor growth inhibition was observed. The concentration of glucuronidase activity in necrotic regions of the tumor may underlie the discrepancy between doxorubicin deposition and efficacy.

C. Prostate-Specific Antigen Activated Doxorubicin

The serine protease, prostate-specific antigen (PSA), is highly expressed in an androgen-dependent manner in prostate cancer cells, and is an effective serological marker for prostate cancer cell growth [24]. Two groups have used PSA activity to activate doxorubicin conjugates. Denmeade et al. [25] linked a seven-residue peptide to doxorubicin to create Mu-His-Ser-Ser-Lys-Leu-Gln-Leu-Dox, which was converted to Leu-Dox by PSA. Prostate cell lines that did not express PSA were at least 10-fold more resistant to cytotoxic effects of this prodrug, which suggested a specific mechanism of activation for this conjugate. This prodrug reduced the growth of tumor xenografts in nude mice, but a direct comparison of its efficacy to that of doxorubicin was not possible because the prodrug was not dosed to MTD [26].

DeFeo-Jones et al., also [27] prepared a PSA-activated doxorubicin conjugate, designated L-377,202. L-377,202 (N-Glutaryl-(4-hydroxyprolyl)Ala-Ser-cyclohexaglycyl-Gln-Ser-Leu-Dox). It was cleaved by PSA to liberate Ser-Leu-Dox, which was subsequently converted to Dox by an undescribed mechanism (Figure 3.1). Like the other PSA-activated conjugate, L-377,202 was at least 10-fold more cytotoxic for cultured cells that expressed PSA than for those that do not express PSA. More important, L-377,202 was about 15-fold more effective at reducing the growth of LNCaP tumor xenografts than doxorubicin. This increased efficacy was consistent with the deposition of doxorubicin in LNCaP tumors from L-377,202. Doxorubicin deposition was probably due to PSA activation because a control compound that could not be cleaved by PSA did not cause tumor accumulation of doxorubicin, and tumor xenografts that did not express PSA were equally susceptible to L-377,202 and doxorubicin.

D. Super-Leu-Doxorubicin

Trouet et al. [28] screened peptide-doxorubicin conjugates for those that were stable in blood, unable to enter cells, and preferentially cleaved by proteases from tumor cells instead of identifying substrates for a known tumor-elevated protease. Using this approach, a conjugate with the structure β-alanyl-Leu-Ala-Leu-Dox was derived (Figure 3.1). Because this conjugate yields Leu-Dox, it was designated Super-Leu-dox. Studies with MCF-7/6 and MAXF-1162 tumor xenografts showed that Super-Leu-dox was more efficacious than doxorubicin at equitoxic doses, although the magnitude of this improvement was not quantified [29].

E. Plasmin-Activated Doxorubicin

Plasminogen, a zymogen, is converted to plasmin, a serine protease, by urokinase plasminogen activator (uPA), a membrane-bound protease that is overexpressed in many tumors (reviewed in reference 30). To exploit the presumed elevated plasmin activity of tumor cells, peptide-doxorubicin conjugates were prepared that were plasmin substrates. One such conjugate, dVal-Leu-Lys-Dox, was about six-fold more cytotoxic for src-transformed chicken embryo fibroblasts than for the corresponding non-transformed cells [31] (Figure 3.1). Unfortunately, the potency of this conjugate was very poor, relative to doxorubicin, probably because of the poor conversion of the conjugate to free doxorubicin. Although the conjugate showed some tumor growth inhibition of implanted B16 tumors in mice, the maximal dose was probably still well below the MTD and, therefore, direct comparisons to doxorubicin were not possible. The poor potency of this conjugate may have been due to steric hindrance of plasmin cleavage of the conjugate by doxorubicin. To reduce this problem, doxorubicin and taxol conjugates with self-immolating linkers were prepared [32, 33]. These conjugates were stable in plasma, rapidly converted to doxorubicin by plasmin, and had greatly reduced cytotoxicity for several cell lines. The characteristics of these conjugates in animal models are unknown.

F. Matrix-Metalloprotease Activated Prodrugs

Matrix-metalloproteases (MMPs) comprise of a family of zinc-dependent endoproteases that participate in several aspects of tissue remodeling, carcinogenesis, and angiogenesis (reviewed in reference 34). A variety of studies have shown that several MMPs are elevated in tumors. To exploit this increased activity, MMP-cleavable peptides were fused with the protective antigen (PA) portion of the anthrax toxin so that the fusion peptides had greatly reduced toxicity [35]. In particular, these fusion peptides had similar cytotoxicity as the PA peptide for HT1080, A2058, and MDA-MB-231 cells, but were much less cytotoxic than PA for Vero and COS-7 cells. These differences in cytotoxicity correlated with the ability of the cell lines to cleave the PA fusion peptide. Cleavage and cytotoxicity were greatly reduced in the susceptible cell lines by MMP inhibitors suggesting that MMPs activated the PA fusion peptide. Interestingly, PA peptides were only cytotoxic for cells that expressed MMPs and did not kill other cells even when co-cultured, suggesting that the PA peptides were only toxic for the cells that processed the fusion proteins.

G. Fibroblast Activation Protein Alpha Activated Prodrugs

Fibroblast activation protein α (FAPα), also known as seprase [36], is a membrane-spanning, serine protease [37, 38]. With the exception of certain pathological conditions, such as wound healing, FAPα is only expressed by the stromal fibroblasts of epithelial cancers [39, 40]. This tumor-selective expression pattern was originally exploited to develop imaging reagents for metastases using ^{131}I-labeled anti-FAPα antibodies [41]. More recently, peptide-doxorubicin conjugates were identified that were cleaved by FAPα, but not by CD26, a closely related protease, or proteases in plasma. Consistent with these properties, one such conjugate, Z-ProAlaGlyPro-Dox, was more cytotoxic for an HT1080 cell line that overexpressed FAPα than for the parental HT1080 cells that did not express detectable FAPα [42] (Figure 3.1).

H. Cathepsin B-Activated Prodrugs

Cathepsin B is a cysteine protease that is primarily found in the lysosomes of normal cells, but it is secreted or associated with the plasma membrane of many transformed cells [43]. Furthermore, the plasma-membrane association of cathepsin B correlates with the experimental metastatic potential of the tumor cells [44]. To exploit this tumor-selective extracellular distribution, peptide-doxorubicin conjugates that are activated by cathepsin B were identified [45]. One such conjugate, Ac-PheLys-PABC-Dox, was cytotoxic for BT-20 cells, which secrete high levels of cathepsin B, and cytotoxicity was reduced about 10-fold by CA-074, an inhibitor of cathepsin B (Figure 3.1). Unfortunately, this conjugate was also cytotoxic for MCF7 cells, which only secrete low levels of cathepsin B, and this cytotoxicity was not affected by CA-074. Whether MCF7 cytotoxicity results from non-cathepsin-B activation or endocytosis and cathepsin B activation in lysosomes is unclear. Activation of the conjugate by lysosomal cathepsin B following endocytosis would limit the utility of this approach.

I. Other Potential Activating Enzymes for Tumor Prodrugs

Several other enzymes could be useful for activating chemotherapeutics. uPA, a membrane-bound protease that activates plasmin, is frequently overexpressed in tumors (reviewed in reference 30). Likewise, other cathepsins, such as cathepsin D and cathepsin L, are overexpressed in some tumor types (reviewed in reference 46). Given the wealth of information about these proteases, testing their ability to activate prodrugs should be straightforward.

In addition to these well-known proteases, some members of an emerging family of type II transmembrane serine proteases are overexpressed in tumors (reviewed in reference 47). In particular, TMPRSS2, TMPRSS3, and hepsin are overexpressed in prostate, pancreatic, and ovarian tumors, respectively [48–50]. Additionally, matripase was found primarily without its kunitz-type inhibitor in some breast cancer lines, which suggested that matripase activity is elevated in breast cancer [51].

A variety of inflammatory cells, including mast cells, neutrophils, and macrophages, supply proteases to tumors that are critical for angiogenesis and other aspects of carcinogenesis [52, 53]. For example, mast cell degranulation releases chymase and tryptase. Unfortunately, a functional screen of protease activity in colorectal carcinoma samples found most chymase activity in normal tissue adjacent to the tumor [54]. Although this localization would be undesirable for activating prodrugs, a tumor-selective localization might be found in other tumors or with other proteases from inflammatory cells.

Finally, TADG14, a member of the kallikrein family of serine proteases, is overexpressed in ovarian cancers [55].

VI. SUMMARY AND FUTURE DIRECTIONS

Since the discovery of chemotherapeutics, efforts to improve the therapeutic index of these drugs by changing their mode of delivery have been investigated. Current efforts are focused in several areas and the two most encouraging are immunoliposomes and enzyme-activated prodrugs. Ongoing clinical trials should reveal whether these impressive preclinical findings translate to the clinic. If either approach is promising, then the explosion of genomic information and mRNA expression profiling may identify new tumor-elevated antigens and enzymes that broaden the applicability of these approaches.

REFERENCES

1. Abeloff M D, Armitage J O, Lichter A S, Niederhuber J E (Eds.) *J. Clinical Oncology (2nd Ed.).* New York, Churchill Livingstone, 2000.
2. Le Coutre P, Mologni L, Cleris L et al. In vivo eradication of human BCR/ABL-positive leukemia cells with an ABL kinase inhibitor. *J. Natl. Cancer Inst.* 1999; 91:163–168.
3. Bagshawe K. Antibody-directed enzyme prodrug therapy. *Clin. Pharmacokinet.* 1994; 27:368–376.
4. Seymour L. Passive tumor targeting of soluble macromolecules and drug conjugates. *Crit. Rev. Ther. Drug* 1992; 9:135–187.
5. Gabizon A, Martin F. Polyethylene glycol-coated (pegylated) liposomal doxorubicin. *Drugs* 1997; 54:15–21.
6. Woessner R, An Z, Li X, Hoffman R, Dix R, Bitonti A. Comparison of three approaches to doxorubicin therapy: Free doxorubicin, liposomal doxorubicin, and β-glucuronidase-activated prodrug (HMR 1826). *Anticancer Res.* 2000; 20:2289–2296.
7. Stewart S, Jablonowski H, Goebel F et al. Randomized comparative trial of pegylated liposomal doxorubicin versus bleomycin and vincristine in the treatment of AIDS-related Kaposi's sarcoma. *J. Clin. Oncol.* 1998; 16:683–691.
8. Northfelt D, Dezube B, Thommes J et al. Pegylated-liposomal doxorubicin versus doxorubicin, bleomycin, and vincristine in the treatment of AIDS-related Kaposi's sarcoma: results of a randomized phase III clinical trial. *J. Clin. Oncol.* 1998; 16: 2445–2451.
9. Frykman G, Williams G, Pazdur R. Conflicting phase II efficacy data for Doxil. *J. Clin. Oncol.* 2001; 19:596–597.
10. Drummond D, Hong K, Park J, Benz C, Kirpotin D. Liposomal targeting to tumors using vitamin and growth factor receptors. *Vitam. Horm.* 2001; 60:285–332.
11. Ladino C, Chari R, Bourret L, Kedersha N, Goldmacher V. Folate-maytansinoids: Target-selective drugs of low molecular weight. *Int. J. Cancer* 1997; 73:859–864.

12. Huang P, Oliff A. Drug-targeting strategies in cancer therapy. *Curr. Biol.* 2001; 11.

13. Trail P, Willner D, Lasch S et al. Cure of xenografted human carcinomas by BR96-doxorubicin immunoconjugates. *Science* 1993; 261:212–215.

14. Liu C, Tadayoni B, Bourret L et al. Eradication of large colon tumor xenografts by targeted delivery of maytansinoids. *Proc. Natl. Acad. Sci. U. S. A.* 1996; 93:8618–8623.

15. Tolcher A, Sugarman S, Gelmon K et al. Randomized phase II study of BR96-doxorubicin conjugate in patients with metastatic breast cancer. *J. Clin. Oncol.* 1999; 17:478–484.

16. Masquelier M, Baurain R, Trouet A. Amino acid and dipeptide derivatives of daunorubicin. 1. Synthesis, physiochemical properties, and lysosomal digestion. *J. Med. Chem.* 1980; 23: 1166–1170.

17. Baurain R, Masquelier M, Deprez-De Campeneere D, Trouet A. Amino acid and dipeptide derivatives of daunorubicin. 2. Cellular pharmacology and antitumor activity on L1210 leukemic cells in vitro and in vivo. *J. Med. Chem.* 1980; 23:1171–1174.

18. Boven E, Hendriks H, Erkelens C, Pinedo H. The anti-tumor effects of the prodrugs N-l-leucyl-doxorubicin and vinblastine-isoleucinate in human ovarian cancer xenografts. *Br. J. Cancer* 1992; 66:1044–1047.

19. Boven E, de Jong J, Kuiper C, Bast A, van der Vijgh W. Relationship between the tumour tissue pharmacokinetics and the antiproliferative effects of anthracyclines and their metabolites. *Eur. J. Cancer* 1996; 32:1382–1387.

20. Breistol L, Hendriks H, Fodstad O. Superior therapeutic efficacy of N-l-leucyl-doxorubicin versus doxorubicin in human melanoma xenografts correlates with higher tumour concentrations of free drug. *Eur. J. Cancer* 1999; 35:1143–1149.

21. de Jong J, Klein I, Bast A, van der Vijgh W. Analysis and pharmacokinetics of N-l-leucyl-doxorubicin and metabolites in tissues of tumour-bearing BALB/c mice. *Cancer Chemother. Pharmacol.* 1992; 31:156–160.

22. Murdter T, Sperker B, Kivisto K et al. Enhanced uptake of doxorubicin into bronchial carcinoma: β-gluronidase mediates release of doxorubicin from a glucuronide prodrug (HMR 1826) at the tumor site. *Cancer Res.* 1997; 57:2440–2445.

23. Bosslet K, Straub R, Blumrich M et al. Elucidation of the mechanism enabling tumor selective prodrug monotherapy. *Cancer Res.* 1998; 58:1195–1201.

24. Levesque M, Yu H, D'Costa M, Diamandis E. Prostate specific antigen expression by various tumors. *J. Clin. Lab. Anal.* 1995; 9:123–128.

25. Denmeade S, Nagy A, Gao J, Lilja H, Schally A, Isaacs J. Enzymatic activation of a doxorubicin-peptide prodrug by prostate-specific antigen. *Cancer Res.* 1998; 58:2537–2540.

26. Khan S, Denmeade S. In vivo activity of a PSA-activated doxorubicin prodrug against PSA-producing human prostate cancer xenografts. *Prostate* 2000; 45:80–83.

27. DeFeo-Jones D, Garsky V, Wong B et al. A peptide-doxorubicin prodrug activated by prostate-specific antigen selectively kill prostate tumor cells positive for prostate-specific antigen *in vivo*. *Nat. Med.* 2000; 6:1248–1252.

28. Trouet A, Baurain R. Tumor-activated prodrug compounds and treatment. United States patent #5, 962, 216, #1999.

29. Trouet A, Passioukov A, Van derpoorten K et al. Extracellularly tumor-activated prodrugs (ETAP) for the selective chemotherapy of cancer: Application to doxorubicin and preliminary *in vitro* and *in vivo* studies. *Cancer Res.* 2001.

30. Andraesen P, Kjoller L, Christensen L, Duffy M. The urokinase-type plasminogen activator system in cancer metastasis: a review. *Int. J. Cancer* 1997; 72:1–22.

31. Charkravarty P, Carl P, Wever M, Katzenellenbogen J. Plasmin-activated prodrugs for cancer chemotherapy. 2. Synthesis and biological activity of peptidyl derivatives of doxorubicin. *J. Med. Chem.* 1983; 26:638–644.

32. de Groot F, de Bart A, Verheijen J, Scheeren H. Synthesis and biological evaluation of novel prodrugs of anthracyclines for selective activation by the tumor-associated protease plasmin. *J. Med. Chem.* 1999; 42:5277–5283.

33. de Groot F, van Berkon L, Scheeren H. Synthesis and biological evaluation of 2′-carbamate-linked and 2′-carbonate linked prodrugs of paclitaxel: Selective activation by the tumor-associated protease plasmin. *J. Med. Chem.* 2000; 43:3093–3102.

34. Nagase J, Woessner J. Matrix metalloproteinases. *J. Biol. Chem.* 1999; 274:21491–21494.

35. Liu S, Netzel-Arnett S, Birkedal-Hansen H, Leppla S. Tumor cell-selective cytotoxicity of matrix metalloproteinase-activated anthrax toxin. *Cancer Res.* 2000; 60:6061–6067.

36. Pineiro-Sanchez M, Goldstein L, Dodt J, Howard L, Yeh Y, Chen W. Identification of the 170-kDa melanoma membrane-bound gelatinase (seprase) as a serine integral membrane protease. *J. Biol. Chem.* 1997; 272:7595–7601.

37. Scanlan M, Raj B, Calvo B et al. Molecular cloning of fibroblast activation protein α, a member of the serine protease family selectively expressed in stromal fibroblasts of epithelial cancers. *Proc. Natl. Acad. Sci. U. S. A.* 1994; 91:5657–5661.

38. Park J, Lenter M, Zimmermann R, Garin-Chesa P, Old L, Rettig W. Fibroblast activation protein, a dual specificity serine protease expressed in reactive human tumor stromal fibroblasts. *J. Biol. Chem.* 1999; 274:36505–36512.

39. Garin C, Old L, Rettig W. Cell surface glycoprotein of reactive stromal fibroblasts as a potential antibody target in human epithelial cancers. *Proc. Natl. Acad. Sci. U. S. A.* 1990; 87:7235–7239.

40. Rettig W, Garin-Chesa P, Healey J et al. Regulation and heteromeric structure of the fibroblast activation protein in normal and transformed cells of mesenchymal and neuroectodermal origin. *Cancer Res.* 1993; 53:3327–3335.

41. Welt S, Divgi C, Scott A et al. Antibody targeting in metastatic colon cancer: A phase I study of monoclonal antibody F19 against a cell-surface protein of reactive tumor stromal fibroblasts. *J. Clin. Oncol.* 1994; 12:1193–1203.

42. Park J, Rettig W, Lenter A et al. FAP-activated antitumor compounds. World Intellectual Property Organization, 2000.

43. Rozhin J, Sameni M, Ziegler G, Sloane B. Pericellular pH affects distribution and secretion of cathepsin B in malignant cells. *Cancer Res.* 1994; 54:6517–6525.

44. Sloane B, Dunn J, Honn K. Lysosomal cathepsin B: Correlation with metastatic potential. *Science* 1981; 212:1151–1153.

45. Firestone R. Hydrolyzable prodrugs for delivery of anticancer drugs to metastatic cells. World Intellectual Property Organization, 1998.

46. Duffy M. Proteases as prognostic markers in cancer. *Clin. Cancer Res.* 1996; 2:613–618.

47. Hooper J, Clements J, Quigley J, Antalis T. Type II transmembrane serine proteases. *J. Biol. Chem.* 2001; 276:857–860.

48. Lin B, Ferguson C, White J et al. Prostate-localized and androgen-regulated expression of the membrane-bound serine protease TMPRSS2. *Cancer Res.* 1999; 59:4180–4184.

49. Wallrapp C, Hahnel S, Muller-Pillasch F et al. A novel transmembrane serine protease (TMPRSS3) overexpressed in pancreatic cancer. *Cancer Res.* 2000; 60:2602–2606.

50. Tanimoto H, Yan Y, Clarke J, Korourian S, Shigemasa K, Parmley T, Parham G, O'Brien T. Hepsin, a cell surface serine protease identified in hepatoma cells, is overexpressed in ovarian cancer. *Cancer Res.* 1997; 57:2884–2887.

51. Lin C, Anders J, Johnson M, Dickson R. Purification and characterization of a complex containing matripase and a kunitz-type serine protease inhibitor from human milk. *J. Biol. Chem.* 1999; 274:18237–18242.

52. Coussens L, Raymond W, Bergers G et al. Inflammatory mast cells up-regulate angiogenesis during squamous epithelial carcinogenesis. *Gene Dev.* 1999; 13:1382–1397.

53. Coussens L, Tinkle C, Hanahan D, Werb Z. MMP-9 supplied by bone marrow-derived cells contributes to skin carcinogenesis. *Cell* 2000; 103:481–490.

54. McKerrow J, Bhargava V, Hansell E et al. A functional proteomics screen of proteases in colorectal cancer. *Mol. Med.* 2000; 6:450–460.

55. Underwood L, Tanimoto H, Wang Y, Shigemasa K, Parmley T, O'Brien T. Cloning of tumor-associated differentially expressed gene-14, a novel serine protease overexpressed in ovarian carcinoma. *Cancer Res.* 1999; 59:4435–4439.

4
QSAR AND PHARMACOPHORE MAPPING STRATEGIES IN NOVEL ANTICANCER DRUG DISCOVERY

JAMES J. KAMINSKI (DECEASED)

Schering-Plough Research Institute
Kenilworth, New Jersey

I. INTRODUCTION
II. PHARMACOPHORE DEFINITION
III. PHARMACOPHORE VALIDATION
IV. CONCLUSIONS

I. INTRODUCTION

Recent advances in combinatorial chemistry and high-throughput screening (HTS) have had a major impact on increasing the number of compounds identified as "hits" against therapeutic targets of interest. However, the number of hits that have been actually transformed into bona fide "leads" and that have ultimately resulted in clinical candidates remains to be credibly defined. Nevertheless, once a lead structure in any therapeutic area of interest has been identified, optimization of its activity profile using a specific armamentarium of selected *in vitro* and *in vivo* pharmacologic assays is customarily accomplished by conducting a systematic structure–activity relationship (SAR) study directed by chemical synthesis. Although the primary goal of the SAR study is to maximize the potency of the potential drug candidate in the various biological models examined, modification of the physical/chemical properties of the drug candidate is considered more often in the discovery phase by the medicinal chemist rather than in the development phase with the design of the dosage form. In most instances, the physical/chemical properties of the drug candidate are modified in an attempt to maximize its efficacy, to maximize its delivery (transport) to the site of action, and to minimize any potential drug safety issues while still satisfying preclinical development criteria. The nature of the modified physical/chemical properties of the drug candidate are determined solely by virtue of the chemical structure of the target compound proposed for synthesis. The process as described above is largely empirical in nature, and the results of such SAR studies, in many cases, are qualitative at best.

In an attempt to more accurately identify promising drug candidates from a series of compounds of interest, approaches to improve the direction provided by such empirical SAR studies have been attempted over the last thirty years by a number of investigators who have incorporated and extended the principles of thermodynamics [1] and physical organic chemistry [2] to biological systems. The results from these initial studies made it possible for Hansch and his co-workers in the early 1960s to develop the most widely used and well-known method of quantitative structure–activity relationships (QSAR) [3–6]. Because the Hansch equations derived attempted to correlate thermodynamic and other related parameters to biological activity without using the formal structure of thermodynamics, this approach to drug design became known as the extrathermodynamic approach and the multiparameter equations that relate the biological activity of an analog to the electronic, steric, and hydrophobic effect of its substituents have been termed extrathermodynamic relationships.

The overall objective of any QSAR study is to identify parameters that will give a statistically significant correlation with the observed biological activity of a series of molecules. Once these parameters have been identified, the resulting equation can be used to predict (calculate) the biological activity of unknown analogs. While this quantitative statistical approach appears to be less empirical, the successful prediction (calculation) of biological activity is more complex and the translation of this information to guide further structural modifications of the lead compound is not readily apparent.

During the last sixty years, it has become more recognized and accepted that the three dimensional (3D) conformation, or shape, of a (bio)molecule is uniquely interrelated with expression of the biological activity and function of the (bio)molecular entity. The interrelationship between the 3D structure of the (bio)molecule and expression of its biological activity and function is so tightly coupled that a better understanding of the molecular conformation and the nature of the intermolecular interactions occurring with a bound substrate might provide the basis for the "rational design" of novel target molecules that could interact with greater precision, affinity, and effect than naturally occurring ligands.

The only known method for precisely determining the 3D structure of any (bio)molecule is by single crystal X-ray analysis. However, relatively few biomolecules that are therapeutic targets have had their solid-state structure successfully determined by X-ray crystallography, and even fewer crystallographic structures exist for biomolecules that also contain their substrate or ligand bound. Thus, in the absence of detailed structural information, alternative approaches have evolved that might mimic investigation of the interactions occurring between biomolecules and substrate molecules. One such approach has its genesis in the generation and utilization of pharmacophore models in the emerging field of 3D QSAR.

II. PHARMACOPHORE DEFINITION

Recently, the discovery of the tricyclic farnesyl protein transferase (FPT) inhibitor 1-(4-pyridylacetyl)-4-(8-chloro-5,6-dihydro-11H-benzo[5,6]cyclohepta-[1,2-b]pyridin-11-ylidene) piperidine, Sch 44342 (see Figure 4.1) **1**, was reported [7]. Sch 44342, **1**, is a unique example of a novel non-peptide, non-sulfhydryl-containing FPT inhibitor that exhibits substantial selectivity against geranyl geranyltransferase-1 (GGPT-1) and kinetically competes with the ras protein, but not with farnesyl pyrophosphate (FPP), in binding to FPT. Significant effort has been expended to optimize the *in vitro* FPT inhibitory potency, and the *in vivo* pharmacologic profile of this series of FPT inhibitors by conducting a systematic structure-FPT inhibitory activity relationship (SAR) study directed by chemical synthesis [8–12]. This effort culminated with the selection for clinical evaluation of R-(+)-4-[2-[4-(3,10-dibromo-8-chloro-6,11-dihydro-5H-benzo[5,6]-cyclohepta[1,2-b]pyridinyl)-2-oxoethyl]-1-piperidine-carboxamide, Sch 66336, **36**, as a potential anticancer agent [13].

Concomitant with this effort has been an analysis of the FPT inhibitory activity data determined *in vitro* for these compounds using Catalyst, a 3D QSAR software program [8,14]. One application of this program is the generation of hypotheses that attempt to correlate the biological activity observed for a series of compounds to their chemical structure [15]. The hypotheses generated are 3D descriptions of a pharmacophore model proposed for the series of compounds examined. The hypotheses are represented by the chemical features that describe the series of compounds, e.g., hydrophobic groups, hydrogen bond donors, hydrogen bond acceptors, positive and negative ionizable groups, etc. The hypotheses generated may be used to estimate the biological activity of proposed targets, which allows a rank ordering of synthetic priorities. In addition, the hypotheses generated may also be used as 3D queries to search databases of proprietary and/or commercially available compounds. These 3D searches could identify structurally novel analogs that might exhibit the biological activity of the prototype. The results obtained from searching our corporate database using a Catalyst generated FPT hypothesis as a 3D query have been reported recently [16, 17] and are discussed further here.

From the analogs prepared to investigate the structure-FPT inhibitory activity relationship of the series exemplified by the prototype 1-(4-pyridyl-acetyl)-4-(8-chloro-5,6-dihydro-11H-benzo[5,6]cyclohepta[1,2-b]pyridin-11-ylidene)piperidine, Sch 44342, **1**, a training set of compounds was selected for Catalyst analysis (Figure 4.1). The compounds in the training set included the most active FPT inhibitors in the series, and each compound possessed something new to teach Catalyst during hypothesis generation. In addition, the compounds in the training set were structurally distinct from a chemical feature point of view and represented the diversity of the series. Each compound in the training set was considered as a collection of energetically reasonable conformations, and in cases where the chirality of an asymmetric center was not specified, Catalyst generated and considered alternative stereoisomers.

The range of *in vitro* FPT inhibitory activity exhibited by these selected compounds spanned four orders of magnitude, i.e., $10^{-1} - 10^3$ µM, and the compound distribution was evenly populated over the activity range. Using this training set, FPT hypotheses (pharmacophore models) were generated. When generating hypotheses, Catalyst tries to minimize a cost function consisting of three terms. One term is a value that increases in a Gaussian form as the feature weight in a model deviates from an idealized value of two, i.e., the weight cost. The second term penalizes the deviation between the estimated activities of the training set and their experimentally determined values, i.e., the error

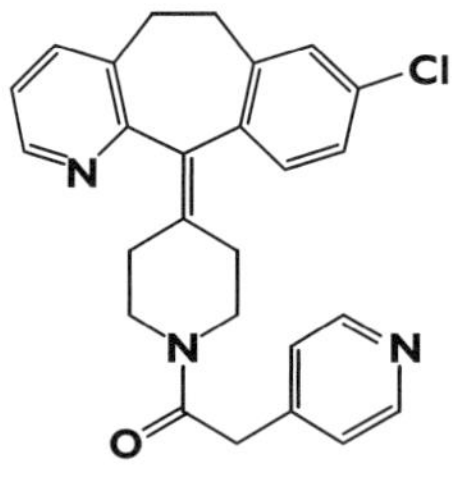

Sch 44342
1, IC_{50} = 0.25 μM

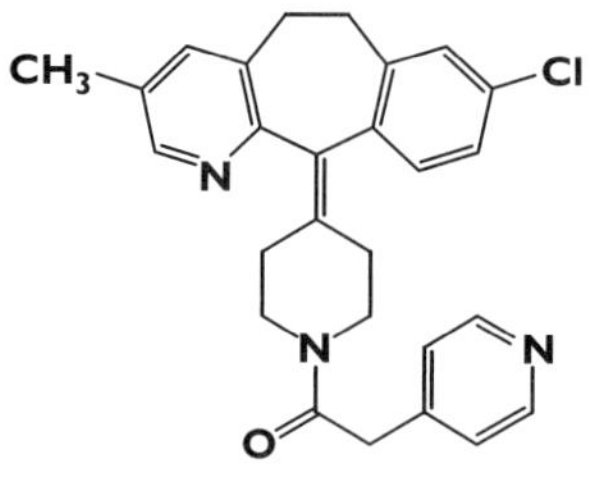

2, IC_{50} = 0.06 μM

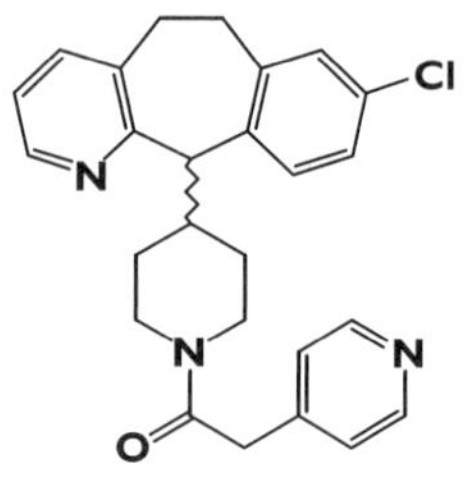

3, IC_{50} = 0.16 μM

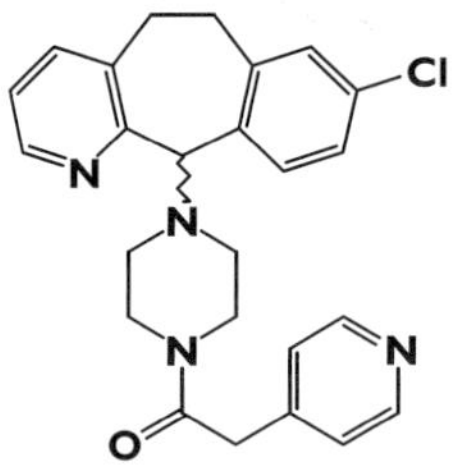

4, IC_{50} = 0.36 μM

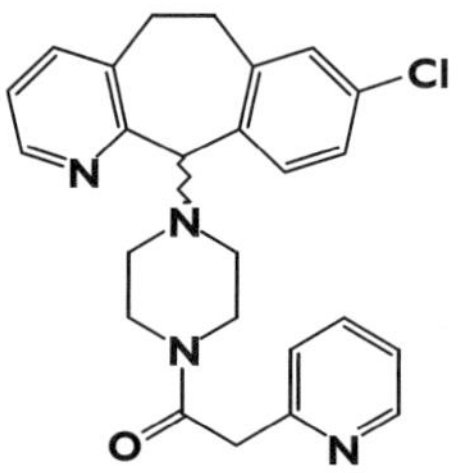

5, IC_{50} = 0.36 μM

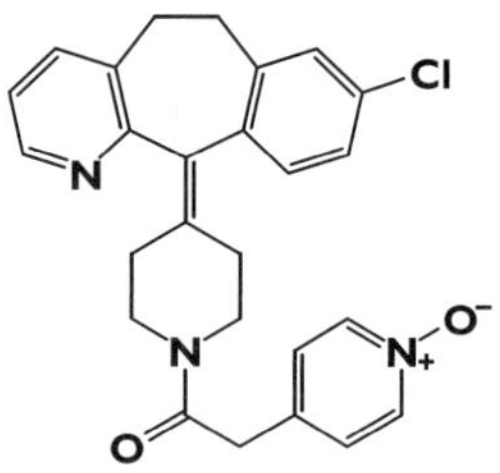

6, IC_{50} = 0.53 μM

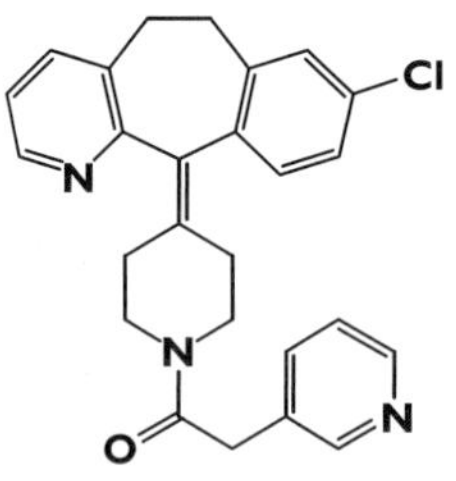

7, IC_{50} = 0.60 μM

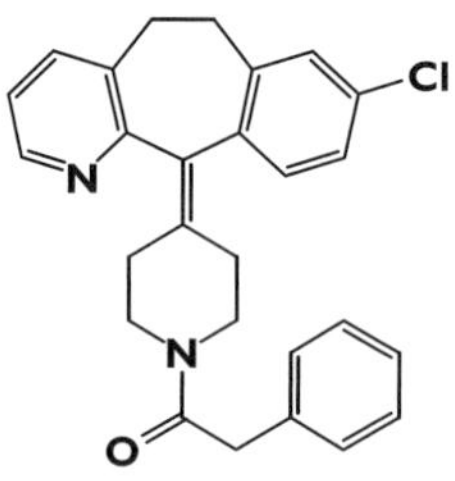

8, IC_{50} = 0.80 μM

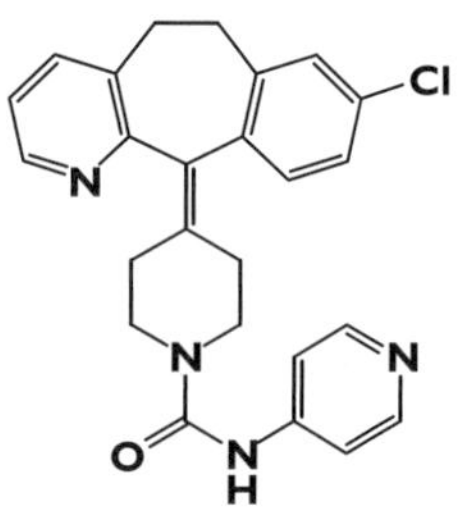

9, IC_{50} = 0.87 μM

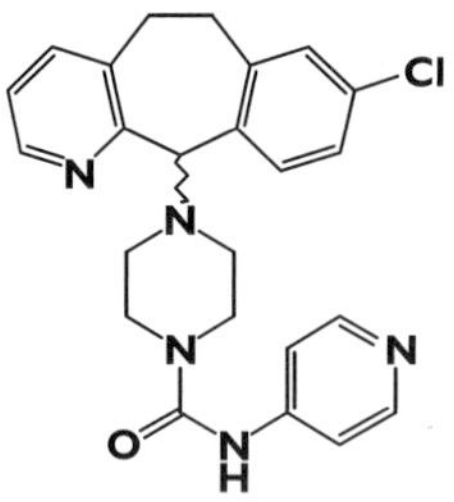

10, IC_{50} = 0.94 μM

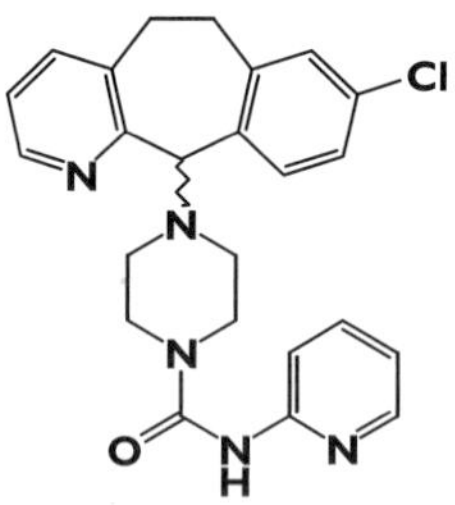

11, IC_{50} = 0.95 μM

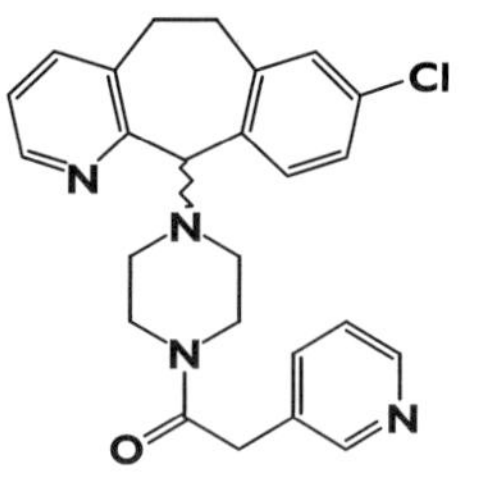

12, IC_{50} = 1.0 μM

FIGURE 4.1 Training set of selected farnesyl protein transferase (FPT) inhibitors and their determined *in vitro* FPT inhibitory activity.

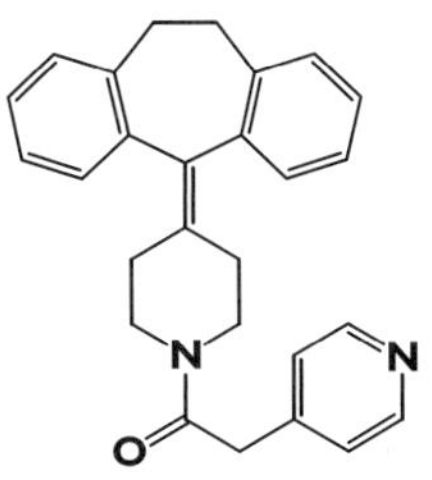

13, IC_{50} = 1.14 μM

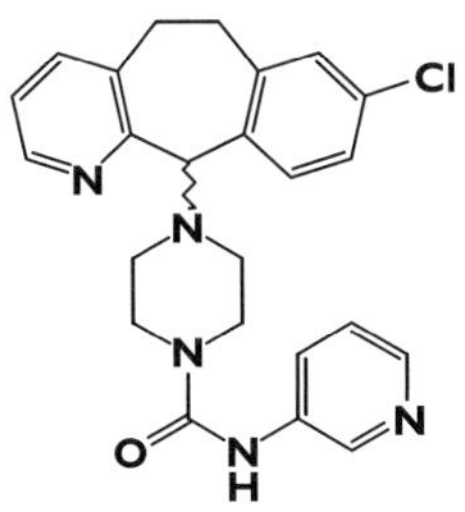

14, IC_{50} = 1.3 μM

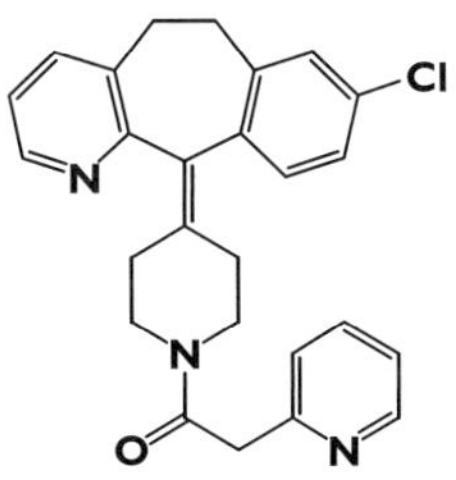

15, IC_{50} = 2.0 μM

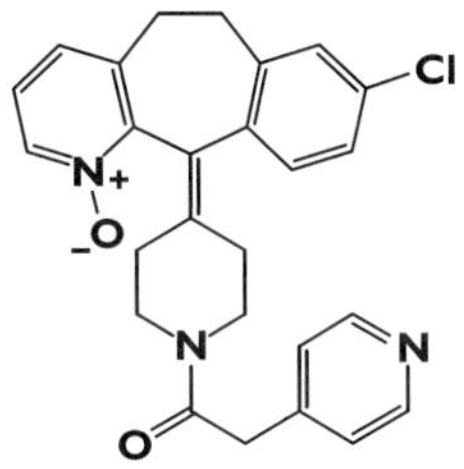

16, IC_{50} = 2.1 μM

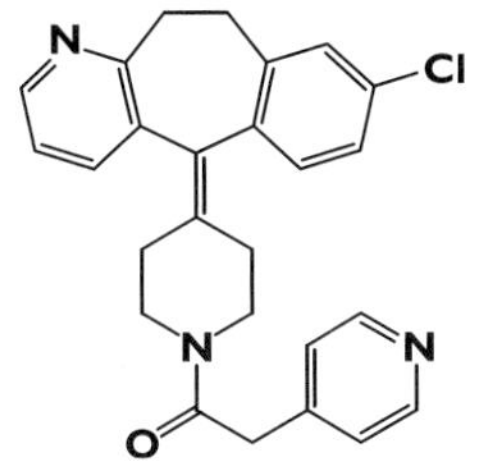

17, IC_{50} = 2.3 μM

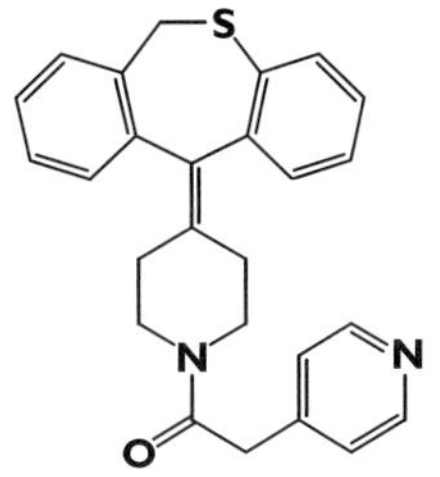

18, IC_{50} = 2.3 μM

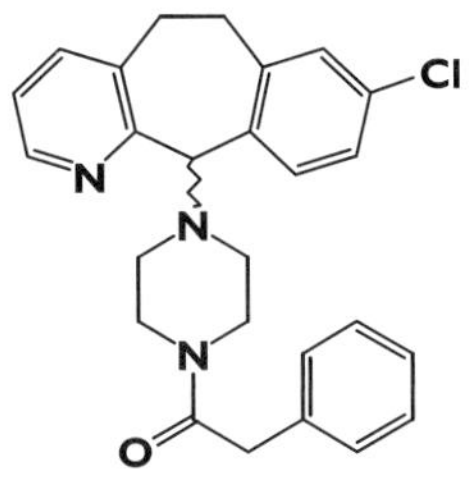

19, IC_{50} = 2.7 μM

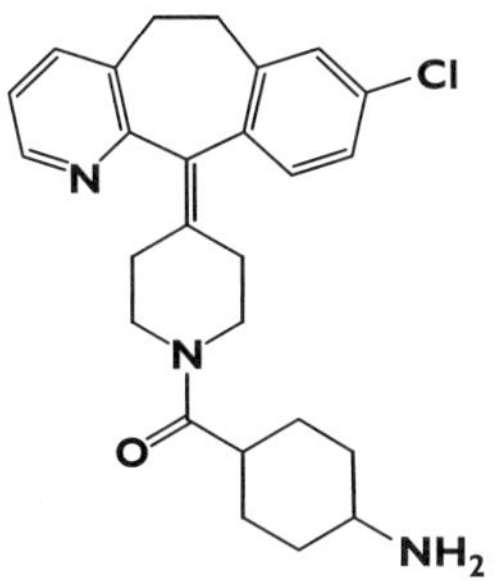

20, IC_{50} = 5.0 μM

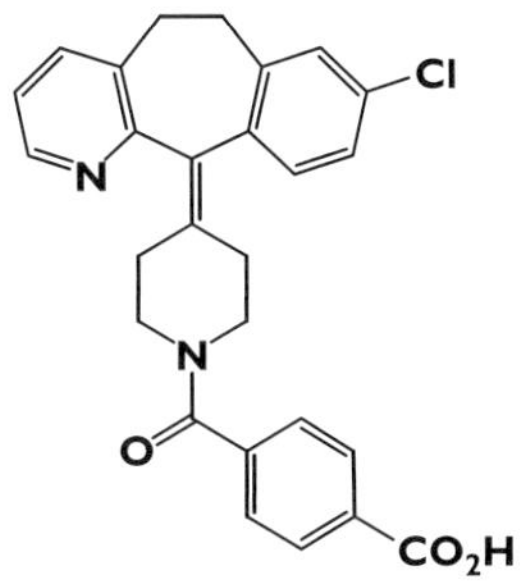

21, IC_{50} = 5.3 μM

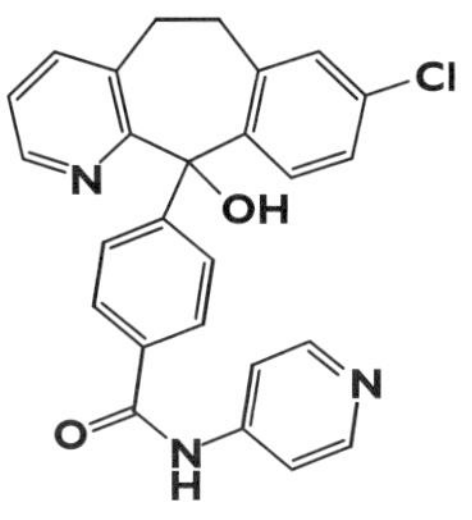

22, IC_{50} = 5.8 μM

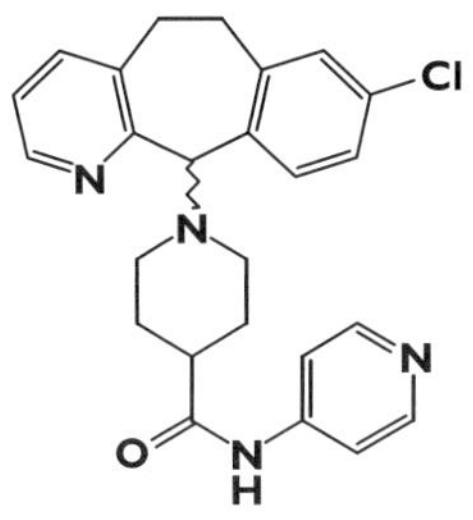

23, IC_{50} = 9.2 μM

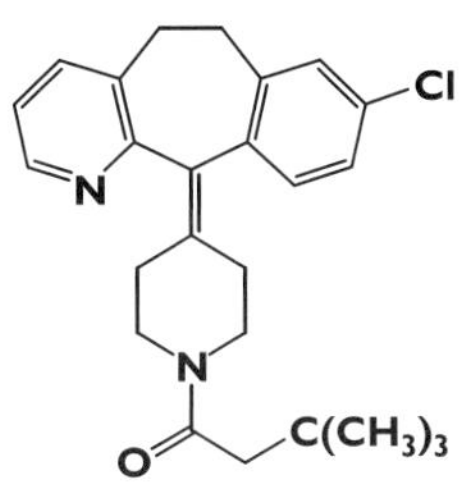

24, IC_{50} = 9.8 μM

FIGURE 4.1 (*Continued*)

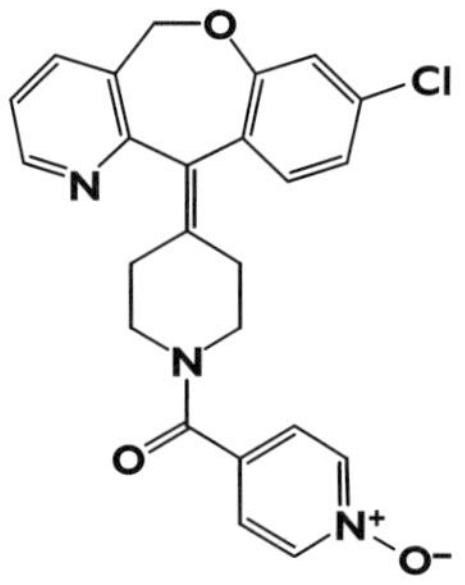

25, IC_{50} = 10.5 µM 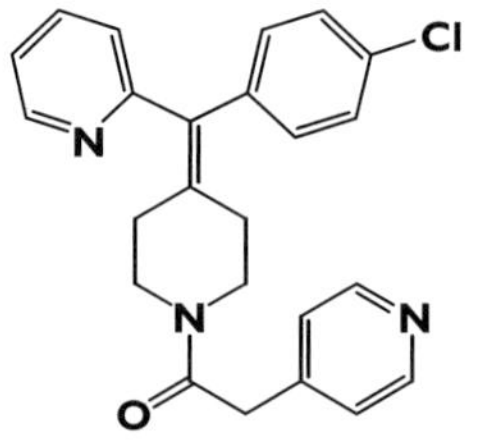   26, IC_{50} = 14.9 µM 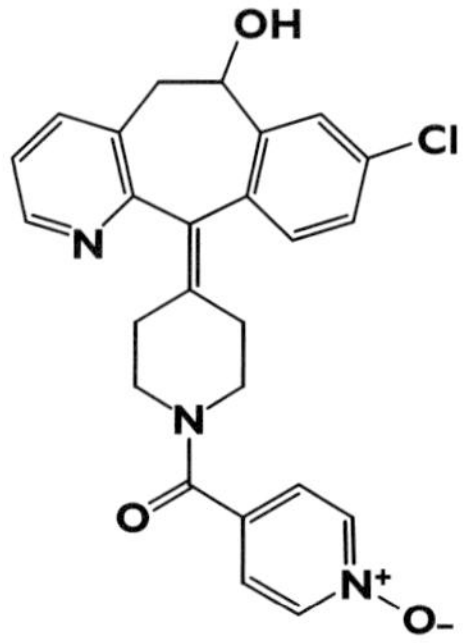   27, IC_{50} = 32.7 µM

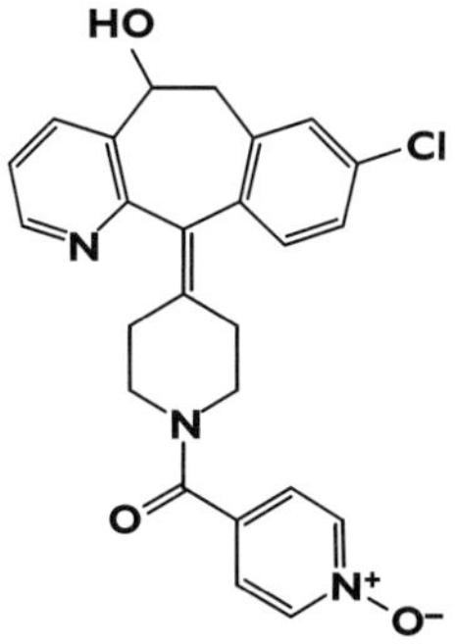

28, IC_{50} = 34.0 µM 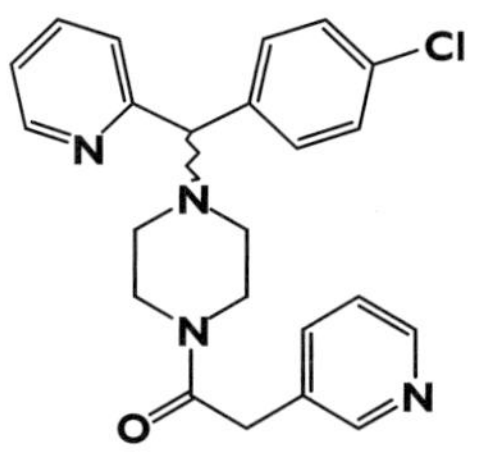   29, IC_{50} = 38.3 µM 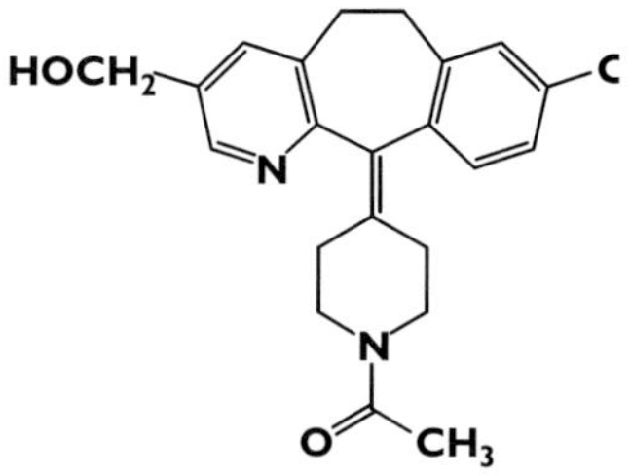   30, IC_{50} = 41.0 µM

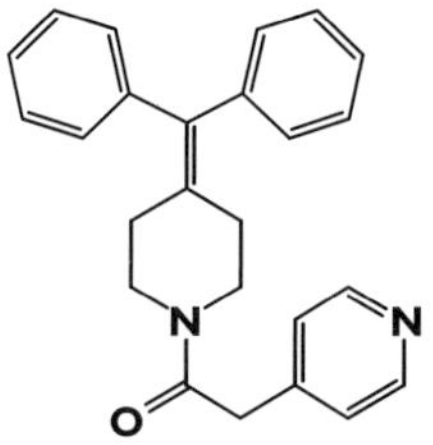

31, IC_{50} = 48.4 µM 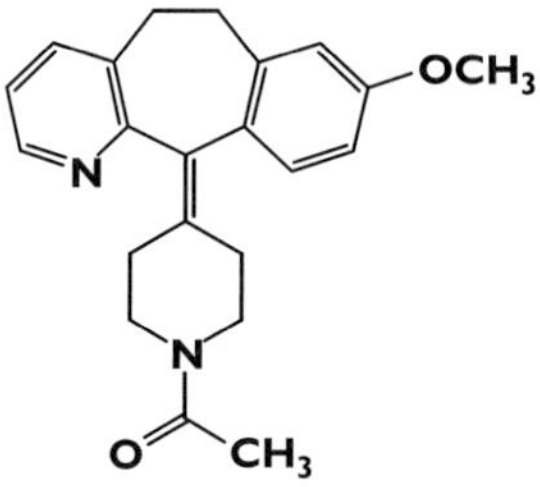   32, IC_{50} = 56 µM 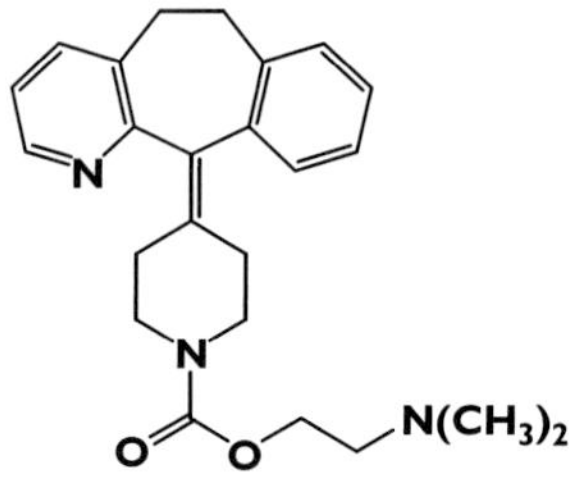   33, IC_{50} = 79 µM

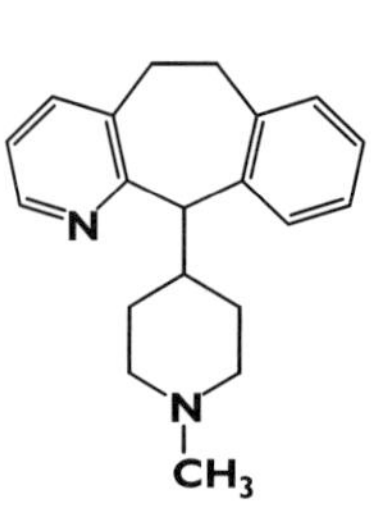

34, IC_{50} = 724 µM 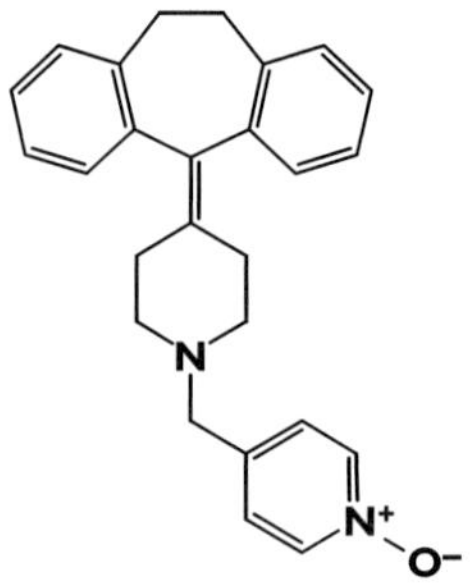   35, IC_{50} = 1832 µM

FIGURE 4.1 (Continued)

cost. The third term penalizes the complexity of the hypothesis, i.e., the configuration cost. This is a fixed cost which is equal to the entropy of the hypothesis space. The overall cost of a hypothesis is calculated by summing over the three cost factors. Of these three, the error cost contributes the most in determining the cost of a hypothesis. During hypothesis generation, Catalyst calculates the cost of two theoretical hypotheses, one in which the error cost is minimal and the slope of the activity correlation line is one, the ideal hypothesis, and one where the error cost is high and the slope of the activity correlation line is zero or the null hypothesis. The greater the difference between these two costs, the higher the probability of generating a useful model.

III. PHARMACOPHORE VALIDATION

The FPT hypothesis chosen from the alternatives generated was the one that exhibited the lowest cost value and resided closest to the ideal hypothesis (Figure 4.2) [15]. The FPT hypothesis is a collection of chemical features distributed in 3D space that is intended to represent groups in the molecule that participate in important binding interactions between drugs and their receptors. The produced pharmacophore model consisted of four hydrophobic regions and one hydrogen bond acceptor site in a specific 3D orientation. Each of the five features in this model were equally weighted. Using **2**, IC_{50} = 0.06 μM, as an example, a flexible fit of the best conformer of this molecule maps to the lowest cost Catalyst generated FPT hypothesis, as described in Figure 4.2. The four hydrophobic regions of the hypothesis are the 3-methyl group on the pyridyl portion of the tricyclic system, the 5,6-ethano bridge of the tricyclic system, the aromatic ring of the 8-chlorophenyl portion of the tricyclic system, and the 4-pyridyl ring of the picolinamide attached to the pendant piperylidenyl ring. The hydrogen bond acceptor identified in the generated FPT hypothesis is the carbonyl group of the γ-picolinamide attached to the pendant piperylidenyl ring.

A regression line of "measured" versus "estimated" FPT inhibitory activity for the training set, expressed as $-\log [IC_{50}]$, based on the lowest cost Catalyst generated FPT hypothesis, exhibited a correlation coefficient (r^2) = 0.91 and a root mean square deviation (RMS) that equaled 0.84 (Figure 4.2). Using these criteria, comparison between the estimated activity of the compounds in the training set relative to their experimentally observed activity is in the worst case, within one order of magnitude, and in most cases, it is within a five-fold difference [16].

In cases where one chiral center is present in the molecule, the generated FPT hypothesis exhibits a preference for the S-stereoisomer relative to the R-stereoisomer, e.g., the estimated FPT inhibitory potency of the S-(−) stereoisomer of **4**, IC_{50} = 0.014 μM, is greater than the estimated FPT inhibitory potency of the R-(+) stereoisomer of **4**, IC_{50} = 0.65 μM. This observation is consistent with the measured FPT inhibitory potency determined for the enantiomers of **4**, the S-(−) stereoisomer, IC_{50} = 0.14 μM relative to the R-(+) stereoisomer, IC_{50} = 0.49 μM [8]. In general, this observation is consistent with the FPT inhibitory potency determined for

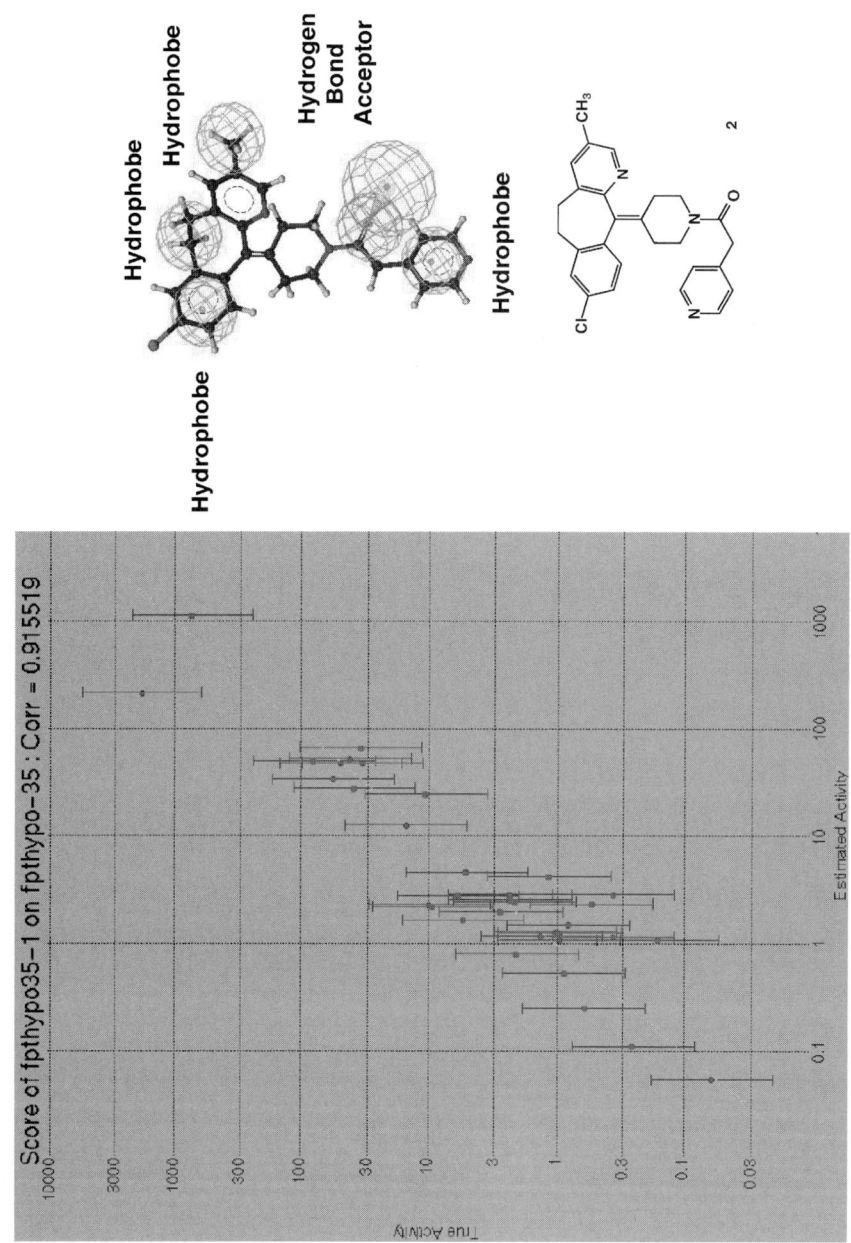

FIGURE 4.2 Best conformation of 2 flexibly fit to the lowest cost Catalyst generated FPT hypothesis (Pharmacophore model). See Color Plate 1.

enantiomers of several other analogs in the series, i.e., the S-stereoisomer exhibits a greater FPT inhibitory potency relative to the R-stereoisomer.

The FPT inhibitory activity predicted for compounds that were not part of the training set, but contain chemical features on which the FPT hypothesis was based, is usually within a four- to five-fold difference. However, consistent with other QSAR methods, activity predictions for compounds outside the training set are inaccurate and can be misleading, for example, the estimated FPT inhibitory activity of the peptide CVWM, $IC_{50} = 0.007$ μM, is approximately two orders of magnitude different from its experimentally measured FPT inhibitory activity, $IC_{50} = 0.525$ μM.

The lowest cost Catalyst generated FPT hypothesis was also used as a 3D query to search the Schering-Plough Research Institute's corporate database and resulted in the identification of 718 compounds. Examination of these compounds revealed that 626 structures were unique, only 330 were available, and determination of their *in vitro* FPT inhibitory activity was initiated.

From the structures examined only five compounds (5/330 = 1.5%), exhibited an *in vitro* FPT inhibitory potency $IC_{50} \leq 5$ μM (Figure 4.3). The 1.5% value obtained from this focused assessment of the corporate database is approximately a two-fold improvement compared to determining the FPT inhibitory activity of a larger subset of the corporate database. HTS of approximately 84,000 structures identified 2468 compounds that exhibited FPT inhibition $\geq 50\%$ at 20 μg/ml. From these compounds, only 22 (22/2468 = 0.9%) exhibited an *in vitro* FPT inhibitory potency $IC_{50} \leq 5$ μM.

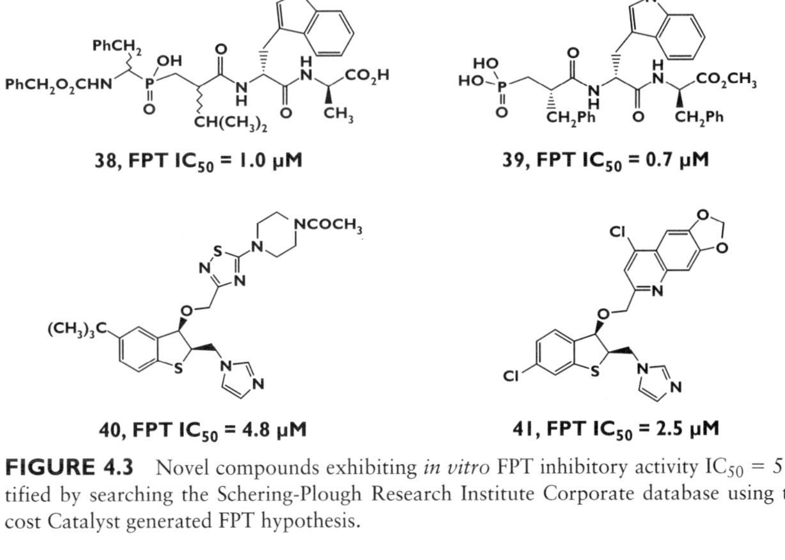

FIGURE 4.3 Novel compounds exhibiting *in vitro* FPT inhibitory activity $IC_{50} = 5$ μM identified by searching the Schering-Plough Research Institute Corporate database using the lowest cost Catalyst generated FPT hypothesis.

Of the five compounds identified, one is steroid-based, **37**; two are peptide-based, **38** and **39**; and two, **40** and **41**, are derived from a series of "azole" antifungals that were clinically investigated as topical agents [18].

From a chemical point of view, the azole antifungals represent a novel class of FPT inhibitors that are structurally distinct from the "tricyclic" series of compounds, as well as other known FPT inhibitors. On that basis, the FPT and GGPT-1 inhibitory activities of these initial leads were profiled further [16].

The FPT inhibitory potency of **40** and **41** was independently confirmed using a secondary assay, i.e., the FPT inhibitory potency of **40** and **41** determined using the FPT Ras/TCA assay was $IC_{50} = 5.3$ μM and $IC_{50} = 3.1$ μM, respectively. Selectivity between FPT and GGPT-1 inhibitory activity for **40** and **41** was also demonstrated, i.e. the GGPT-1 inhibitory potency of **40** and **41** was $IC_{50} > 39$ μM and $IC_{50} = 1.4$ μM, respectively. In addition, the lack of significant FPT inhibitory activity exhibited by other azole antifungal agents– such as ketoconazole ($IC_{50} > 46$ μM) and fluconazole (% Inhibition = 3 at 20 μg/ml), suggested that the FPT inhibitory activity of these compounds may not be coupled to their antifungal activity. These observations encouraged the determination of the *in vitro* FPT inhibitory potency of other available analogs from this series [16].

The structure-FPT inhibitory activity relationships determined from the preliminary study are summarized in Figure 4.4, and the most active FPT inhibitors identified from the initial leads were **42** and **43**.

While the FPT inhibitory potency of **42**, FPT $IC_{50} = 0.2$ μM and GGPT-1 $IC_{50} = 16.8$ μM, and **43**, FPT $IC_{50} = 0.3$ μM and GGPT-1 $IC_{50} = 0.7$ μM, are comparable to each other, the FPT to GGPT-1 selectivity of **42** (84) is greater than the FPT to GGPT-1 selectivity of **43** (2).

Using one of the initial lead compounds, **40**, as an example, a flexible fit of the *cis*-isomer of this molecule maps to the lowest cost Catalyst generated

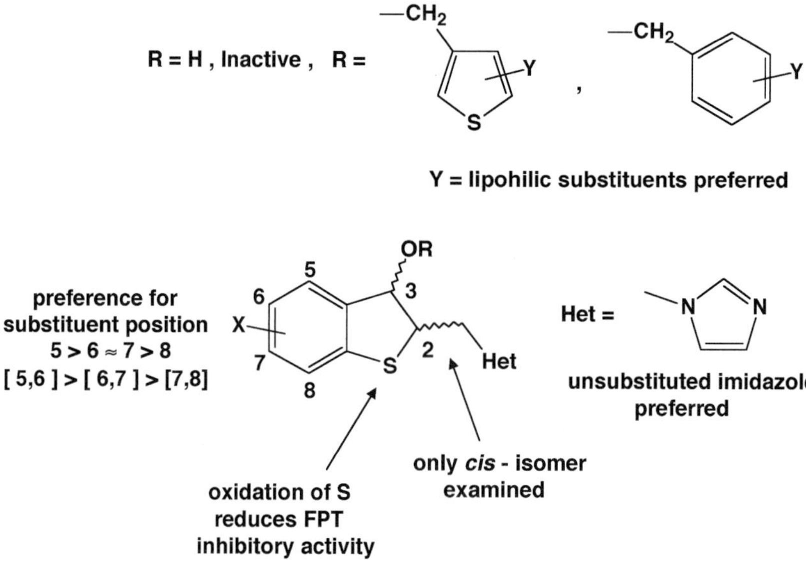

FIGURE 4.4 Preliminary structure–FPT inhibitor activity relationships of the substituted dihydrobenzothiophenes.

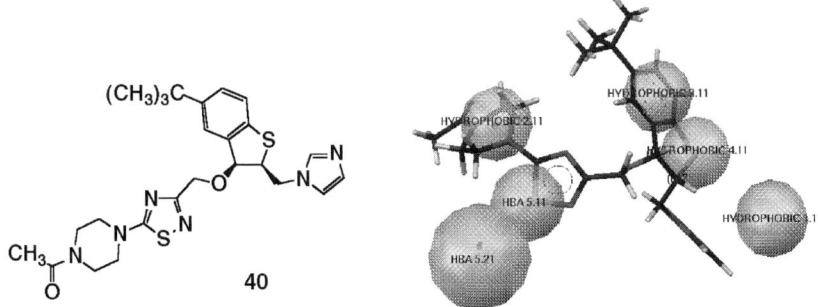

FIGURE 4.5 Best conformation of **40**, *cis*-isomer, flexibly fit to the lowest cost Catalyst generated FPT hypothesis. See Color Plate 2.

FPT hypothesis as described in Figure 4.5. Only three of the four possible hydrophobic regions of the FPT hypothesis map to the molecule, i.e., the piperazine ring of the side chain, and the aromatic ring and sulfur atom of the dihydrobenzothiophene ring system. The hydrogen bond acceptor in the generated FPT hypothesis is identified as the sulfur atom in the thiadiazine ring system [19]. The estimated FPT inhibitory activity for the *cis*-isomer of **40**, $IC_{50} = 3.8$ μM, based on the generated FPT hypothesis is in excellent agreement with its experimentally measured FPT inhibitory activity, $IC_{50} = 4.8$ μM. This observation is particularly surprising because only four of the five features of the FPT hypothesis map to the molecule.

Interestingly, the *trans*-isomer of **40**, flexibly fit to the lowest cost Catalyst generated FPT hypothesis, maps to all five features of the hypothesis (Figure 4.6). More important, an estimate of the FPT inhibitory activity of

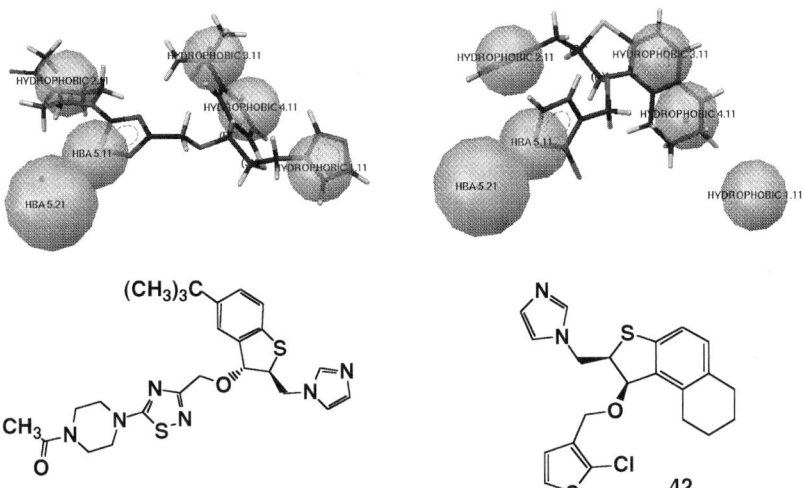

FIGURE 4.6 A conformation of the *trans*-isomer of **40** and the best conformation of **42** flexibly fit to the lowest cost Catalyst generated FPT hypothesis. See Color Plate 3.

this isomer based on the model, $IC_{50} = 0.18$ μM, suggests that the *trans*-isomer could be as potent as **42**, the best compound identified from the structure FPT inhibitory relationship study, $IC_{50} = 0.2$ μM. In addition, the FPT inhibitory potency of **42** might also be improved by further analog synthesis. Because **42** maps to only four of the five features of the lowest cost Catalyst generated FPT hypothesis (Figure 4.6), introduction of functionality in **42** that might interact with the fifth feature of the hypothesis could impart enhanced FPT inhibitory activity to the compound.

IV. CONCLUSIONS

Using a training set of novel FPT inhibitors, exemplified by the prototype 1-(4-pyridylacetyl)-4-(8-chloro-4-(8-chloro-5,6-dihydro-11H-benzo[5,6]cyclohepta[1,2-b]pyridin-11-ylidene)piperidine, Sch 44342, **1**, a 3D pharmacophore model (hypothesis) was generated that successfully correlated the FPT inhibitory activity observed for this series of these compounds to their chemical structure. Using the lowest cost Catalyst generated FPT hypothesis as a 3D query to search a database of compounds identified several other structurally novel analogs that exhibited the biological activity of the prototype. Investigating the structure-FPT inhibitory activity relationships of one of the identified series using the lowest cost Catalyst generated FPT hypothesis demonstrated that it was useful for assessing the relative merits of proposed synthetic targets prior to their synthesis. In addition, the lowest cost Catalyst generated FPT hypothesis was useful in the conceptual design of other novel FPT inhibitor targets in the series.

REFERENCES

1. Ferguson J. The use of chemical potentials as indices of toxicity. *Proc. R. Soc. London Ser. B* 1939; 127:387–403.
2. Hammett LP. *Physical Organic Chemistry*, McGraw-Hill, New York, 1940.
3. Hansch C, Muir RM, Fujita T, Maloney PP, Geiger F, Streich M. The correlation of biological activity of plant growth regulators and chloromycetin derivatives with hammett constants and partition coefficients. *J. Am. Chem. Soc.* 1963; 85:2817–2824.
4. Fujita T, Iwasa J, Hansch C. A new substituent constant, π, derived from partition coefficients. *J. Am. Chem. Soc.* 1964; 86:5175–5180.
5. Martin YC. *Quantitative Drug Design* Marcel Dekker, New York, 1978.
6. Ramsden CA. Quantitative drug design. In *Comprehensive Medicinal Chemistry, Vol. 4* (Hansch, C., eds.),. Pergamon Press, New York, 1990.
7. Bishop WR, Bond R, Petrin J et al. Novel tricyclic inhibitors of farnesyl protein transferase. *J. Biol. Chem.* 1995; 270:30611–30618.
8. Mallams AK, Njoroge FG, Doll RJ et al. Antitumor 8-chlorobenzocycloheptapyridines: A new class of selective, nonpeptidic, nonsulfhydryl inhibitors of Ras farnesylation. *Bioorg. Med. Chem.* 1997; 5:93–99.
9. Njoroge FG, Doll RJ, Vibulbhan B et al. Discovery of novel nonpeptide tricyclic inhibitors of ras farnesylation. *Bioorg. Med. Chem.* 1997; 5:101–114.
10. Njoroge FG, Vibulbhan B, Rane DF et al. Structure — activity relationship of 3-substituted N-(pyridinylacetyl)-4-(8-chloro-5,6-dihydro-11H-benzo[5,6]cyclohepta[1,2-b]pyridin-11-ylidene)piperidine inhibitors of farensyl protein transferase: design and synthesis of in vivo active antitumor compounds. *J. Med. Chem.* 1997; 40:4290–4301.

11. Mallams AK, Rossman RR, Doll RJ et al. Inhibitors of farnesyl protein transferase. 4-amido, 4-carbamoyl, and 4-carboxamido derivatives of 1-(8-chloro-6,11-dihydro-5H-benzo[5,6]-cyclohepta[1,2-b]pyridin-11-yl)piperazine and 1-(3-bromo-8-chloro-6,11-dinyhdro-5H-benzo[5,6]-cyclohepta[1,2-b]-pyridin-11-yl)piperazine. *J. Med. Chem.* 1998; 41:877–893.

12. Njoroge FG, Vibulbhan B, Pinto P et al. Potent, selective, and orally bioavailable tricyclic pyridylacetamide *N*-oxide inhibitors of farnesyl protein transferase with enhanced in vivo antitumor activity. *J. Med. Chem.* 1998; 41:1561–1567.

13. Njoroge G, Taveras A, Kelly J et al. (+)-4-[2-[4-(3,10-dibromo-8-chloro-6,11-dihydro-5H-benzo[5,6]-cyclohepta[1,2-b]pyridinyl)-2-oxoethyl]-1-piperidinecarboxamide (Sch 66336): A very potent farnesyl protein transferase inhibitor as a novel antitumor agent. *J. Med. Chem.* 1998; 41:4890–4902.

14. Catalyst v2.1. Molecular Simulations, Inc., Burlington, MA.

15. Sprague PW. Automated chemical hypothesis generation and database searching with catalyst. *Perspect. Drug Discov. Design* 1995; 3:1–20.

16. Kaminski JJ, Rane DF, Snow ME et al. Identification of novel farnesyl protein transferase inhibitors using three — dimensional database searching methods. *J. Med. Chem.* 1997; 40:4103–4112.

17. Kaminski JJ, Rane DF, Rothofsky ML. Database mining using pharmacophore models to discover novel structural prototypes. In Guner OF, eds. *Pharmacophore Perception, Development and Use in Drug Design* (Guner, O.F., eds.), International University Line, La Jolla, CA, 2000; pp. 251–268.

18. Rane DF, Pike RE, Puar MS, Wright JJ, McPhail AT. A novel synthesis of *Cis*-1-[[6-Chloro-3-[(2-chloro-3-thienyl)methoxy]-2,3-dihydrobenzo[b]thien-2-yl]methyl]-1H-imidazole: a new class of azole antifungal agents. *Tetrahedron* 1988; 44:2397–2402.

19. Allen FH, Bird CM, Rowland RS, Raithby PR. Hydrogen-bond acceptor and donor properties of divalent sulfur. *Acta Crystallogr. Sect. B* 1997; *Struct. Sci. B* 53(4):696–701.

5

APPLICATIONS OF NUCLEAR MAGNETIC RESONANCE AND MASS SPECTROMETRY TO ANTICANCER DRUG DISCOVERY

ROBERT POWERS

Department of Chemistry
University of Nebraska Lincoln
Lincoln, Nebraska

MARSHALL M. SIEGEL

Discovery Analytical Chemistry
Wyeth Research
Pearl River, New York

I. INTRODUCTION
II. NMR IN ANTICANCER DRUG DISCOVERY
III. MS IN ANTICANCER DRUG DISCOVERY
IV. MS/NMR SCREENING ASSAY
V. CONCLUSIONS

I. INTRODUCTION

A fundamental component of the drug discovery process is the identification of a lead chemical whose biological activity is further optimized by a combination of medicinal chemistry and structure-based drug design methodologies [1–4]. The beneficial impact of structure-based design efforts on the drug discovery process is evident from the continuing success in delivering novel drugs for clinical evaluation [1, 2, 5–10]. The structure-based drug design process is composed of two key stages: (1) identification of a small molecule that binds the protein of interest in a biologically relevant location (active site) and (2) determination of the structure of the protein-ligand complex for further iteration of the drug-design cycle. Nuclear magnetic resonance (NMR) spectroscopy and mass spectrometry (MS) are now routinely applied at all stages of the design process to facilitate the identification, evaluation, and optimization of chemical leads [7, 11–19].

Traditionally, high-throughput screening (HTS) approaches have been utilized to identify chemical leads based on observed affects on the biological activity of the protein of interest [20–25]. The optimization of these compounds would proceed through standard medicinal chemistry methods where positive feedback is based on improved activity in the biological assay [26–28]. Unfortunately, this historical approach to drug discovery has a number of pitfalls that may result in the expenditure of vast amounts of resources chasing after false leads [29]. The problem arises from the nature of an HTS effort and the methodology of monitoring an affect on the activity of the protein target. To reasonably mimic the cellular function of a target protein an assay may require a relatively complex *in vitro* system. The assay may be membrane-based, cell-based, or contain multiple proteins in addition to other components necessary to monitor the protein activity (monoclonal antibodies, radiolabels, fluorescent tag, scintillation beads, etc.). The end result of the necessary complexity is the ambiguous nature of a positive hit because the molecular interaction between a target protein and a small molecule is not readily correlated to an observed biological response. It is very plausible that the source of the observed response in the assay is not a result of a small molecule interacting with the protein of interest, but rather the result of an interaction with another component of the assay. Even more troubling is the observation that there are numerous undesirable mechanisms resulting from poor physical behavior of the compound that will result in a positive response in an HTS screen. These poor properties of the compound may include insolubility, reactivity, impurities, aggregation, instability, and non-specific binding. Relying simply on a biological response to drive the chemistry effort would evidently lead to compounds with either an increase in poor physical behavior or activity against the wrong target. A structure-based approach to drug design has been a widely applied remedy to the difficulties associated with relying strictly on HTS and biological assay results to drive a drug discovery program [1, 2, 5–10]. Clearly, visualizing a small-molecule complexed in the active site of the protein of interest provides a wealth of information to validate the lead compound and rationalize approaches to optimize the compound. X-ray crystallography has historically been a major source for obtaining three-dimensional structures of protein-ligand complexes for the iterative drug design cycle [30], whereas the use of NMR is a relatively recent addition to the structure-based drug design approach [12, 31]. The use of HTS assays still plays a vital role in the drug discovery process by efficiently filtering millions of compounds for potential biological activity and generating initial starting points for the structure-based approach [20–25].

The structure-based approach also has inherent limitations that impact a drug discovery program. A primary shortcoming is the current difficulty in obtaining structural information of membrane-bound proteins, which corresponds to an active area of research [32–35]. Additionally, the success of X-ray-based drug design programs is dependent on ready access to high-quality crystals that diffract to a high resolution for each protein-ligand complex [36, 37]. Similarly, NMR requires that proteins be well-behaved, isotope-labeled, and soluble up to concentrations of ~1 mM. Additionally, NMR is restricted by the molecular-weight (MW) of the protein, where the current upper limit is ~40 kDa. Extending the protein MW upper limit amenable to NMR is a very active area of research where current developments may increase the MW limit to between 100 and 500 kDa [38–43]. Furthermore, both NMR and X-ray are relatively resource intensive and time-consuming methodologies, which greatly limits the number of structures that may be obtained in a given time-period. A variety of factors such as personnel, instrumentation, methodology, and protein properties will contribute to the absolute number of structures that may be determined for a particular project. Nevertheless, this number will typically represent a very small fraction of the number of "hits" identified from an HTS assay. Exacerbating this inequity is the continued progress in HTS technology that is allowing more compounds (1–10 million) to be screened more efficiently (weeks to months). Clearly a need has evolved to filter HTS hits prior to initiating a structure-based program in order to increase the likelihood of successfully obtaining a co-structure. Numerous applications of NMR and MS are being developed and implemented for the sole purpose of screening compounds for their ability to bind to a protein target of interest.

NMR and MS are playing increasingly important and diverse roles in most structure-based drug design programs where the analytical techniques are used to identify and validate chemical leads, determine structures of protein and protein-ligand complexes, and analyze the dynamics of these interactions [11]. An overview of the approaches currently employed and investigated in our laboratories will be discussed in this chapter. In addition, the complementary usage of NMR and MS will be described in terms of the development of the MS/NMR assay.

II. NMR IN ANTICANCER DRUG DISCOVERY

Some of the earliest biological applications of NMR have been in the investigation of biomolecular (protein-protein, protein-DNA/RNA) and biomolecular-ligand interactions [44–47]. Because structural information on protein-ligand complexes is a fundamental necessity for the rational design of new drug candidates [1, 2, 4, 48], NMR has evolved to be an essential component of drug discovery programs. A number of these research projects target proteins with functionality and activity directly related to cancer including growth factors, interleukins/cytokines, kinases, matrix metalloproteinases, and proteins involved in signaling pathways and apoptosis. In addition, ligand binding to DNA and RNA sequences associated with cancer have been routinely investigated by NMR [49, 50]. The abundance of structural information readily obtained by NMR for these various targets has provided a means to develop a variety of anticancer therapeutics.

Excitingly, NMR continues to rapidly expand and redefine its role in the drug design process. In recent years, there have been a number of notable milestones in the development of NMR methodologies that have significantly impacted and expanded the application of NMR in structural biology and, correspondingly, structure-based drug design. These have included the application of multidimensional Nuclear Magnetic Resonance (NMR), routine availability of isotope (^{2}H, ^{13}C, ^{15}N) labeled proteins, deuterium NMR, TROSY (Transverse Relaxation Optimized Spectroscopy) NMR, NMR-based screening methods, and the measurement of residual dipolar coupling constants [42, 51–53]. Additionally, there is extensive effort in the development and implementation of NMR-based software that integrates these methodologies in an effort to automate and expedite the analysis of NMR data to rapidly and efficiently obtain structural information [54–60]. The full impact of these advancements has yet to be realized, but the expectations are that NMR will make significant contributions to the ongoing structural genomics effort while continuing to play an increasingly valuable function in structure-based drug design programs [14, 61]. A recent application that has had a dramatic impact on how NMR is utilized in the pharmaceutical industry has been the implementation of NMR-based screening methods.

A. NMR Screening

From its earliest implementation, NMR has been used to investigate the binding interaction of small molecules with proteins [11, 12, 62–64]. This has occurred because of the relatively unique ability of NMR to provide direct evidence for binding between the ligand and protein target through a variety of responses based on the nature of the NMR experiment [44, 45]. Observation of a binding event by NMR may occur through changes in line width and/or peak intensity (T_1 and T_2 relaxation changes) [65, 66], changes in the measured diffusion coefficient for the ligand [67–69], chemical shift perturbations for either the ligand or protein [44, 45, 70], induced transferred Nuclear Overhauser Effect (NOE) (trNOE) for the ligand [71, 72], a saturation transfer difference (STD) between either the protein or bulk solvent to the ligand [73, 74], appearance of new NOEs, and/or intermolecular NOEs between the ligand and protein [75, 76]. In addition, the information obtained from the NMR analysis may be used to identify the binding site and determine a co-structure of the protein with the ligand [12, 75, 77, 78].

An extremely valuable benefit of NMR is the additional ability to obtain critical information on the viability of a compound to be identified as a quality lead candidate in a very simple manner. From extensive experience analyzing hits from an HTS assay, there are numerous undesirable mechanisms resulting from poor physical behavior of the compound that will result in a positive response in an HTS screen. These poor properties of the compound may include insolubility, reactivity, impurities, aggregation, instability, and non-specific binding. As a result, depending on the nature of the assay and the protein target, only a small percentage of the identified hits actually bind the protein target of interest in a desirable manner. NMR is unique because it can provide direct evidence of the ligand's correct structure, purity, and solubility by rapidly obtaining a simple ^{1}H NMR spectrum of the compound collected under appropriate buffer conditions. Although the solubility of the compound is readily inferred by peak intensities relative to an internal standard (3-(Trimethylsilyl)-Propionic acid, TSP) at a defined concentration, the absence of aggregation or micelle-like behavior is implied from the compound's line widths. The line widths observed in NMR spectra are directly related to the tumbling rate (correlation time, τ_c), which in turn is related to the molecule's apparent MW. Therefore, a small molecule that either aggregates or forms micelles will exhibit extremely broad NMR lines relative to a well-behaved compound. It is very plausible that the NMR lines may be broadened beyond the point of detection such that an NMR sample will simultaneously exhibit both the absence of a precipitate and an NMR spectrum. Similarly, the proposed structure and sample purity may be verified by comparing the number and intensity of observed peaks to a predicted NMR spectrum. In practice, rapid examination of the aromatic region of the ^{1}H NMR spectra for the correct number of peaks with the expected intensity and splitting from J-couplings yields a qualitative measure of the structural integrity and purity of the NMR sample.

As a result of the versatility and unique information content, NMR has routinely been used in structure-based drug design programs as an approach to further validate lead compounds. The observation of specific binding to a target protein with reasonable aqueous solubility corresponds to "good" physical properties from an NMR perspective. Readily and rapidly obtaining this information is a crucial component of a structure-based drug design project, since a high correlation between compounds that show "good" physical properties by NMR and the resulting success rate in obtaining a co-structure have been empirically observed.

The application of NMR to validate leads is typically applied to a small set of compounds. An influential manuscript by Fesik and co-workers describes the "SAR by NMR" method, which elegantly illustrates the application of NMR to screen a library of small molecules for their ability to bind proteins from observed chemical shift perturbations [79]. The resulting impact of this manuscript has been the explosive effort in academia and industry to design and implement a number of novel approaches for screening compound libraries using NMR [11, 12, 62–64]. These NMR screening methods can be readily classified into two general categories; one-dimensional (1D) or two-dimensional (2D) NMR techniques.

1. 2D NMR Screening Techniques

HTS and biological assays have provided a traditional approach for the initial identification of chemical classes for a drug design program. The results of these screens generally imply a biological activity associated with the compound, which is usually demonstrated through a decrease in the functional activity of the protein of interest. Nevertheless, there exists a potential disconnect between the observed inhibition of the protein and a productive interaction of the compound with the protein. Clearly, the most fundamental and valuable information necessary to identify a lead compound is verification that the compound actually binds the protein of interest in a beneficial mechanism. NMR provides a relatively unique approach to ascertain this information while providing additional information on the quality of the chemical series.

a. SAR by NMR

The structure-activity relationship (SAR) by NMR method described by Fesik and co-workers illustrates the use of NMR for screening a small-molecule library as an approach to design inhibitors against stromelysin (MMP-3) [80] (Figure 5.1). Stromelysin is involved in the degradation of the extracellular matrix that is associated with normal tissue remodeling. The loss in regulation of this activity may result in the pathological destruction of connective tissue associated with tumor metastases [81, 82]. A key structural

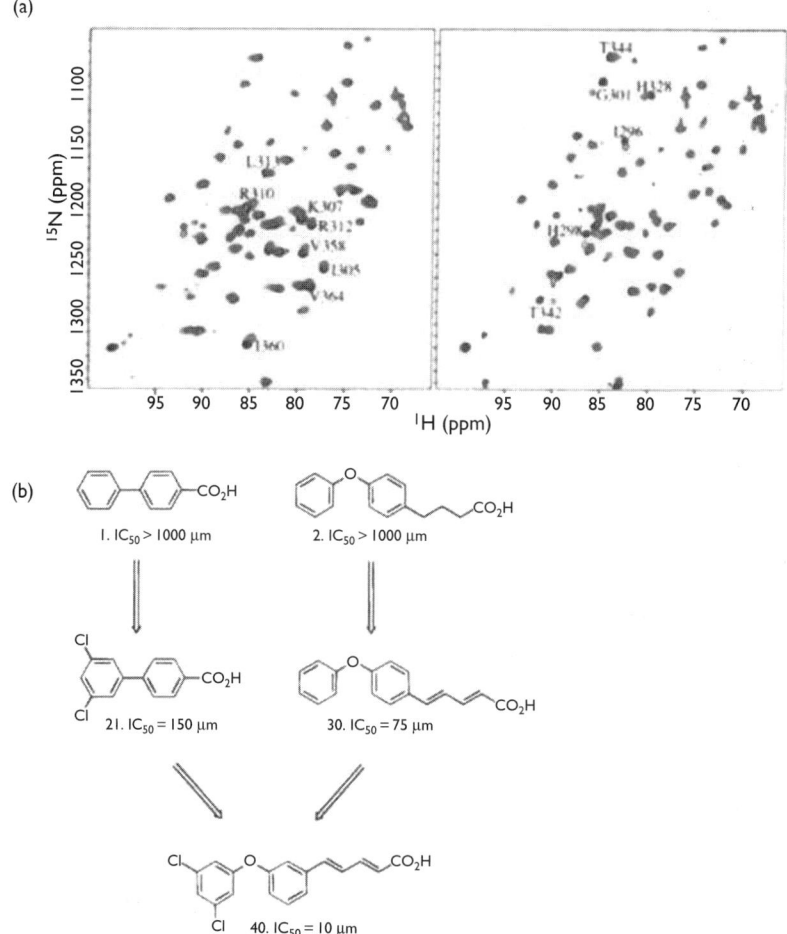

FIGURE 5.1 Examples of the application of the SAR by NMR screening approach with human papillomaviruses (HPV) DNA binding protein E2 and stromelysin. (a) Two examples of ^1H-^{15}N HSQC spectra of E2 in the absence of added ligand (black) and the presence of added ligand (red). Some residues that exhibit chemical shift changes upon binding are labeled. (b) Summary of the discovery of a 10-μM inhibitor of E2 starting from mM leads identified using SAR by NMR. (c) Ribbons depiction of (left) stromelysin complexed with acetohydroxamic acid and a biphenyl compound; (right) the stromelysin linked compound complex (green) superimposed with a collagenase:inhibitor complex (cyan). (d) A summary of the SAR by NMR approach applied to the discovery of stromelysin inhibitors. (Reprinted with permission from references [79, 80]. Copyright 1997 by American Chemical Society.) See Color Plate 4.

feature of matrix metalloproteinases (MMPs) is the presence of an S1' pocket proximal to the catalytic Zn. A typical approach to the design of MMP inhibitors incorporates functionality into the compound to chelate the active site Zn while optimizing the fit in the S1' pocket.

The SAR by NMR method employs 2D ^1H-^{15}N HSQC spectra [79, 80, 83, 84] and more recently 2D ^1H-^{13}C HSQC spectra [85] to monitor chemical shift changes to identify a binding event (Figure 5.1a). Chemical shifts provide

(c)

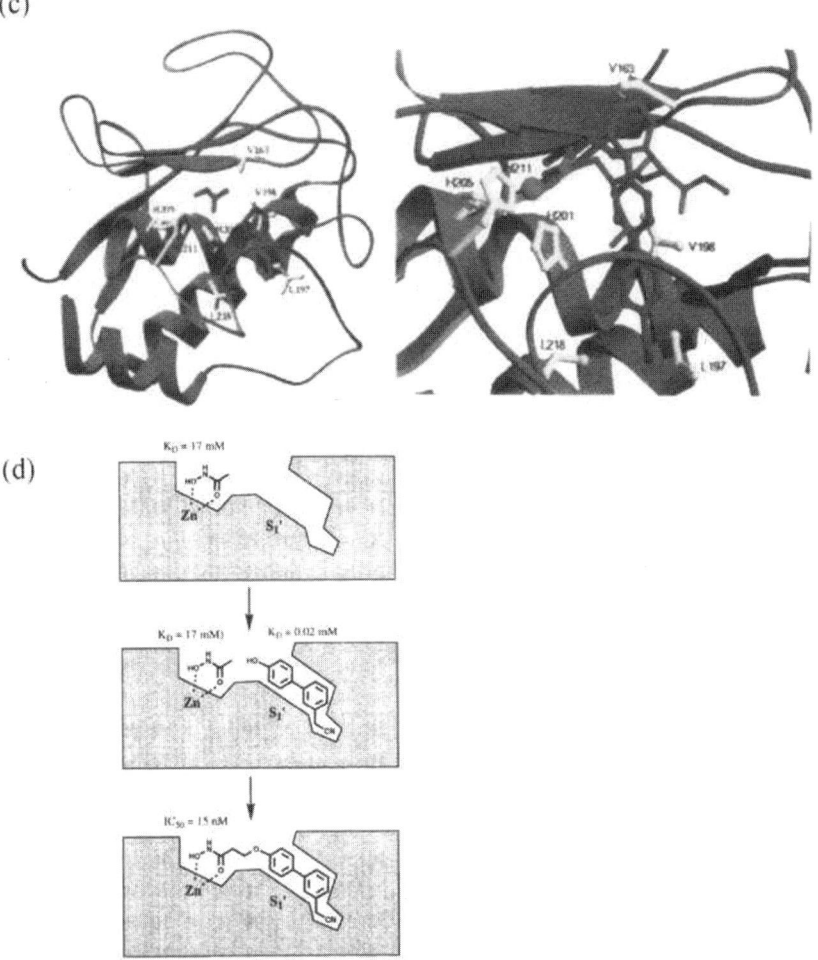

(d)

FIGURE 5.1 (*Continued*)

a wealth of information because of their direct correlation with the local environment of the probed nuclei. A 2D ^{1}H-^{15}N HSQC spectrum correlates the ^{1}H chemical shift of the proton attached to the backbone amide nitrogen with the corresponding ^{15}N chemical shift of the same amide nitrogen. The end result is a 2D plot of peaks with X,Y-coordinates corresponding to the ^{1}H and ^{15}N chemical shifts for the backbone amides of each amino acid residue in the protein sequence. In general, each residue will generate a unique peak in the 2D ^{1}H-^{15}N HSQC spectrum consistent with its own local environment. Of course, some overlap in peak locations will occur for residues in comparable environments and the occurrence of overlap will increase proportional to the size of the protein.

Through the application of isotope labeling (^{13}C, ^{15}N) of the protein and 3D triple-resonance NMR experiments, it is routinely possible to assign each observed peak in a 2D ^{1}H-^{15}N HSQC spectra with a specific amino acid in the protein sequence [40, 86]. Briefly, the protein assignment protocol utilizes a series of triple-resonance experiments where each experiment correlates a subset of the protein backbone atoms through J-coupling. By combining overlapping information between the various experiments, it is possible to "walk" down the protein backbone and complete the resonance assignments. As an example, two typical triple-resonance experiments are the HNCA and HN(CO)CA experiments. The HNCA experiment correlates the ^{1}H and ^{15}N chemical shifts of the backbone amide with the ^{13}C chemical shift of the Cα for both the I and I-1 residues. Similarly, the HN(CO)CA experiment correlates the ^{1}H and ^{15}N chemical shifts of the backbone amide with the ^{13}C chemical shift of the Cα for the I-1 residue. Thus, an I and I-1 residue pair will be identified by correlating a backbone amide from the HN(CO)CA spectrum with a particular Cα_{I-1} resonance with the corresponding Cα_I resonance associated with a particular backbone amide in the HNCA spectrum. The assignments are completed by sequentially joining these residue pairs. Typically multiple pairs of NMR experiments are collected that correlate distinct components of the backbone and side-chain (C', Hα, Cβ) because of peak overlap and potential chemical shift degeneracy. This assignment approach is generally limited to proteins with a MW limit of 20–25 kDa. To assign proteins with larger MW requires the addition of deuterium labeling and the application of TROSY-based experiments [42, 87].

A compound interacting specifically with a protein will result in a significant change in the local environment at the binding site. Furthermore, any induced conformational changes that result from the formation of the ligand-protein complex, even distal from the binding site, will result in a de facto environment change. Because backbone amide chemical shifts are very sensitive to the local environment, a binding event will manifest itself by perturbations in peak positions in the 2D ^{1}H-^{15}N HSQC spectrum. The observation of the chemical shift perturbations is readily obtained by simply overlaying the 2D ^{1}H-^{15}N HSQC spectrum of the free protein with the 2D ^{1}H-^{15}N HSQC spectrum of the protein-ligand complex. Furthermore, because each peak in the 2D ^{1}H-^{15}N HSQC has been assigned to a particular residue in the protein sequence, the identity of the binding site is determined by mapping the residues that incurred a chemical shift perturbation onto the molecular surface of the protein. A specific binding site for the compound will be apparent from the appearance of a cluster of residues that exhibits chemical shift changes on the protein's surface. Conversely, non-specific interactions or a detrimental impact to the protein (denaturation, aggregation) will be apparent by either a random distribution of residues exhibiting chemical shift perturbations or from the observation that the vast majority of residues exhibit significant chemical shift changes or reduction in signal intensity.

Another feature exploited in the SAR by NMR approach is based on the ability of the 2D ^{1}H-^{15}N HSQC spectra to both verify that the compound binds to the protein of interest and to readily identify the binding site on the protein surface. This information may then be used to identify distinct compounds that bind to the protein in proximal binding sites (Figures 5.1c and d). It may then be feasible to chemically link two or more compounds and design a compound with a significant increase in binding affinity (Figures 5.1b and d).

The identification and effective linking of compounds that bind proximally to each other on a protein surface was illustrated in the SAR by NMR screen for stromelysin. Acetohydroxamic acid (K_D = 17 mM) and 3-(cyanomethyl)-4'-hydroxybiphenyl (K_D = 0.02 mM) that bind to the catalytic Zn and in the S1' pocket, respectively, were identified [80]. Linking these two fragments resulted in a compound with a dramatic improvement in affinity (K_D = 15 nM) (Figures 5.1c and d). A similar SAR by NMR screen was conducted using the human papillomavirus (HPV) DNA binding protein E2 as a target [79], where certain strains of HPV have been implicated in cancer [88, 89]. Biphenyl and biphenyl ether compounds containing a carboxylic acid were observed to interact with the DNA binding site on E2 (IC_{50} > 1000 μM). The binding sites for both classes of compounds were similar, as indicated by the fact that both compounds perturbed the same set of amide NMR resonances (Figure 5.1a). By combining features from both classes of the E2 binders, a hybrid structure [5-(3'-(3', 5'-dichlorophenoxy)-phenyl)-2,4-pentadienoic acid], was synthesized with an IC_{50} of 10 μM (Figure 5.1b).

The application of the SAR by NMR screening methodology as a complimentary approach to HTS assay or even as an alternative to standard HTS assay has great potential. Nevertheless, there are a number of caveats that may limit the application of the methodology. NMR is an inherently insensitive technique that requires relatively high quantities of isotope-labeled protein (hundreds of milligrams to grams per screen) and data acquisition times (>10 minutes per sample). The problem is partially addressed by conducting the NMR screen using mixtures instead of single compounds, where a positive hit would require deconvolution of the mixture. Of course, there are practical limits to the size of the mixtures based on the anticipated hit rate, because a point will eventually be reached where deconvolution of the mixture would be equivalent to the analysis of individual compounds. Additionally, mixtures may pose potential problems such as reduced solubility, reactivity, and cooperative binding, i.e., a compound only exhibits binding in the presence of the mixture.

Another potential problem arises from the inherent strength of the technique, the relative sensitivity of the amide chemical shifts to the environment. In an HTS format, maintaining consistency of sample preparation is a non-trivial exercise. It is especially difficult predicting the affect of the compounds or mixtures on the sample. Specifically, changes in pH or solvent concentration upon addition of the compounds to the protein sample may induce chemical shift changes not associated with a binding event. Proper controls will aid in identifying potential false positives.

Finally, the quality of the 2D ^{1}H-^{15}N HSQC spectra and the ability to take advantage of the NMR assignments to identify ligand binding sites is limited by the MW of the protein. Proteins in the less than 20- to 25-kDa range are routinely assigned and amenable to the SAR by NMR approach assuming the protein is reasonably soluble and stable. For larger MW proteins, it is necessary to employ deuterium labeling in conjunction with TROSY-based experiments. It is important to note that the 2D ^{1}H-^{15}N HSQC screening is not dependent on the protein assignments. Chemical shift perturbations in the absence of assignments will still identify a potential binder to the protein, whereas comparison of chemical shift perturbation patterns to known ligands may generate some information on the binding site for the unknown ligand. The unavoidable fact is that the nature of the protein will dictate the feasibility of the application of the SAR by NMR approach to drug screening.

b. 2D- trNOE

An alternative to the 2D ^{1}H-^{15}N HSQC approach described in detail above is the 2D-transferred NOE experiment [71, 90, 91]. The 2D-trNOE experiment addresses some of the issues that are raised by the 2D ^{1}H-^{15}N HSQC experiment, particularly the protein MW limit and the quantity of isotope-labeled protein. An NOE occurs from a through-space transfer of magnetization through a dipole-dipole interaction. This transfer is strongly distant dependent ($1/r^6$) and provides the fundamental source of structural information in NMR analysis. The trNOE is the extension of the NOE phenomena to a biological system under exchange. Essentially, two protons in close contact in the bound conformation of ligand will give rise to an NOE. This NOE will be transferred to the free ligand's resonance through chemical exchange. Thus, it is possible to observe an NOE arising from the ligand's bound conformation by observing the free ligand's NMR spectrum (Figure 5.2). To be able to observe a trNOE, the off-rate between the free and bound forms of the ligand must be much faster then the cross-relaxation rate (which gives rise to the NOE) and the spin-lattice relaxation rate. The result of these requirements is that the trNOE experiment increases in efficiency and sensitivity for weak binding ligands ($K_D > 10$ μM) and large MW proteins (>20 kDa).

In practice, a 2D-trNOE experiment requires a minimal amount of unlabeled protein because the sample preparation requires the ligand be in 10- to 20-fold excess. Significant excess of the ligand relative to the protein accomplishes the objective of observing the NMR spectrum of the free ligand while maximizing the number of exchange events that occur during the NMR experiment. Briefly, a 2D-trNOE experiment correlates ^{1}H chemical shifts that are separated by 6 Å in the bound state of the ligand. A 2D-trNOE spectrum would contain diagonal peaks consistent with the 1D ^{1}H spectrum of the ligand where same-sign off-diagonal peaks would indicate resonances that exhibit a trNOE (Figure 5.2c). Additionally, the relative intensity of the trNOE cross-peaks is related to the distance separation between the two correlated protons. This information may then be used to determine the bound conformation of the ligand. Obviously, the structure of the bound form of the ligand is only of interest if the compound is inherently flexible. If the compound does not bind the target protein, the 2D-trNOE experiment will be void of off-diagonal peaks or the peaks will be the opposite sign (Figure 5.2b). The 2D-trNOE does not provide any structural information relative to the protein or the identity of the ligand-binding site. Furthermore, the 2D trNOE experiment requires relatively long data acquisition times (>1 h per sample) that limit its utility in a high-throughput format.

Thus, the 2D-trNOE may be a preferred alternative to the 2D ^{1}H-^{15}N HSQC experiment for the analysis of a small library of ligands that bind weakly to large MW proteins. Additionally, the 2D-trNOE may be used in combination with the 2D ^{1}H-^{15}N HSQC experiment to identify both the binding conformation of the ligand and its binding site on the protein target.

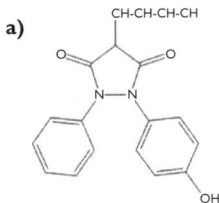

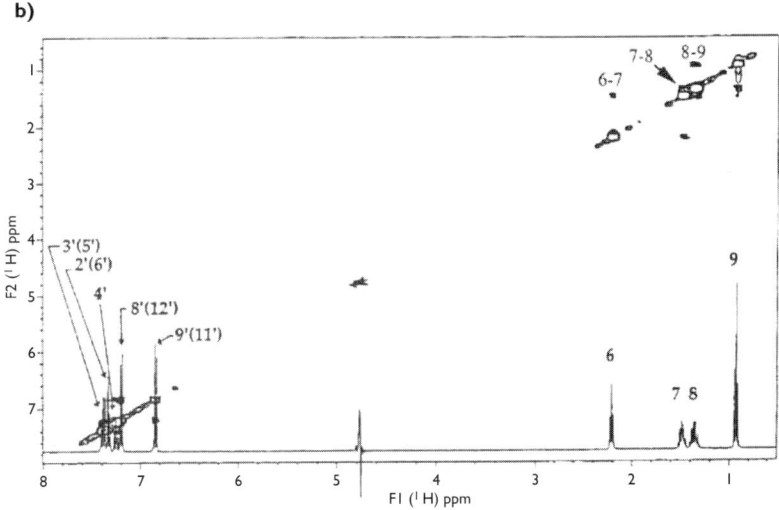

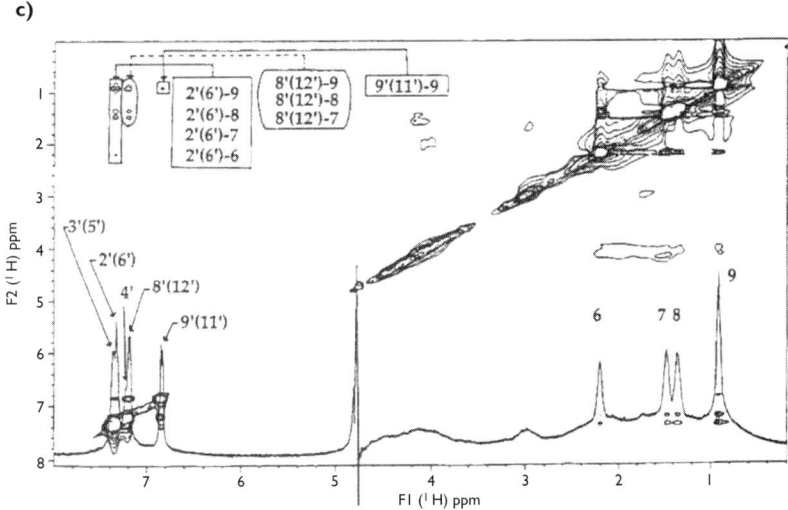

FIGURE 5.2 Example of the 2D-trNOE experiment to identify binders to a protein target. (a) Chemical structure of OXY. (b) 2D ^{1}H NOESY spectra of OXY (5 mM) and a corresponding 1D ^{1}H trace. (c) spectra of OXY (5 mM) in the presence of 0.083 mM of human serum albumin. The observed trNOEs for OXY upon binding human serum albumin are boxed and labeled. (Reprinted with permission from reference [91]. Copyright 1998 by John Wiley & Sons, Inc.) See Color Plate 5.

This information may be useful in generating a rapid model of the protein-ligand complex in lieu of a high-resolution structure. The advantage of this approach would be a combination of speed and overcoming difficulties in obtaining a high-resolution structure of the complex.

2. 1D NMR Screening Techniques

The obvious benefits identified in the SAR by NMR screen and its illustrated success in designing stromelysin inhibitors combined with the inherent limitations described above has fostered an interest in identifying alternative NMR screening approaches. There exists a variety of NMR techniques utilized in the evaluation of ligand binding that exhibit inherent strengths and weakness associated with the amount of material required, experiment time, ability to differentiate between non-specific and stoichiometric binders, and the ability to identify the ligand binding site. All of these factors will contribute to the effectiveness and utility of a particular approach in an NMR-based screen.

a. 1D Line-Broadening

The 2D ^{1}H-^{15}N HSQC experiments described in detail above take advantage of one principle property of an NMR experiment, the chemical shift, to monitor the interaction of a ligand with a protein target. Another fundamental property of an NMR spectrum is the inherent line width of an NMR resonance. NMR line widths are dependent on T_2 relaxation, which is directly correlated with the MW of the molecule. Thus, the inherent NMR line widths for a molecule increase or broaden proportionally to its MW. This provides a simple mechanism to monitor the binding of a low MW ligand to a relatively large MW protein. Upon binding the protein, the ligand will experience an increase in line width proportional to the MW of the protein (Figure 5.3). The observed increase in the line width for the ligand will depend on a number of factors including K_D, concentration of the ligand and

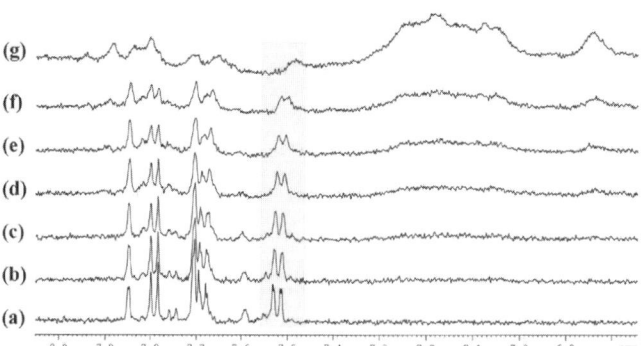

FIGURE 5.3 Illustration of the application of 1D line-broadening to identify binders [423]. (a) The 1D-NMR spectrum of the free compound (50 μM). (b–g) Addition of 2 μM to 50 μM of ER-α to the compound in (a). The observed line-broadening indicates the compound binds ER-α. The resonances centered around 7.52 ppm are outlined in yellow to highlight the observed line-broadening and chemical shift changes upon the addition of ER-α. See Color Plate 6.

protein, exchange rates, dynamics, and the MW of the protein. In general, the observed change in the ligand's line width (ν_{obs}) will follow:

$$\nu_{obs} = f_{free} \cdot \nu_{free} + f_{bound} \cdot \nu_{bound}$$

where f_{free} and f_{bound} are the fraction free and bound, respectively, and ν_{free} and ν_{bound} are the line widths for the free and bound states of the ligand, respectively. Thus, the increase in line width for the ligand will depend directly on the fraction bound and the line width of the complex. Obviously, the fraction bound (f_{bound}) will be dependent on the K_D of the complex and the concentration of both the ligand and protein, where the line width of the complex will be primarily dependent on the MW of the protein. For a ligand with an unknown affinity for the protein target, an experiment is designed based on an estimate of the K_D's upper limit and practical considerations such as the solubility of the compound and the NMR detection limit. Also, the protein target should be >20 kDa to obtain noticeable line-broadening effects.

The analysis of line-broadening effects may also be complicated by exchange rates (k_{ex}), where effects on the NMR spectra are only observable if $k_{ex}^{-1} \sim T_2$. There are effectively three regimes of exchange on the NMR timescale, fast ($k_{ex} \gg 2\pi\Delta\delta$), slow ($k_{ex} \ll 2\pi\Delta\delta$), and intermediate ($k_{ex} \sim 2\pi\Delta\delta$) that are differentiated by the chemical shift difference ($\Delta\delta$) between the free and bound forms of the ligand. For fast exchange, the increase in line width for the bound ligand will be dominated by the line width of the protein. In the slow exchange regime, two different resonances will be observed that correspond to the bound and free forms of the ligand where the line widths will correlate with the MWs of the complex and the free ligand, respectively. In practice for a large MW protein, the intensity of the NMR resonance for the ligand will appear to decrease upon binding the protein, because the ligand resonances associated with complex formation will typically be broadened into the baseline. In the intermediate regime, the peak shape and line width will follow a complex function resulting in a more dramatic broadening of the peak relative to either the fast or slow exchange regime.

The dynamics of localized regions within the protein may further complicate the impact on the observed line-width change for the ligand upon binding the protein. In a similar analysis to the exchange rate for the complex formation, the region of the protein that interacts with the ligand may also be undergoing a conformational exchange. Thus, the apparent impact of the line-width change on the ligand may be greater then the effective MW difference because of the additional exchange broadening that results from the local protein dynamics. Of course, the formation of the complex may alter the local protein dynamics and potentially eliminate this contribution.

Also contributing to the ligand's observed line-width increase would be non-stoichiometric binding behavior of the ligand. If the ligand binds non-specifically with multiple modes of interaction then the effective fraction bound will be much greater relative to a stoichiometric binder. The observed result is a large increase in the line width of the ligand at relatively high ligand-to-protein ratios (20–10:1). Therefore, in the absence of protein dynamics and intermediate exchange, monitoring line-width changes as a function of protein concentration may provide a qualitative indication of non-stoichiometric behavior. Identifying compounds with non-specific protein binding is a very valuable tool, because these compounds tend to be undesirable lead candidates and problematic in the structure determination of protein-ligand complexes. An important caveat is verifying that the NMR binding analysis is done under conditions comparable to the ligands K_D or IC_{50}. If the NMR experiments are done at concentrations well above the K_D, the observed non-stoichiometric binding may be irrelevant and may mask a specific tight binding interaction.

Unknown factors in the practical application of 1D line-broadening experiments to screen for potential binders of a protein target of interest are the K_D for the complex, the NMR regime for the exchange rate, the stoichiometry or specificity of binding, and compound solubility or whether the compound actually binds the protein. Nevertheless, at the start of a drug discovery effort the initial leads are expected to be weak binders that would most likely bind in the fast exchange regime on the NMR timescale. Additionally, $IC_{50}s$ obtained from biological assays provide an approximation of the potential K_D of the complex, and the inherent aqueous solubility of the compound will dictate limits on the experiment. In addition, unusual protein dynamics may be discerned from structural information, dynamic analysis, or the observed behavior of known stoichiometric binders. The 1D line-broadening experiments have the advantage of being relatively rapid (requiring a few minutes per spectra) while avoiding the need for an isotope-labeled protein. Additionally, the approach does not require any NMR information on the protein (assignments, structure) to fully analyze the data. Furthermore, the utility of the 1D line-broadening experiment increases with large MW proteins that are typical pharmaceutical and cancer targets. The gain in speed relative to the 2D trNOE or 2D ^1H-^{15}N HSQC spectra is based on collecting one (~1:1 ligand-protein ratio) or two titration points (additional high ligand-to-protein ratio) instead of a full titration experiment. Also, there is only a modest savings in protein usage relative to the 2D ^1H-^{15}N HSQC because a significant change in line width is usually observed close to a 1:1 ratio. This is due to a combination of factors including the typical solubility range of the organic compounds in aqueous buffers, the weak K_Ds of the complex, NMR sensitivity, and the desire for fast acquisition times. Nevertheless, 1D line-broadening experiments provide a rapid means for determining if an identified lead binds to the protein target of interest while obtaining qualitative information of the relatively stoichiometry of binding. This binding information is critical for a successful structure-based drug design effort.

b. 1D STD

While the 1D line-broadening experiment described in detail above is a very robust and routine approach for validating potential lead molecules, the optimal application of the methodology requires collecting a full titration over a range of protein concentrations. This effectively limits the application in a screening approach. For screening large libraries of compounds by NMR, the desire is to minimize protein requirements while increasing the speed of acquiring the NMR spectra. Furthermore, it would be ideal for the methodology to be applicable to a wide MW range of proteins while eliminating the requirement for labeled protein. The 1D-STD experiment effectively addresses these issues. The 1D-STD experiment is analogous to the 2D-trNOE previously described.

The basic idea of the 1D-STD experiment is to transfer the saturation of magnetization from the protein target to the ligand through a binding event (Figure 5.4). The experiment is conducted by alternatively subtracting a 1D spectrum with on- and off-resonance irradiation of protein resonances. In practice, this is accomplished by selectively irradiating a region of the ^{1}H NMR spectra that is devoid of ligand resonances, but contains protein resonances. The edge of the methyl region (0.3 to −0.3 ppm) is typically chosen for these experiments. With sufficient pulse strength and duration, a majority of the protein NMR signals will be saturated through spin diffusion. Then, if the ligand binds the protein, the effective saturation will be transferred to the ligand. The result is a reduction in the intensity of the ligand NMR spectrum during the on-resonance irradiation compared to the off-resonance irradiation cycle. Because the spectrum is being alternatively subtracted, the difference spectra should yield the 1D NMR spectrum of the ligand (Figure 5.4). Conversely, if the ligand does not bind the protein, no change in the ligand's intensity occurs for either the on- or off-resonance irradiation cycle, thus the end result is a null spectrum.

Similar to the 2D-trNOE experiment, the 1D-STD experiment is more sensitive to weak binding compounds with fast off-rates. By maximizing the number of exchange events that take place during the on-resonance irradiation time, a maximal number of ligand molecules will incur a decrease in signal intensity. Again, similar to the 2D-trNOE experiment, the 1D-STD experiment is conducted at a high ratio of ligand to protein (20–50:1). Also, the sensitivity of the 1D-STD experiment will depend on the proton density at the ligand-protein interface. The higher the density of protons at the binding site the more efficient is the saturation transfer. A comparable experiment to the 1D-STD is the WaterLOGSY experiment, which uses the transfer of magnetization from the water shell instead of the protein [92, 93]. The WaterLOGSY experiment is particularly beneficial for compounds binding to DNA/RNA that have a relatively low proton density but a more defined water shell in the minor and major grooves.

The 1D-STD experiment provides a rapid approach to screening compounds that bind proteins while significantly reducing the protein requirement (from µM–mM to nM–µM) and acquisition times (<15 mins. per spectrum) relative to other NMR experiments previously described. Also, the methodology does not require isotope labeling and is not limited by the MW of the protein. The protein size will affect the sensitivity of the experiment since spin diffusion is more efficient at higher MWs. One significant caveat to the approach is the higher likelihood of false positives, because the approach does not differentiate between specific and non-specific binding events. In fact, weak non-stoichiometric binding may generate a strong STD response, which suggests the approach may be more susceptible to identifying non-specific binders. Conversely, the methodology may miss very tight binders ($K_D \sim$ nM) with slow off-rates, which may be problematic because ultimately these are the compounds of interest. Of course, at the early stages of a drug discovery project, identifying a low nanomolar binder is highly unusual.

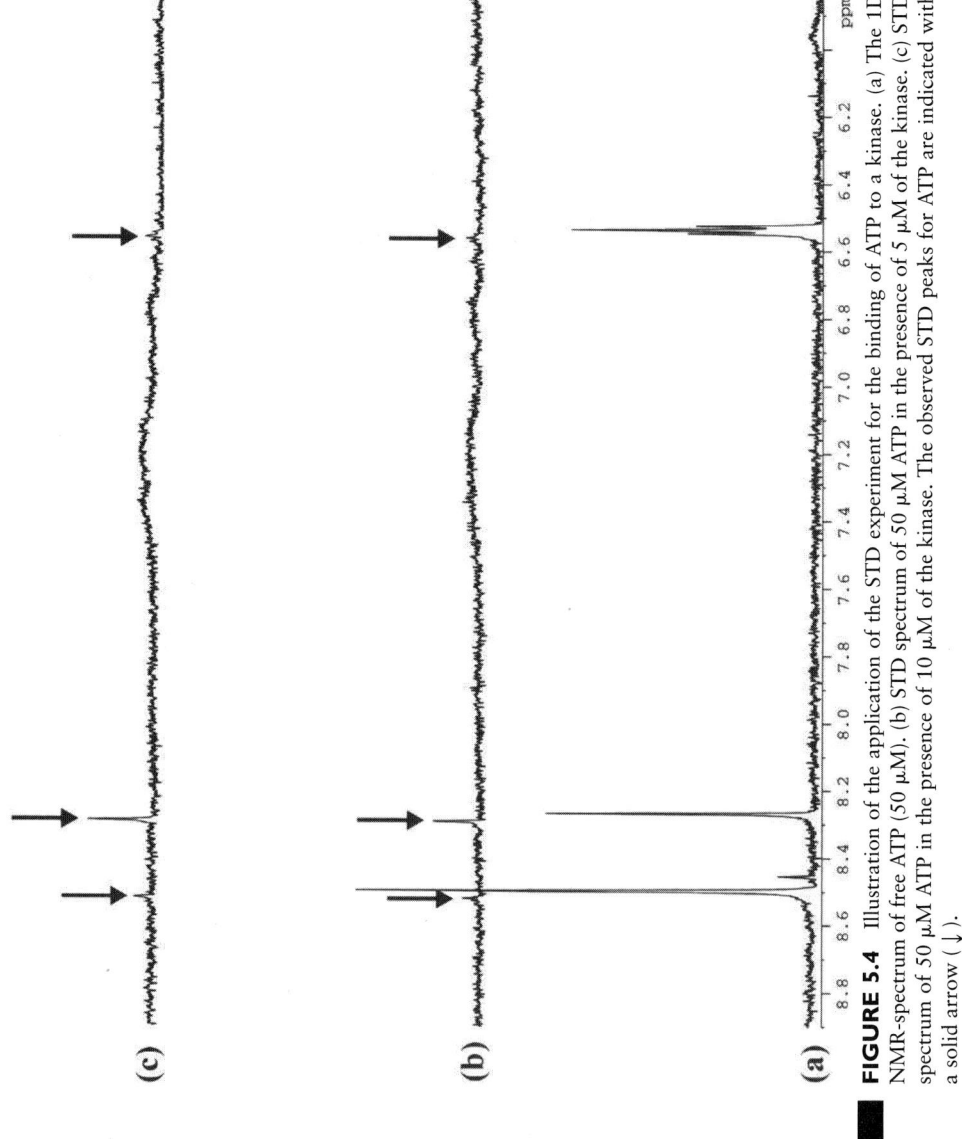

FIGURE 5.4 Illustration of the application of the STD experiment for the binding of ATP to a kinase. (a) The 1D NMR-spectrum of free ATP (50 µM). (b) STD spectrum of 50 µM ATP in the presence of 5 µM of the kinase. (c) STD spectrum of 50 µM ATP in the presence of 10 µM of the kinase. The observed STD peaks for ATP are indicated with a solid arrow (↓).

Effectively, the 1D-STD experiment determines the presence of relatively weak binding interactions, is amenable to HTS, and provides a good starting point for further evaluation of compounds.

c. SHAPES Approach

Given the ability of traditional high-throughput approaches to screen a library containing upwards of a million compounds, where this limit continues to expand as the technology advances, NMR-based screens will tend to pale in comparison to the total number of compounds screened in an HTS assay. Thus, the composition of a library screened by NMR becomes a very important consideration. There are numerous and equally acceptable approaches to designing a chemical library utilized in an NMR screen. The variety of possible compound library designs has been described at length [94–98]. A common approach is to design a chemical library that focuses on specific properties of the compounds, such as solubility, "drug-like" properties, and structural diversity [99, 100].

The design and composition of the chemical library is a major component of the SHAPES approach to screening by NMR [101] (Figure 5.5). Briefly, the compounds in the comprehensive medicinal chemistry (CMC) database (MDL Information Systems, San Leandro, CA) were classified into frameworks, a system consisting of rings and linkers [102]. Side-chains attached to the frameworks of known drugs in the CMC database were also identified. The 41 most frequently occurring frameworks and 30 common side chains were used to search the available chemical directory (ACD). The resulting hits from the ACD were filtered for aqueous solubility, availability, ease of synthesis, representative drug class from the CMC, and quality of the NMR spectra. The end result is a library consisting of about 200 compounds that can be readily and quickly screened by NMR. The screening for binders in the SHAPES approach is typically accomplished by either 1D line-broadening or 2D-trNOE experiments as described in detail above (Figure 5.5a). The positive hits are then used as starting points for ligand design by using the compounds as the basis for structure-based searches of compound databases, which direct the design of compound libraries for HTS assays or for guiding the synthesis of combinatorial libraries. In effect, a small compound library that can be screened quickly and efficiently by NMR while requiring minimal amounts of protein can be used as a surrogate to obtain information for a large database containing millions of compounds.

The SHAPES method has been applied to a number of protein targets including p38 MAP kinase (Figure 5.5). The p38 MAP kinase signaling pathway transmits cytokine- and stress-induced apoptosis, which is associated with a number of cancers including breast, stomach, liver, and prostrate [103]. Fejzo et al., illustrated the design of a p38 MAP kinase inhibitor starting from weak binders (K_D = 1–7 mM) identified in the SHAPES screen [101]. By fusing fragments with common scaffolds, the affinity of the compounds increased to a K_D of 200–300 μM and eventually to a compound with a K_D of ~200 nM (Figure 5.5b). The tight binding compound designed from the SHAPES initial lead is in the same structural class as the SmithKline Beecham SB-203580 compound, which is a well-characterized and potent

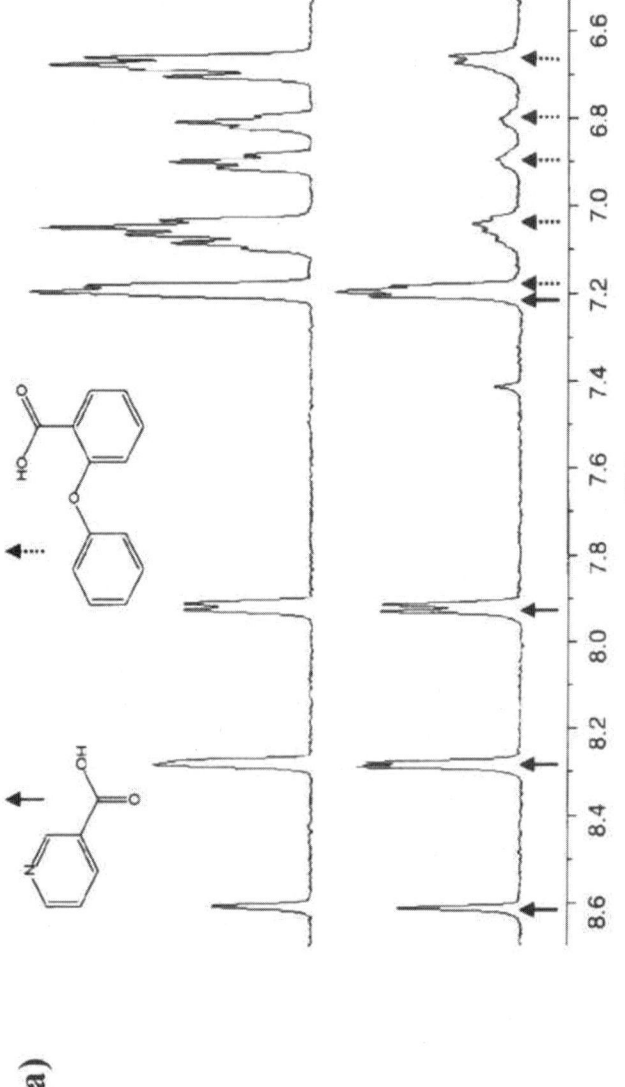

FIGURE 5.5 Example of the application of the SHAPES approach to NMR screening for the design of p38 MAP kinase inhibitors (from [101]). (a) Comparison of the 1D ¹H spectra of a mixture of two ligands in the absence (top) and presence (bottom) of p38 MAP kinase. The broadening of the 2-phenoxy benzoic acid NMR resonances indicates binding to p38 MAP kinase. (↑). No broadening was observed in the nicotinic acid (↑). (b) An example showing how fusion of fragments identified from the SHAPES screen with a common scaffold lead to a potent inhibitor of p38 MAP kinase that was structurally similar to a previously identified and well-studied inhibitor. (Reprinted with permission from reference [101]. Copyright 1999 by Elsevier Science.)

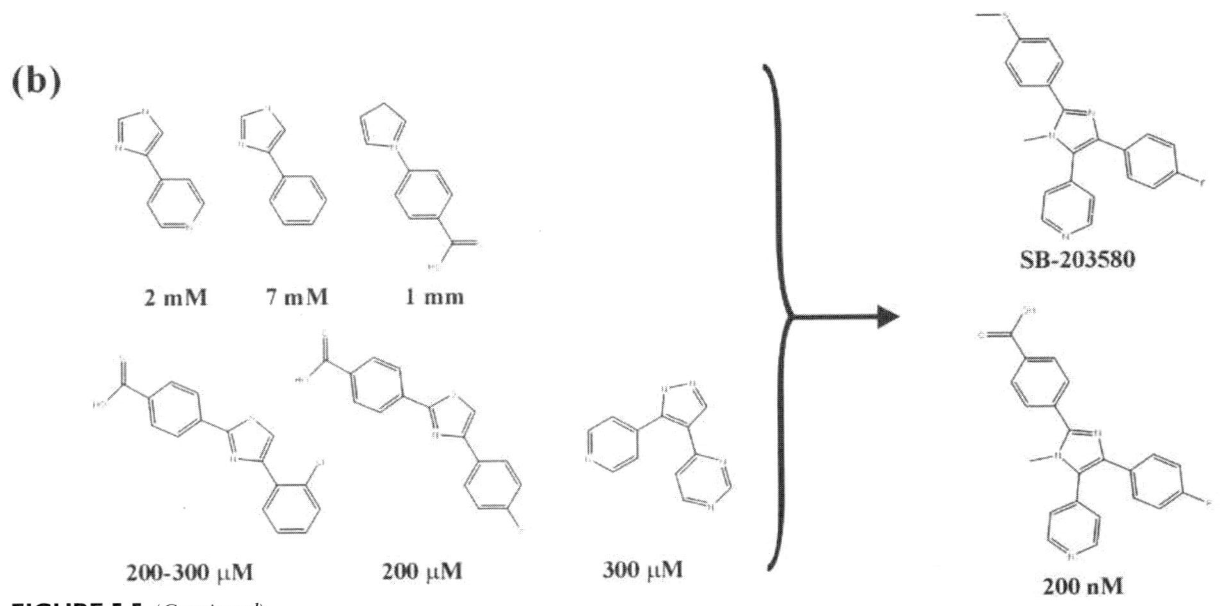

(b)

2 mM   7 mM   1 mm

200 µM

200–300 µM

300 µM

SB-203580

200 nM

FIGURE 5.5 (*Continued*)

p38 MAP kinase inhibitor. This result provides further credence to the SHAPES approach of lead discovery and drug design.

d. Other NMR Screening Approaches

Some of the major and routinely used applications of NMR in a screening effort have been described in some detail, but this is far from complete. This is especially true because the list is continually evolving and expanding as new techniques become available. Additional NMR approaches that have been applied to screening compound libraries include diffusion-edited [66, 68, 104], relaxation-edited [66], and NOE-pumping techniques [76]. These approaches fall into the 1D NMR class of techniques, which are similar to the 1D-STD and 1D-line broadening methods. What fundamentally differentiates these techniques is the NMR property associated with the binding event. Similar to the other approaches described herein, there are inherent advantages and disadvantages associated with each method that will determine its appropriate utility in a particular screen.

B. Protein Structures by NMR

Essential to a structure-based drug design program is the availability of a high-quality structure of the protein of interest (Figure 5.6). X-ray crystallography has historically been a major source for obtaining 3D structures of proteins [30], where the use of NMR is a relatively recent addition to the structure-based drug design approach [12]. A number of barriers exist that have sometimes limited the application of NMR. Specifically, NMR requires extensive isotope labeling of the protein and may take six months to a year using standard methodology to determine a high-resolution structure for proteins <40 kDa. Conversely, X-ray crystallography routinely solves protein-ligand structures in weeks to months and in some cases as fast as a few days. Furthermore, there is generally no limit to the size of the protein that may be solved by X-ray crystallography and no dependency on isotope labeling. Nevertheless, X-ray crystallography is highly dependent on the ability to obtain crystals that exhibit reasonable diffraction (<2.5 Å). In addition, because NMR determines a solution structure of the protein, information concerning dynamics is obtained while avoiding issues associated with crystal packing interactions. In essence, NMR and X-ray crystallography are complementary approaches to ascertain as much structural information about a protein as possible. A number of analyses have demonstrated that protein structures determined by both NMR and X-ray are generally quite similar [105–107], and that it is feasible to determine a protein structure by combining both NMR and X-ray data [108–110]. The total number of X-ray and NMR structures determined and deposited in the protein database [111] continue to expand at an impressive rate. To date, ~4600 and ~27,000 biomolecular structures have been determined by NMR and X-ray, respectively. These numbers are sure to increase rapidly with the burgeoning role of structural genomics [52, 61]. The NMR structures determined cover a wide range of therapeutic targets where cancer has been a primary area of exploration. A few select examples will be summarized.

1. Growth Factors

Growth factors have been a prominent target for the development of cancer therapeutics as a result of their proliferative response, modulation of cell motility, cell differentiation, and survival. Additionally, some growth factors have been identified as oncogenic whereas others transform cells *in vivo*. Correspondingly, the structures of a number of growth factors have been determined as an aid to understand their mechanism of activity and as part of a drug development program. A prime example of a growth factor family that has been extensively studied is the fibroblast growth factors (FGF) [112] where a number of NMR [113–117] and X-ray structures [118] have been determined (Figure 5.6a).

Basic fibroblast growth factor (FGF-2) exhibits angiogenic and a variety of growth and differentiation activities with involvement in tumor growth and cancer [119–122]. A common feature of FGF family members is their high affinity toward heparin sulfate proteoglycans (HSPG) [119]. The interaction of FGF-2 with HSPG is required for high-affinity binding to its cell surface tyrosine kinase receptor (FGFR) and essential for mediating internalization and intracellular targeting through a ternary complex [123]. As a result of the importance of the role of heparin in the function of FGF-2 and a minimal understanding of its mechanism of action, structural effort on FGF-2 has focused on the heparin interaction with FGF-2 and FGFR. NMR and X-ray structures have determined the interaction of FGF-2 with heparin and its role in forming the ternary complex with the receptor (Figure 5.7). Both FGF-2 and FGFR contain defined heparin binding sites composed of spatially clustered Arg and Lys residues, which interact through salt bridges with sequence-specific sulfates from heparin. Heparin stabilizes the FGF-2:FGFR complex by simultaneously binding the heparin binding site on both FGF-2 and FGFR. The exact mechanism of receptor-induced dimerization is still uncertain as a number of distinct models exist based on multiple X-ray structures of FGF-FGFR-heparin complex [124, 125]. NMR and X-ray have also suggested that the role of heparin is to form a biological active form of an FGF-2 dimer as a precursor to receptor dimerization [114, 126] (Figure 5.7). The resulting complexity of the FGF-FGFR ternary complex implies an extreme difficulty in designing a small molecule that may effectively inhibit the interaction of FGF-2 with its receptor. Nevertheless, suramin and suramin analogs, which mimic heparin and bind to the FGF-2 heparin binding site, have presented one approach to inhibiting the FGF-2-FGFR receptor interaction [127].

Additional growth factors have been explored structurally by NMR in an effort to further our understanding of their function and activity; these have included vascular endothelial growth factor (VEGF) [128, 129], epidermal growth factor (EGF) [130–132], transforming growth factor (TGF) [130, 133–135], and insulin-like growth factor (IGF) [136].

2. Cytokines

Analogous to growth factors, cytokines have also been an extremely active area of structural effort [137]. In fact, some of the first applications of NMR to determine high-resolution solution structures of protein based on the combined utilization of multidimensional NMR and protein isotope labeling

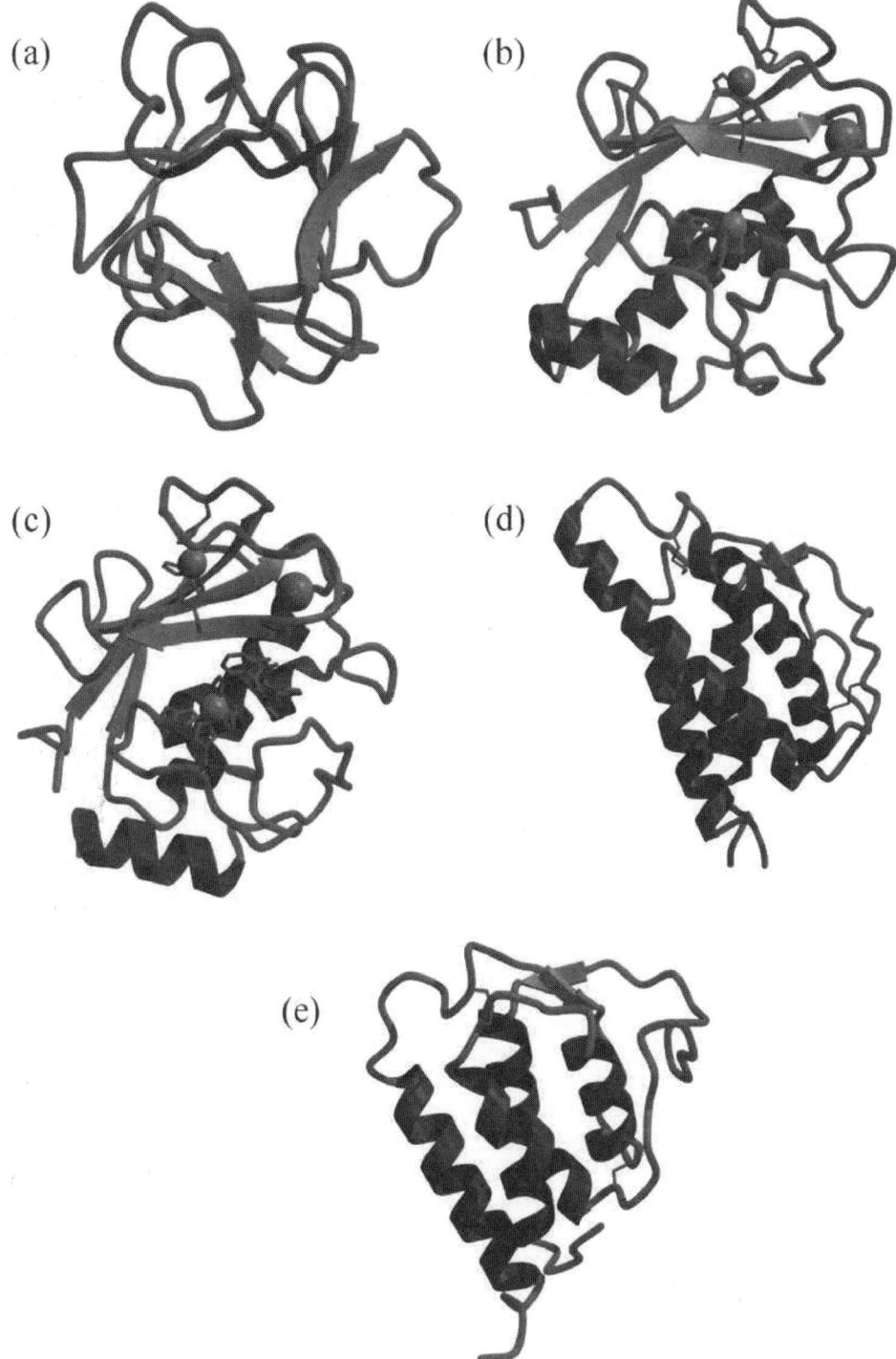

FIGURE 5.6 Ribbon diagrams of the NMR solution structures of (a) FGF-2, (b) MMP-1, (c) MMP-13:CPD-693, (d) IL-4, and (e) IL-13 (from [113, 150, 151, 161]). (Reprinted with permission from references [154, 167]. Copyright 2001 and 2000 by Elsevier Science.) See Color Plate 7.

(a)

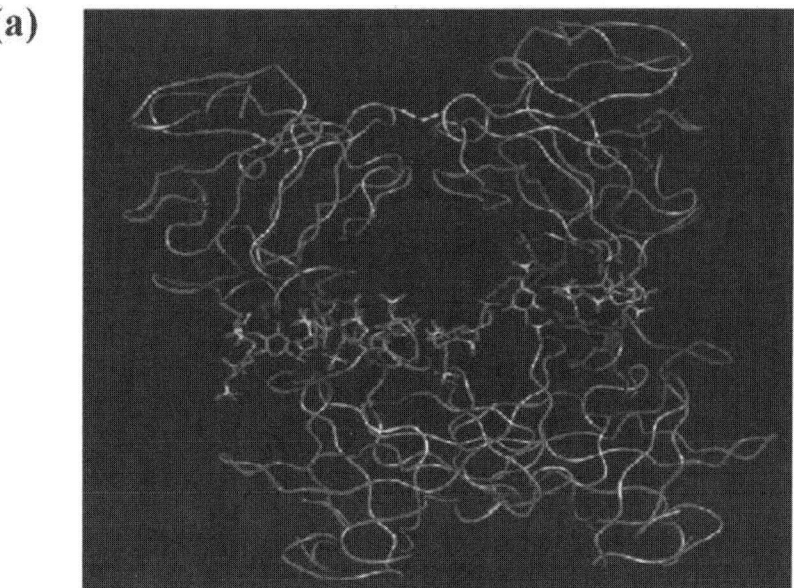

(b)

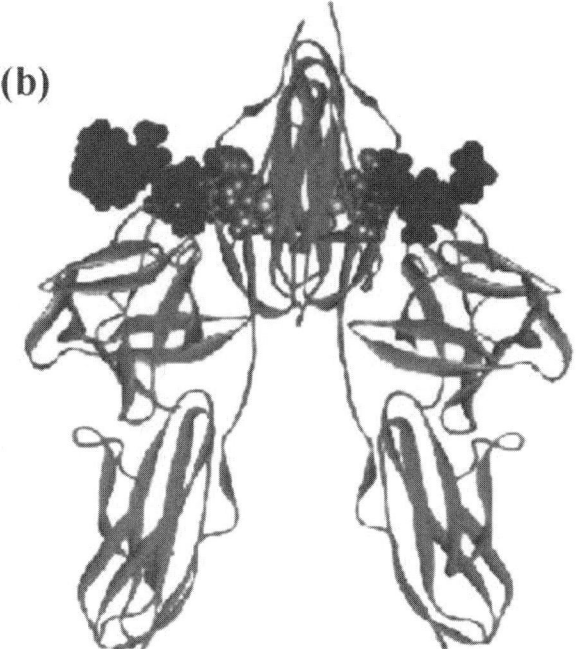

FIGURE 5.7 (a) NMR model of the heparin-induced oligomerization of FGF-2 as a prerequisite to receptor binding. FGF-2 is shown as a ribbon where side chains for residues involved in heparin binding are illustrated. Heparin is shown as a licorice bond representation colored by atom type. The putative receptor binding site is colored red and residues that incur chemical shift changes in the heparin-binding site from heparin-binding site are colored blue. (Reprinted with permission from reference [114], Copyright 1997 by American Chemical Society.) (b) X-ray model of an FGF2-FGFR1-heparin complex with 2:2:2 stoichiometry. FGFR (green) and FGF (cyan) are in ribbon representation and heparin is in a spacefill representation. (Reprinted with permission from reference [118]. Copyright 2001 by Elsevier Science.) See Color Plate 8.

has been applied to cytokines. Specifically, both the structures of interleukin-8 (IL-8) [138, 139] and interleukin-1β (IL-1β) [140] were determined early on by NMR. Again, this interest originates from the observation that cytokines are able to stimulate the proliferation and differentiation of a number of different cell types. This activity arises from the binding interaction of the cytokine with its specific receptor, where the cytokine-receptor binding interaction generates the intracellular signal. A variety of cancer cell lines are differentiated by the specific overexpression of a particular cytokine receptor that provides a potential opportunity for a therapeutic treatment for cancer [141–144].

Interleukin-4 (IL-4) [145, 146] and interleukin-13 (IL-13) [147, 148] are two cytokines of recent interest because of their overlapping biological function and important roles in asthma, allergy, and inflammatory response as well as their activity in cancer. IL-13 shares many functional properties with IL-4 as a result of the common IL-4Rα component in their receptors [146, 149]. Comparison of the solution structures of IL-4 [150–153] and IL-13 [154, 155] indicates a similarity in the overall fold of the proteins with the adoption of the short chain left-handed four-helix bundles observed in a number of cytokines [137] (Figures 5.6d and e). Based on the available structural and mutational data for IL-4 and IL-13, an IL-13/IL-4Rα model and a sequential mechanism for forming the signaling heterodimer has been proposed for IL-13. IL-4 binds the IL-4Rα chain of the IL-4R with high affinity and only binds the common γ_C chain after the complex with the IL-4Rα chain. Conversely, IL-13 does not bind the IL-4Rα chain until after the complex with IL-13Rα1 is formed. From the similarity of the IL-4 and IL-13 structure, a model for IL-13 complexed to IL-4Rα was based on the IL-4/IL-4Rα X-ray structure (Figure 5.8). The IL-13/IL-4Rα model indicates a suboptimal interaction between the two proteins consistent with the corresponding weak affinity. The model also suggests that a conformational change in IL-13 probably occurs upon the formation of the IL13/IL-13Rα1 complex as a prerequisite to recruit IL-4Rα to the ternary complex. The analysis of IL-4 and IL-13 represents a prime example of the complementary nature of NMR, X-ray, and mutagenesis data to further our understanding of protein function. In addition to IL-1β, IL-4, IL-8, and IL-13, solution structures for IL-2 [156], IL-6 [157], and IL-16 [158] have been determined by NMR.

3. Matrix-Metalloproteases

An exceptionally active area of research has been in the design of inhibitors against various matrix-metalloproteases (MMPs) for use as therapeutic agents in the treatment of cancer [81, 82] (Figures 5.6b and c). The MMP family consists of more than 25 enzymes, which in total are capable of hydrolyzing the major components of the extracellular matrix including collagens, elastins, proteoglycans, and matrix glycoproteins. The degradation of the extracellular matrix is associated with normal tissue remodeling and, as result, MMP expression and activity is highly controlled by tissue inhibitor of metalloendoproteases (TIMP). A number of biochemical stimuli, including oncogene products and tumor promoters, also affect the synthesis and activation of MMPs, which may contribute to the loss in MMP regulation and result in the pathological destruction of connective tissue and an ensuing disease state [159, 160]. The process

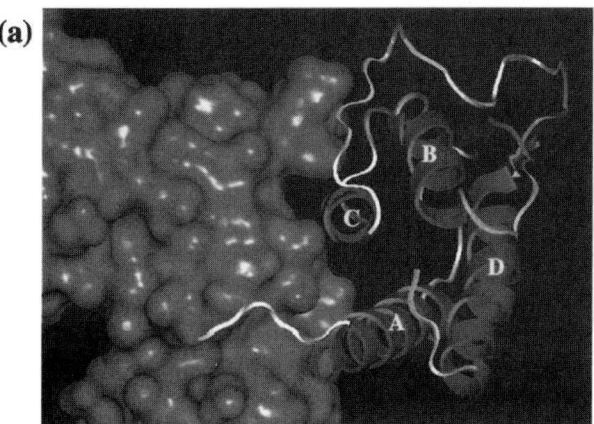

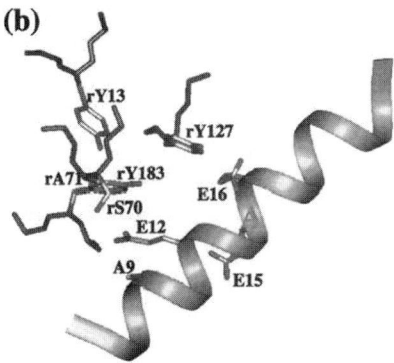

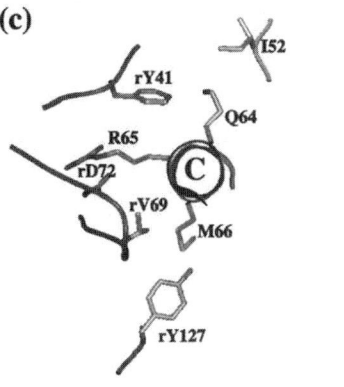

FIGURE 5.8 Interaction of IL-13 with its receptor. (a) IL-13/IL-4Rα model based on the IL-4/IL-4Rα X-ray structure (PDB ID:1IRA) [422]. IL-13 replaced IL-4 in the IL-4/IL-4Rα X-ray structure by overlaying IL-13 onto IL-4 based on the common secondary structure elements and cysteines. IL-4Rα is shown as a molecular surface (green) and IL-13 as a ribbon diagram colored by secondary structure, where the helices are colored purple and the β-sheets are colored yellow. Only the IL-13/IL-4Rα interface is illustrated. The secondary structure elements are labeled. (b) Expanded view of the IL-13/IL-4Rα binding site indicating the interaction with helix αA from IL-13. (c) Expanded view of the IL-13/IL-4Rα binding site illustrating the interaction with helix αC from IL-13. The side chains for critical residues based on the IL-4/IL-4Rα X-ray structure and mutational data are shown and labeled. Residues from IL-4Rα are labeled with the prefix "r." The side chains are colored by element type; the backbone atoms for IL-13 and IL-4Rα are colored magenta and blue, respectively. (Reprinted with permission from reference [154]. Copyright 2001 by Elsevier Science.) See Color Plate 9.

of cell metastasis inherently requires the tumorigenic cell to extradite itself from its current location, travel to a new destination, and integrate itself into its new surroundings. This process necessitates the degradation of the extracellular matrix at both cellular locations, which implicates the MMPs as being a critical component of metastasis and angiogenesis. As a result, extensive structural data has been collected for the MMP family [82] where NMR structures have been determined for MMP-1 (collagenase-1) [161, 162], MMP-2 (gelatinase A) [163], MMP-3 (stromelysin-1) [164–166], and MMP-13 (collagenase-3) [167, 168]. The MMPs are multi-domain proteins composed of a pre-domain involved in enzyme secretion, a pro-domain that is autoinhibitory, a catalytic domain responsible for enzyme activity, and a hemopexin-like domain involved in substrate recognition. A preponderance of the structural effort has focused on the catalytic domain based on the interest in drug design. The resulting availability of an abundance of MMP structural information has been successfully applied to the design of a plethora of MMP inhibitors that have successfully advanced to clinical trials. [169–172, 81, 82].

C. Protein-Ligand Complexes by NMR

The availability of the structure of the protein of interest provides an abundance of information critical to understanding the function and activity of the therapeutic target. As previously described, the structures for FGF-2, IL-13, and the MMPs have furthered our understanding of the role of heparin, the mechanism of protein-receptor complex formation, and the mechanism of peptide bond hydrolysis. Of course, access to the protein structure provides the groundwork for the design process for the development of inhibitors against the therapeutic targets. Fundamental to the structure-based drug design approach is the iterative cycle of obtaining a structure of the protein-ligand complex with each improvement in the compound's affinity. Obtaining structural information on a protein-ligand complex by NMR may arise from a number of novel approaches: high-resolution structure of the complex, conformation of the bound ligand from 2D trNOEs, or a hybrid-model approach combining specific structural information for a protein-ligand complex with a prior protein structure.

The NMR methodology for determining high-resolution protein structures has been previously described in detail [31, 39, 173]. Briefly, a prerequisite to the structure determination process is the availability of complete or nearly complete NMR resonance assignments for the protein as described in Section II.A.1.a. First, the regular secondary structure elements are identified from a qualitative analysis of sequential and inter-strand NOEs, NH exchange rates (hydrogen-bond restraints), $^3J_{HN\alpha}$-coupling constants, and the $^{13}C\alpha$ and $^{13}C\beta$ secondary chemical shifts. NOE distance restraints defining the protein structure are then identified from 3D ^{15}N-edited NOESY and ^{13}C-edited NOESY experiments. Also, φ, ψ, and χ torsion angle restraints are obtained from coupling constants, approximate distance restraints for intra-residue and sequential NOEs, and from chemical shift analysis using the TALOS program [174]. Also, a conformational database [175, 176] and radius of gyration [177] potential have been added to the structure calculation procedure to improve the quality of structures and increase the number of restraints. Recently, residual dipolar coupling constants obtained from proteins in aligned media have been incorporated into the refinement protocol [178] and have demonstrated the capability of significantly improving the quality of NMR structures with minimal restraints [179–182]. The total of available restraints and structural information are utilized to calculate structures of the protein using a hybrid distance geometry-dynamical simulated annealing method [138, 183–185].

To incorporate the ligand into the protein structure requires obtaining additional intermolecular NOEs between the protein and ligand and intramolecular NOEs for the ligand itself. This is accomplished by taking advantage of the different isotope labeling between the protein and ligand. In general, the protein is ^{13}C and ^{15}N labeled while the small molecule is unlabeled or natural abundance. By applying appropriate isotope-filtering and -editing techniques it is possible to selectively observe NMR resonances originating from either the protein or small molecule. Thus, traditional 2D-NOESY, COSY, and TOCSY spectra of a compound in the presence of the protein are obtained from 2D ^{12}C-filtering experiments [186–188] where only cross-peaks between protons attached to ^{12}C carbons are observed. These experiments efficiently filter all protein resonances and allow for the straightforward analysis of the compound spectrum in the presence of the protein. This information is then used to determine the bound conformation of the ligand. Intermolecular NOEs between the compound and the protein are obtained similarly by employing 3D ^{13}C-edited/^{12}C-filtered NOESY in combination with 3D ^{15}N-edited NOESY [189, 190]. The 3D ^{13}C-edited/^{12}C-filtered NOESY experiment only exhibits NOEs from protons directly attached to ^{13}C labeled carbons to protons attached to ^{12}C unlabeled carbons. Thus, NOEs are only observed between the labeled protein and the unlabeled compound; protein-protein and ligand-ligand NOEs are effectively filtered. This is not the case for the 3D ^{15}N-edited NOESY experiment. The protein-ligand NOEs have to be differentiated from the protein-protein NOEs. This is accomplished from comparison to the free protein spectra and/or focusing on protein amides associated with the ligand binding site identified from the 3D ^{13}C-edited/^{12}C-filtered NOESY and 2D ^{1}H-^{15}N HSQC spectra. The resulting ligand intramolecular NOEs and the ligand-protein intermolecular NOEs are added to the protein structural restraints to determine the structure of the complex.

The standard approach to determining a high-resolution solution structure of a protein-ligand complex lends itself to a hybrid method to expedite the data analysis process and refinement protocol [162]. The concept is based on merging the specific ligand intermolecular and intra-residue NOEs observed for a new compound with the complete data set previously used to determine a high-resolution solution structure of a protein. The complete restraint files for the protein are subsequently edited or filtered to remove restraints that are consistently violated in the structure calculation of the new complex. In this manner, preference is given to the new experimental restraints unique to the complex permitting the details of the binding site to be preferentially determined by the intermolecular NOES. The approach is equally applicable to either an inhibitor-free or protein-ligand complex as the reference structure. For a protein-ligand complex, the previous inter- and intra-molecular NOEs associated with the original inhibitor are simply replaced with the data for the new inhibitor.

The MMPs have been a very active and successful target for structure-based drug design programs, whereas the compounds identified from these efforts have potential utility as cancer therapies. The MMPs are involved in the degradation of the extracellular matrix, and the loss of control of their activity may contribute to metastasis and angiogenesis. The MMPs contain a catalytic domain that has been the focus of the structural effort for drug design based on the presentation of a "classic" enzymatic active site. This is in contrast to the more difficult challenge of identifying small MW compounds that may effectively inhibit protein-protein interactions such as observed in FGF-2 and IL-13.

Members of the MMP family exhibit a high similarity in the overall structural fold of the catalytic domain while maintaining a number of key features. In general, the protein is comprised of a five-stranded mixed parallel and anti-parallel β-sheet, three α-helices, and structural Zn and Ca ions. The enzyme active site contains a catalytic Zn coordinated by three histidines proximal to a variable sized S1′ pocket. The active site is bordered by β-strand IV, the Ca^{+2} binding loop, helix B, and a random coil region and contains additional shallow solvent exposed S2′, S3′ and unprimed S subsites.

It has been postulated that the toxicity demonstrated by many MMP inhibitors in clinical trials may result from non-specific inhibition. Thus, the current approach relies on structure-based design of inhibitors of specific MMPs, where selectivity against MMP-1 may be a desirable trait. The extensive structural data available for the MMPs [82] has enabled the identification of an obvious approach for designing specificity by taking advantage of the sequence difference and the distinct size and shape of the S1′ pocket (Figure 5.9). The high-resolution solution structures for inhibitor-free MMP-1 [161], MMP-1 complexed with CGS-27023A, and MMP-13 complexed with CPD-693 [167] readily illustrate this point (Figures 5.6b and c).

Comparison of the sequences in the active site between MMP-1 and MMP-13 indicates only three significant changes: an Arg to Leu, Asn to Leu, and Ile to Ser, respectively. The close sequence similarity in the active site between various MMPs is a common theme that makes it difficult to design selectivity into inhibitors based strictly on sequence differences. The most distinct structural difference between the MMPs that is readily amenable to incorporating specificity in drug design is the relative size and shape of the S1′ pocket. This is clearly evident by comparison of the S1′ pockets for MMP-13 and MMP-1 where the large difference in size of the pockets is striking (Figure 5.9). The S1′ pocket for MMP-13 nearly reaches the outer surface of the protein and is greater then twice the size of the MMP-1 pocket. The additional size of the MMP-13 S1′ pocket relative to MMP-1 is further illustrated by the filling capacity of the two inhibitors. In the MMP-1:CGS-27023A structure the p-methoxyphenyl effectively fills the available S1′ pocket for MMP-1. Conversely, in the MMP-13:CPD-693 complex, the p-methoxyphenyl only partially fills the available space. This structural difference suggests a ready approach for designing specificity between MMPs by taking advantage of the significant size difference of the S1′ pockets. Based on these structural differences, a novel, potent, and selective inhibitor for MMP-13 was designed from a weak HTS lead [191] (Figure 5.10). CPD-198 was identified as

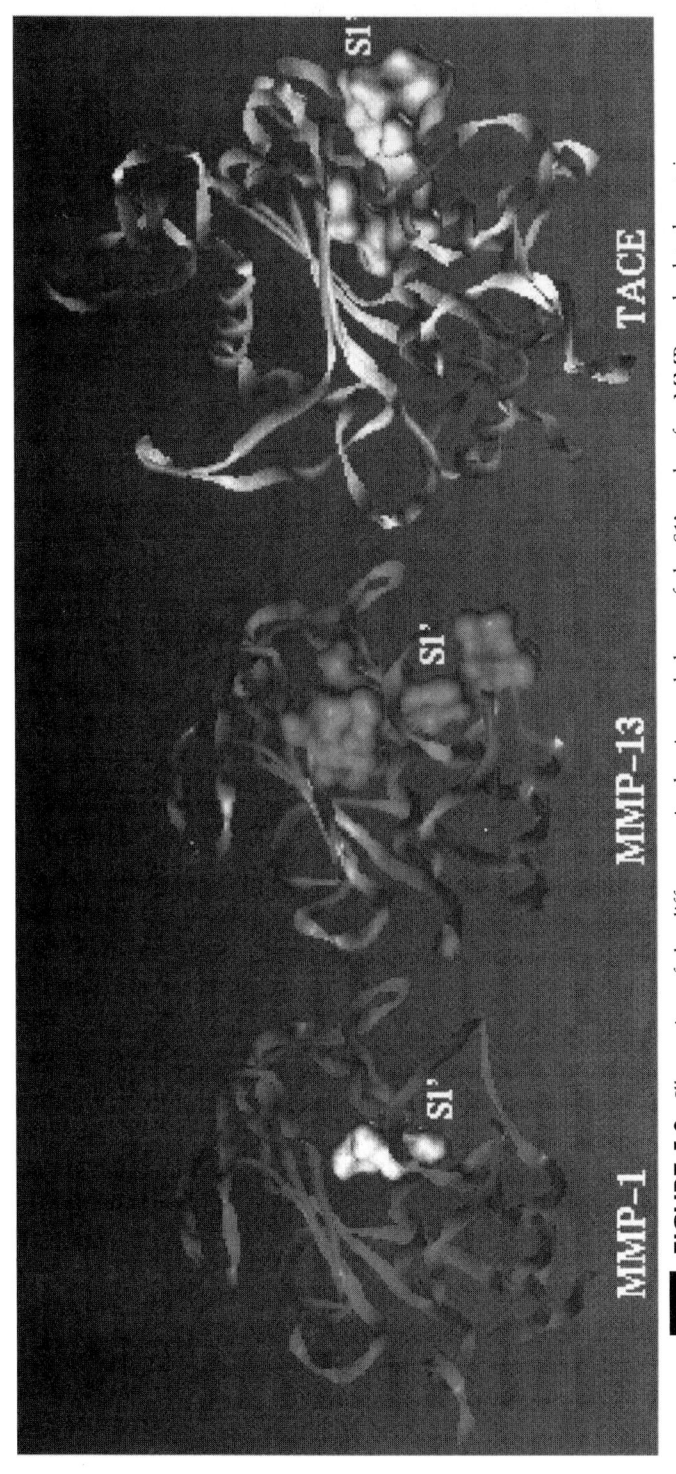

FIGURE 5.9 Illustration of the differences in the size and shape of the S1' pocket for MMPs and related proteins. Ribbon diagrams and S1' pockets for MMP-1, MMP-13, and TACE. See Color Plate 10.

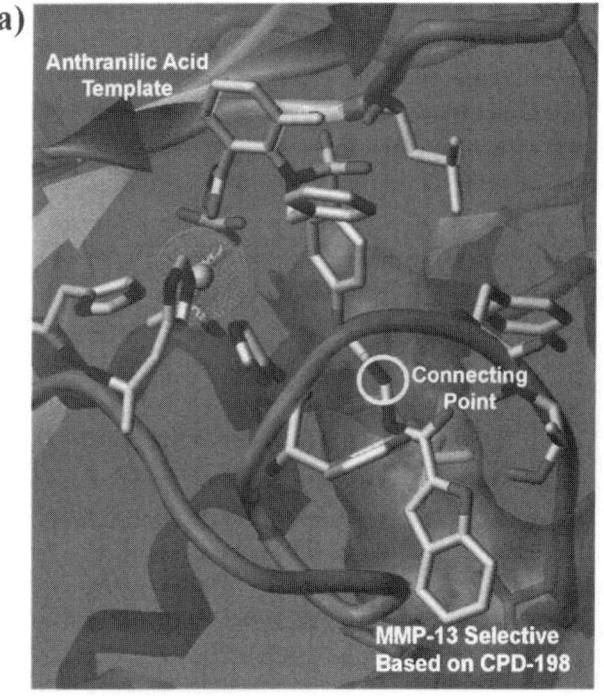

MMP-13	MMP-1	MMP-9	TACE
17nM	16%(10μM)	945 nM	19% (1μM)
selectivity	>5800x	56x	>500x

FIGURE 5.10 Application of the MMP NMR structures for the design of a novel, potent, and selective inhibitor for MMP-13. (a) Expanded view of the NMR MMP-13:CPD-198 complex overlaid with the MMP-13:CPD-177 model. This demonstrates the approach to forming the hybrid inhibitor CPD-523 where the MMP-13 active site is shown as a grid surface with CPD-198 and CPD-177 are shown with licorice bonds. (b) Design scheme showing the flow from CPD-198 and CPD-062 to CPD-523. The observed IC_{50} and selectivity against MMPs and TACE for inhibitor CPD-523 are listed below the design scheme. (Reprinted with permission from reference [191]. Copyright 2000 by American Chemical Society.) See Color Plate 11.

a weak (10 μM) inhibitor against MMP-13 while demonstrating no activity against MMP-1, MMP-9, or the related enzyme TACE. The structure of CPD-198 did not contain a Zn-chelating moiety and its binding interaction with MMP-13 was not obvious. An NMR structure for MMP-13 complexed with CPD-198 was determined by combining ^{1}H-^{15}N HSQC chemical shift perturbation data with intra- and inter-molecular NOEs from NMR-filtering/editing experiments. The model for MMP-13:CPD-198 complex was generated using the hybrid approach, described above, using the MMP-13:CPD-693 high-resolution solution structure as the reference structure. Standard molecular modeling and dynamics approaches were used to refine the resulting structure. The MMP-13:CPD-198 NMR structure indicates that morpholine binds proximal to the catalytic zinc where the oxygen forms a hydrogen bond with the backbone amide group of Leu-82 and the benzofuran group packs deep in the hydrophobic region of the S1' pocket with the peptide bond linker portion forming hydrogen bonds with protein backbone groups. The structure was then used as a template for the design of a chimera structure containing the MMP-13 selectivity features of CPD-198 combined with the high MMP-13 affinity of CPD-177. As anticipated, the resulting structure, CPD-523, maintained its high selectivity for MMP-13 while substantially increasing its affinity for the protein. CPD-523 exhibited an IC_{50} of 17 nM for MMP-13 while demonstrating a >5800, 56, and >500-fold selectivity against MMP-1, MMP-9, and TACE, respectively. The success of the MMP-13 inhibitor design effort validates the hybrid approach of protein-ligand structure determination by NMR and the design of inhibitor selectivity based on the size and shape of the S1' pocket. The MMP-13 inhibitor project is only one of a number of examples of the utilization of NMR as an aid in the drug discovery and design process [7, 12, 13, 15].

D. Dynamics Analysis by NMR

A unique feature of NMR that has significant potential and is generally underutilized in aiding the drug design process is the analysis of protein-ligand dynamics. Protein and ligand dynamics may have profound and unexpected impact on the effectiveness of a designed compound's activity that is not readily apparent from a static model of the protein [13]. Protein dynamics are generally monitored by NMR by measuring heteronuclear relaxation parameters (T_1, T_2, and NOE), where ^{15}N and ^{13}C relaxation values generally yield information about the protein's backbone and side-chain dynamics, respectively [192–194]. This arises from the relationship between the proteins correlation time (τ_c), the average time for a molecule to progress through one radian, and the mechanisms of the NMR relaxation process. For typical proteins, T_1 increases proportionally with τ_c, T_2 is inversely proportional to τ_C, and the magnitude of the NOE is proportional to the distance between the spin pair and a function of the correlation time ($1/r^6 \times f(\tau_c)$). In practice, the overall correlation time (τ_C) is ascertained from the T_1/T_2 ratio from each residue in the protein. While the τ_c provides a measure of the overall protein motion, local per residue motion is determined by the variation of measured T_1, T_2, and NOE values from the expected values based on the measured τ_c:

$$1/\tau = 1/\tau_c + 1/\tau_e$$

where τ_e is an effective correlation time describing the rapid internal motions associated with a particular residue. A model-free analysis of the relaxation data provides information on τ_e, the order parameter (S^2), and exchange rate (R_{ex}) [195, 196]. S^2 provides information about the angular amplitude of the internal motion of the bond vector studied and varies from 0 to 1. In general, order parameters close to one are consistent with a rigid structure, whereas low-order parameters are consistent with dynamic regions of the protein. In practice, regions of the protein that exhibit significantly lower order parameters relative to the average are usually characterized as a dynamic region of the protein structure. A residue exhibiting an exchange rate implies an additional slow motion on the millisecond timescale, which further implies a dynamic region of the protein.

As previously described, the abundance of structural data available for the MMPs has provided a mechanism for the structure-based design of numerous MMP inhibitors. A focal point of this effort has been the goal of designing compounds with selective affinity to a particular MMP. To accomplish this goal, the design effort has primarily taken advantage of distinct size and shape differences in the S1' pocket between various MMPs (Figure 5.9). The underlying assumption of this approach is a relatively static image of the MMP active site. NMR dynamic analysis of the MMPs has actually indicated that the active site of the proteins is inherently dynamic [161, 167, 197–199] (Figure 5.11). Furthermore, the nature of the inhibitor and its interaction with the protein can have differential affects on the active-site dynamics. The impact of the active-site mobility on drug design was clearly illustrated in recent MMP X-ray structures that demonstrated the ability of side chains in the active site to undergo conformational changes to accommodate a bound inhibitor [82, 200]. These inhibitors would be predicted to have a low affinity based on a poor fit in the active site from prior static images of the protein. Similarly, the dynamic behavior of a bound ligand may result in unexpected protein-affinity [424]. A series of hydroxamic acid compounds containing a butynyl P1' group were predicted not to bind MMP-1 because of strong steric clashes in the MMP-1 S1' pocket. Nevertheless, a number of these compounds exhibited high (5–40 nM) affinity that was attributed to both a slow exchange between two bound conformations and a second fast exchange between two additional bound conformations. Thus, the poor fit of the butynyl group in the MMP-1 S1' pocket is compensated by the compound maintaining a significant entropic contribution to its free energy of binding. Clearly, knowledge of the MMP active-site and ligand dynamics will influence design features of new compounds synthesized for MMP selectivity.

The analysis of MMP dynamics by NMR also illustrates an important caveat with interpreting X-ray structures from a dynamics perspective. It is generally accepted that regions of mobility in an X-ray structure are evident by relatively higher B factors [201]. Nevertheless, a correlation between

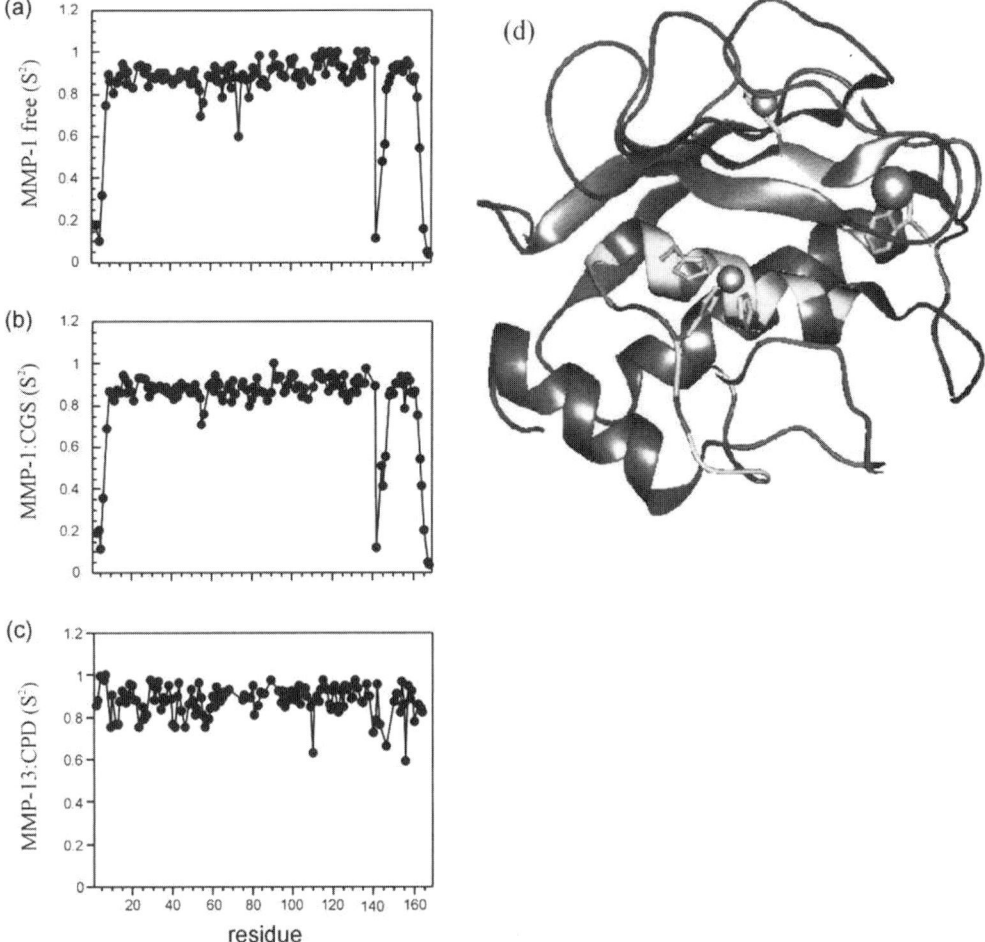

FIGURE 5.11 Residue plot of the order parameters (S^2) for (a) MMP-1 free, (b) MMP-1 complexed with CGS-27023A, and (c) MMP-13 complexed with CPD-693, which illustrates the mobility of the MMP active site and the effect of inhibitors on the mobility (from [167, 197]). (d) Ribbon diagram of MMP-1 with residues exhibiting doubling of peaks in the ^{1}H-^{15}NHSQC colored yellow, which indicates slow exchange, and the mobile active site loop is colored red. (Reprinted with permission from reference [167]. Copyright 2000 by Elsevier Science. Also reprinted with permission from reference [197]. Copyright 1997 by Kluwer Academic Publishers.) See Color Plate 12.

X-ray B factors and NMR order parameters does not always occur, because other factors such as crystal packing interactions may induce artificially low or high B factors [202–207]. The lack of a correlation between B factors and order parameters is evident in the MMP structures where a majority of the MMP X-ray structures exhibit low B factors for active-site residues [82]. Again, the utility of NMR for the analysis of protein dynamics validates the complementary roles of X-ray and NMR techniques in structural biology programs.

III. MASS SPECTROMETRY IN ANTICANCER DRUG DISCOVERY

MS is a powerful tool in cancer research. This became possible within the last quarter century with the advent of very soft ionization techniques and the availability of tandem MS. With soft-ionization techniques, molecular ions of thermally unstable materials can be reliably generated enabling materials of pharmaceutical and biological origin to be readily identified and characterized. These ionization techniques include FAB, ESI, and MALDI. (See Table 5.1 for definitions of MS and related terms.) By collisionally activating the molecular

TABLE 5.1   Mass Spectrometry and Related Terms and Definitions

Term	Definition-description	Ref.
Ionization methods		
EI	Electron impact ionization: electrons used to ionize gas-phase analytes under vacuum	[399]
CI	Chemical ionization: ionized reagent gas molecules used to ionize analytes by ion-molecule reactions	[400]
FI	Field ionization: high-electric fields (generated using emitters consisting of carbon dendrites) ionize gaseous analytesunder vacuum	[401]
FD	Field desorption: high-electric fields ionize condensed-phase analytes residing on the emitter dendrites	[401, 402]
CfPD	Californium plasma desorption: high-energy fission fragments of Californium-252 used to ionize condensed-phase analytes	[403]
SIMS	Secondary ionization mass spectrometry: ion beams used to produce secondary ions from condensed-phase analytes	[404]
FAB	Fast atom bombardment: high-energy ion or neutral gas beams used to ionized analytes residing in a liquid matrix (also referred to as liquid-SIMS)	[405]
TSP	Thermospray: thermally vaporizing a solution often inthe presence of a volatile buffer (ammonium acetate) to aid in ionization	[406, 407]
ESI	Electrospray ionization: spraying (often with nebulization) of a liquid solution through a capillary maintained at high voltage to create charged analytes	[408, 409]
APCI	Atmospheric pressure chemical ionization: the use of a corona discharge to ionize gaseous analytes at atmospheric pressure	[409]
MALDI	Matrix-assisted laser desorption/ionization: analyte residing ina solid matrix is desorbed and ionized by a high-energy laser pulse	[410, 411]
SELDI	Surface-enhanced laser desorption ionization: the MALDI probe surface is modified to affinity capture analytes of interest for MALDI analysis	[412]
LD/PI	Two step laser desorption/laser photoionization: the use of two lasers serially to desorb/volatilize (IR) and photoionize (UV) analytes of interest	[413]
ICP	Inductively coupled plasma mass spectrometry: used principally for the generation of ions from inorganic and organometallic materials for qualitative and quantitative analysis	[414]

(Continues)

TABLE 5.1 (*Continued*)

Term	Definition-description	Ref.
Methods for ion activation and ion monitoring		
CID	Collision-induced dissociation: fragmentation of gaseous analytes induced by collisions of parent ions with neutral reagent gas to produce product ions	[415–417]
MRM, SRM	Multiple (selected) ion reaction monitoring: the monitoring in time of the product ion abundances produced by CID and used generally for analyte quantitation	[415]
TIC, SIC	Total (selected) ion current chromatogram: the monitoring in time of the total or selected ion currents produced in mass spectra and displayed as a mass chromatogram	
MS chromatographic inlets		
GC	Gas chromatography	[418]
HPLC	High performance liquid chromatography	[407, 419]
SCF	Super critical fluid chromatography	[420]
CZE	Capillary zone electrophoresis	[421]

ions into interpretable fragment ions using tandem MS, the structures of anticancer agents and their reaction products can be elucidated. With modern instrumentation, the processes of molecular ion production and their induced fragmentation can be achieved with very high sensitivity and high resolution. Selected applications of MS in the field of cancer research will be covered. The principal illustrations include the use of MS for the discovery and structure elucidation of anticancer drugs and natural products, mechanisms of action of selected anticancer drugs studied by MS, metabolic profiling of selected anticancer drugs, diagnostic applications of MS in cancer detection and the screening of chemical libraries for anticancer agents. Two extensive reviews have been authored by John Roboz covering this broad subject; the most recent review consists of a comprehensive book titled *Mass Spectrometry in Cancer Research* [208, 209].

B. MS Structure Determination and Characterization of Anticancer Agents

The developments in MS and its selected applications to anticancer chemotherapeutic agents are presented in historical order. The earliest work illustrated corresponds to the efforts in discovering general chemotherapeutic agents that targeted DNA and the corresponding efforts by MS to discover ionization methods capable of producing molecular ions and biomechanistic information for these general anticancer agents. In more recent work, new ionization techniques that are quite universal, sensitive, and capable of analyzing both small molecules and high MW biomolecules have been used to facilitate the development of significantly more complex therapeutic agents, which include specific chemical reagents capable of targeting specific cancers.

1. Thiotepa

Thiotepa (N,N′,N″-triethylenethiophosphoramide, MW 189) is an older chemotherapeutic anticancer agent that acts by alkylating DNA and is prescribed for treating solid tumors and various leukemias often at high doses and in combination with other anticancer agents. Mass spectrometric methods were developed for characterizing the structure of thiotepa and related therapeutic agents. A battery of mass spectral ionization techniques has been used to study thiotepa and related agents and their fragmentation processes. The ionization methods include EI [210], FI [211–214], HPLC-thermospray [215], SCF-CI [216], FD [212, 217], FAB [217, 218], CfPD [219], and HPLC-ESI [220–222]. These mass spectral ionization techniques were used to characterize degradation products and metabolites from animal and human origin. The reported degradation products include triethylenephosphamide (Tepa) and the addition of up to three HCl molecules with one to each of the aziridine rings forming 2-chloro ethyl moieties [211, 223–225]. All of these molecules were also observed as metabolites [226, 227]. Another metabolite reported was a thiotepa-mercapturate conjugate [218, 220, 228]. Model metabolites prepared and analyzed were a thiotepa-glutathione conjugate [221, 229] and a thiotepa-hemoglobin conjugate [221]. Also studied was the effect of hydrazine sulfate on inhibiting thiotepa metabolite formation [230] and metabolite stability [231].

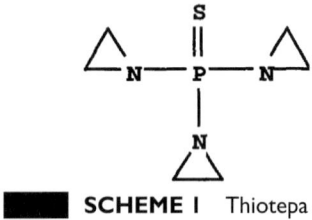

SCHEME 1   Thiotepa

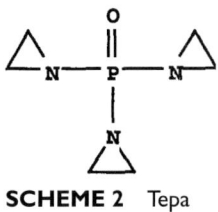

SCHEME 2   Tepa

The interaction of thiotepa with alkylating reagents was studied extensively by MS to understand the reaction chemistry and to model the biological activity of thiotepa. Among the studies conducted was the evaluation of the alkylation reaction of thiotepa with four different nucleic acid bases and the determination of the site of alkylation [213, 215, 219, 232–238].

2. Methotrexate

Methotrexate is an established anticancer agent employed in the treatment of solid tumors and leukemias and more recently as an immunosuppressive agent. As an anticancer agent, methotrexate inhibits dihydrofolate reductase in the biosynthesis of nucleic acids thereby blocking the synthesis of DNA. Methotrexate cannot be analyzed directly by EI but as the permethylated derivative instead [239, 240]. The general application of MS to methotrexate-related analytical problems was restrained until the advent of soft ionization techniques. Molecular ions of methotrexate and related metabolites can be directly generated by DCI [241], FD [242–244], CfPD [245], FAB [246], SIMS [247, 248], and ESI [249–252]. ESI/MS and ESI/MS/MS coupled with HPLC have been utilized in high-throughput sampling modes for the quantitative analysis of methotrexate and its metabolites in human urine and plasma [249–252] and for quantitating methotrexate in wipe and air environmental samples for monitoring human exposure in a hospital setting [253]. Some impurities in methotrexate parenteral dosage forms were characterized by GC/MS [254]. A MALDI/MS method was reported for the determination of the average number of methotrexate molecules covalently conjugated to a protein useful for eliciting antibody responses from drugs [255]. A pulsed ultrafiltration technique coupled with ESI/MS was developed for the screening and detection of receptor-bound ligands to dihydrofolate reductase. The method identified methotrexate and aminopterin as the two compounds with the highest affinity from a compound library consisting of 22 components [256].

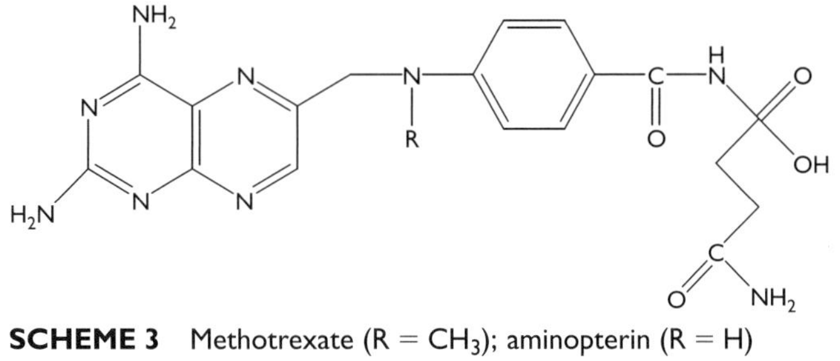

SCHEME 3   Methotrexate (R = CH$_3$); aminopterin (R = H)

3. Mitoxantrone

Mitoxantrone is an anticancer anthraquinone agent often used to treat leukemias and solid tumors, and its activity is due to its ability to intercalate with DNA. Its popularity stems from its low cardiac toxicity. The majority of work reported using MS is related to the identification and characterization of low-level metabolites present in biological fluids. Further verification and elucidation by NMR and synthesis followed the MS analysis. Isolation techniques have been demonstrated utilizing sequential and different combinations of adsorption on glass wool, C18-Sep-Pak cartridges, HPLC, preparative HPLC, HPLC/MS, and HPLC/MS-MS [251–255]. These approaches are routinely used in MS laboratories specializing in metabolism studies.

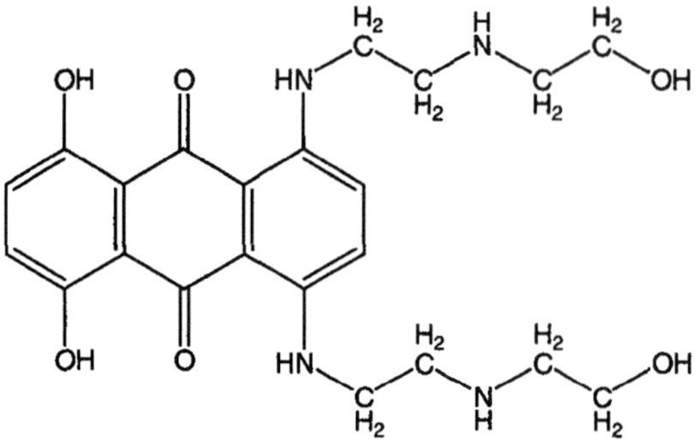

SCHEME 4   Mitoxantrone

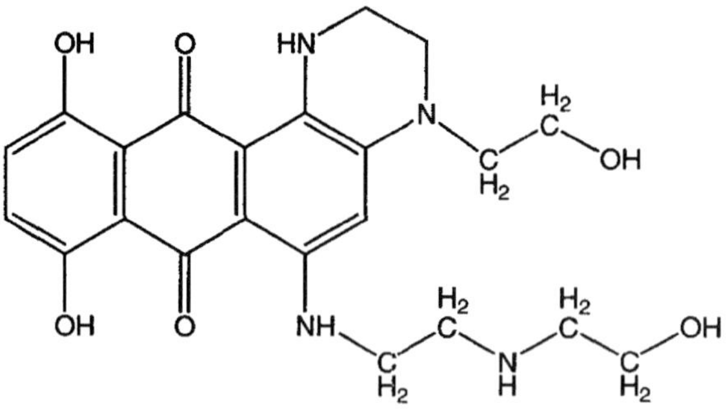

SCHEME 5   Mitoxantrone oxidation metabolite

Among the mitoxantrone urinary metabolites observed are the mono- and di-carboxylic acids resulting from the oxidation of the terminal hydroxyl groups of the side chains [257, 258], oxidation products of the phenylene diamine moiety [259], and glucuronic acid metabolites [258, 259]. Three thioether biliary metabolites of mitoxantrone were observed in addition to the above oxidation metabolites [260, 261].

A useful mass spectral analysis tool was demonstrated using mitoxantrone where the number of labile hydrogen atoms in the molecule could be routinely determined from condensed phase thermospray MS studies [262]. This approach also can be extended to the condensed phase ionization techniques of FAB [263], electrospray [264], and MALDI [265].

4. Cisplatin and Analogs

Cisplatin and related analogs — potent anticancer agents for ovarian, testicular, and bladder cancers — have historically been difficult samples to analyze. A routine analytical method for obtaining the FAB mass spectra of cisplatin, $Pt(NH_3)_2(Cl)_2$, and its analogs of the type PtL_ACl_2 and PtL_AL_B, where L_A is a bidentate amine ligand and L_B is a bidentate carboxylate ligand, utilized a mixed solvent system of dimethylsulfoxide:thioglycerol 1:3 v/v as the FAB matrix [266]. Prominent ions observed for cisplatin in the positive ion mode were $[M + H + DMSO]^{1+}$ and $[M\text{-}Cl + DMSO]^{1+}$, whereas in the negative mode the prominent ion observed was $[M + Cl]^{1-}$. For PtL_ACl_2, abundant positive ions observed were $[M + H + DMSO]^{1+}$, $[M\text{-}Cl + DMSO]^{1+}$, and $[L_A + H]^{1+}$, whereas in the negative mode $[M + Cl]^{1-}$ and $[M\text{-}H + Thioglycerol]^{1-}$ were observed. For PtL_AL_B, abundant positive ions observed were $[M + H + DMSO]^{1+}$, $[M + H]^{1+}$, and $[L_A + H]^{1+}$, whereas in the negative mode $[M\text{-}H]^{1-}$, $[M\text{-}H + Thioglycerol]^{1-}$, and $[(L_B + 2H)\text{-}H]^{1-}$ were observed. The mixed solvent system served as a solvation and reaction medium for efficiently producing reliable FAB mass spectra and for the partial displacement of the ligands for ease in their identification. FAB-MS has been a popular soft-ionization technique for the analysis of cisplatin analogs [267–270].

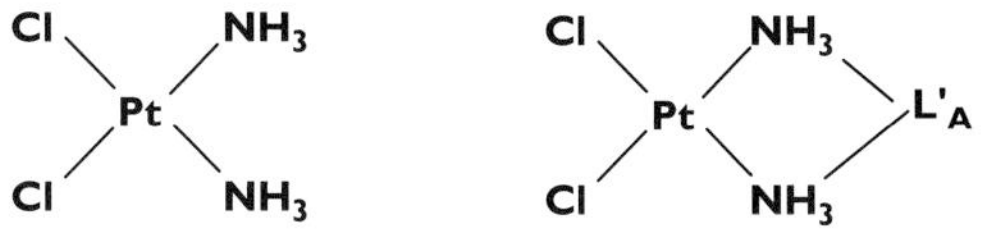

SCHEME 6   Cisplatin

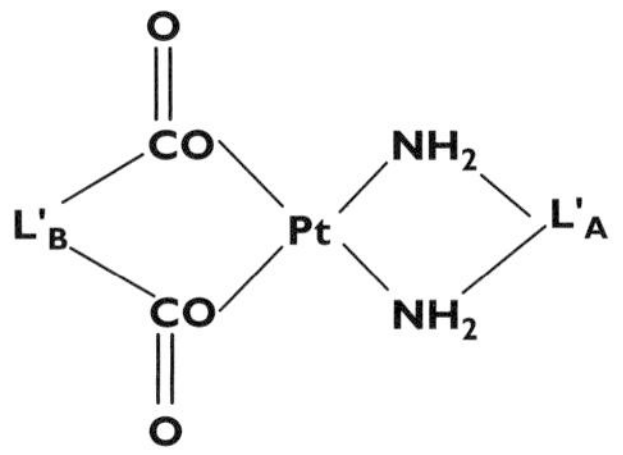

SCHEME 7   Cisplatin analogs

Recent work with more soluble cisplatin analogs has been performed using ESI-MS [271, 272], ESI-MS-MS [273], and ICP-MS [274] with and without HPLC and CZE interfaces. To a lesser extent UV- and IR-MALDI-MS [275, 276] have also been investigated in studies of cisplatin analogs. In all cases, the results suggest that these techniques are more sensitive than that of FAB-MS.

The mechanism of action of cisplatin and its analogs is to bind with cellular DNA. This reaction has been extensively modeled by studying the reaction products of cisplatin and its analogs with short representative strands of DNA using MS. In FAB-MS studies [277], intact molecular ions in the positive and negative ionization modes were observed as well as fragments arising from the loss of one or two ammonia groups. Under FAB-MS-MS high-energy, collision-induced dissociation conditions, fragment ions consistent with the DNA platinum binding site were observed that corresponded to platinum adducts with one and two nucleobases (B_x, B_y), viz. $Pt(NH_3)_{0-2}(B_x$ or $B_y)$ and $Pt(NH_3)_{0-2}(B_xB_y)$. Model DNA-cisplatin analog association constants were determined using ESI-MS [278] and platination rate constants were determined using ESI-MS and MALDI-MS [279]. Side effects of cisplatin therapy are believed to arise from the formation of protein-platinum complexes. Studies of the reaction of cisplatin and its analogs with ubiquitin by ESI-MS exhibited a variety of platinum-containing ubiquitin adducts where the platinum was bound to the ubiquitin at from one to three sites [280].

Other modeling studies of the reactions of cisplatin and analogs with endogenous compounds using mass spectrometric detection include interactions with cysteine [281], glutathione [281], 5′-guanosine mono phosphate [282, 283], dipeptides [284], selenomethionine [285], nucleotides [286], and metabolite formation [274, 287, 288].

5. Enediyne Antibiotics/Anticancer Drugs Conjugated to Antibodies and Proteins

The enediyne structural class of antibiotics has potent anti-tumor activity. These antibiotics contain a cyclic enediyne moiety, protein, or novel sugars and a substructure that serves as a chemical trigger to activate the molecule. The protein or sugars serve as a vehicle for protecting the enediyne and for DNA-binding. Upon chemically activating the trigger mechanism, a free diradical is generated from the enediyne moiety that acts as a warhead to induce DNA damage. The subject of enediyne antibiotics as anti-tumor agents has been extensively reviewed in a text edited by Borders and Doyle [289]. For the enediyne antibiotics, MS has been used extensively to initially characterize the overall structures and degradation products, whereas NMR and X-ray crystallography have been used to elucidate the connectivities of the substructures. From this work the structures of the enediyne antibiotics were determined.

Calicheamicin is a very potent anti-tumor antibiotic and the only enediyne compound presently used commercially as an anticancer agent. The elemental formula for the N-acetyl-calicheamicin γ_1^I and its degradation products were determined by high-resolution exact-mass FAB-MS. From this information together with NMR and X-ray crystallographic substructure data, the overall structure for calicheamicin was determined [290–293]. Figure 5.12 illustrates the exact masses obtained using FAB-MS for the molecular ion of N-acetyl-calicheamicin γ_1^I (Figure 5.12A) and its reacted form (Figure 5.12b) as well as all the observed fragment ions. From these exact masses, the molecular formula as well as the elemental formulas for the chemical substructures were determined. The chemical trigger for this molecule is the allylic methyl trisulfide group, which when chemically reduced to an allylic sulfhydryl group, triggers the warhead to undergo the reaction of N-acetyl-calicheamicin γ_1^I (Figure 5.12A) to its reacted form (Figure 5.12B) via the formation of a diradical with the abstraction of two hydrogen atoms from DNA or in its absence from the local chemical environment. The number of labile hydroxyl groups present in the fragment ions of calicheamicin degradation products was confirmed by acetylation. The structures of the esperamicin enediyne antibiotics were elucidated in a fashion similar to that of the calicheamicins [294]. One novel set of mass spectrometric experiments used to confirm the esperamicin A_{1c} structure and the biosynthetic origin of the sulfur atoms in the molecule was performed when the molecule was produced in a broth enriched in media containing sodium sulfate where the sulfur was enriched as sulfur 34. By comparing the nominal masses of the fragment ions of the natural and enriched esperamicin A_{1c}, the sites containing sulfur were confirmed and clearly defined the presence of the methyl trisulfide moiety [295] (Figure 5.13).

N-Acetyl Calicheamicin $\gamma_1{}^I$: High Resolution FAB Data

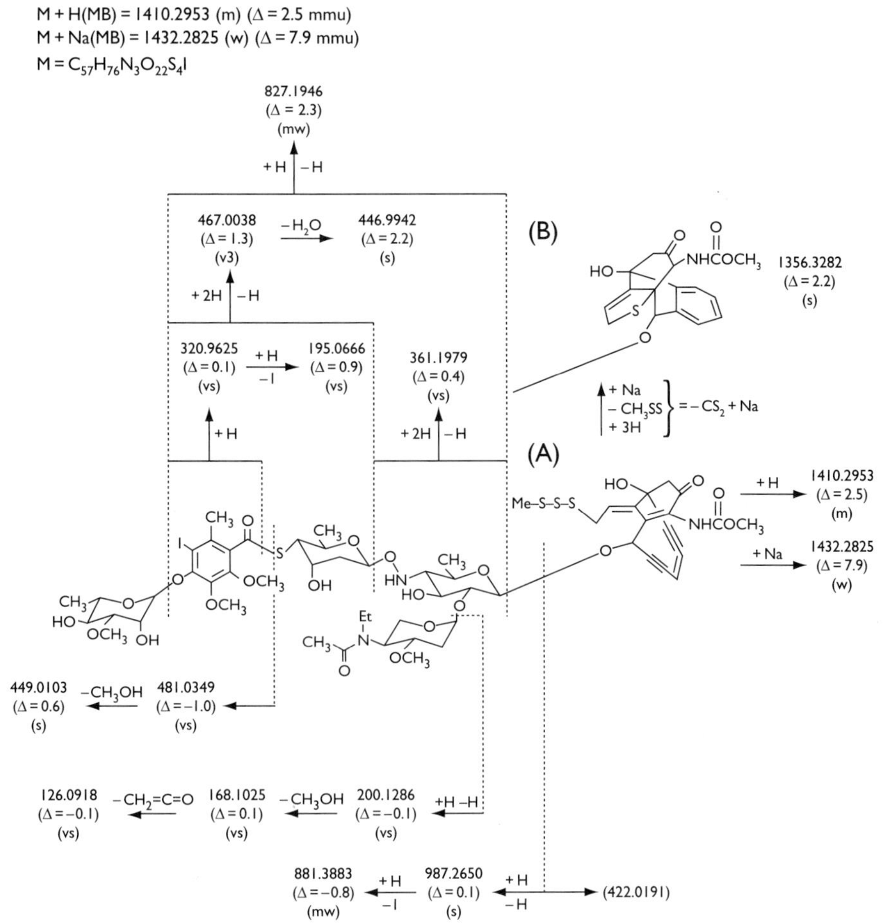

$M + H(MB) = 1410.2953$ (m) ($\Delta = 2.5$ mmu)
$M + Na(MB) = 1432.2825$ (w) ($\Delta = 7.9$ mmu)
$M = C_{57}H_{76}N_3O_{22}S_4I$

FIGURE 5.12 FAB-MS exact-mass fragment ion structural assignments for (A) N-acetyl-calicheamicin $\gamma_1{}^I$, and (B) its reacted form. The trigger corresponds to the methyl trisulfide group, the warhead to the unit corresponding to mass of 422 containing the enediyne group and the body of the molecule corresponding to linked polysaccharide groups. The mass errors (Δ) are in millimass units.

Mass spectrometry has been applied to assist in the elucidation of the mechanism of action of the core structure of the enediyne protein antibiotic neocarzinostatin [296]. Figure 5.14a illustrates the FAB tandem mass spectrum for the neocarzinostatin core structure. After activation of the enediyne with NaBH$_4$ in the presence of H$_2$O/CH$_3$OH, the observed FAB tandem mass spectrum and fragment ion assignments are as illustrated in Figure 5.14b. Note that the naphthoate group is missing and that the cyclic enediyne moiety has been converted to a fused tricyclic ring system. When the same experiment was performed with an excess of DNA present with NaBD$_4$ in D$_2$O, only one

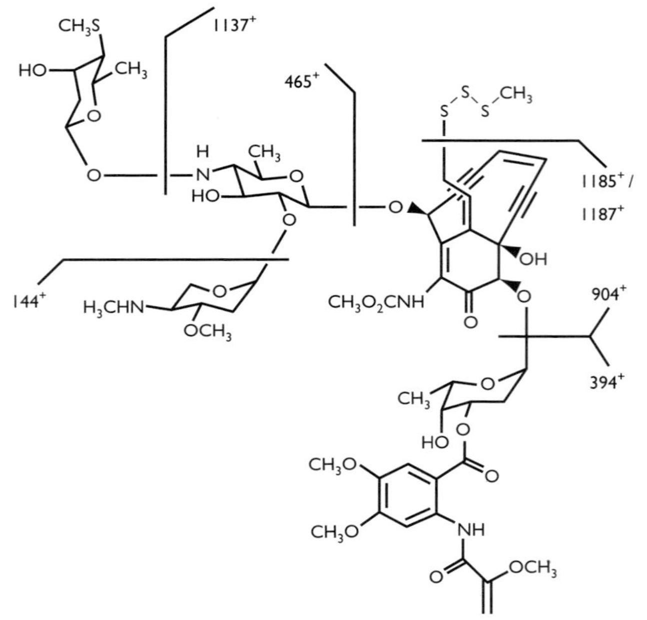

^{32}S – Esperamicin A_{1c}

Accurate Mass : 1296.3860 ($C_{57}H_{76}N_4O_{22}S_4$, 2.0 ppm)

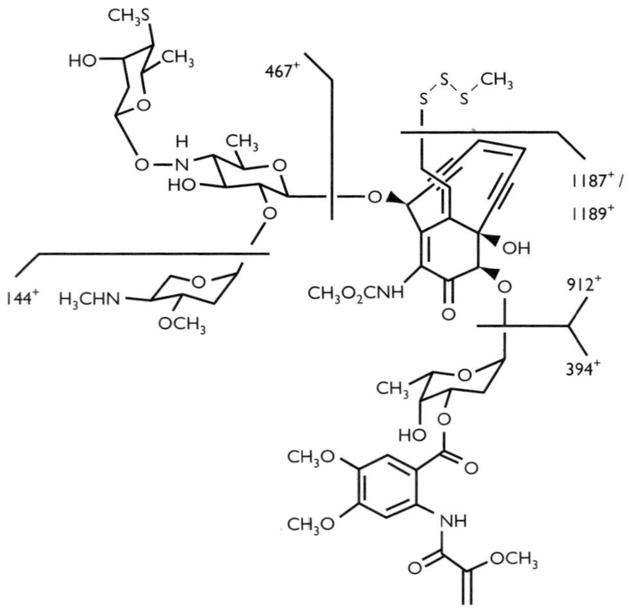

^{34}S – Esperamicin A_{1c}

Accurate Mass : 1304.3630 ($C_{57}H_{76}N_4O_{22}{}^{34}S_4$, 2.6 ppm)

FIGURE 5.13 Comparison of the fragment ion structural assignments for unenriched ^{32}S-esperamicin A_{1c} (MW 1296) and biosynthetically enriched ^{34}S-esperamicin A_{1c} (MW 1304). The mass shifts between similar substructures identify the numbers of sulfur atoms present in each substructure. The most unique feature of the data is the presence of the methyl trisulfide group deduced from the mass differences between the parent and highest mass fragment ions for the enriched and unenriched samples, respectively. (Reprinted with permission from reference [295]. Copyright 1995 by Marcel Dekker, Inc.)

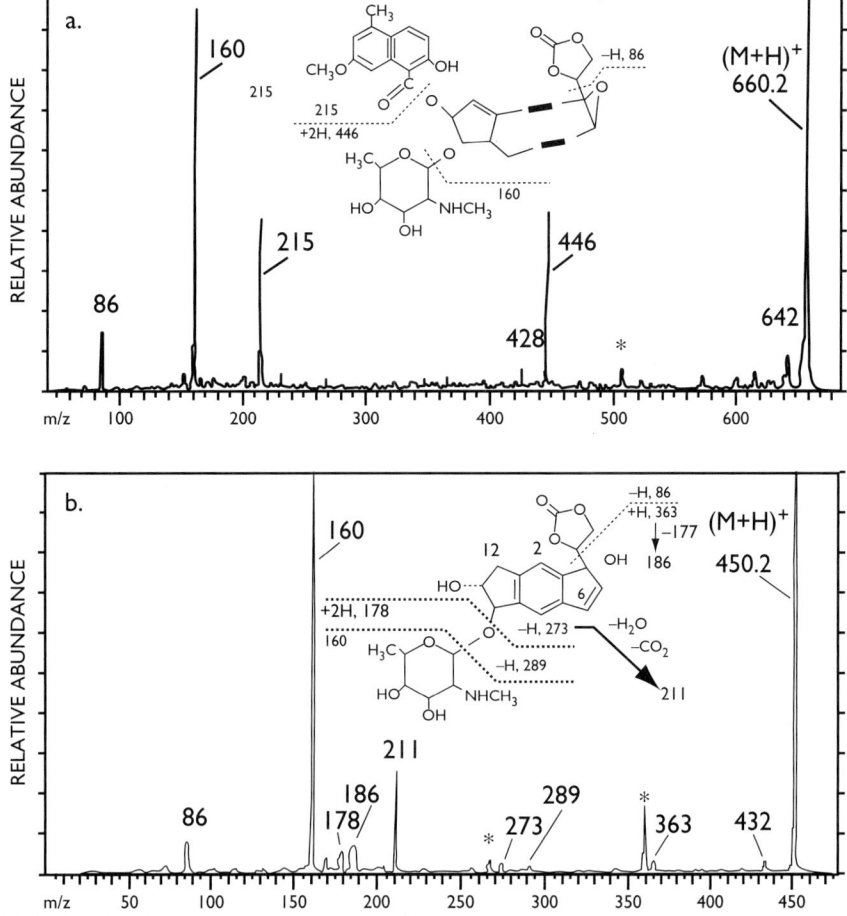

FIGURE 5.14 FAB-MS-MS spectrum of (a) the neocarzinostatin core structure $[M+H]^{1+}$ parent ion m/z 660.2, and (b) after activation by reduction with $NaBH_4$ with $[M+H]^{1+}$ parent ion m/z 450.2. When reduction is performed with $NaBD_4$ in D_2O with excess DNA present, only one deuterium atom was incorporated into the core structure as indicated by the mass shift in the m/z 211 fragment ion to m/z 212. NMR demonstrated that the site of incorporation was C-12 and corresponded to the trigger site for the reaction. Peaks marked with an asterisk are FAB matrix related. (Reprinted with permission from reference [296]. Copyright 1998 by the American Chemical Society.)

deuterium atom was incorporated into the activated neocarzinostatin core structure as indicated in the spectrum by the shift in the mass of the fragment ion initially from m/z 211 to m/z 212. This reversed isotope-labeling experiment indicates that one deuterium was incorporated into the molecule upon activating the trigger of the molecule while two hydrogen atoms were extracted from the DNA and not the sample solvent. NMR data confirmed that the deuterium atom was at C-12 (the trigger point) and that C-2 and C-6 are the sites of the free radicals. ESI-MS non-covalent binding studies of the neocarzinostatin chromophores (R = H and CH_2OH) demonstrated that a bulged 22-mer DNA bound as a 1:1 complex only when R = H and not when R = CH$_2$OH which indicated the specificity of this binding and the ability of ESI-MS to detect this small structural difference [297].

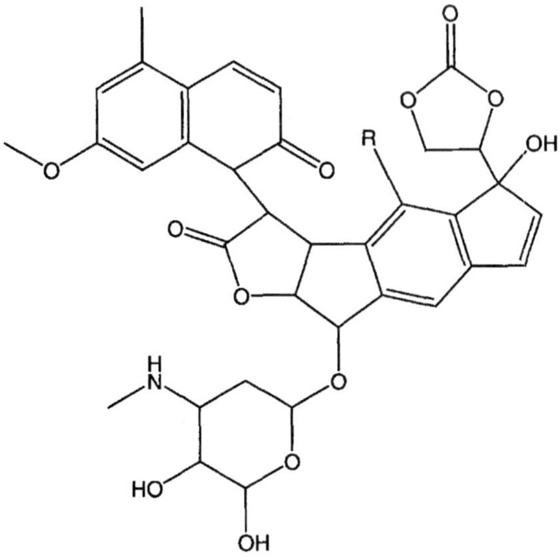

SCHEME 8   Neocarzinostatin chromophores [R = H or CH$_2$OH]

For anticancer therapy, the enediyne antibiotic calicheamicin is administered covalently attached to a cancer-seeking antibody via a chemical linker. In this way, the antibody targets the cancer cells and delivers to that site a known anticancer agent. Mylotarg (gemtuzumab ozogamicin) is a compound where N-acetyl-calicheamicin γ_1^I is covalently linked with AcBut, a hydrolyzable linker, to hP67.6 antibody, a humanized murine antibody that targets cells with the CD33 myeloid antigen, common with cells of acute myeloid leukemia (AML) [298, 299]. Infrared MALDI-MS has been used to determine the average number and distribution of conjugated calicheamicin [300]. Figure 5.15 illustrates a bimodal distribution of drug and the deconvoluted peaks corresponding to the addition of a drug molecule for each peak of increasing mass with an average drug loading of 5.54 calicheamicin molecules per antibody. Note that these measurements covered the mass range up to 400,000 Da and utilized laser irradiation in the IR region where calicheamicin is stable as opposed to the UV region where it is unstable. Similar drug-loading studies of other anticancer drugs (mitoxantrone, doxorubicin, methotrexate, aminopterin, and vincristine) as well as metal chelators (for delivering imaging or radioactive reagents to sites of tumors) covalently conjugated to cancer-seeking antibodies [255, 301] and proteins [301, 302] have been reported utilizing UV-MALDI-MS and ESI-MS. The use of MS for characterizing pure monoclonal antibodies for treating cancers such as Herceptin (for advanced breast cancer), Retuxan (for B-cell non-Hodgkin's lymphoma), and 17–1A (for intestinal cancer) have not yet been reported.

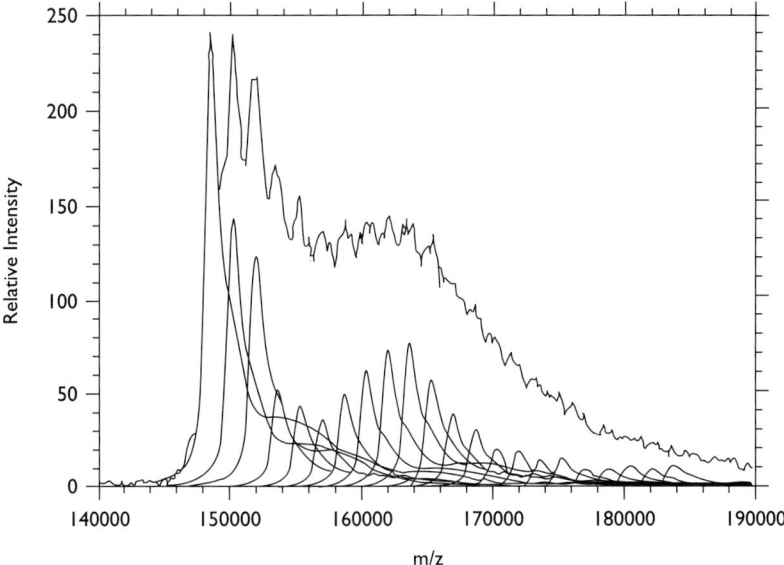

FIGURE 5.15 IR-MALDI mass spectrum of N-acetyl-calicheamicin conjugated to monoclonal antibody hP67.6 for the singly charged parent ions in the *m/z* range of 140,000–190,000. The experimental and mathematically fitted peak profiles are illustrated. A bimodal distribution is illustrated with an average loading of 5.54 calicheamicin molecules per antibody. (Reprinted with permission from reference [300]. Copyright 1997 by the American Chemical Society.)

6. Photofrin

Photodynamic treatment of cancer is based on the ability of a non-toxic sensitizer to accumulate more selectively in tumors than surrounding tissues. Irradiation of treated tumors with light produces singlet oxygen that ultimately leads to tumor necrosis. Photofrin is the first commercially developed non-toxic sensitizer used for anticancer photodynamic therapy. Photofrin is prepared from hematoporphyrin, which after undergoing a series of reactions and purifications, is isolated as a high MW fraction by a diafiltration process. A variety of mass spectral ionization techniques were used independently to characterize Photofrin. The methods used included FAB, UV-MALDI, IR-MALDI, ESI, and LD/PI. The results of these studies demonstrated that Photofrin consists of a distribution of porphyrin oligomers with an average oligomer number of about 2.8 porphyrin units [303, 304] (Figure 5.16). The unique feature of these measurements is that similar oligomer distributions were obtained using vastly different mass spectral ionization techniques that provided confidence in the validity of these independent measurements. The reaction products of analogs of hematoporphyrin were characterized by MS, which demonstrated that the porphyrin oligomers observed in Photofrin are linked by ether and ester bonds [304].

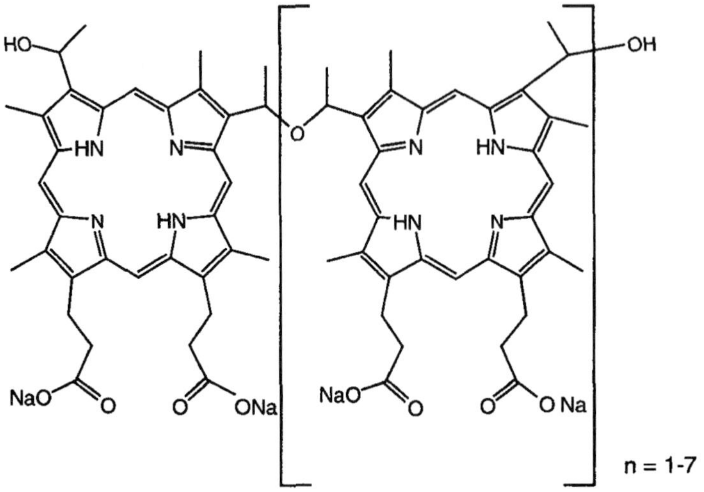

SCHEME 9   Photofrin (ether linkage)

While previous compounds used in photodynamic therapy were mixtures, researchers are presently developing newer photosensitizing agents that are pure materials that absorb radiation in the 660–800 nm range; a more penetrating region that is longer than the 630-nm absorption wavelength of Photofrin. Also, work is under way to understand the chemistry of the photosensitizing agents upon irradiation with laser light that is referred to as photobleaching. MS is playing a crucial role in analyzing and characterizing these new photosensitizing agents and the products of photobleaching; for example, temoporfin is being developed as a single compound photosensitizer. MS has been used to study the metabolism of temoporfin (no metabolites were observed) [305], to characterize the conjugate of polyethylene glycol 2000 with temoporfin [306], and to identify the photobleaching products of temoporfin [307–309].

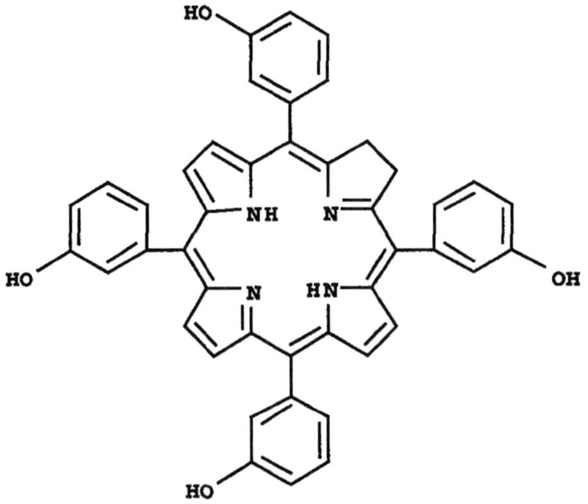

SCHEME 10   Temoporfin

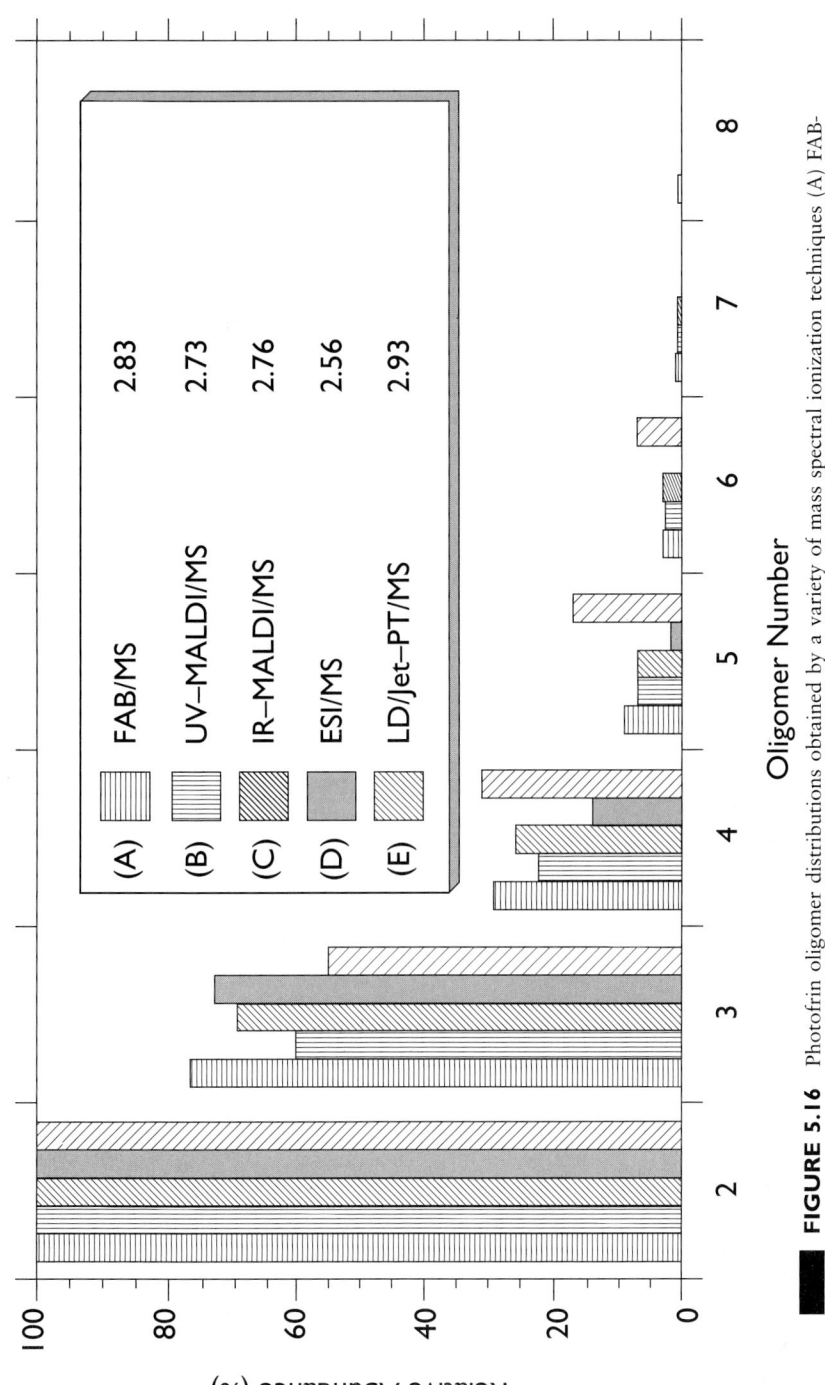

FIGURE 5.16 Photofrin oligomer distributions obtained by a variety of mass spectral ionization techniques (A) FAB-MS, (B) UV-MALDI-MS, (C) IR-MALDI-MS, (D) ESI-MS, and (E) LD/jet-PI-MS. The calculated average oligomer numbers for each ionization mode are indicated in the inset. The overall average oligomer number is 2.76. (Reprinted with permission from reference [303]. Copyright 1997 by John Wiley & Sons, Ltd.)

7. Taxol and Related Taxanes

Taxol and related taxanes have a unique mechanism of action in that they bind to tubulin protein thereby inhibiting cell division. The discovery, isolation, elucidation, characterization, and manufacture of these small anticancer natural products have occurred during a period of rapid development and acceptance of MS for the analysis of small molecules and the general availability of the technique as a highly sensitive, specific detector for the identification and characterization of new chemical entities. During this time, the coupling of an HPLC to ESI mass spectrometer has become a standard tool for the analysis of complex mixtures. Furthermore, the coupling of HPLC with UV detection and tandem MS has been a very powerful means for the multidimensional analysis of unknown materials because very high degrees of specificity and sensitivity can be achieved. However, MS has not played a significant role in the determination of the biological reaction mechanisms of taxol and related materials in their interactions with tubulin. In this area, biochemical methods have prevailed in spite of the fact that MS is a powerful tool for protein analysis and proteomics.

Mass spectrometry was not used extensively in the original determination of the taxol structure; however, its use has become more prominent in determining the structures of analogs in leaves, roots, and stems of Pacific yew [310–312] and the structures of metabolites [313–323]. This has been achieved using a variety of ionization techniques to produce parent ions such as EI [324, 325], CI [324, 325], DCI [326, 327], thermospray [327, 328], FAB [324, 325, 329, 330], ESI [331–333], APCI [316], and MALDI [334] often coupled to an HPLC with fragmentation produced in the source (EI, CI, FAB, ESI) or by CID utilizing tandem MS(ESI, APCI). Three series of fragment ions have been observed and are related to losses from the parent ion, the taxane ring, and the C-13 side chain [324, 325, 335–337]. Figure 5.17 illustrates the ESI-MS-MS spectrum of the $[M+NH_4]^{1+}$ parent ion of taxol, m/z 871, and the fragment ions associated with the taxol structure.

MS has played a key role in detecting molecular ions of taxol and its analogs by their identification in fungal growths [317, 338–340], genetically modified plants [341], plant tissue cultures [342, 343], rat tissues [344], human serum [345], environmental samples [346], production issues [347], and related quantitation [348–350]. MS was crucial in the development of taxol by profiling the taxanes for ease in their identification [337] and in the characterization of their degradation products [351]. Assays related to the fundamental understanding of taxol where MS was utilized include biosynthesis studies [352], taxo uptake in normal and multiple-drug-resistant cell strains [353], MALDI analysis of taxol-BSA conjugates [346], gas-phase drug complexes studied by H/D exchange [354], the calcium content of native and taxol-treated cells determined by SIMS [355], and the use of a MALDI microprobe to investigate the distribution of taxol in liver slices [356].

8. Gleevec

Gleevec (imatinib mesylate) is a protein-tyrosine kinase inhibitor used for treating chronic myeloid leukemia. Gleevec inhibits an abnormal protein (Ber-Abl oncoprotein) in the blood marrow from participating in the massive production of white blood cells. Gleevec represents a major breakthrough in

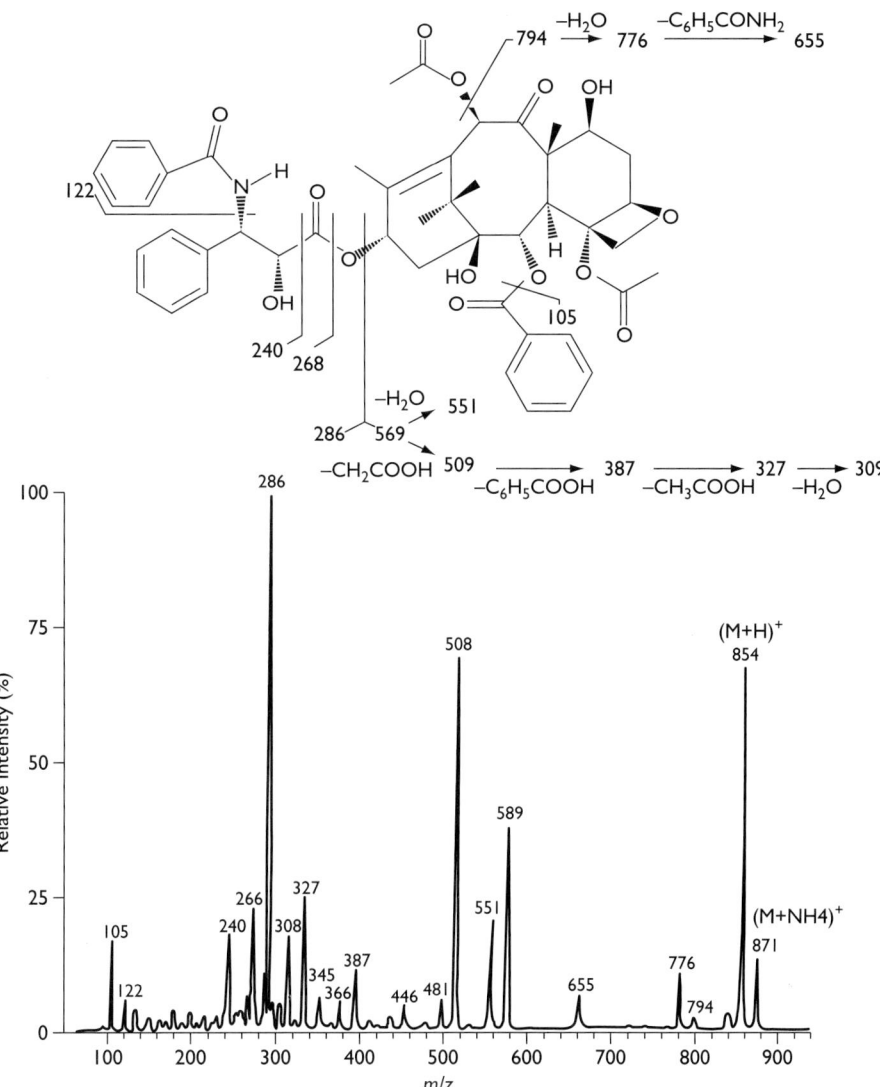

FIGURE 5.17 ESI-MS-MS mass spectrum of the taxol [M + NH₄]$^{1+}$ parent ion, m/z 871. The fragment ion assignments are indicated and are templates for elucidating minor components and degradation products in taxol. (Reprinted with permission from reference [337]. Copyright 1994 by the American Chemical Society.)

treating a specific cancer and is one of the first successful methods in which a targeted drug has competitively inhibited a cancer-producing mechanism. The quantitation of drug metabolites in human plasma using HPLC-ESI tandem MS has become a standard analytical procedure. Gleevec (STI571, MW 493) and its main metabolite CGP 74588 (MW 479) in human plasma was recently quantitated in a high-throughput assay using a deuterium-enriched (D₈) analog of Gleevec ([D₈]-STI571, MW 501) as the internal standard [357]. Figure 5.18 illustrates these chemical structures and the product ion at m/z 394 common to all the structures. Quantitation was achieved with

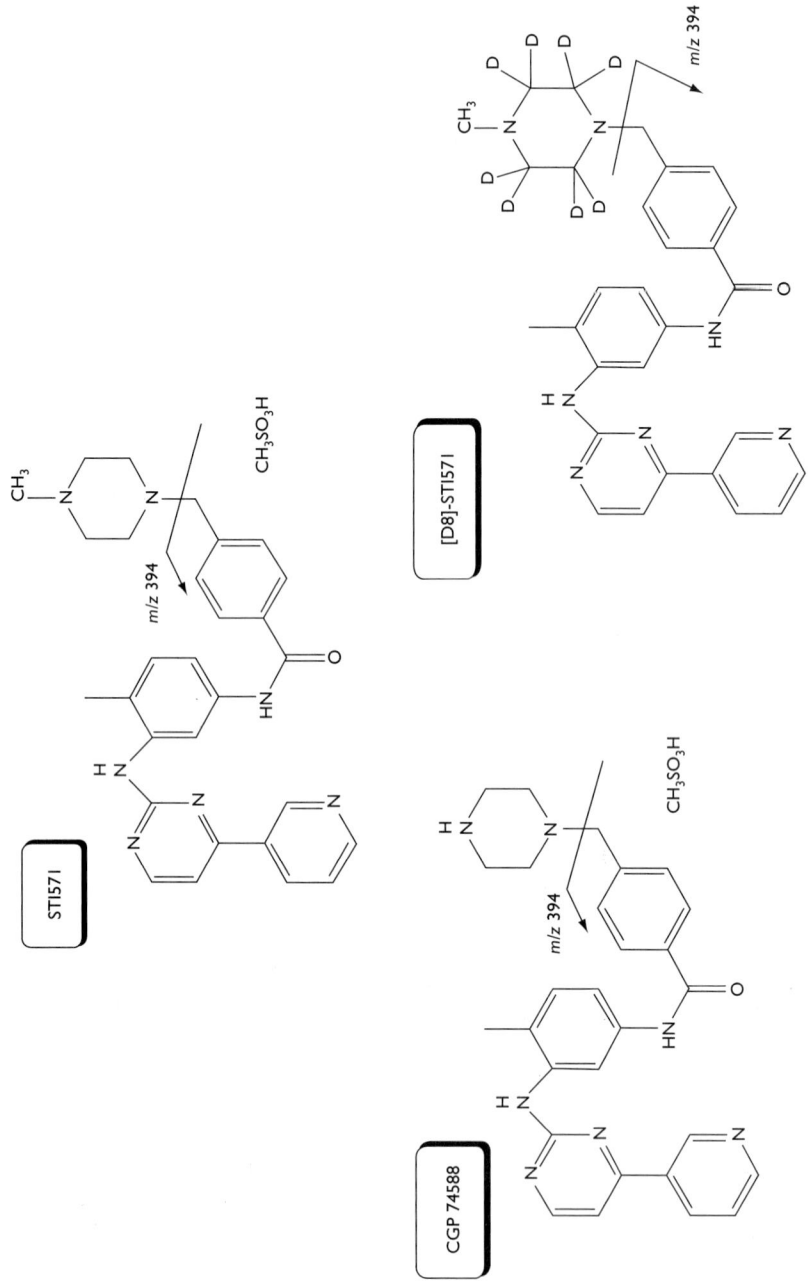

FIGURE 5.18 The structures of Gleevec (STI571), its main metabolite CGP74588, and the deuterated internal standard [D8]-STI571 used to quantitate Gleevec and its main metabolite. The APCI-MS-MS product ion at m/z 394 was selected for quantitation in the HPLC multiple-reaction monitoring experiments. (Reprinted with permission from reference [357]. Copyright 1997 by Elsevier Science B.V.)

monitoring by HPLC-ESI-tandem MS in the multiple-reaction monitoring mode the intensities of the transitions between the $[M+H]^{1+}$ ion and the m/z 394 ion for each of the three components. A semi-automated procedure was developed to remove protein from human plasma by precipitation and centrifugation for the analysis of the supernate. The assay for the three Gleevec components exhibited linearity from 4 to 10,000 ng/ml and was very rapid because each component had retention times of about 1 minute.

B. Diagnostic Applications of MS in Cancer Detection

MALDI-MS has been used principally for the characterization of peptides and proteins. Due to the high sensitivity and relative insensitivity to buffer and salt contamination, MALDI-MS has been the preferred technique for proteomics studies viz. the characterization of the protein content of cells. An embodiment of MALDI-MS ideally suited for proteomics studies, referred to as SELDI-MS, is where the MALDI probe tips have been modified by activating the metal surface with chemicals or biomolecules that serve as affinity targets for proteins and peptides and from which buffers, salts, detergents, and organics can be easily washed away for optimum sensitivity. SELDI-MS has been found to be a powerful tool for unearthing diagnostic markers in the cancer proteome and as a clinical tool for monitoring tumor progression. Ultimately, SELDI-MS may become a rapid and simple tool for the early detection and diagnosis of cancers not easily identified with present analytical and biological technologies [358, 359]. This can become even more significant when SELDI-MS is used to analyze small numbers of isolated cells obtained by using a laser capture microdissection microscope [359–361].

An early example in the application of SELDI-MS was demonstrated by Wright and co-workers [360] for prostate cancer biomarkers from tissues, serum, and seminal plasma. The four prostate cancer-associated biomarkers studied were prostate specific peptide (PSP; 10.7 kDa), prostrate-specific antigen (PSA; 28 kDa), prostate acid phosphatase (PAP; 47 kDa), and prostate-specific membrane antigen (PSMA; 100 kDa). Peaks associated with the four prostate cancer-associated biomarkers were confirmed by SELDI-MS for serum and seminal plasma proteins bound to the chemically modified probes. To rule out possible protein contamination, the probe tips were treated with specific antibodies to capture the prostate cancer-associated biomarkers in serum and seminal plasma. This approach has validated the earlier results. From lysed cells isolated by laser capture microdissection, three upregulated proteins (3.5, 18, and 33 kDa) were observed in SELDI mass spectra from prostate cancer epithelial cells, but were absent from normal prostate epithelial cells. Figure 5.19 clearly indicates the upregulation of the 3.5 kDa protein in three prostate cancer epithelial cell lysates and its absence in normal prostate epithelial cell lysates. These novel proteins may represent unique prostate cancer biomarkers easily identified using SELDI-MS that are useful for early diagnosis of prostate cancer.

New technologies for the early detection of ovarian cancer are urgently needed to reduce morbidity due to this high-risk disease. Recently, Petricoin and co-workers [361] demonstrated that proteomic patterns in SELDI mass spectra of sera from patients with and without ovarian cancer could be classified and used to identify early-stage ovarian cancer. Statistical methods were employed to

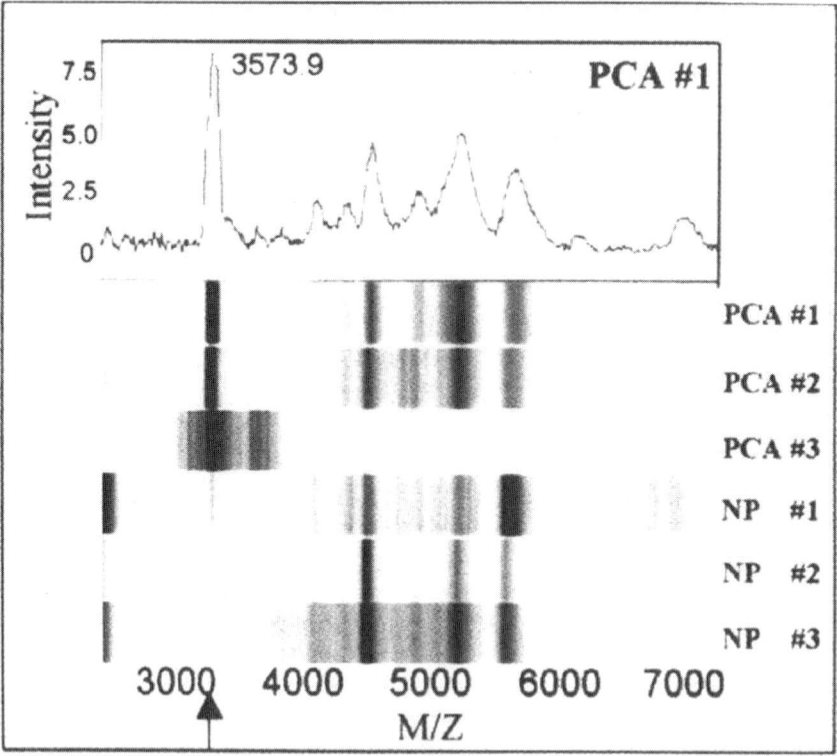

FIGURE 5.19 SELDI-MS analysis of proteins bound to a hydrophobic ProteinChip originating from prostate cancer-associated (PCA) and normal prostate (NP) cell lysates. The top panel is the observed mass spectrum and the lower panels are gel representations of the mass spectra. A potential prostate cancer biomarker is suggested by the presence of the protein at m/z 3573.9 in the three PCA samples and its absence in the three NP samples. (Reprinted with permission from reference [360]. Copyright 1999 by Macmillan Publishers Ltd.) See color insert.

identify in the mass spectra 5 to 20 key proteins that best distinguish ovarian cancer spectra from non-ovarian cancer spectra. This signature pattern from the training sets was then statistically matched with spectra of the unknowns to predict the presence or absence of ovarian cancer. It was found that the abundances of the peptide/protein peaks at m/z 534, 989, 2111, 2251, and 2465 corresponded to an optimum discriminatory pattern for ovarian cancer. Figure 5.20 illustrates the presence of a weak peak at m/z 2111 in sera of patients without ovarian cancer (top three panels and top two subpanels of lower two panels), while this same peak is absent in patients with ovarian cancer (lower two subpanels of lower two panels). Based on the mass spectral pattern information from 100 diagnosed patients, the clustering algorithm was applied to the spectra of 116 patients. The program correctly predicted the 50 patients with ovarian cancer and 63 out of 66 patients without cancer. The three cases incorrectly diagnosed with cancer corresponded to a correct diagnosis of 95% of the patients. This SELDI-MS technique appears to be a very promising method for diagnosing early-stage ovarian cancer.

Proteomic approaches utilizing MS have also been applied to the identification of markers for lung cancer [362], breast cancer [363, 364], hepatocellular

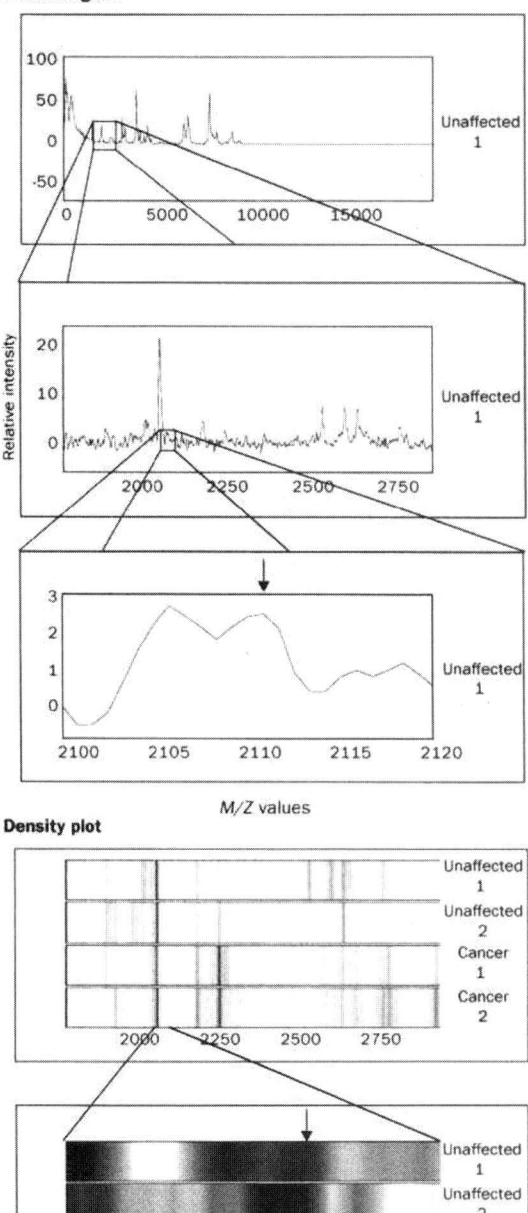

FIGURE 5.20 SELDI mass spectra of sera obtained from patients without (Unaffected) and diagnosed with ovarian cancer (Cancer). The top three panels illustrate the exploded regions in a SELDI mass spectrum where a protein biomarker was identified using statistical methods at *m/z* 2111 to be present in patients free of ovarian cancer. Similar exploded views are illustrated in the bottom two panels indicating the presence of the *m/z* 2111 protein in patients without ovarian cancer but absent in patients with ovarian cancer. Statistical analyses of similar SELDI mass spectral data were instrumental in identifying spectral patterns for diagnosing ovarian cancer. (Reprinted with permission from reference [361]. Copyright 2002 by the Lancet Publishing Group.) See Color Plate 13.

carcinoma [365], and tumor-specific antigens [366]. A MALDI-MS method for identifying principally glycolipid, ganglioside, and oligosaccharide cancer markers in blood and serum has also been described [367].

C. Exploratory/Early Discovery Drug Screening for Anticancer Agents Using MS

The role of early discovery drug screening is to uncover in a high-throughput manner those compounds in a library that selectively inhibit or activate a protein to produce a desired pharmaceutical outcome. Typically the desired compounds bind to the active site of a biopolymer (protein, DNA, RNA) either covalently or non-covalently. Potentially MS is slated to play a major role in screening programs because of its high sensitivity and specificity, especially when only limited quantities of biopolymer are available. A number of techniques have been developed to screen chemical libraries for biologically active compounds and they have recently been reviewed [368]. Although the screening methods can be applied generally to a variety of biochemical processes, in this section the primary focus will be on those mass spectral screening techniques that can or have been applied specifically to the identification of anticancer agents.

Three strategies can be used for screening covalent and non-covalent biopolymer-ligand complexes. One strategy is the direct sampling and analysis from the condensed phase of a biopolymer-ligand complex via gas-phase ESI-MS studies. The second strategy utilizes a condensed phase separation technique prior to or coupled with ESI-MS. The third strategy is a solid-phase analysis utilizing MALDI-MS. The first two strategies have become popular methods for early drug discovery screening while the third method has not become popular due to matrix and background problems, but it has gained importance for cancer diagnostic purposes by use of affinity probes for MALDI-MS, as described above in section III.B.

1. MS Screening by Gas-Phase ESI-MS Sampling of Condensed Phase Systems

Because ESI-MS can be performed under very gentle conditions, molecular ions of non-covalently as well as covalently bound complexes can be detected. It is believed that often the gas-phase non-covalently bound complexes mimic the condensed-phase properties of the ligand-biopolymer complex in spite of the absence of the condensed-phase solvent. The Src SH2 (Src homology 2) domain protein is critical in the signal transduction pathways of the tyrosine kinase. Inhibition of this pathway can prevent the uncontrolled growth of cancer cells. The non-covalent binding of various peptide inhibitors to Src SH2 domain protein was studied by ESI-MS [369, 370]. In addition, under competitive binding conditions where mixtures of the peptide inhibitors with Src SH2 domain protein were analyzed by ESI-MS, the relative abundances of the peptide-protein complexes were consistent with the solution-phase binding constants. This approach for screening chemical libraries could be applied in general to find small molecule inhibitors of the Src SH2 domain protein or any protein involved in signal transduction that may become an anticancer agent. A similar gas-phase ESI-MS screening approach can be taken to find small molecules, which inhibit the RAS proteins that serve as signal transducers to control cell proliferation or differentiation [371–374]. A gas-phase ESI-MS screening protocol has recently been described to identify pharmaceutical leads with the undesirable property of binding to DNA and thereby behaving as an anticancer agent with potential cytotoxic properties [375]. This same approach has been used to study the non-covalent binding of anti-tumor agents to model DNAs and the methodology can be expanded for the screening of chemical libraries to the model DNAs [376–380]. Likewise, the same gas-phase ESI-MS screening methodology has been applied to non-covalent ligand-RNA interactions [376, 381, 382], but no applications to screening for anticancer agents has been reported. An example of gas-phase ESI-MS screening for ligands that covalently bind to proteins and behave as anticancer agents was illustrated for the epidermal growth factor receptor (EGFr) protein that covalently binds to ligands via a Michael addition reaction at the active-site cysteine of the protein. With available EGFr protein, chemical libraries can be screened for compounds that covalently bind to EGFr by observing a mass shift in the protein signals in the ESI mass spectra [383, 384]. The amino acid residue sites in the protein that react can be confirmed by the analysis of the protein digestion products or by a "top down approach" [385] where the protein is degraded in the mass spectrometer and the reactive sites identified by comparison with a similarly treated pure protein. These approaches for screening covalently and non-covalently bound ligands to proteins can be routinely implemented using very small amounts of protein and ligands in an automated fashion. For even higher throughput, mixtures of ligands can be analyzed in a competitive fashion with the protein of interest to identify the strongest bound ligands. However, in general, the non-covalent studies are conducted by nanoelectrospray at elevated pHs under native conditions where the data is signal averaged over long periods of time to improve signal-to-noise ratios. On the other hand, the covalent studies are normally conducted by ESI-MS at low pHs where sensitivities are much greater.

2. ESI-MS Screening of Chromatographically Prepared Components

A number of condensed-phase separation procedures coupled with ESI-MS for detection have been developed for HTS of compounds covalently and non-covalently bound to biopolymers. Typically, a single component or mixture is incubated with a biopolymer and the final products are resolved chromatographically under native conditions followed by ESI-MS under denaturing conditions. As reviewed recently [368], the separation techniques, all capable of being coupled either on- or off-line to ESI-MS include: affinity chromatography and extraction, frontal affinity chromatography, affinity capillary electrophoresis, centrifugal and pulsed ultrafiltration, and gel permeation chromatography (GPC, also referred to as size-exclusion chromatography; SEC). Because all of these separation methods are generally applicable to all types of compounds and biopolymers, the methods are applicable for discovering substances that inhibit proteins involved in activating or inhibiting cancer-causing processes or that disrupt the DNA of cancer cells.

One of the more popular screening methods is the use of GPC materials in a variety of permutations coupled with MS. A unique feature of GPC, when applied to an incubated ligand-biopolymer mixture, is that the retention times of the biopolymer-ligand complexes are shorter and resolvable from the lower

MW ligands, thereby permitting the separation of ligand-biopolymer complexes from uncomplexed ligands for screening purposes. The simplest approach in performing GPC is in the spin column format where a short column packed with GPC material is centrifuged to achieve separation and isolation of the biopolymer and ligand-biopolymer complex from the unreacted ligand. The isolated complex is then analyzed by ESI-MS to identify the low MW ligand(s) present in the complex [386, 387]. Other variations on this theme include GPC in tandem with reverse-phase HPLC with ESI-MS detection [388–390] and GPC-ultrafiltration-reverse phase HPLC with ESI-MS detection [391]. Recently, the GPC-spin column/ESI-MS method was applied to the screening of drug candidates that could potentially disrupt cell growth by non-covalently binding to RNA and DNA [392]. Compounds that elute and bind non-covalently to the RNA or DNA are thereby eliminated as potential drug candidates.

IV. MS/NMR SCREENING ASSAY

A principal component of a drug discovery effort is the identification and validation of a chemical lead for its ability to bind the protein target in a biologically relevant manner. HTS techniques have traditionally filled the role of identifying potential binders from a large compound library. Unfortunately, there are numerous mechanisms by which a compound may interfere with a protein's function distinct from a stoichiometric binding interaction with the active site of the protein. The impact of compound aggregation on the activity of a number of proteins from a number of drug discovery programs has recently been illustrated [29]. The unfortunate ramification of non-productive chemical leads is a considerable loss of time and resources in attempts to optimize these compounds. Toward this end, there has been a concerted effort to develop alternate approaches to identify potential lead compounds where the technique intrinsically substantiates a binding interaction between the small molecule and the protein target. In particular, NMR and MS, as described in detail above, have evolved as alternative methods for the screening and the evaluation of chemical leads. Although both NMR and MS have inherent strengths and provide critical information for identifying and validating potential lead compounds, each technique also has shortcomings that limit its application in an HTS protocol. Among these are low sensitivity, throughput, and high protein sample requirements with isotope labeling of NMR and the lack of information on the binding site, stoichiometry, of binding and verification that the binding of the ligand is at the active site of the protein obtained from MS-based assays. What became apparent from comparison of NMR- and MS-based screening efforts was that the strengths and weaknesses of the two methods are very complementary to each other. This observation lead to the development of a hybrid MS/NMR screening assay [393].

A flow-diagram of the MS/NMR screening assay is depicted in Figure 5.21 where small-molecule binding to MMP-1 is used to illustrate the approach. The MS/NMR screen combines the inherent strengths of SEC, MS, and NMR spectroscopy. Briefly, compound(s) are incubated with the protein target of interest and passed through a size-exclusion column where low MW compounds are retained on the column. In this manner, only compounds that interact with the

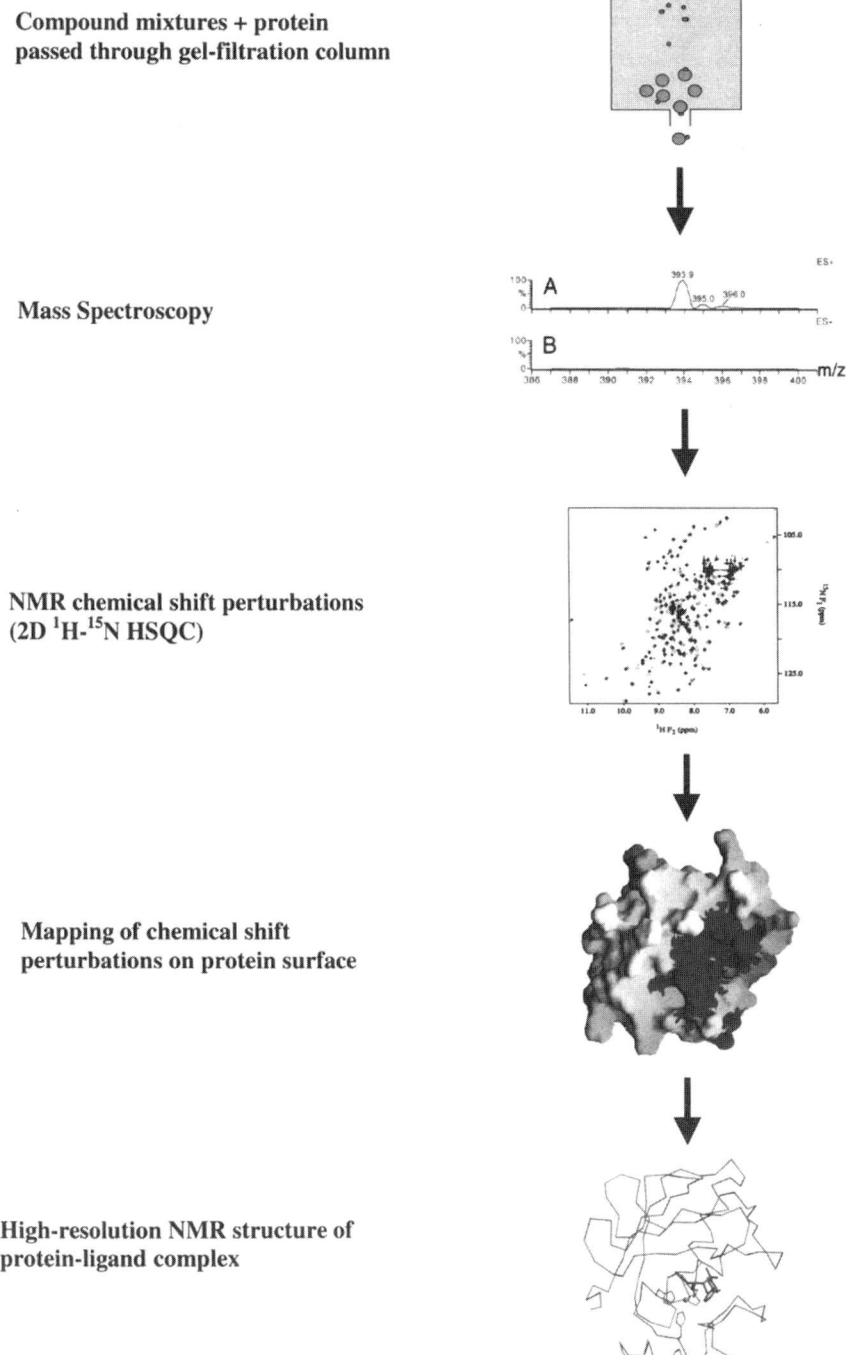

Compound mixtures + protein
passed through gel-filtration column

Mass Spectroscopy

NMR chemical shift perturbations
(2D ^{1}H-^{15}N HSQC)

Mapping of chemical shift
perturbations on protein surface

High-resolution NMR structure of
protein-ligand complex

FIGURE 5.21 Pictorial flow diagram of MS/NMR assay using data from the MMP-1 binding assay. (Reprinted with permission from reference [393]. Copyright 2001 by American Chemical Society.) See Color Plate 14.

protein will be present in the eluant. The eluant is then evaluated by ESI/MS for the presence of molecular ion(s) consistent with the compound(s) in the protein mixture. To verify that the presence of a molecular ion in the eluant is a result of an interaction with the protein and not an undesirable mechanism, the compound(s) are also run through the SEC column in the absence of the protein. In this case, the absence of a molecular ion peak in the ESI mass spectrum supports a binding interaction when a molecular ion peak is observed in the presence of the protein. The MS/NMR assay is amenable to using mixtures without incurring a necessary deconvolution step because the MW of each compound in a mixture acts as a molecular tag to identify the molecule. The MS/NMR assay has been applied utilizing mixtures of ten compounds with MW differences of ~3 Da. Following identification of a molecular ion consistent with a compound in the mixture, a 2D ^{1}H-^{15}N HSQC NMR spectrum is obtained for the appropriate compound-protein complex. The observation of chemical shift perturbations clustered in the vicinity of the protein's active site verifies a binding interaction between the compound and protein while simultaneously identifying the binding site and implying a specific interaction that probably has biological activity. Conversely, the absence of chemical shift perturbations or a random distribution of chemical shift changes on the protein surface would imply a lack of an interaction of the compound with the protein or potentially the existence of non-specific binding. Also, a binding site identified from the cluster of chemical shift changes on the protein's surface distinct from the active site of the protein may imply a specific binding interaction of the compound with the protein that may not be biologically relevant. The MS/NMR assay was developed utilizing MMP-1 and a small compound library containing compounds known to inhibit MMP-1, compounds known not to bind the protein, and 230 soluble and structurally diverse compounds with unknown activity against MMP-1. MMP-1 (collagenase), a matrix metalloproteinase, is an enzyme that hydrolyzes the extracellular matrix to which cells adhere. MMP-1 in excessive amounts has been implicated as a contributor to cancer metastasis and angiogenesis.

To validate the proposed MS/NMR screen, the behavior of a number of known MMP-1 inhibitors with an IC_{50} range of 9 nM to 100 μM were evaluated in the various steps of the assay. Figure 5.22 illustrates examples of both the MS and NMR results for a few select inhibitors. It is clearly evident that the molecular ion peak for each compound is only observed in the presence of MMP-1. Furthermore, each compound exhibits a similar pattern of chemical shift perturbations in the 2D ^{1}H-^{15}N HSQC spectra, which confirms the binding interaction of these compounds with MMP-1. Residues in the vicinity of the catalytic Zn and the S1' pocket in the MMP-1 active site exhibit chemical shift changes in the presence of these inhibitors. Particularly, residues 80–83, 114–119, and 136–142 exhibited the largest chemical shift changes. These results further establish that the compound is binding specifically to MMP-1 in a biologically relevant manner consistent with the previously observed inhibitory activity. In addition, the magnitude and number of chemical shift perturbations observed correlate to the observed IC_{50} values for each of the compounds. Compounds with lower IC_{50} values (stronger binders) correlate with larger numbers of protein residues undergoing larger chemical shift changes relative to compounds with higher IC_{50} values (weaker binders).

To further evaluate the application of SEC coupled with ESI/MS as a valid approach to identify potential protein binders in the MS/NMR assay, dose-response titrations and the behavior of compounds in mixtures were analyzed. Figure 5.23 illustrates the expected dose response of a known MMP-1 inhibitor. It is clearly evident that the abundance of the molecular ion at m/z 457.9 increases as a function of an increase in MMP-1 concentration. The behavior of compounds in mixtures was explored by two approaches. First, the impact of a response in the MS of a known MMP-1 inhibitor was evaluated in

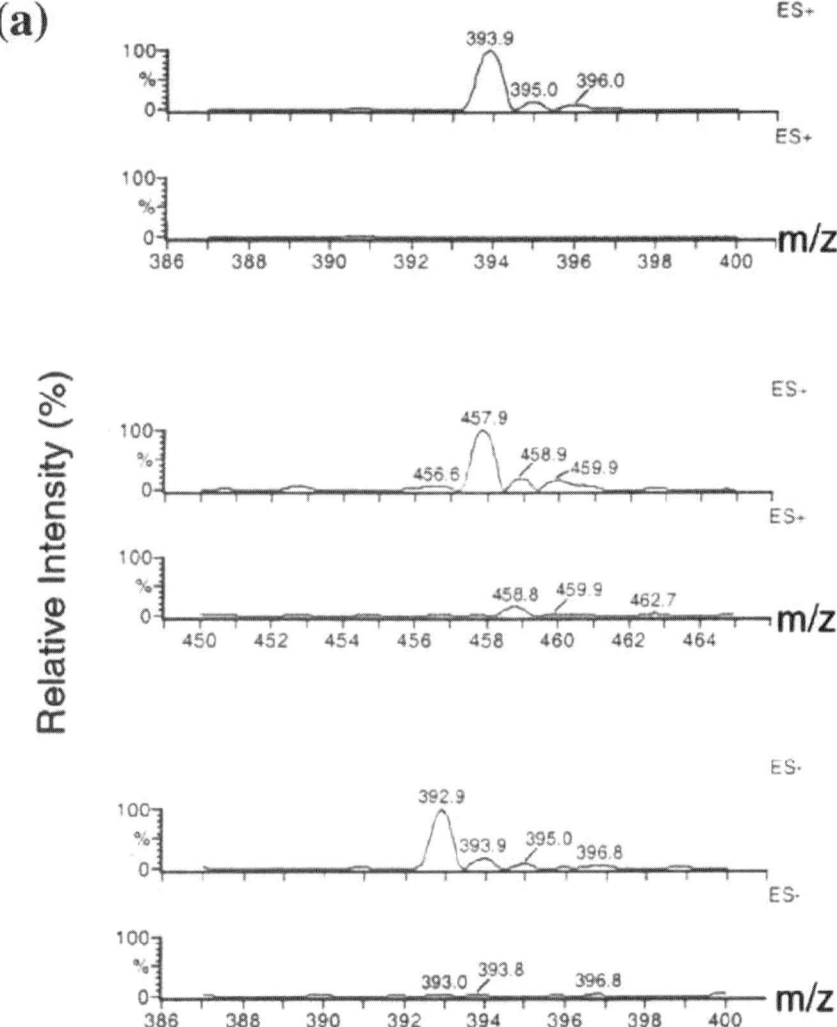

FIGURE 5.22 (a) ESI mass spectral analysis of the filtrate after passing MMP-1 inhibitors through Sephedex G-25 columns in the presence and absence of MMP-1. (Top) compound **1** (MW 393, IC_{50} 9 nM) and MMP-1 and compound **1** alone; (middle) compound **2** (MW 457, IC_{50} 9.9 μM) and MMP-1 and compound **2** alone; (bottom) compound **3** (MW 394, IC_{50} 89 μM) and MMP-1 and compound **3** alone. (b) Overlay of the free MMP-1 2D ^{1}H-^{15}N HSQC spectra (solid peaks) with the MMP-1 complex 2D ^{1}H-^{15}N HSQC spectra (1–2 contours) for compound **1** (top), compound **2** (middle), and compound **3** (bottom). (Reprinted with permission from reference [393]. Copyright 2001 by American Chemical Society.)

(b)

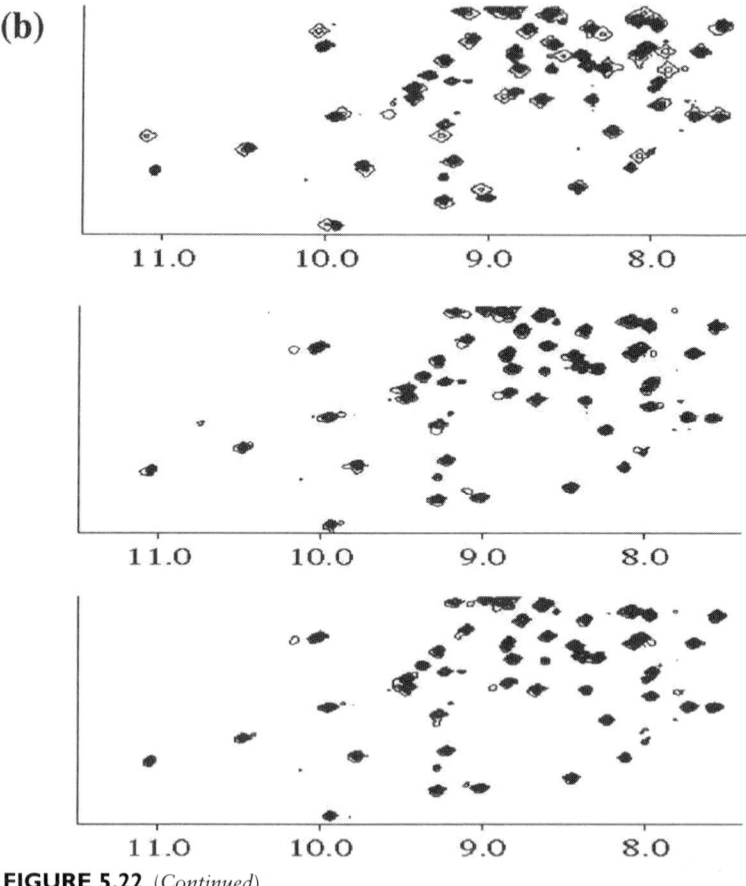

FIGURE 5.22 *(Continued)*

a mixture with nine compounds known not to bind MMP-1. These results were compared to the spectra obtained for the compound alone. No significant impact on the ability to observe a positive response for known inhibitors in a mixture was detected for the set of compounds. A more dramatic example of the reliability of the SEC-MS component of the MS/NMR assay was the analysis of a mixture of ten known inhibitors with an IC_{50} range of 9 nm to 100 μM (Figure 5.24). Despite the wide range of IC_{50}s, all ten compounds were clearly observed in the MS in the presence of MMP-1. None of the compounds were observed when MMP-1 was not present.

To demonstrate the screening of compounds for a potential anticancer discovery program, a small chemical library of 230 compounds, selected based on MW, solubility, structural diversity, availability, and stability, was screened to identify those components that non-covalently bind to MMP-1. The samples were prepared as 23 mixtures, each composed of 10 compounds. The components in each mixture were selected to produce solutions that had minimal impact on the pH of the sample by balancing the number of acids and bases in each mixture. The mixtures were incubated with MMP-1 and analyzed using the GPC-spin column/ESI-MS flow injection approach. The resulting data were

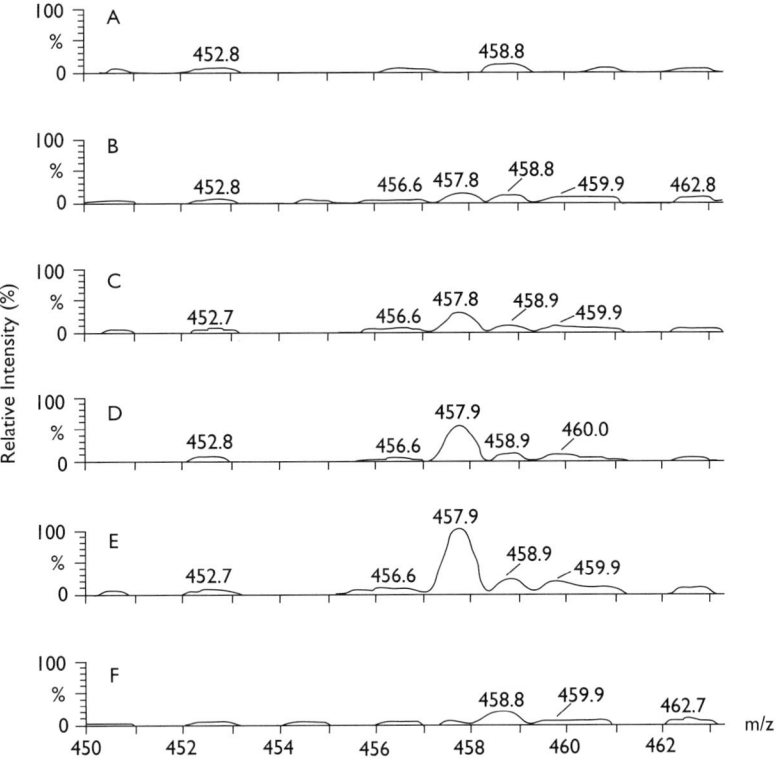

FIGURE 5.23 ESI (positive ionization mode) mass spectral analysis of the filtrate from the gel-filtration titration of compound **2** (MW 457) with MMP-1. (A) MMP-1 alone at 50 μM and (F) compound **2** alone at 250 μM, respectively; (B–E) increasing amount of MMP-1 (B) 20 μM, (C) 30 μM, (D) 40 μM, and (E) 50 μM and increasing amount of compound **2** from (B) 100 μM, (C) 150 μM, (D) 200 μM, and (E) 250 μM. (Reprinted with permission from reference [393]. Copyright 2001 by American Chemical Society.)

analyzed in two dimensions. The ESI mass spectra of the mixtures, analyzed before and after the mixture of interest, were compared to identify background peaks and new peaks associated with the mixture of interest. The second dimension analyzed was the evolution in time of the mass chromatograms for each of the components of the mixture to verify that they were components of the mixture and not from the background. Figure 5.25 illustrates a total of five mass spectra sequentially acquired, two from mixtures immediately prior to the mixture of interest (Figures 5.25A and B), the mixture of interest (Figure 5.25C), and two from mixtures immediately following the mixture of interest (Figures 5.25D and E). Note that most of the mass spectral peaks in the mixture of interest, Figure 5.25C, are present in most of the other spectra except for peaks at m/z 145.8 and 155.7. Figure 5.26 illustrates the total ion chromatogram for the mixture of interest (Figure 5.26A) and the mass chromatograms for the ions with m/z 145.8 (Figure 5.26B) and 155.7 (Figure 5.26C). Note that in both cases mass chromatographic peaks evolve in time, which confirms the fact that these two components with MWs 145 and 155, respectively, most likely passed through the GPC-spin column non-covalently bound to the MMP-1. These two

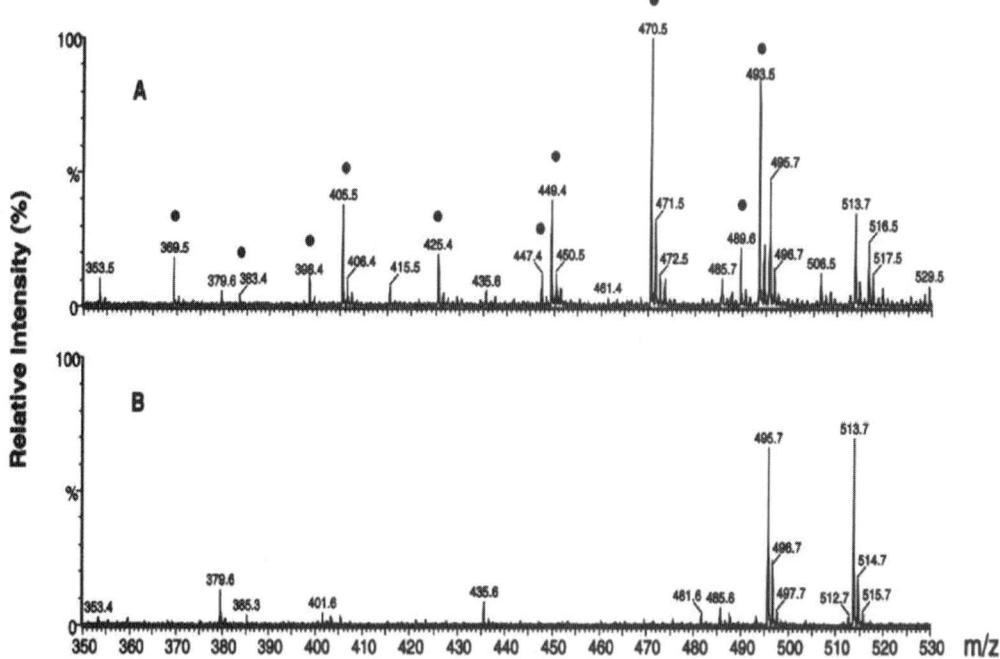

FIGURE 5.24   ESI (negative ionization mode) mass spectral analysis of the filtrate from the gel-filtration analysis of a mixture containing ten known MMP-1 inhibitors. (A) with MMP-1 and (B) without MMP-1. The [M-H]$^{1-}$ ions for the ten compounds are indicated by solid circles (•) on the spectra. (Reprinted with permission from reference [393]. Copyright 2001 by American Chemical Society.)

compounds, when analyzed in the same manner but in the absence of MMP-1 by GPC-spin column/ESI-MS, did not produce any detectable mass spectral peaks. This further verified that the compounds were non-covalently bound to MMP-1.

The two compounds with MWs of 145 and 155, identified by GPC/MS as non-covalent binders to MMP-1, were then each analyzed in the presence of MMP-1 by 2D ^{1}H-^{15}N HSQC NMR (Figure 5.27). Chemical shift perturbations associated with the active-site amide amino acid residue(s) were not observed for the MW 145 compound but were observed for the MW 155 compound. The NMR data verify the fact that the MW 155 compound, corresponding to a *p*-phenyl pyridine compound, was specifically bound to the MMP-1 active site while the MW 145 compound, corresponding to 8-hydroxyquinoline, was non-specifically bound to MMP-1. The *p*-phenyl pyridine compound was independently found by NMR studies to bind to stromelysin (MMP-3) [80], which provided further support for the reliability of the MS/NMR assay.

The MS/NMR assay was automated and successfully applied to a 32,000 compound library that was screened for compounds non-covalently bound to the RGS4 protein [393]. Regulators of G-protein signaling (RGS)

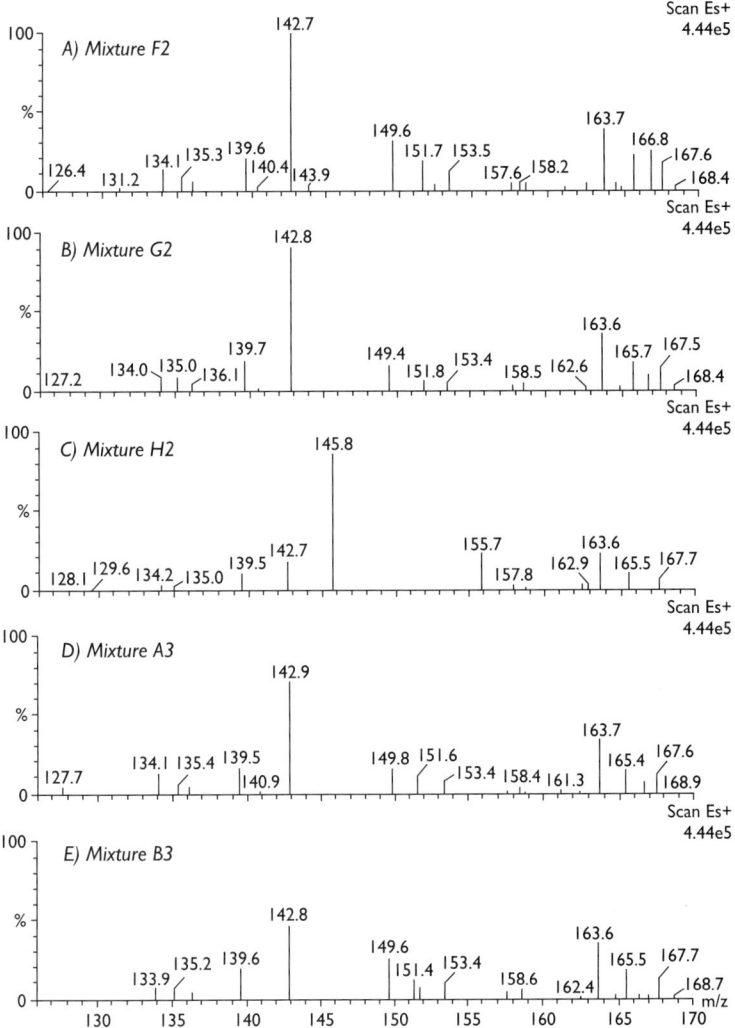

FIGURE 5.25 ESI mass spectra acquired from five consecutive samples (A–E) prepared from the eluates of GPC-spin columns. The spin column eluates were each obtained from mixtures of 10 components incubated with MMP-1 to screen for compounds non-covalently bound to the protein. The ESI mass spectra shown in panels A, B and D, E serve as background spectra for the ESI spectrum of the sample of interest (panel C), mixture H2. Nearly all the ions are from the protein, buffer, and solvent background except for the ions at *m/z* 145.8 and 155.7, These two ions are protonated molecular ions for compounds with MWs of 145 and 155 that bind to MMP-1.

act as attenuators of the G-protein signal cascade by binding to the Gα subunit of G-proteins and inducing a 30-fold increase in the intrinsic Gα GTPase activity (for reviews see references 394 through 398). The MS/NMR assay successfully identified a low MW compound that has demonstrated direct binding to RGS4 and inhibition of the interaction of RGS4 with Gα.

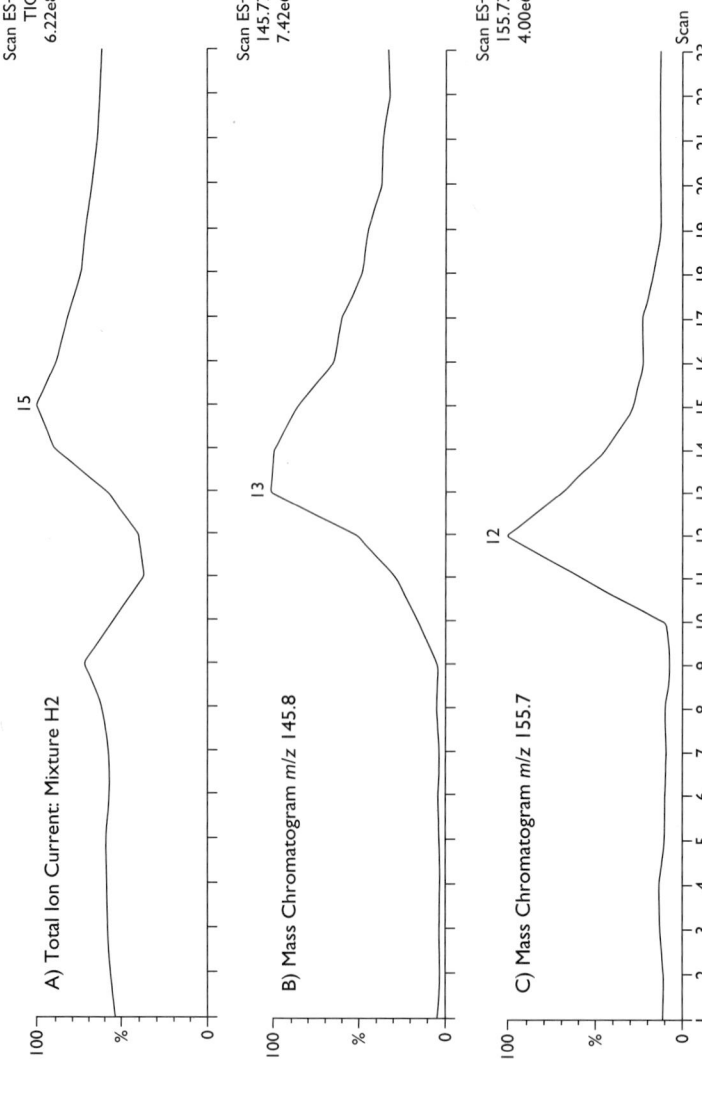

FIGURE 5.26 (A) ESI total ion chromatogram from mixture H2. Mass chromatograms for the components with (B) *m/z* 145.8 and (C) *m/z* 155.7 from the GPC-spin-column eluate originating from mixture H2 of 10 components incubated with MMP-1. (The ESI mass spectrum for this mixture is illustrated as Figure 5.25C.) The evolution of these peaks with time (scan numbers) demonstrates that these are unique components that eluted from the mixture while the other eight components were retained by the spin-column and not observed in the ESI mass spectrum.

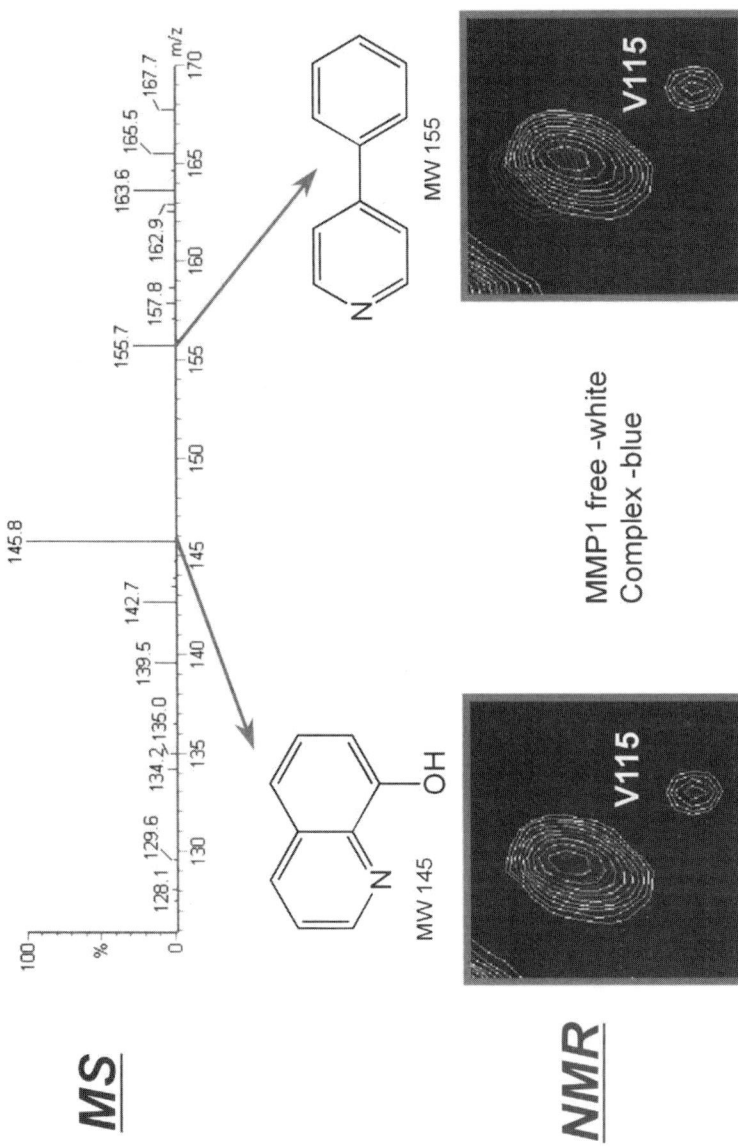

FIGURE 5.27 Illustration of the complementary nature of NMR and MS in the MS/NMR MMP-1 assay. (Top) MS shows the presence of molecular ions for both compounds (MW 145 and 155) after passing through the size-exclusion column in the presence of MMP-1, which indicates binding to the protein. (Bottom) Expanded 2D ^{1}H-^{15}N HSQC NMR spectra which indicates that the *p*-phenyl pyridine induces a chemical shift change for V115 in the MMP-1 active site. See Color Plate 15.

V. CONCLUSIONS

The process of identifying and developing chemical leads prior to submitting drugs for clinical trials for cancer and other therapeutic uses is undergoing a significant evolution with NMR and MS making critical contributions to these advancements. The traditional roles of HTS screening and medicinal chemistry are augmented with NMR and MS applications to screen, identify, and validate potential lead compounds as part of a structure-based drug discovery program utilizing both NMR and X-ray techniques.

NMR provides a plethora of tools that can be applied to address a number of issues or questions that typically occur during a drug development program. NMR is routinely used to determine high-resolution structures of proteins and protein-ligand complexes. Additionally, NMR can provide valuable information on the dynamic behavior of the same proteins and protein-ligand complexes. These data are essential to a structure-based drug discovery program. More recently, NMR has been used to address a fundamental issue associated with the drug discovery process, namely, to verify that a chemical lead actually binds in a biologically relevant manner to the protein target of interest. A variety of NMR techniques, including 2D HSQCs, STDs, and 1D line-broadening, have been successfully applied to screening compound libraries by NMR. Similarly, a variety of MS techniques have been used for structure elucidation, analysis of metabolism, diagnostics, and drug screening. In fact, the parallel development of MS as a technique to screen libraries for compounds that bind biomolecules and the complementary nature of NMR and MS lead to the development of the MS/NMR assay by combining the inherent strengths of these analytical techniques.

NMR and MS, coupled with chromatographic techniques, are now poised to contribute extensively to the progress in cancer research, especially with advances in the field of proteomics and the developing area of structural genomics. Subjects such as signal transduction, apoptosis, angiogenesis, cell metastasis, cancer diagnostics, and screening will develop rapidly with the insights provided by NMR and MS. By identifying, characterizing, elucidating, and quantifying biomolecules in disease states, NMR and MS represent the fundamental tools that will facilitate our understanding of the basic cellular processes of cancer at a molecular level. This will lead to an understanding of the mechanisms responsible for cancer and ultimately the development of a new generation of therapeutic agents for the treatment and eventual cure of cancer.

ACKNOWLEDGEMENTS

We would like to thank Franklin J. Moy for his extensive contributions to the various projects described within the manuscript. The authors appreciate the suggestions and comments of Michelle A. Markus, Ravindra K. Pandey, Michael Pastel, John Roboz, Paul D. Schnier, and Joel I. Siegel for preparing and improving this manuscript.

REFERENCES

1. Gubernator K, Boehm HJ. Examples of active areas of structure based-design. *Methods Princ. Med. Chem.* 1998; 6:15–36.
2. Kubinyi H. Structure-based design of enzyme inhibitors and receptor ligands. *Curr. Opin. Drug Disc. Dev.* 1998; 1:4–15.
3. Li J, Murray CW, Waszkowycz B, Young SC. Targeted molecular diversity in drug discovery: Integration of structure-based design and combinatorial chemistry. *Drug Disc. Today* 1998; 3:105–112.
4. Gane PJ, Dean PM. Recent advances in structure-based rational drug design. *Curr. Opin. Struct. Biol.* 2000; 10:401–404.
5. Morris PE, Jr., Omura GA. Inhibitors of the enzyme purine nucleoside phosphorylase as potential therapy for psoriasis. *Curr. Pharm. Des.* 2000; 6:943–959.
6. Maignan S, Mikol V. The use of 3D structural data in the design of specific Factor Xa inhibitors. *Curr. Top. Med. Chem.* 2001; 1:161–174.
7. Craik DJ, Scanlon MJ. Pharmaceutical applications of NMR. *Annu. Rep. NMR Spectrosc.* 2000; 42:115–174.
8. Colacino JM, Staschke KA, Laver WG. Approaches and strategies for the treatment of influenza virus infections. *Antiviral Chem. Chemother.* 1999; 10:155–185.
9. Mihelich ED, Schevitz RW. Structure-based design of a new class of anti-inflammatory drugs: secretory phospholipase A2 inhibitors, SPI. *Biochim. Biophys. Acta* 1999; 1441:223–228.
10. Sintchak MD, Nimmesgern E. The structure of inosine 5′-monophosphate dehydrogenase and the design of novel inhibitors. *Immunopharmacology* 2000; 47:163–184.
11. Sem DS, Pellecchia M. NMR in the acceleration of drug discovery. *Curr. Opin. Drug Disc. Dev.* 2001; 4:479–492.
12. Roberts GCK. Applications of NMR in drug discovery. *Drug Disc. Today* 2000; 5:230–240.
13. Roberts GCK. NMR spectroscopy in structure-based drug design. *Curr. Opin. Biotechnol.* 1999; 10:42–47.
14. Prestegard JH, Valafar H, Glushka J, Tian F. Nuclear magnetic resonance in the era of structural genomics. *Biochemistry* 2001; 40:8677–8685.
15. Craik DJ, Nielsen KJ, Higgins KA. Pharmaceutical applications of NMR. *Annu. Rep. NMR Spectrosc.* 1996; 32:143–213.
16. Feeney J. NMR studies of protein-ligand and protein-protein interactions involving proteins of therapeutic interest. *NATO ASI Ser., Ser C* 1999; 526:281–300.
17. Dunayevskiy YM, Lai J-J, Quinn C, Talley F, Vouros P. Mass spectrometric identification of ligands selected from combinatorial libraries using gel filtration. *Rapid Commun. Mass Spectrom.* 1997; 11:1178–1184.
18. Siegel MM, Tabei K, Bebernitz GA, Baum EZ. Rapid methods for screening low molecular mass compounds non-covalently bound to proteins using size exclusion and mass spectrometry applied to inhibitors of human cytomegalovirus protease. *J. Mass Spectrum* 1998; 33:264–273.
19. Siegel MM. Early discovery drug screening using mass spectrometry. *Curr. Top. Med. Chem.* 2002; 2:13–33.
20. Armstrong JW. A review of high-throughput screening approaches for drug discovery. *Am. Biotechnol. Lab.* 1999; 17:26–28.
21. Gonzalez JE, Negulescu PA. Intracellular detection assays for high-throughput screening. *Curr. Opin. Biotechnol.* 1998; 9:624–631.
22. Oldenburg KR. Current and future trends in high throughput screening for drug discovery. *Annu. Rep. Med. Chem.* 1998; 33:301–311.
23. Fernandes PB. Technological advances in high-throughput screening. *Curr. Opin. Chem. Biol.* 1998; 2:597–603.
24. Kenny BA, Bushfield M, Parry-Smith DJ, Fogarty S, Treherne JM. The application of high-throughput screening to novel lead discovery. *Prog. Drug Res.* 1998; 51:245–269.
25. Silverman L, Campbell R, Broach JR. New assay technologies for high-throughput screening. *Curr. Opin. Chem. Biol.* 1998; 2:397–403.
26. Schreiber SL. Target-oriented and diversity-oriented organic synthesis in drug discovery. *Science* 2000; 287:1964–1969.

27. Nicolaou KC, Vourloumis D, Winssinger N, Baran PS. The art and science of total synthesis at the dawn of the twenty-first century. *Angew Chem. Int. Ed.* 2000; 39:44–122.

28. Chakraborty TK. Future directions in organic synthesis. *J. Indian Chem. Soc.* 2001; 78:211–223.

29. McGovern SL, Caselli E, Grigorieff N, Shoichet BK. A common mechanism underlying promiscuous inhibitors from virtual and high-throughput screening. *J. Med. Chem.* 2002; 45:1712–1722.

30. Oakley AJ, Wilce MCJ. Macromolecular crystallography as a tool for investigating drug, enzyme and receptor interactions. *Clin. Exp. Pharmacol. Physiol.* 2000; 27:145–151.

31. Ferentz AE, Wagner G. NMR spectroscopy: a multifaceted approach to macromolecular structure. *Q. Rev. Biophys.* 2000; 33:29–65.

32. Nogi T, Miki K. Structural basis of bacterial photosynthetic reaction centers. *J. Biochem.* 2001; 130:319–329.

33. Tsukihara T, Aoyama H. Membrane protein assemblies — towards atomic resolution analysis: commentary. *Curr. Opin. Struct. Biol.* 2000; 10:208–212.

34. Baleja JD. Structure determination of membrane-associated proteins from nuclear magnetic resonance data. *Anal. Biochem.* 2001; 288:1–15.

35. Fernandez C, Hilty C, Bonjour S, Adeishvili K, Pervushin K, Wüthrich K. Solution NMR studies of the integral membrane proteins OmpX and OmpA from *Escherichia coli. FEBS Lett.* 2001; 504:173–178.

36. Powell HR. Molecular structure from X-ray diffraction. *Annu. Rep. Prog. Chem.*, Section C: Physical Chemistry 2000; 96:139–175.

37. Smyth MS, Martin JHJ. X-ray crystallography. *Mol. Pathol.* 2000; 53:8–14.

38. Gardner KH, Kay LE. The use of ^{2}H, ^{13}C, ^{15}N multidimensional NMR to study the structure and dynamics of proteins. *Annu. Rev. Biophys. Biomol. Struct.* 1998; 27:357–406.

39. Kay LE, Gardner KH. Solution NMR spectroscopy beyond 25 kDa. *Curr. Opin. Struct. Biol.* 1997; 7:722–731.

40. Clore GM, Gronenborn AM. NMR structure determination of proteins and protein complexes larger than 20 kDa. *Curr. Opin. Chem. Biol.* 1998; 2:564–570.

41. Arrowsmith CH, Wu Y-S. NMR of large (>25 kDa) proteins and protein complexes. *Prog. Nucl. Magn. Reson. Spectrosc.* 1998; 32:277–286.

42. Pervushin K. Impact of transverse relaxation optimized spectroscopy (TROSY) on NMR as a technique in structural biology. *Q. Rev. Biophys.* 2000; 33:161–197.

43. Riek R, Pervushin K, Wüthrich K. TROSY and CRINEPT: NMR with large molecular and supramolecular structures in solution. *Trends Biochem. Sci.* 2000; 25:462–468.

44. Wüthrich K. *NMR of Proteins and Nucleic Acids.* John Wiley & Sons, New York, 1986.

45. Otting G. Experimental NMR techniques for studies of protein-ligand interactions. *Curr. Opin. Struct. Biol.* 1993; 3:760–768.

46. Whittle PJ, Blundell TL. Protein structure-based drug design. *Annu. Rev. Biophys. Biomol. Struct.* 1994; 23:349–375.

47. Blundell TL. Structure-based drug design. *Nature* 1996; 384:(Suppl):23–26.

48. Joseph-McCarthy D. Computational approaches to structure-based ligand design. *Pharmacol. Ther.* 1999; 84:179–191.

49. Gmeiner WH. NMR spectroscopy as a tool to investigate the structural basis of anticancer drugs. *Curr. Med. Chem.* 1998; 5:115–135.

50. Pindur U, Fischer G. DNA complexing minor groove-binding ligands: Perspectives in antitumor and antimicrobial drug design. *Curr. Med. Chem.* 1996; 3:379–406.

51. Fowler CA, Tian F, Al-Hashimi HM, Prestegard JH. Rapid determination of protein folds using residual dipolar couplings. *J. Mol. Biol.* 2000; 304:447–460.

52. Prestegard JH. Orientational constraints of polypeptide folds: The role of NMR in structural genomics. *Polym. Prepr.* 2001; 42:60.

53. Tjandra N, Bax A. Direct measurement of distances and angles in biomolecules by NMR in a dilute liquid crystalline medium. *Science* 1997; 278:1111–1114.

54. Moseley HNB, Montelione GT. Automated analysis of NMR assignments and structures for proteins. *Curr. Opin. Struct. Biol.* 1999; 9:635–642.

55. Linge JP, O'Donoghue SI, Nilges M. Automated assignment of ambiguous nuclear Overhauser effects with ARIA. *Methods Enzymol.* 2001; 339:71–90.

56. Greenfield NJ, Huang YJ, Palm T et al. Solution NMR structure and folding dynamics of the n terminus of a rat non-muscle α-tropomyosin in an engineered chimeric protein. *J. Mol. Biol.* 2001; 312:833–847.

57. Xu Y, Jablonsky MJ, Jackson PL, Braun W, Krishna NR. Automatic assignment of NOESY cross peaks and determination of the protein structure of a new world scorpion neurotoxin using NOAH/DIAMOD. *J. Magn. Reson.* 2001; 148:35–46.

58. Xu Y, Wu J, Gorenstein D, Braun W. Automated 2D NOESY assignment and structure calculation of crambin(S22/I25) with the self-correcting distance geometry based NOAH/DIAMOD programs. *J. Magn. Reson.* 1999; 136:76–85.

59. Bowers PM, Strauss CEM, Baker D. De novo protein structure determination using sparse NMR data. *J. Biomo. NMR* 2000; 18:311–318.

60. Rohl CA, Baker D. De novo determination of protein backbone structure from residual dipolar couplings using rosetta. *J. Am. Chem. Soc.* 2002; 124:2723–2729.

61. Montelione GT, Zheng D, Huang YJ, Gunsalus KC, Szyperski T. Protein NMR spectroscopy in structural genomics. *Nat. Struct. Biol.* 2000; 7:982–985.

62. Moore JM. NMR techniques for characterization of ligand binding: Utility for lead generation and optimization in drug discovery. *Biopolymers* 1999; 51:221–243.

63. Moore JM. NMR screening in drug discovery. *Curr. Opin. Biotechnol.* 1999; 10:54–58.

64. Peng JW, Lepre CA, Fejzo J, Abdul-Manan N, Moore JM. Nuclear magnetic resonance-based approaches for lead generation in drug discovery. *Methods Enzymol.* 2001; 338:202–230.

65. Rossi C, Donati A, Sansoni MR. Nuclear magnetic resonance as a tool for the identification of specific DNA-ligand interaction. *Chem. Phys. Lett.* 1992; 189:278–280.

66. Hajduk PJ, Olejniczak ET, Fesik SW. One-dimensional relaxation- and diffusion-edited NMR methods for screening compounds that bind to macromolecules. *J. Am. Chem. Soc.* 1997; 119:12257–12261.

67. Lin M, Shapiro MJ, Wareing JR. Diffusion-edited NMR-affinity NMR for direct observation of molecular interactions. *J. Am. Chem. Soc.* 1997; 119:5249–5250.

68. Lin M, Shapiro MJ, Wareing JR. Screening mixtures by affinity NMR. *J. Org. Chem.* 1997; 62:8930–8931.

69. Waldeck AR, Kuchel PW, Lennon AJ, Chapman BE. NMR diffusion measurements to characterize membrane transport and solute binding. *Prog. Nucl. Magn. Reson. Spectrosc.* 1997; 30:39–68.

70. Shirakawa M, Lee SJ, Takimoto M, Matsuo H, Akutsu H, Kyogoku Y. Interaction of the λ-cro repressor protein with operator DNA fragments monitored as to amide proton magnetic resonances. *J. Mol. Struct.* 1991; 242:355–366.

71. Ni F. Recent developments in transferred NOE methods. *Prog. Nucl. Magn. Reson. Spectrosc.* 1994; 26:517–606.

72. Vogtherr M, Peters T. Application of NMR based binding assays to identify key hydroxy groups for intermolecular recognition. *J. Am. Chem. Soc.* 2000; 122:6093–6099.

73. Mayer M, Meyer B. Characterization of ligand binding by saturation transfer difference NMR spectroscopy. *Angew Chem. Int. Ed.* 1999; 38:1784–1788.

74. Dalvit C, Pevarello P, Tato M, Veronesi M, Vulpetti A, Sundstrom M. Identification of compounds with binding affinity to proteins via magnetization transfer from bulk water. *J. Biomol. NMR* 2000; 18:65–68.

75. Clore GM, Gronenborn AM. Structures of larger proteins, protein-ligand and protein-DNA complexes by multidimensional heteronuclear NMR. *Protein Sci.* 1994; 3:372–390.

76. Chen A, Shapiro MJ. NOE Pumping: A novel NMR technique for identification of compounds with binding affinity to macromolecules. *J. Am. Chem. Soc.* 1998; 120:10258–10259.

77. Cooke RM. Protein NMR extends into new fields of structural biology. *Curr. Opin. Chem. Biol.* 1997; 1:359–364.

78. Kay LE. NMR methods for the study of protein structure and dynamics. *Biochem. Cell Biol.* 1997; 75:1–15.

79. Hajduk PJ, Dinges J, Miknis GF et al. NMR-based discovery of lead inhibitors that block DNA binding of the human papillomavirus E2 protein. *J. Med. Chem.* 1997; 40:3144–3150.

80. Hajduk PJ, Sheppard G, Nettesheim DG et al. Discovery of potent nonpeptide inhibitors of stromelysin using SAR by NMR. *J. Am. Chem. Soc.* 1997; 119:5818–5827.

81. Zask A, Levin JI, Killar LM, Skotnicki JS. Inhibition of matrix metalloproteinases: Structure based design. *Curr. Pharm. Des.* 1996; 2:624–661.

82. Skiles JW, Gonnella NC, Jeng AY. The design, structure, and therapeutic application of matrix metalloproteinase inhibitors. *Curr. Med. Chem.* 2001; 8:425–474.

83. Shuker SB, Hajduk PJ, Meadows RP, Fesik SW. Discovering high-affinity ligands for proteins: SAR by NMR. *Science* 1996; 274:1531–1534.

84. Hajduk PJ, Gerfin T, Boehlen J-M, Haeberli M, Marek D, Fesik SW. High-throughput nuclear magnetic resonance-based screening. *J. Med. Chem.* 1999; 42:2315–2317.

85. Hajduk PJ, Augeri DJ, Mack J et al. NMR-based screening of proteins containing ^{13}C-labeled methyl groups. *J. Am. Chem. Soc.* 2000; 122:7898–7904.

86. Clore GM, Gronenborn AM. Determining the structures of large proteins and protein complexes by NMR. *Trends Biotechnol.* 1998; 16:22–34.

87. Salzmann M, Wider G, Pervushin K, Senn H, Wüthrich K. TROSY-type triple-resonance experiments for sequential NMR assignments of large proteins. *J. Am. Chem. Soc.* 1999; 121:844–848.

88. Pfister H. Human papillomaviruses and skin cancer. *Cancer Biol.* 1992; 3:263–271.

89. Garcia-Carranca A, Gariglio PV. Molecular aspects of human papillomaviruses and their relation to uterine cervix cancer. *Rev. Invest. Clin.* (Mexico) 1993; 45:85–92.

90. Meyer B, Weimar T, Peters T. Screening mixtures for biological activity by NMR. *Eur. J. Biochem.* 1997; 246:705–709.

91. Matsushita Y, Gouda H, Tsujishita H, Hirono S. Determination of binding conformations of drugs to human serum albumin by transferred nuclear Overhauser effect measurements and conformational analyses using high-temperature molecular dynamics calculations. *J. Pharm. Sci.* 1998; 87:379–386.

92. Dalvit C, Fogliatto G, Stewart A, Veronesi M, Stockman B. WaterLOGSY as a method for primary NMR screening: practical aspects and range of applicability. *J. Biomol. NMR* 2001; 21:349–359.

93. Dalvit C, Pevarello P, Tato M, Veronesi M, Vulpetti A, Sundstrom M. Identification of compounds with binding affinity to proteins via magnetization transfer from bulk water. *J. Biomol. NMR* 2000; 18:65–68.

94. Xue L, Bajorath J. Molecular descriptors in chemoinformatics, computational combinatorial chemistry, and virtual screening. *Comb. Chem. High Throughput Screen* 2000; 3:363–372.

95. Lewis RA, Pickett SD, Clark DE. Computer-aided molecular diversity analysis and combinatorial library design. *Rev. Comput. Chem.* 2000; 16:1–51.

96. Willett P. Chemoinformatics — similarity and diversity in chemical libraries. *Curr. Opin. Biotechnol.* 2000; 11:85–88.

97. Spellmeyer DC, Grootenhuis PDJ. Recent developments in molecular diversity. Computational approaches to combinatorial chemistry. *Annu. Rep. Med. Chem.* 1999; 34:287–296.

98. Gorse D, Lahana R. Functional diversity of compound libraries. *Curr. Opin. Chem. Biol.* 2000; 4:287–294.

99. Lipinski CA, Lombardo F, Dominy BW, Feeney PJ. Experimental and computational approaches to estimate solubility and permeability in drug discovery and development settings. *Adv. Drug Deliver. Rev.* 1997; 23:3–25.

100. Lipinski CA. Drug-like properties and the causes of poor solubility and poor permeability. *J. Pharmacol. Toxicol. Methods* 2001; 44:235–249.

101. Fejzo J, Lepre CA, Peng JW et al. The SHAPES strategy: An NMR-based approach for lead generation in drug discovery. *Chem. Biol.* 1999; 6:755–769.

102. Bemis GW, Murcko MA. The properties of known drugs. 1. Molecular frameworks. *J. Med. Chem.* 1996; 39:2887–2893.

103. Matsuzawa A, Ichijo H. Molecular mechanisms of the decision between life and death: Regulation of apoptosis by apoptosis signal-regulating kinase 1. *J. Biochem.* 2001; 130:1–8.

104. Altieri AS, Hinton DP, Byrd RA. Association of biomolecular systems via pulsed field gradient NMR self-diffusion measurements. *J. Am. Chem. Soc.* 1995; 117:7566–7567.

105. Luxon BA, Gorenstein DG. Comparison of x-ray and NMR-determined nucleic acid structures. *Methods Enzymol.* 1995; 261:45–73.

106. Wagner G, Hyberts SG, Havel TF. NMR structure determination in solution: A critique and comparison with x-ray crystallography. *Annu. Rev. Biophys. Biomol. Struct.* 1992; 21:167–198.

107. Billeter M. Comparison of protein structures determined by NMR in solution and by x-ray diffraction in single crystals. *Q. Rev. Biophys.* 1992; 25:325–377.

108. Hoffman DW, Cameron CS, Davies C, White SW, Ramakrishnan V. Ribosomal protein L9: A structure determination by the combined use of x-ray crystallography and NMR spectroscopy. *J. Mol. Biol.* 1996; 264:1058–1071.

109. Shaanan B, Gronenborn AM, Cohen GH et al. Combining experimental information from crystal and solution studies: joint x-ray and NMR refinement. *Science* 1992; 257:961–964.

110. Braun W, Epp O, Wüthrich K, Huber R. Solution of the phase problem in the x-ray diffraction method for proteins with the nuclear magnetic resonance solution structure as initial model. Patterson search and refinement for the α-amylase inhibitor Tendamistat. *J. Mol. Biol.* 1989; 206:669–676.

111. Berman HM, Westbrook J, Feng Z et al. The protein data bank. *Nucleic Acids Res.* 2000; 28:235–242.

112. Coombes RC, Marsh S, Gomm J, Johnston C. Fibroblast growth factors and their receptors in breast and prostate cancer. *Endo. Oncol.* 2000; 237–254.

113. Moy FJ, Seddon AP, Boehlen P, Powers R. High-resolution solution structure of basic fibroblast growth factor determined by multidimensional heteronuclear magnetic resonance spectroscopy. *Biochemistry* 1996; 35:13552–13561.

114. Moy FJ, Safran M, Seddon AP et al. Properly oriented heparin-decasaccharide-induced dimers are the biologically active form of basic fibroblast growth factor. *Biochemistry* 1997; 36:4782–4791.

115. Ogura K, Nagata K, Hatanaka H et al. Solution structure of human acidic fibroblast growth factor and interaction with heparin-derived hexasaccharide. *J. Biomol. NMR* 1999; 13:11–24.

116. Pineda-Lucena A, Jimenez MA, Lozano RM et al. Three-dimensional structure of acidic fibroblast growth factor in solution: effects of binding to a heparin functional analog. *J. Mol. Biol.* 1996; 264:162–178.

117. Pineda-Lucena A, Jimenez MA, Nieto JL, Santoro J, Rico M, Gimenez-Gallego G. 1H-NMR assignment and solution structure of human acidic fibroblast growth factor activated by inositol hexasulfate. *J. Mol. Biol.* 1994; 242:81–98.

118. Pellegrini L. Role of heparan sulfate in fibroblast growth factor signalling: A structural view. *Curr. Opin. Struct. Biol.* 2001; 11:629–634.

119. Miyamoto M, Naruo K-I, Seko C, Matsumoto S, Kondo T, Kurokawa T. Molecular cloning of a novel cytokine cDNA encoding the ninth member of the fibroblast growth factor family, which has a unique secretion property. *Mol. Cell Biol.* 1993; 13:4251–4259.

120. Folkman J, Klagsbrun M. Angiogenic factors. *Science* 1987; 235:442–447.

121. Baird A, Bohlen P. Peptide growth factors and their receptors. In *Handbook of Experimental Pharmacology* (Sporn MRA, ed.), Springer-Verlag, New York, 1990; 369–418.

122. Basilico C, Moscatelli D. The FGF family of growth factors and oncogenes. *Adv. Cancer Res.* 1992; 59:115–165.

123. Ornitz DM. FGFs, heparan sulfate and FGFRs: complex interactions essential for development. *BioEssays* 2000; 22:108–112.

124. Schlessinger J, Plotnikov AN, Ibrahimi OA et al. Crystal structure of a ternary FGF-FGFR-heparin complex reveals a dual role for heparin in FGFR binding and dimerization. *Mol. Cell* 2000; 6:743–750.

125. Pellegrini L, Burke DF, Von Delft F, Mulloy B, Blundell TL. Crystal structure of fibroblast growth factor receptor ectodomain bound to ligand and heparin. *Nature* 2000; 407:1029–1034.

126. DiGabriele AD, Lax I, Chen DI et al. Structure of a heparin-linked biologically active dimer of fibroblast growth factor. *Nature* 1998; 393:812–817.

127. Manetti F, Corelli F, Botta M. Fibroblast growth factors and their inhibitors. *Curr. Pharm. Des.* 2000; 6:1897–1924.

128. Fairbrother WJ, Champe MA, Christinger HW, Keyt BA, Starovasnik MA. Solution structure of the heparin-binding domain of vascular endothelial growth factor. *Structure* 1998; 6:637–648.

129. Starovasnik MA, Christinger HW, Wiesmann C, Champe MA, de Vos AM, Skelton NJ. Solution structure of the VEGF-binding domain of Flt-1: Comparison of its free and bound states. *J. Mol. Biol.* 1999; 293:531–544.

130. Campbell ID, Cooke RM. Structure function relationships in EGF, TGF-α and IGFI. *J. Cell Sci. Suppl.* 1990; 13:5–10.

131. Montelione GT, Wuethrich K, Burgess AW et al. Solution structure of murine epidermal growth factor determined by NMR spectroscopy and refined by energy minimization with restraints. *Biochemistry* 1992; 31:236–249.

132. Kohda D, Inagaki F. Three-dimensional nuclear magnetic resonance structures of mouse epidermal growth factor in acidic and physiological pH solutions. *Biochemistry* 1992; 31:11928–11939.

133. Schlunegger MP, Guretter MG. Refined crystal structure of human transforming growth factor b2 at 1.95 Å resolution. *J. Mol. Biol.* 1993; 231:445–458.

134. Harvey TS, Wilkinson AJ, Tappin MJ, Cooke RM, Campbell ID. The solution structure of human transforming growth factor α. *Eur. J. Biochem.* 1991; 198:555–562.

135. Hinck AP, Archer SJ, Qian SW et al. Transforming growth factor β1: Three-dimensional structure in solution and comparison with the x-ray structure of transforming growth factor β2. *Biochemistry* 1996; 35:8517–8534.

136. Baxter RC. Insulin-like growth factor (IGF)-binding proteins: Interactions with IGFs and intrinsic bioactivities. *Am. J. Physiol.* 2000; 278:E967–E976.

137. Sprang SR, Bazan JF. Cytokine structural taxonomy and mechanisms of receptor engagement. *Curr. Opin. Struct. Biol.* 1993; 3:815–827.

138. Clore GM, Appella E, Yamada M, Matsushima K, Gronenborn AM. Three-dimensional structure of interleukin 8 in solution. *Biochemistry* 1990; 29:1689–1696.

139. Gronenborn AM, Clore GM. The three dimensional structure of interleukin-8. *Challenges Mod. Med.* 1994; 3:13–24.

140. Clore GM, Wingfield PT, Gronenborn AM. High-resolution three-dimensional structure of interleukin 1b in solution by three- and four-dimensional nuclear magnetic resonance spectroscopy. *Biochemistry* 1991; 30:2315–2323.

141. Xie K. Interleukin-8 and human cancer biology. *Cytokine Growth Factor Rev.* 2001; 12:375–391.

142. Smith PC, Hobisch A, Lin D-L, Culig Z, Keller ET. Interleukin-6 and prostate cancer progression. *Cytokine Growth Factor Rev.* 2001; 12:33–40.

143. Mekhail T, Wood L, Bukowski R. Interleukin-2 in cancer therapy: Uses and optimum management of adverse effects. *BioDrugs* 2000; 14:299–318.

144. Gurjal A, Philip PA. Interleukin-2 in cancer. *Emerging Drugs* 2000; 5:273–285.

145. Maher DW, Davis I, Boyd AW, Morstyn G. Human interleukin-4: An immunomodulator with potential therapeutic applications. *Prog. Growth Factor Res.* 1991; 3:43–56.

146. Gessner A, Rollinghoff M. Biologic functions and signaling of the interleukin-4 receptor complexes. *Immunobiology* 2000; 201:285–307.

147. Murata T, Obiri NI, Debinski W, Puri RK. Structure of IL-13 receptor: analysis of subunit composition in cancer and immune cells. *Biochem. Biophys. Res. Commun.* 1997; 238:90–94.

148. Mintz A, Debinski W. Cancer genetics/epigenetics and the X chromosome. Possible new links for malignant glioma pathogenesis and immune-based therapies. *Crit. Rev. Oncog.* 2000; 11:77–95.

149. Callard RE, Matthews DJ, Hibbert L. IL-4 and IL-13 receptors: Are they one and the same? *Immunol. Today* 1996; 17:108–110.

150. Powers R, Garrett DS, March CJ, Frieden EA, Gronenborn AM, Clore GM. Three-dimensional solution structure of human interleukin-4 by multidimensional heteronuclear magnetic resonance spectroscopy. *Science* 1992; 256:1673–1677.

151. Powers R, Garrett DS, March CJ, Frieden EA, Gronenborn AM, Clore GM. The high-resolution, three-dimensional solution structure of human interleukin-4 determined by multidimensional heteronuclear magnetic resonance spectroscopy. *Biochemistry* 1993; 32:6744–6762.

152. Redfield C, Smith LJ, Boyd J et al. Analysis of the solution structure of human interleukin-4 determined by heteronuclear three-dimensional nuclear magnetic resonance techniques. *J. Mol. Biol.* 1994; 238:23–41.

153. Redfield C, Smith LJ, Boyd J et al. Secondary structure and topology of human interleukin 4 in solution. *Biochemistry* 1991; 30:11029–11035.

154. Moy FJ, Diblasio E, Wilhelm J, Powers R. Solution structure of human IL-13 and implication for receptor binding. *J. Mol. Biol.* 2001; 310:219–230.

155. Eisenmesser EZ, Horita DA, Altieri AS, Byrd RA. Solution structure of interleukin-13 and insights into receptor engagement. *J. Mol. Biol.* 2001; 310:231–241.

156. Mott HR, Baines BS, Hall RM et al. The solution structure of the F42A mutant of human interleukin 2. *J. Mol. Biol.* 1995; 247:979–994.

157. Xu G-Y, Yu H-A, Hong J et al. Solution structure of recombinant human interleukin-6. *J. Mol. Biol.* 1997; 268:468–481.

158. Muhlhahn P, Zweckstetter M, Georgescu J et al. Structure of interleukin 16 resembles a PDZ domain with an occluded peptide binding site. *Nat. Struct. Biol.* 1998; 5:682–686.

159. Woessner JF, Jr. Matrix metalloproteinases and their inhibitors in connective tissue remodeling. *FASEB J.* 1991; 5:2145–2154.

160. Ries C, Petrides E. Cytokine regulation of matrix metalloproteinase activity and its regulatory dysfunction in disease. *Biol. Chem. Hoppe-Seyler* 1995; 376:345–355.

161. Moy FJ, Chanda PK, Cosmi S et al. High-resolution solution structure of the inhibitor-free catalytic fragment of human fibroblast collagenase determined by multidimensional NMR. *Biochemistry* 1998; 37:1495–1504.

162. Moy FJ, Chanda PK, Chen JM et al. NMR solution structure of the catalytic fragment of human fibroblast collagenase complexed with a sulfonamide derivative of a hydroxamic acid compound. *Biochemistry* 1999; 38:7085–7096.

163. Feng Y, Likos J, Zhu L et al. ^{1}H, ^{13}C and ^{15}N resonance assignments for a truncated and inhibited catalytic domain of matrix metalloproteinase-2. *J. Biomol. NMR* 2000; 17:85–86.

164. Li Y-C, Zhang X, Melton R, Ganu V, Gonnella NC. Solution structure of the catalytic domain of human stromelysin-1 complexed to a potent, nonpeptidic inhibitor. *Biochemistry* 1998; 37:14048–14056.

165. Van Doren SR, Kurochkin AV, Hu W et al. Solution structure of the catalytic domain of human stromelysin complexed with a hydrophobic inhibitor. *Protein Sci.* 1995; 4:2487–2498.

166. Gooley PR, O'Connell JF, Marcy AI et al. The NMR structure of the inhibited catalytic domain of human stromelysin-1. *Nat. Struct. Biol.* 1994; 1:111–118.

167. Moy FJ, Chanda PK, Chen JM et al. High-resolution solution structure of the catalytic fragment of human collagenase-3 (MMP-13) complexed with a hydroxamic acid inhibitor. *J. Mol. Biol.* 2000; 302:671–689.

168. Zhang X, Gonnella NC, Koehn J et al. Solution structure of the catalytic domain of human collagenase-3 (MMP-13) complexed to a potent non-peptidic sulfonamide inhibitor: Binding comparison with stromelysin-1 and collagenase-1. *J. Mol. Biol.* 2000; 301:513–524.

169. Morphy JR, Millican TA, Porter JR. Matrix metalloproteinase inhibitors: Current status. *Curr. Med. Chem.* 1995; 2:743–762.

170. Drummond AH, Beckett P, Brown PD et al. Preclinical and clinical studies of MMP inhibitors in cancer. *Ann. N.Y. Acad. Sci.* 1999; 878:228–235.

171. Belotti D, Paganoni P, Giavazzi R. MMP inhibitors: Experimental and clinical studies. *Int. J. Biol. Markers* 1999; 14:232–238.

172. De B, Natchus MG, Cheng M et al. The next generation of MMP inhibitors: Design and synthesis. *Ann. N.Y. Acad. Sci.* 1999; 878:40–60.

173. Clore GM, Gronenborn AM. New methods of structure refinement for macromolecular structure determination by NMR. *Proc. Natl. Acad. Sci. U. S. A.* 1998; 95:5891–5898.

174. Cornilescu G, Delaglio F, Bax A. Protein backbone angle restraints from searching a database for chemical shift and sequence homology. *J. Biomol. NMR* 1999; 13:289–302.

175. Kuszewski J, Gronenborn AM, Clore GM. Improving the quality of NMR and crystallographic protein structures by means of a conformational database potential derived from structure databases. *Protein Sci.* 1996; 5:1067–1080.

176. Kuszewski J, Gronenborn AM, Clore GM. Improvements and extensions in the conformational database potential for the refinement of NMR and x-ray structures of proteins and nucleic acids. *J. Magn. Reson.* 1997; 125:171–177.

177. Kuszewski J, Gronenborn AM, Clore GM. Improving the packing and accuracy of NMR structures with a pseudopotential for the radius of gyration. *J. Am. Chem. Soc.* 1999; 121:2337–2338.

178. Tjandra N, Bax A. Direct measurement of distances and angles in biomolecules by NMR in a dilute liquid crystalline medium [see comments] [published erratum appears in *Science* 1997 Dec 5; 278(5344):1697]. *Science* 1997; 278:1111–274.

179. Clore GM, Starich MR, Bewley CA, Cai M, Kuszewski J. Impact of residual dipolar couplings on the accuracy of NMR structures determined from a minimal number of NOE restraints. *J. Am. Chem. Soc.* 1999; 121:6513–6514.

180. Gardner KH, Rosen MK, Kay LE. Global folds of highly deuterated, methyl-protonated proteins by multidimensional NMR. *Biochemistry* 1997; 36:1389–1401.

181. Huang X, Moy F, Powers R. Evaluation of the utility of NMR structures determined from minimal NOE-based restraints for structure-based drug design, using MMP-1 as an example. *Biochemistry* 2000; 39:13365–13375.

182. Brunner E. Residual dipolar couplings in protein NMR. *Concepts Magnetic Res.* 2001; 13:238–259.

183. Nilges M, Gronenborn AM, Bruenger AT, Clore GM. Determination of three-dimensional structures of proteins by simulated annealing with interproton distance restraints. Application to crambin, potato carboxypeptidase inhibitor and barley serine proteinase inhibitor 2. *Protein Eng.* 1988; 2:27–38.

184. Brunger AT. X-PLOR Version 3.1 Manual. Yale University, New Haven, CT, 1993.

185. Kuszewski J, Qin J, Gronenborn AM, Clore GM. The impact of direct refinement against $^{13}C\alpha$ and $^{13}C\beta$ chemical shifts on protein structure determination by NMR. *J. Magn. Reson. Ser. B* 1995; 106:92–96.

186. Petros AM, Kawai M, Luly JR, Fesik SW. Conformation of two non-immunosuppressive FK506 analogs when bound to FKBP by isotope-filtered NMR. *FEBS Lett.* 1992; 308:309–314.

187. Ikura M, Bax A. Isotope-filtered 2D NMR of a protein-peptide complex: Study of a skeletal muscle myosin light chain kinase fragment bound to calmodulin. *J. Am. Chem. Soc.* 1992; 114:2433–2440.

188. Gemmecker G, Olejniczak ET, Fesik SW. An improved method for selectivity observing protons attached to carbon-12 in the presence of proton-carbon-13 spin pairs. *J. Magn. Reson.* 1992; 96:199–204.

189. Marion D, Driscoll PC, Kay LE et al. Overcoming the overlap problem in the assignment of proton NMR spectra of larger proteins by use of three-dimensional heteronuclear proton-nitrogen-15 Hartmann-Hahn-multiple quantum coherence and nuclear Overhauser-multiple quantum coherence spectroscopy: Application to interleukin 1β. *Biochemistry* 1989; 28:6150–6156.

190. Zuiderweg ERP, Fesik SW. Heteronuclear three-dimensional NMR spectroscopy of the inflammatory protein C5a. *Biochemistry* 1989; 28:2387–2391.

191. Chen JM, Nelson FC, Levin JI et al. Structure-based design of a novel, potent, and selective inhibitor for MMP-13 utilizing NMR spectroscopy and computer-aided molecular design. *J. Am. Chem. Soc.* 2000; 122:9648–9654.

192. Palmer AG, III. Probing molecular motion by NMR. *Curr. Opin. Struct. Biol.* 1997; 7:732–737.

193. Kay LE. Protein dynamics from NMR. *Biochem. Cell Biol.* 1998; 76:145–152.

194. Ishima R, Torchia DA. Protein dynamics from NMR. *Nat. Struct. Biol.* 2000; 7:740–743.

195. Lipari G, Szabo A. Model-free approach to the interpretation of nuclear magnetic resonance relaxation in macromolecules. 1. Theory and range of validity. *J. Am. Chem. Soc.* 1982; 104:4546–4559.

196. Lipari G, Szabo A. Model-free approach to the interpretation of nuclear magnetic resonance relaxation in macromolecules. 2. Analysis of experimental results. *J. Am. Chem. Soc.* 1982; 104:4559–4570.

197. Moy FJ, Pisano MR, Chanda PK et al. Assignments, secondary structure and dynamics of the inhibitor-free catalytic fragment of human fibroblast collagenase. *J. Biomol. NMR* 1997; 10:9–19.

198. Yuan P, Marshall VP, Petzold GL, Poorman RA, Stockman BJ. Dynamics of stromelysin/inhibitor interactions studied by ^{15}N NMR relaxation measurements: Comparison of ligand binding to the S1-S3 and S1'-S3' subsites. *J. Biomol. NMR* 1999; 15:55–64.

199. Zhang X, Gonnella NC, Koehn J et al. Solution structure of the catalytic domain of human collagenase-3 (MMP-13) complexed to a potent non-peptidic sulfonamide inhibitor: Binding comparison with stromelysin-1 and collagenase-1. *J. Mol. Biol.* 2000; 301:513–524.

200. Lovejoy B, Welch AR, Carr S et al. Crystal structures of MMP-1 and -13 reveal the structural basis for selectivity of collagenase inhibitors. *Nat. Struct. Biol.* 1999; 6:217–221.

201. Ringe D, Petsko GA. Study of protein dynamics by x-ray diffraction. *Methods Enzymol.* 1986; 131:389–433.

202. Powers R, Clore GM, Garrett DS, Gronenborn AM. Relationships between the precision of high-resolution protein NMR structures, solution-order parameters, and crystallographic B factors. *J. Magn. Reson. Ser. B* 1993; 101:325–327.

203. Sahu SC, Bhuyan AK, Majumdar A, Udgaonkar JB. Backbone dynamics of barstar: A ^{15}N NMR relaxation study. *Proteins Struct. Funct. Genet.* 2000; 41:460–474.

204. Pang Y, Buck M, Zuiderweg ERP. Backbone dynamics of the ribonuclease binase active site area using multinuclear (^{15}N and [13]CO) NMR relaxation and computational molecular dynamics. *Biochemistry* 2002; 41:2655–2666.

205. Uhrinova S, Smith MH, Jameson GB, Uhrin D, Sawyer L, Barlow PN. Structural changes accompanying pH-induced dissociation of the β-lactoglobulin dimer. *Biochemistry* 2000; 39:3565–3574.

206. Zhang P, Dayie KT, Wagner G. Unusual lack of internal mobility and fast overall tumbling in oxidized flavodoxin from Anacystis nidulans. *J. Mol. Biol.* 1997; 272:443–455.

207. Constantine KL, Friedrichs MS, Goldfarb V, Jeffrey PD, Sheriff S, Mueller L. Characterization of the backbone dynamics of an anti-digoxin antibody VL domain by inverse detected proton-nitrogen-15 NMR: Comparisons with x-ray data for the Fab. *Proteins Struct. Funct. Genet.* 1993; 15:290–311.

208. Roboz J. Mass spectrometry in cancer research. *Adv. Cancer Res.* 1978; 27:201–267.

209. Roboz J. *Mass Spectrometry in Cancer Research.* CRC Press, Boca Raton, FL, 2002.

210. Chistyakov VV, Anisimova OS, Sheinker YN, Safonova TS. Mass spectra of antitumor drugs containing phosphoric and thiophosphoric acid ethylenimides. *Khim. Farm. Zh.* 1984; 18:1290–1294.

211. Pyatigorskaya TL, Zhil'kova OY, Shelkovskii VS, Arkhangelova NM, Grizodub AI, Sukhodub LF. Hydrolysis of 1,1,1"-phosphinothioylidinetrisaziridine thiotepa in aqueous solution. *Biomed. Environ. Mass Spectrom.* 1987; 14:143–148.

212. Kosevich MV, Shelkovskii VS. On the formation of doubly charged fragment and cluster ions of oxygen- and sulfur-containing substances in field ionization and field desorption mass spectrometry. *Rapid Commun. Mass Spectrom.* 1990; 4:493–494.

213. Sukhodub LF. Soft-ionization mass spectrometry study of deoxynucleoside bioclusters and deoxynucleoside-antitumor medicinal preparation clusters. *Mass Spectrom. Rev.* 1996; 14:235–254.

214. Kosevich MV, Shelkovsky VS, Stepanian SG. Dependence of the biological activity and mass spectrometric pattern on the structure peculiarities of the molecule of alkylating drug thiotepa. *Biophys. Chem.* 1996; 57:123–131.

215. Musser SM, Pan SS, Callery PS. Liquid chromatography-thermospray mass spectrometry of DNA adducts formed with mitomycin C, porfiromycin and thiotepa. *J. Chromatogr.* 1989; 474:197–207.

216. Musser SM, Callery PS. Supercritical fluid chromatography/chemical ionization/mass spectrometry of some anticancer drugs in a thermospray ion source. *Biomed. Environ. Mass Spectrom.* 1990; 19:348–352.

217. Sukhodub LF, Kosevich MV, Shelkovskii VS, Pyatigorskaya TL, Zhilkova OY. Direct detection of nitrogen base-thiotepa adducts by mild ionization mass spectrometry. *Biofizika* 1990; 35:549–551.

218. Van Maanen MJ, Tijhof IM, Damen JMA et al. A search for new metabolites of N,N',N"-triethylenethiophosphoramide. *Cancer Res.* 1999; 59:4720–4724.

219. Sukhodub LF, Chivanov VD, Grebenik LI, Bondarenko PV, Zubarev RA, Knysh AN. Study of triethylenethiophosphamide interaction with nucleotides by mass spectrometry with ionization by fission fragments californium-252. *Ukr. Biokhim. Zh.* 1992; 64:41–49.

220. van Maanen MJ, Beijnen JH. Liquid chromatographic-mass spectrometric determination of the novel, recently identified thioTEPA metabolite, thioTEPA-mercapturate, in urine. *J. Chromatogr. B: Biomed. Sci. Appl.* 1999; 732:73–79.

221. Bakhtiar R. In vitro exposure of human hemoglobin to the antineoplastic drug thiotepa. *Rapid Commun. Mass Spectrom.* 2000; 14:534–537.

222. van Maanen MJ, Doesburg Smits K, Damen JMA, Heck AJR, Beijnen JH. Stability of thioTEPA and its metabolites, TEPA, monochloroTEPA and thioTEPA-mercapturate, in plasma and urine. *Int. J. Pharm.* 2000; 200:187–194.

223. van Maanen MJ, Brandt AC, Damen JMA, Beijnen JH. Degradation study of thiotepa in aqueous solutions. *Int. J. Pharm.* 1999; 179:55–64.

224. Cohen BE, Egorin MJ, Nayar MSB, Gutierrez PL. Effects of pH and temperature on the stability and decomposition of N,N',N''-triethylenethiophosphoramide in urine and buffer. *Cancer Res.* 1984; 44:4312–4316.

225. Pyatigorskaya TL, Zhilkova OY, Shelkovskii VS et al. Analysis of the products of thiophosphamide transformation in aqueous solutions using thin-layer chromatography and mass spectrometry. *Khim. Farm Zh.* 1985; 19:1235–1241.

226. Chistyakov VV, Anisimova OS, Presnova ZF et al. Study on the metabolism of the antineoplastic agent thiophosphamide in rats. *Khim. Farm Zh.* 1988; 22:1158–1162.

227. Van Maanen RJ, Van Ooijen RD, Zwikker JW, Huitema ADR, Rodenhuis S, Beijnen JH. Determination of N,N'N''-triethylenethiophosphoramide and its active metabolite N,N'N''-triethylenephosphoramide in plasma and urine using capillary gas chromatography. *J. Chromatogr. B: Biomed. Sci. Appl.* 1998; 719:103–112.

228. Van Maanen MJ, Huitema ADR, Rodenhuis S, Beijnen JH. Urinary excretion of thioTEPA and its metabolites in patients treated with high-dose cyclophosphamide, thioTEPA and carboplatin. *Anticancer Drugs* 2001; 12:519–524.

229. Srivastava SK, Singhal SS, Hu X, Awasthi YC, Zimniak P, Singh SV. Differential catalytic efficiency of allelic variants of human glutathione S-transferase Pi in catalyzing the glutathione conjugation of thiotepa. *Arch. Biochem. Biophys.* 1999; 366:89–94.

230. Chistyakov VV, Anisimova OS, Losev GA, Chernov VA, Sheinker YN. Hydrazine sulfate, an oxidative desulfation inhibitor for thiophosphamide and thiodipin. *Khim. Farm. Zh.* 1989; 23:1291–1294.

231. Huitema ADR, Tibben MM, Kerbusch T, Den Bosch JJK-V, Rodenhuis S, Beijnen JH. High performance liquid chromatographic determination of the stabilized cyclophosphamide metabolite 4-hydroxycyclophosphamide in plasma and red blood cells. *J. Liq. Chromatogr. Relat. Technol.* 2000; 23:1725–1744.

232. Sukhodub LF, Shelkovskii VS, Kosevich MV, Pyatigorskaya TL, Zhilkova OY. Nucleic acid base complexes with thiotepa as revealed by field ionization mass spectrometry. *Biomed. Environ. Mass Spectrom.* 1986; 13:167–170.

233. Sukhodub LF, Shelkovskii VS, Kosevich MV, Pyatigorskaya TL, Zhilkova OI. Mass-spectrometric study of the interaction between thiophosphamide and nucleic acid bases. *Dokl. Akad. Nauk. SSSR* 1985; 283:714–716.

234. Andrievskii GV, Nikolaeva MI, Serebryanyi AM, Tantsyrev GD, Sharova OL. Analysis of canonical and modified components of nucleic acids by fast-atom-bombardment secondary-ion mass spectrometry. *Zh. Anal. Khim.* 1988; 43:1850–1856.

235. Sukhodub LF, Andrievskii GV, Pyatigorskaya TL, Kosevich MV, Zhilkova OY. Identification of DNA-thiotepa adducts by fast atom bombardment mass spectrometry. *Bioorg. Khim.* 1988; 14:1698–1699.

236. Sukhodub LF, Chivanov VD, Grebenik LI, Bondarenko PV, Zubarev RA, Knysh AN. Observation of thiotepa deoxyguanosine 5'-phosphate modification products by PDMS. *Bioorg. Khim.* 1991; 17:999–1001.

237. Andrievskii GV, Sukhodub LF, Pyatigorskaya TL, Boryak OA, Limanskaya OY, Shelkovskii VS. Direct observation of the alkylation products of deoxyguanosine and DNA by fast atom bombardment mass spectrometry. *Biol. Mass Spectrom.* 1991; 20:665–668.

238. Voloshchuk TP, Patskovsky YV, Potopalsky AI. Alkylation of nucleic acid components by ethylenimine derivatives. 2. Alkylation of nucleosides. *Bioorg. Khim.* 1993; 19:484–493.

239. Hignite CE, Azarnoff DL. Identification of methotrexate and folic acid analogs by mass spectrometry. *Biomed. Mass Spectrom.* 1978; 5:161–163.

240. Smith RG, Pegues JC, Farquhar D, Loo TL, Wang Y-M. Mass spectrometry of permethylated folic acid analogs. *Biomed. Mass Spectrom.* 1981; 8:144–148.

241. Cheung HTA, Tattam BN, Antonjuk DJ, Boadle DK. Ammonia and methane chemical ionization mass spectra of methotrexate and its amide and ester analogs. *Biomed. Mass Spectrom.* 1985; 12:11–18.

242. Przybylski M. Identification of metabolism pathways of anticancer drugs by high-pressure liquid chromatography in combination with field desorption mass spectrometry. *Biomed. Mass Spectrom.* 1982; 9:995–1012.

243. Przybylski M, Preiss J, Dennebaum R, Fischer J. Identification and quantitation of methotrexate and methotrexate metabolites in clinical high-dose therapy by high-pressure liquid chromatography and field desorption mass spectrometry. *Biomed. Mass Spectrom.* 1982; 9:22–32.

244. Morris HR, Riddoch A, Chapman JR, Aspinal ML, Compson KR, McDowell RA. Field desorption and chemical ionization analysis using a double beam mass spectrometer. *Adv. Mass Spectrom.* 1978; 7B:832–837.

245. Tatischeff I, Spiro M, Della Negra S et al. Plasma desorption mass spectrometry (PDMS) of folic acid and derivatives. *Int. J. Mass Spectrom. Ion Phys.* 1983; 48:165–168.

246. Cairnes DA, Evans WE. A simple preparation of the methotrexate metabolites 7-hydroxymethotrexate and 4-deoxy-4-amino-N10-methylpteroic acid. *Ther. Drug Monit.* 1983; 5:363–366.

247. Eicke A, Anders V, Junack M, Sichtermann W, Benninghoven A. Secondary ion mass spectrometry of folic acid analogs. *Int. J. Mass Spectrom. Ion Phys.* 1983; 46:479–482.

248. Eicke A, Anders V, Junack M, Sichtermann W, Benninghoven A. Secondary ion mass spectrometry of folic acid analogs. *Anal. Chem.* 1983; 55:178–182.

249. Deng Y, Zeng H, Unger SE, Wu J-T. Multiple-sprayer tandem mass spectrometry with parallel high flow extraction and parallel separation for high-throughput quantitation in biological fluids. *Rapid Commun. Mass Spectrom.* 2001; 15:1634–1640.

250. Rule G, Chapple M, Henion J. A 384-well solid-phase extraction for LC/MS/MS determination of methotrexate and its 7-hydroxy metabolite in human urine and plasma. *Anal. Chem.* 2001; 73:439–443.

251. Widemann BC, Sung E, Anderson L et al. Pharmacokinetics and metabolism of the methotrexate metabolite 2,4-diamino-N10-methylpteroic acid. *J. Pharmacol. Exp. Ther.* 2000; 294:894–901.

252. Steinborner S, Henion J. Liquid-liquid extraction in the 96-well plate format with SRM LC/MS quantitative determination of methotrexate and its major metabolite in human plasma. *Anal. Chem.* 1999; 71:2340–2345.

253. Turci R, Micoli G, Minoia C. Determination of methotrexate in environmental samples by solid phase extraction and high performance liquid chromatography: Ultraviolet or tandem mass spectrometry detection. *Rapid Commun. Mass Spectrom.* 2000; 14:685–691.

254. Hignite CE, Shen DD, Azarnoff DL. Separation and identification of impurities in parenteral methotrexate dosage forms. *Cancer Treat. Rep.* 1978; 62:13–18.

255. Siegel MM, Hollander IJ, Hamann PR et al. Matrix-assisted UV-laser desorption/ionization mass spectrometric analysis of monoclonal antibodies for the determination of carbohydrate, conjugated chelator, and conjugated drug content. *Anal. Chem.* 1991; 63:2470–2481.

256. Nikolic D, van Breemen RB. Screening for inhibitors of dihydrofolate reductase using pulsed ultrafiltration mass spectrometry. *Comb. Chem. High Throughput Screen* 1998; 1:47–55.

257. Chiccarelli FS, Morrison JA, Cosulich DB et al. Identification of human urinary mitoxantrone metabolites. *Cancer Res.* 1986; 46:4858–4861.

258. Blanz J, Mewes K, Ehninger G et al. Isolation and structure elucidation of urinary metabolites of mitoxantrone. *Cancer Res.* 1991; 51:3427–3433.

259. Blanz J, Mewes K, Ehninger G et al. Evidence for oxidative activation of mitoxantrone in human, pig, and rat. *Drug Metab. Dispos.* 1991; 19:871–880.

260. Mewes K, Blanz J, Ehninger G, Gebhardt R, Zeller KP. Cytochrome P-450-induced cytotoxicity of mitoxantrone by formation of electrophilic intermediates. *Cancer Res.* 1993; 53:5135–5142.

261. Mewes K, Blanz J, Freund S, Ehninger G, Zeller KP. Synthesis and structural elucidation of biliary excreted thioether derivatives of mitoxantrone. *Xenobiotica* 1994; 24:199–213.

262. Siegel MM. Hydrogen-deuterium exchange studies utilizing a thermospray mass spectrometer interface. *Anal. Chem.* 1988; 60:2090–2095.

263. Reddy AM, Mykytyn VV, Schram KH. Deuterium-labeled 3-nitrobenzyl alcohol as a matrix for fast atom bombardment mass spectrometry. *Biomed. Environ. Mass Spectrom.* 1989; 18:1087–1095.

264. Sepetov NF, Issakova OL, Lebl M, Swiderek K, Stahl DC, Lee TD. The use of hydrogen-deuterium exchange to facilitate peptide sequencing by electrospray tandem mass spectrometry. *Rapid Commun. Mass Spectrom.* 1993; 7:58–62.

265. Spengler B, Luetzenkirchen F, Kaufmann R. On-target deuteration for peptide sequencing by laser mass spectrometry. *Org. Mass Spectrom.* 1993; 28:1482–1490.

266. Siegel MM, Bitha P, Child RG, Hlavka JJ, Lin YI, Chang TT. Fast atom bombardment mass spectrometry of cisplatin analogs. *Biomed. Environ. Mass Spectrom.* 1986; 13:25–32.

267. Martin LB, III, Schreiner AF, Van Breemen RB. Characterization of cisplatin adducts of oligonucleotides by fast atom bombardment mass spectrometry. *Anal. Biochem.* 1991; 193:6–15.

268. Cetini G, Operti L, Vaglio GA, Bandini AL, Banditelli G, Minghetti G. Fast atom bombardment mass spectrometry of neutral methanide and ionic carbene platinum (II) derivatives. *Org. Mass Spectrom.* 1989; 24:479–484.

269. Claerboudt J, De Spiegeleer B, Lippert B, De Bruijn EA, Claeys M. Fast atom bombardment and tandem mass spectrometry for the structural characterization of cisplatin analogs and bis-nucleobase adducts with cisplatin. *Spectroscopy (Ottawa)* 1989; 7:91–112.

270. Bruce DW, Cole-Hamilton DJ, Cottee FH, Page JA. A fast atom bombardment mass spectrometric investigation of some triethylphosphine complexes of platinum (II) in aqueous solution. *J. Organomet. Chem.* 1987; 320:249–255.

271. Burns RB, Burton RW, Albon SP, Embree L. Liquid chromatography-mass spectrometry for the detection of platinum antineoplastic complexes. *J. Pharm. Biomed. Anal.* 1996; 14:367–372.

272. Poon GK, Mistry P, Lewis S. Electrospray ionization mass spectrometry of platinum anticancer agents. *Biol. Mass Spectrom.* 1991; 20:687–692.

273. Bergamini P, Bortolini O, Curcuruto O, Hamdan M. Investigation of bisdiphenylphosphinomethane Pt (II) complexes by electrospray and fast atom bombardment mass spectrometry. *J. Mass Spectrom.* 1995;Spec. Issue:S77–S84.

274. Allain P, Heudi O, Cailleux A et al. Early biotransformations of oxaliplatin after its intravenous administration to cancer patients. *Drug Metab. Dispos.* 2000; 28:1379–1384.

275. Costello CE, Nordhoff E, Hillenkamp F. Matrix-assisted UV and IR laser desorption-ionization time-of-flight mass spectrometry of diamminoplatinum (II) oligodeoxyribonucleotide adducts and their unplatinated analogs. *Int. J. Mass Spectrom. Ion Proc.* 1994; 132:239–249.

276. Guittard J, Pacifico C, Blais JC, Bolbach G, Chottard JC, Spassky A. Matrix-assisted laser desorption ionization time-of-flight mass spectrometry of DNA-PtII complexes. *Rapid Commun. Mass Spectrom.* 1995; 9:33–36.

277. Costello CE, Comess KM, Plaziak AS, Bancroft DP, Lippard SJ. Fast atom bombardment and high performance tandem mass spectrometry of platinum (II) oligodeoxyribonucleotide fragments. *Int. J. Mass Spectrom. Ion Proc.* 1992; 122:255–279.

278. Carte N, Legendre F, Leize E et al. Determination by electrospray mass spectrometry of the outersphere association constants of DNA/platinum complexes using 20-mer oligonucleotides and $[Pt(NH_3)4]^{2+}$, $2Cl^-$ or $[Pt(py)4]^{2+}$, $2Cl^-$. *Anal. Biochem.* 2000; 284:77–86.

279. Gonnet F, Kocher F, Blais JC, Bolbach G, Tabet JC, Chottard JC. Kinetic analysis of the reaction between d(TTGGCCAA) and $[Pt(NH_3)_3H2O]^{2+}$ by enzymatic degradation of the products and ESI and MALDI mass spectrometries. *J. Mass Spectrom.* 1996; 31:802–809.

280. Gibson D, Costello CE. A mass spectral study of the binding of the anticancer drug cisplatin to ubiquitin. *Eur. Mass Spectrom.* 1999; 5:501–510.

281. Heudi O, Brisset H, Cailleux A, Allain P. Chemical instability and methods for measurement of cisplatin adducts formed by interactions with cysteine and glutathione. *Int. J. Clin. Pharmacol. Ther.* 2001; 39:344–349.

282. Zollner P, Zenker A, Galanski M, Keppler BK, Lindner W. Reaction monitoring of platinum (II) complex-5′-guanosine monophosphate adduct formation by ion exchange liquid chromatography/electrospray ionization mass spectrometry. *J. Mass Spectrom.* 2001; 36:742–753.

283. Kung A, Strickmann DB, Galanski M, Keppler BK. Comparison of the binding behavior of oxaliplatin, cisplatin and analogues to 5′-GMP in the presence of sulfur-containing molecules by means of capillary electrophoresis and electrospray mass spectrometry. *J. Inorg. Biochem.* 2001; 86:691–698.

284. Styles ML, O'Hair RAJ, McFadyen WD. Evaluating the role of the ligand in the fragmentation reactions of platinum (II) complexes of aliphatic dipeptides. Electrospray ionization tandem mass spectrometry of $[Pt(L3)M]^{2+}$ and $[Pt(L3)M-H]^+$ ions [L3 = $H_3N)_3$], diethylenetriamine and terpyridine M = gly-gly, ala-gly and gly-ala]. *Eur. J. Mass Spectrom.* 2001; 7:69–78.

285. Liu Q, Zhang J, Ke X, Mei Y, Zhu L, Guo Z. ESMS and NMR investigations on the interaction of the anticancer drug cisplatin and chemopreventive agent selenomethionine. *J. Chem. Soc. Dalton Trans.* 2001; 6:911–916.

286. Warnke U, Gysler J, Hofte B et al. Separation and identification of platinum adducts with DNA nucleotides by capillary zone electrophoresis and capillary zone electrophoresis coupled to mass spectrometry. *Electrophoresis* 2001; 22:97–103.

287. Mio T, Sumino K. FAB mass spectrometry of carboplatin and its metabolite in the urine. *Iyo Masu Kenkyukai Koenshu* 1987; 12:207–210.

288. Poon GK, Mistry P, Raynaud FI, Harrap KR, Murrer BA, Barnard CFJ. Determination of metabolites of a novel platinum anticancer drug JM216 in human plasma ultrafiltrates. *J. Pharm. Biomed. Anal.* 1995; 13:1493–1498.

289. Borders DB, Doyle TW, eds. *Enediyne Antibiotic Antitumor Agents*. Dekker, New York, 1995.

290. Lee MD, Dunne TS, Siegel MM, Chang CC, Morton GO, Borders DB. Calicheamicins, a novel family of antitumor antibiotics. 1. Chemistry and partial structure of calichemicin γ1I. *J. Am. Chem. Soc.* 1987; 109:3464–3466.

291. Lee MD, Dunne TS, Chang CC et al. Calicheamicins, a novel family of antitumor antibiotics. 2. Chemistry and structure of calicheamicin γ 1I. *J. Am. Chem. Soc.* 1987; 109:3466–3468.

292. Lee MD, Dunne TS, Chang CC et al. Calicheamicins, a novel family of antitumor antibiotics. 4. Structure elucidation of calicheamicins β1Br, γ1Br, α2I, α3I, β1I, γ1I, and δ1I. *J. Am. Chem. Soc.* 1992; 114:985–997.

293. Lee MD. Identification, isolation, and structure determination [of Calecheamicins]. In *Enediyne Antibiotic Antitumor Agents* (Borders DB and Doyle TD, eds.), Dekker, New York, 1995.

294. Golik J. Structure determination of the esperamicins. In *Enediyne Antibiotic Antitumor Agents* (Borders DB and Doyle TW, eds.), Dekker, New York, 1995; 187–215.

295. Lam KS, Veitch JA. Biosynthesis of esperamicin. In *Enediyne Antibiotic Antitumor Agents* (Borders DB and Doyle TW, eds.), Dekker, New York, 1995; 217–237.

296. Chin DH, Zeng CH, Costello CE, Goldberg IH. Sites in the diyne-ene bicyclic core of neocarzinostatin chromophore responsible for hydrogen abstraction from DNA. *Biochemistry* 1988; 27:8106–8114.

297. Gao Q, Cheng X, Smith RD, Yang CF, Goldberg IH. Binding specificity of post-activated neocarzinostatin chromophore drug-bulged DNA complex studied using electrospray ionization mass spectrometry. *J. Mass Spectrom.* 1996; 31:31–36.

298. Hamann PR, Hinman LM, Hollander I et al. Gemtuzumab ozogamicin, a potent and selective anti-CD33 antibody-calicheamicin conjugate for treatment of acute myeloid leukemia. *Bioconjugate Chem.* 2002; 13:47–58.

299. Hamann PR, Hinman LM, Beyer CF et al. An anti-CD33 antibody-calicheamicin conjugate for treatment of acute myeloid leukemia. Choice of linker. *Bioconjugate Chem.* 2002; 13:40–46.

300. Siegel MM, Tabei K, Kunz A et al. Calicheamicin derivatives conjugated to monoclonal antibodies: Determination of loading values and distributions by infrared and UV matrix-assisted laser desorption/ionization mass spectrometry and electrospray ionization mass spectrometry. *Anal. Chem.* 1997; 69:2716–2726.

301. Siegel MM. Determination of loading values and distributions for drugs conjugated to proteins and antibodies by MALDI-MS and ESI-MS. *Methods Mol. Biol. (Totowa NJ)* 1996; 61:211–226.

302. Siegel MM, Tsou HR, Lin B et al. Determination of the loading values for high levels of drugs and sugars conjugated to proteins by matrix-assisted ultraviolet laser desorption/ionization mass spectrometry. *Biol. Mass. Spectrom* 1993; 22:369–376.

303. Siegel MM, Tabei K, Tsao R et al. Comparative mass spectrometric analyses of photofrin oligomers by fast atom bombardment mass spectrometry, UV and IR matrix-assisted laser desorption/ionization mass spectrometry, electrospray ionization mass spectrometry and laser desorption/jet-cooling photoionization mass spectrometry. *J. Mass Spectrom.* 1999; 34:661–669.

304. Pandey RK, Siegel MM, Tsao R, McReynolds JH, Dougherty TJ. Fast atom bombardment mass spectral analyses of Photofrin II and its synthetic analogs. *Biomed. Environ. Mass Spectrom.* 1990; 19:405–414.

305. Cai H, Wang Q, Luo J, Lim CK. Study of temoporfin metabolism by HPLC and electrospray mass spectrometry. *Biomed. Chromatogr.* 1999; 13:354–359.

306. Lord GA, Cai H, Luo JL, Lim CK. HPLC-electrospray mass spectrometry for the analysis of temoporfin-polyethylene glycol conjugates. *Analyst (Cambridge, UK)* 2000; 125:605–608.

307. Angotti M, Maunit B, Muller J-F, Bezdetnaya L, Guillemin F. Characterization by matrix-assisted laser desorption/ionization Fourier transform ion cyclotron resonance mass spectrometry of the major photoproducts of Temoporfin μ-THPC and bacteriochlorin μ-THPBC. *J. Mass Spectrom.* 2001; 36:825–831.

308. Angotti M, Maunit B, Muller J-F, Bezdetnaya L, Guillemin F. Matrix-assisted laser desorption/ionization coupled to Fourier transform ion cyclotron resonance mass spectrometry: A method to characterize temoporfin photoproducts. *Rapid Commun. Mass Spectrom.* 1999; 13:597–603.

309. Jones RM, Wang Q, Lamb JH, Djelal BD, Bonnett R, Lim CK. Identification of photochemical oxidation products of 5,10,15,20-tetram-hydroxyphenyl)chlorin by online HPLC-electrospray ionization tandem mass spectrometry. *J. Chromatogr. A* 1996; 722:257–265.

310. Miller RW, Powell RG, Smith CR, Jr., Arnold E, Clardy J. Antileukemic alkaloids from Taxus wallichiana Zucc. *J. Org. Chem.* 1981; 46:1469–1474.

311. Ringel I, Horwitz SB. Taxol is converted to 7-epitaxol, a biologically active isomer, in cell culture medium. *J. Pharmacol. Exp. Ther.* 1987; 242:692–698.

312. Zamir LO, Nedea ME, Zhou Z-H, et al. Taxus canadensis taxanes: Structures and stereochemistry. *Can. J. Chem.* 1995; 73:655–665.

313. Monsarrat B, Mariel E, Cros S et al. Taxol metabolism. Isolation and identification of three major metabolites of taxol in rat bile. *Drug Metab. Dispos.* 1990; 18:895–901.

314. Walle T, Kumar GN, McMillan JM, Thornburg KR, Walle UK. Taxol metabolism in rat hepatocytes. *Biochem. Pharmacol.* 1993; 46:1661–1664.

315. Monsarrat B, Alvinerie P, Gares M et al. Hepatic metabolism and biliary excretion of taxol. *Cell Pharmacol.* 1993; 1:S77–S81.

316. Royer I, Alvinerie P, Armand JP, Ho LK, Wright M, Monsarrat B. Paclitaxel metabolites in human plasma and urine: identification of 6α-hydroxytaxol, 7-epitaxol and taxol hydrolysis products by liquid chromatography/atmospheric-pressure chemical ionization mass spectrometry. *Rapid Commun. Mass Spectrom.* 1995; 9:495–502.

317. Sparreboom A, Huizing MT, Boesen JJB, Nooijen WJ, van Tellingen O, Beijnen JH. Isolation, purification, and biological activity of mono- and dihydroxylated paclitaxel metabolites from human feces. *Cancer Chemother. Pharmacol.* 1995; 36:299–304.

318. Royer I, Monsarrat B, Sonnier M, Wright M, Cresteil T. Metabolism of docetaxel by human cytochromes P450: interactions with paclitaxel and other antineoplastic drugs. *Cancer Res.* 1996; 56:58–65.

319. Poon GK, Bloomer JW, Clarke SE, Maltas J. Rapid screening of taxol metabolites in human microsomes by liquid chromatography/electrospray ionization-mass spectrometry. *Rapid Commun. Mass Spectrom.* 1996; 10:1165–1168.

320. Sottani C, Minoia C, Colombo A, Zucchetti M, D'Incalci M, Fanelli R. Structural characterization of mono- and dihydroxylated metabolites of paclitaxel in rat bile using liquid chromatography/ion spray tandem mass spectrometry. *Rapid Commun. Mass Spectrom.* 1997; 11:1025–1032.

321. Hauck C. Structure elucidation of taxol metabolites by liquid chromatography/mass spectrometry and species differences in taxol metabolism. *Rapid Commun. Mass Spectrom.* 1997; 11:1823.

322. Sottani C, Minoia C, Colombo T, Zucchetti M, D'Incalci M, Fanelli R. Structure elucidation of taxol metabolites by liquid chromatography/mass spectrometry and species differences in taxol metabolism. Reply. *Rapid Commun. Mass Spectrom.* 1997; 11:1824.

323. Dierks EA, Stams KR, Lim H-K, Cornelius G, Zhang H, Ball SE. A method for the simultaneous evaluation of the activities of seven major human drug-metabolizing cytochrome P450s using an in vitro cocktail of probe substrates and fast gradient liquid chromatography tandem mass spectrometry. *Drug Metab. Dispos.* 2001; 29:23–29.

324. McClure TD, Schram KH, Reimer MLJ. The mass spectrometry of taxol. *J. Am. Soc. Mass Spectrom.* 1992; 3:672–679.

325. McClure TD, Schram KH, Reimer MLJ. The mass spectrometry of taxol. *J. Am. Soc. Mass Spectrom.* 1993; 4:85.

326. Hoke SH, II, Wood JM, Cooks RG, Li XH, Chang CJ. Rapid screening for taxanes by tandem mass spectrometry. *Anal. Chem.* 1992; 64:2313–2315.

327. Griffini A, Peterlongo F, De Bellis P, Pace R. Desorption chemical ionization and thermospray mass spectra of taxol and related compounds. *Fitoterapia* 1993; 64:53–81.

328. Auriola SOK, Lepisto AM, Naaranlahti T, Lapinjoki SP. Determination of taxol by high-performance liquid chromatography-thermospray mass spectrometry. *J. Chromatogr.* 1992; 594:153–158.

329. Madhusudanan KP. Formation of radical anion adduct between Paclitaxel and matrix under fast-atom bombardment. *Rapid Commun. Mass Spectrom.* 1997; 11:295–297.

330. Takayama M, Kataoka H, Katagi T et al. A new versatile matrix for fast atom bombardment mass spectrometry. *J. Mass Spectrom. Soc. Jpn.* 1998; 46:143–149.

331. Ishida T, Fenselau C, Kaltashov I, Yu X. Evaluation of electrospray for drug analysis. *Nippon Iyo Masu Supekutoru Gakkai Koenshu* 1992; 17:275–276.

332. Blay PKS, Thibault P, Thiberge N, Kiecken B, Lebrun A, Mercure C. Analysis of taxol and related taxanes from *Taxus canadensis* using liquid chromatography combined with mass spectrometry or tandem mass spectrometry. *Rapid Commun. Mass Spectrom.* 1993; 7:626–634.

333. Liu J, Volk KJ, Mata MJ, Kerns EH, Lee MS. Miniaturized HPLC and ionspray mass spectrometry applied to the analysis of Paclitaxel and taxanes. *J. Pharm. Biomed. Anal.* 1997; 15:1729–1739.

334. Gimon ME, Kinsel GR, Edmondson RD, Russell DH, Prout T, Ewald HA. Matrix-assisted laser desorption/ionization time-of-flight mass spectrometry of paclitaxel and related taxanes. *J. Nat. Prod.* 1994; 57:1404–1410.

335. Bitsch F, Ma W, Macdonald F, Nieder M, Shackleton CHL. Analysis of taxol and related diterpenoids from cell cultures by liquid chromatography-electrospray mass spectrometry. *J. Chromatogr. Biomed. Appl.* 1993; 615:273–280.

336. Bitsch F, Shackleton CHL, Ma W, Park G, Nieder M. Taxoid side-chain structure determination by electrospray ionization tandem mass spectrometry. *Rapid Commun. Mass Spectrom.* 1993; 7:891–894.

337. Kerns EH, Volk KJ, Hill SE, Lee MS. Profiling taxanes in Taxus extracts using LC/MS and LC/MS/MS techniques. *J. Nat. Prod.* 1994; 57:1391–1403.

338. Stierle A, Strobel G, Stierle D. Taxol and taxane production by *Taxomyces andreanae*, an endophytic fungus of Pacific yew. *Science* 1993; 260:214–217.

339. Stierle A, Strobel G, Stierle D, Grothaus P, Bignami G. The search for a taxol-producing microorganisms among the endophytic fungi of the Pacific yew, *Taxus brevifolia*. *J. Nat. Prod.* 1995; 58:1315–1324.

340. Noh M-J, Yang J-G, Kim K-S et al. Isolation of a novel microorganism, *Pestalotia heterocornis*, producing paclitaxel. *Biotechnol. Bioeng.* 1999; 64:620–623.

341. Han KH, Fleming P, Walker K et al. Genetic transformation of mature Taxus: An approach to genetically control the in vitro production of the anticancer drug, taxol. *Plant Sci.* 1994; 95:187–196.

342. Zhiri A, Jaziri M, Guo Y et al. Tissue cultures of Taxus baccata as a source of 10-deacetyl-baccatin III, a precursor for the hemisynthesis of taxol. *Biol. Chem. Hoppe-Seyler* 1995; 376:583–586.

343. Theodoridis G, Laskaris G, Van Rozendaal ELM, Verpoorte R. Analysis of taxines in Taxus plant material and cell cultures by HPLC photodiode array and HPLC-electrospray mass spectrometry. *J. Liq. Chromatogr. Relat. Technol.* 2001; 24:2267–2282.

344. Cavaletti G, Cavalletti E, Oggioni N et al. Distribution of paclitaxel within the nervous system of the rat after ed intravenous administration. *Neurotoxicology* 2000; 21:389–393.

345. Schellen A, Ooms B, Van Gils M et al. High throughput on-line solid phase extraction/tandem mass spectrometric determination of paclitaxel in human serum. *Rapid Commun. Mass Spectrom.* 2000; 14:230–233.

346. Blitzke T, Baranovsky A, Schneider B. Synthesis and protein binding of 4-carboxybutylcarbamoyl-substituted taxoids. *Helv. Chim. Acta* 2001; 84:1989–1995.

347. Xu QA, Trissel LA, Davis MR. Compatibility of paclitaxel in 5% glucose and 0.9% sodium chloride injections with EVA minibags. *Aust. J. Hosp. Pharm.* 1998; 28:156–159.

348. Hoke SH, II, Cooks RG, Chang CJ et al. Determination of taxanes in *Taxus brevifolia* extracts by tandem mass spectrometry and high-performance liquid chromatography. *J. Nat. Prod.* 1994; 57:277–286.

349. Theodoridis G, Laskaris G, de Jong CF, Hofte AJP, Verpoorte R. Determination of paclitaxel and related diterpenoids in plant extracts by high-performance liquid chromatography with UV detection in high-performance liquid chromatography-mass spectrometry. *J. Chromatogr. A* 1998; 802:297–305.

350. Sottanil C, Minoia C, D'Incalci M, Paganini M, Zucchetti M. High-performance liquid chromatography tandem mass spectrometry procedure with automated solid phase extraction sample preparation for the quantitative determination of paclitaxel (taxol) in human plasma. *Rapid Commun. Mass Spectrom.* 1998; 12:251–255.

351. Volk KJ, Hill SE, H. Kerns E, Lee MS. Profiling degradants of paclitaxel using liquid chromatography-mass spectrometry and liquid chromatography-tandem mass spectrometry substructural techniques. *J. Chromatogr. B: Biomed. Sci. Appl.* 1997; 696:99–115.

352. Fleming PE, Floss HG, Haertel M et al. Biosynthetic studies on taxol. *Pure Appl. Chem.* 1994; 66:2045–2048.

353. Kerns EH, Hill SE, Detlefsen DJ et al. Cellular uptake profile of paclitaxel using liquid chromatography tandem mass spectrometry. *Rapid Commun. Mass Spectrom.* 1998; 12:620–624.

354. Lorenz SA, Maziarz EP, Wood TD. Using solution phase hydrogen/deuterium (H/D) exchange to determine the origin of non-covalent complexes observed by electrospray ionization mass spectrometry: In solution or in vacuo. *J. Am. Soc. Mass Spectrom.* 2001; 12:795–804.

355. Chandra S, Lorey DR, II. SIMS ion microscopy in cancer research: Single cell isotopic imaging for chemical composition, cytotoxicity and cell cycle recognition. *Cell. Mol. Biol.* 2001; 47:503–518.

356. Troendle FJ, Reddick CD, Yost RA. Detection of pharmaceutical compounds in tissue by matrix-assisted laser desorption/ionization and laser desorption/chemical ionization Tandem mass spectrometry with a quadruple ion trap. *J. Am. Soc. Mass Spectrom.* 1999; 10:1315–1321.

357. Bakhtiar R, Lohne J, Ramos L, Khemani L, Hayes M, Tse F. High-throughput quantification of the anti-leukemia drug STI571 (Gleevec) and its main metabolite (CGP 74588) in human plasma using liquid chromatography-tandem mass spectrometry. *J. Chromat. B: Anal. Tech. Biomed. Life Sci.* 2002; 768:325–340.

358. Rai AJ, Chan DW. Cancer proteomics: New developments in clinical chemistry. *Laboratoriumsmedizin* 2001; 25:399–403.

359. Verma M, Wright GL, Jr., Hanash SM, Gopal-Srivastava R, Srivastava S. Proteomic approaches within the NCI early detection research network for the discovery and identification of cancer biomarkers. *Ann. N. Y. Acad. Sci.* (Circulating Nucleic Acids in Plasma or Serum II) 2001; 945:103–115.

360. Wright GL, Jr., Cazares LH, Leung S-M et al. ProteinChip surface enhanced laser desorption/ionization (SELDI) mass spectrometry: A novel protein biochip technology for detection of prostate cancer biomarkers in complex protein mixtures. *Prostate Cancer Prostate Dis.* 2000; 2:264–276.

361. Petricoin EF, Ardekani AM, Hitt BA et al. Use of proteomic patterns in serum to identify ovarian cancer. *Lancet* 2002; 359:572–577.

362. Hanash S, Brichory F, Beer D. A proteomic approach to the identification of lung cancer markers. *Dis. Markers* 2001; 17:295–300.

363. Paweletz CP, Trock B, Pennanen M et al. Proteomic patterns of nipple aspirate fluids obtained by SELDI-TOF: Potential for new biomarkers to aid in the diagnosis of breast cancer. *Dis. Markers* 2001; 17:301–307.

364. Harris RA, Yang A, Stein RC et al. Cluster analysis of an extensive human breast cancer cell line protein expression map database. *Proteomics* 2002; 2:212–223.

365. Shalhoub P, Kern S, Girard S, Beretta L. Proteomic-based approach for the identification of tumor markers associated with hepatocellular carcinoma. *Dis. Markers* 2001; 17:217–223.

366. Barnea E, Beer I, Patoka R et al. Analysis of endogenous peptides bound by soluble MHC class I molecules: a novel approach for identifying tumor-specific antigen. *Eur. J. Immunol.* 2002; 32:213–222.

367. Parish CR, Cabalda-Crane VM. Method of identifying cancer markers by mass spectrometry and uses therefore in the diagnosis of cancer. *PCT Int. Appl.* 2002; 55.

368. Siegel MM. Early discovery drug screening using mass spectrometry. *Curr. Top. Med. Chem.* 2002; 2:13–33.

369. Loo JA, Hu P, Thanbal V. Studying noncovalent protein-peptide interactions by electrospray ionization mass spectrometry. Proceedings of the 43rd ASMS Conference on Mass Spectrometry and Allied Topics. Atlanta, GA, 1995; p.35.

370. Loo JA. Bioanalytical mass spectrometry: many flavors to choose. *Bioconjugate Chem.* 1995; 6:644–665.

371. Ganguly AK, Pramanik BN, Tsarbopoulos A, Covey TR, Huang E, Fuhrman SA. Mass spectrometric detection of the noncovalent GDP-bound conformational state of the human H-ras protein. *J. Am. Chem. Soc.* 1992; 114:6559–6560.

372. Huang EC, Pramanik BN, Tsarbopoulos A et al. Application of electrospray mass spectrometry in probing protein-protein and protein-ligand noncovalent interactions. *J. Am. Soc. Mass Spectrom.* 1993; 4:624–630.

373. Ganguly AK, Pramanik BN, Huang EC, Tsarbopoulos A, Girijavallabhan VM, Liberles S. Studies of the ras-GDP and ras-GTP noncovalent complexes by electrospray mass spectrometry. *Tetrahedron* 1993; 49:7985–7996.

374. Taveras AG, Remiszewski SW, Doll RJ et al. Ras oncoprotein inhibitors: the discovery of potent, ras nucleotide exchange inhibitors and the structural determination of a drug-protein complex. *Bioorg. Med. Chem.* 1997; 5:125–133.

375. Grieg M, Robinson J. Detection of oligonucleotide ligand complexes by ESI-MS (DOLCE-MS) as a component of high throughput screening. CPSA 2000 — 3rd Annual Symposium on Chemical and Pharmaceutical Structure Analysis, Sept. 26–28, 2000; Princeton, NJ.

376. Hofstadler SA, Griffey RH. Analysis of Noncovalent Complexes of DNA and RNA by Mass Spectrometry. *Chem. Rev.* 2001; 101:377–390.

377. Wan KX, Shibue T, Gross ML. Non-covalent complexes between DNA-binding drugs and double-stranded oligodeoxynucleotides: A study by ESI ion-trap mass spectrometry. *J. Am. Chem. Soc.* 2000; 122:300–307.

378. Shibue T, Wan KX, Gross ML. A study of non-covalent interaction between DNA-binding drugs and double-stranded oligodeoxynucleotides by ESI ion trap mass spectrometry. *J. Mass Spectrom. Soc. Jpn.* 2000; 48:221–227.

379. Wan KX, Gross ML, Shibue TJ. Gas-phase stability of double-stranded oligodeoxynucleotides and their noncovalent complexes with DNA-binding drugs as revealed by collisional activation in an ion trap. *J. Am. Soc. Mass Spectrom.* 2000; 11:450–457.

380. Gabelica V, De Pauw E, Rosu F. Interaction between antitumor drugs and a double-stranded oligonucleotide studied by electrospray ionization mass spectrometry. *J. Mass Spectrom.* 1999; 34:1328–1337.

381. Hofstadler SA, Griffey RH. Mass spectrometry as a drug discovery platform against RNA targets. *Curr. Opin. Drug Disc. Dev.* 2000; 3:423–431.

382. Griffey RH, Sannes-Lowery KA, Drader JJ, Mohan V, Swayze EE, Hofstadler SA. Characterization of low-affinity complexes between RNA and small molecules using electrospray ionization mass spectrometry. *J. Am. Chem. Soc.* 2000; 122:9933–9938.

383. Fry DW, Bridges AJ, Denny WA et al. Specific, irreversible inactivation of the epidermal growth factor receptor and erbB2, by a new class of tyrosine kinase inhibitor. *Proc. Natl. Acad. Sci. U. S. A.* 1998; 95:12022–12027.

384. Smaill JB, Rewcastle GW, Loo JA et al. Tyrosine kinase inhibitors. 17. Irreversible inhibitors of the epidermal growth factor receptor: 4-(phenylamino)quinazoline- and 4-(Phenylamino)pyrido[3,2-d]pyrimidine-6-acrylamides bearing additional solubilizing functions. *J. Med. Chem.* 2000; 43:1380–1397.

385. Kelleher NL, Lin HY, Valaskovic GA, Aaserud DJ, Fridriksson EK, McLafferty FW. Top down versus bottom up protein characterization by tandem high-resolution mass spectrometry. *J. Am. Chem. Soc.* 1999; 121:806–812.

386. Siegel MM, Tabei K, Bebernitz GA, Baum EZ. Rapid methods for screening low molecular mass compounds non-covalently bound to proteins using size exclusion and mass spectrometry applied to inhibitors of human cytomegalovirus protease. *J. Mass Spectrom.* 1998; 33:264–273.

387. Dunayevskiy YM, Lai J-J, Quinn C, Talley F, Vouros P. Mass spectrometric identification of ligands selected from combinatorial libraries using gel filtration. *Rapid Commun. Mass Spectrom.* 1997; 11:1178–1184.

388. Blom KF, Larsen BS, McEwen CN. Determining affinity-selected ligands and estimating binding affinities by online size exclusion chromatography/liquid chromatography-mass spectrometry. *J. Comb. Chem.* 1999; 1:82–90.

389. Annis A. An affinity selection-mass spectral method for the identification of small molecule ligands from self-encoded combinatorial libraries. Greater Boston Mass Spectrometry Discussion Group, Dec. 13, 2000. www. neogenesis. com.

390. Hsieh YF, Gordon N, Regnier F, Afeyan N, Martin SA, Vella G. Multidimensional chromatography coupled with mass spectrometry for target-based screening. *J. Mol. Diversity* 1997; 2:189–196.

391. Dunayevskiy YM, Hughes DE. High throughput size-exclusive method of screening complex biological materials for affinity ligands. *PCT Int. Appl.* 2000; 33. WO 0047999 A1 20000817.

392. Tong H, Tabei K, Amin A, Olson M, Bebernitz G, Siegel MM. Identification of compounds non-covalently bound to RNA using GPC spin columns with ESI MS. Proceedings of the 49th American Society of Mass Spectrometry Conference on Mass Spectrometry & Allied Topics. Chicago IL, 2001; Poster Th 274.

393. Moy FJ, Haraki K, Mobilio D, Walker G, Powers R and Tabei K, Tong H, Siegel MM. MS/NMR: A structure-based approach for discovering protein ligands and for drug design by

coupling size exclusion chromatography, mass spectrometry, and nuclear magnetic resonance spectroscopy. *Anal. Chem.* 2001; 73:571–581.

394. Dohlman HG, Thorner J. RGS proteins and signaling by heterotrimeric G proteins. *J. Biol. Chem.* 1997; 272:3871–3874.

395. Kehrl JH. Heterotrimeric G protein signaling: roles in immune function and fine-tuning by RGS proteins. *Immunity* 1998; 8:1–10.

396. Arshavsky VY, Pugh EN, Jr. Lifetime regulation of G protein-effector complex: Emerging importance of RGS proteins. *Neuron* 1998; 20:11–14.

397. Zerangue N, Jan LY. G-protein signaling: fine-tuning signaling kinetics. *Curr. Biol.* 1998; 8:R313–R316.

398. De Vries L, Farquhar MG. RGS proteins: More than just GAPs for heterotrimeric G proteins. *Trends Cell Biol.* 1999; 9:138–144.

399. McLafferty FW, Turecek F. *Interpretation of Mass Spectra; An Introduction.* University Science Books, Mill Valley CA, 1993.

400. Harrison AG. *Chemical Ionization Mass Spectrometry.* CRC Press, Boca Raton, FL, 1992.

401. Schulten HR. Biochemical, medical, and environmental applications of field-ionization and field-desorption mass spectrometry. *Int. J. Mass Spectrom. Ion Phys.* 1979; 32:97–283.

402. Prokai L. *Field Desorption Mass Spectrometry.* Marcel Dekker, New York, 1990.

403. Sundqvist B, Macfarlane RD. Californium-252-plasma desorption mass spectrometry. *Mass Spectrom. Rev.* 1985; 4:421–460.

404. Benninghaven A, Rudenauer FG, Werner HW. *Secondary Ion Mass Spectrometry.* Wiley-Interscience, New York, 1987.

405. Seifert WEJ, Caprioli RM. Fast atom bombardment mass spectrometry. *Methods Enzymol.* 1996; 270:453–486.

406. Vestal ML. Ionization techniques for nonvolatile molecules. *Mass Spectrom. Rev.* 1983; 2:447–480.

407. Niessen WMA. *Liquid Chromatography-Mass Spectrometry.* Marcel Dekker, New York, 2000.

408. Cole RB, ed. *Electrospray Ionization Mass Spectrometry.* John Wiley, New York, 1997.

409. Pramanik BN, Ganguly AK, Gross ML, eds. *Applied Electrospray Mass Spectrometry.* Marcel Dekker, New York, 2000.

410. Zenobi R, Knochenmuss R. Ion formation in MALDI mass spectrometry. *Mass Spectrom. Rev.* 1999; 17:337–366.

411. Bahr U, Karas M, Hillenkamp FF. Analysis of biopolymers by matrix-assisted laser desorption/ionization (MALDI) mass spectrometry. *Fresenius' J. Anal. Chem.* 1994; 348:783–791.

412. Merchant M, Weinberger SR. Recent advancements in surface-enhanced laser desorption/ionization-time of flight-mass spectrometry. *Electrophoresis* 2000; 21:1164–1177.

413. Lubman DM, ed. *Lasers and Mass Spectrometry.* Oxford University Press, New York, 1990.

414. Montaser A, ed. *Inductively Coupled Plasma Mass Spectrometry.* Wiley-VCH, New York, 1998.

415. Busch KL, Glish GL, McLuckey SA. *Mass Spectrometry/Mass Spectrometry.* VHC, New York, 1988.

416. McLafferty FW, ed. *Tandem Mass Spectrometry.* John Wiley, New York, 1983.

417. Cooks RG, ed. *Collision Spectroscopy.* Plenum Press, New York, 1978.

418. Niessen WMA, ed. *Current Practice of Gas Chromatography-Mass Spectrometry.* Marcel Dekker, New York, 2001.

419. Lee MS. *LC/MS Applications in Drug Development.* John Wiley, New York, 2002.

420. Combs MT, Ashraf-Khorassani M, Taylor LT. Packed column supercritical fluid chromatography-mass spectroscopy: A review. *J. Chromatogr.* 1997; 785:85–100.

421. Cherkaoui S. Combining capillary electrophoresis with electrospray ionization mass spectrometry. In *Clinical and Forensic Applications of Capillary Electrophoresis* (Petersen JR and Mohammad AA, eds.), Humana Press Inc., Totowa, New Jersey, 2001:285–313.

422. Hage T, Sebald W, Reinemer P. Crystal structure of the interleukin-4/receptor a chain complex reveals a mosaic binding interface. *Cell* 1999; 97:271–281.

423. Shao D, et al. Identification of novel estrogen receptor & antagonist. *J. Steroid Biochem. Mol. Biol.* 2004; 88(4–5), 351–360.

424. Moy F, et al. Impact of mobility on structure based drug design for MMPs. *JACS* 2002; 124(43), 12658–12659.

6

ANTISENSE STRATEGIES FOR THE DEVELOPMENT OF NOVEL CANCER THERAPEUTICS

RUIWEN ZHANG

HUI WANG

Department of Pharmacology and Toxicology
Cancer Pharmacology Laboratory, Comprehensive Cancer Center, and Gene Therapy Center
University of Alabama at Birmingham
Birmingham, Alabama

I. INTRODUCTION
II. DESIGN AND EVALUATION OF ANTISENSE
   OLIGONUCLEOTIDES
III. CONCLUSION

Antisense therapy delivers antisense molecules that target to mRNA to the target cells with which they can hybridize and specifically inhibit the expression of target genes. Antisense oligonucleotides have been widely used in investigating gene functions and regulation. There now has been a large body of evidence from preclinical and clinical studies supporting the idea that antisense oligonucleotides offer the possibility of specific, rational, genetic-based drug design. In this chapter, approaches to developing these drugs from preclinical to clinical settings will be discussed. Examples will illustrate the progress in this field and emphasize the importance of target selection and advanced antisense chemistry in the development of antisense therapeutics.

I. INTRODUCTION

It is widely accepted that the majority of human cancers are derived from single somatic cells that undergo a series of genetic and epigenetic changes, which leads to changes in gene activity, loss of control of proliferation, and development of cancer phenotypes. These cancer cell phenotypes include the disregard of signals to differentiate and to stop proliferating; the capacity of sustained proliferation; and the loss of apoptosis, invasion, and angiogenesis [1]. Two factors that influence the evolution of cancer are oncogenes and tumor suppressor genes. In the last two decades, significant progress has been made in identifying, cloning, sequencing, and characterizing pathogenic genes important to cancer development, which has lead to the development of genetic-based therapy. One of the approaches, antisense therapy, delivers to the target cells antisense molecules that can hybridize and specifically inhibit the expression of pathogenic genes.

Antisense nucleic acids are single-stranded oligonucleotides that are complementary to the sequence of a target RNA or DNA. Zamecnik and colleagues [2] first introduced antisense therapy over 20 years ago. In addition, naturally occurring antisense RNA was found to be a means of regulation of gene expression in living cells [3]. However, the development of antisense therapeutics experienced a slow period in the 1970s and 1980s. After a major breakthrough in automated oligonucleotide synthesis, which yielded high-quality oligonucleotides in sufficient amounts for *in vitro* and *in vivo* studies, antisense techniques are rapidly developed and widely applied for investigating gene function and regulation, modulation of gene expression, and validation of new drug targets. There is a large body of published studies that suggests the potential use of antisense oligonucleotides in the treatment of various human diseases such as hypertension and other cardiovascular diseases, cancer, genetic disorders, and viral infections [4–9]. The first antisense drug, Vitravene, has been approved for the treatment of patients with cytomegalovirus-induced retinitis [10]. Several other antisense oligonucleotides have entered phases I–III clinical trials as

TABLE 6.1 Examples of Anticancer Antisense Oligonucleotides in Clinical Trials

Target	Oligonucleotide sequence[a]	Patient population
Phosphorothioate oligonucleotides		
bcl-2	5′-TCTCCCAGCGTGCGCCAT-3′	Lymphoma, prostate, cancer, melanoma
c-raf-1	5′-TCCCGCCTGTGACATGCATT-3′	Colon cancer, renal carcinoma, ovarian cancer, pancreatic cancer
Ha-ras	5′-GGGACTCCTCGCTACTGCCT-3′	Sarcoma, pancreatic cancer, colon cancer, melanoma
PKC-α	5′-GTTCTCGCTGGTGAGTTTCA-3′	Lymphoma, non-small cell lung cancer, ovarian cancer
bcr-abl	5′-CGCTGAAGGGCTTCTTCCTTATTGAT-3′	Chronic myeloid leukemia
bcr-abl	5′-CGCTGAAGGGCTTTTGAACTGTGCTT-3′	Chronic myeloid leukemia
c-myb	5′-TATGCTGTGCCGGGGTCTTCGGGC-3′	Chronic myeloid leukemia
c-myc	5′-GCTAACGTTGAGGGGCAT-3′	Restenosis
IGF-IR	5′-GGACCCTCCTCCGGAGCC-3′	Malignant astrocytomas
p53	5′-CCCTGCTCCCCCCTGGCTCC-3′	Acute myeloid leukemia, myelodysplastic syndrome
Mixed-backbone oligonucleotides		
PKA-RIα	5′-**GCG**UGCCTCCTCAC**UGGC**-3′	Solid tumors

[a]All the sequences contain phosphorothioate internucleotide linkages; plain and bold letters indicate deoxy- and 2′-O-methyl-ribonucleosides, respectively.

anticancer agents administered alone or in combination with conventional chemotherapy [4, 5, 9, 11–15] (Table 6.1).

II. DESIGN AND EVALUATION OF ANTISENSE OLIGONUCLEOTIDES

Like any other chemical drugs, antisense oligonucleotide therapeutics need to undergo an extensive, systematic evaluation in various preclinical and clinical settings (Figures 6.1 and 6.2). In theory, the concept and rationale of antisense

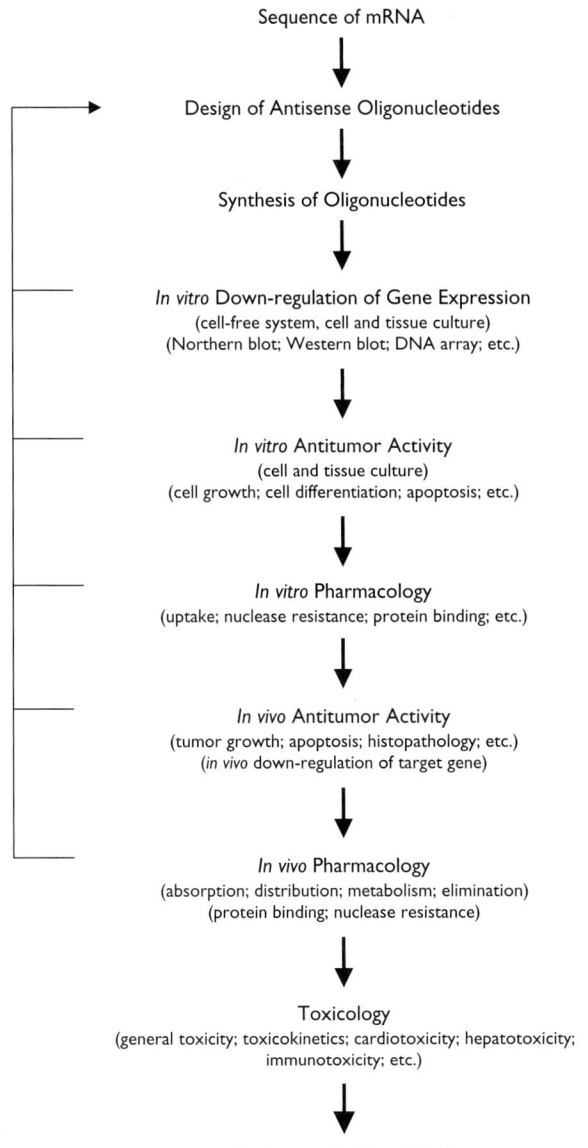

Sequence of mRNA

↓

Design of Antisense Oligonucleotides

↓

Synthesis of Oligonucleotides

↓

In vitro Down-regulation of Gene Expression
(cell-free system, cell and tissue culture)
(Northern blot; Western blot; DNA array; etc.)

↓

In vitro Antitumor Activity
(cell and tissue culture)
(cell growth; cell differentiation; apoptosis; etc.)

↓

In vitro Pharmacology
(uptake; nuclease resistance; protein binding; etc.)

↓

In vivo Antitumor Activity
(tumor growth; apoptosis; histopathology; etc.)
(*in vivo* down-regulation of target gene)

↓

In vivo Pharmacology
(absorption; distribution; metabolism; elimination)
(protein binding; nuclease resistance)

↓

Toxicology
(general toxicity; toxicokinetics; cardiotoxicity; hepatotoxicity;
immunotoxicity; etc.)

↓

Application for Clinical Trials

FIGURE 6.1 Outline of preclinical evaluation of anitsense oligonucleotides as therapeutic agents.

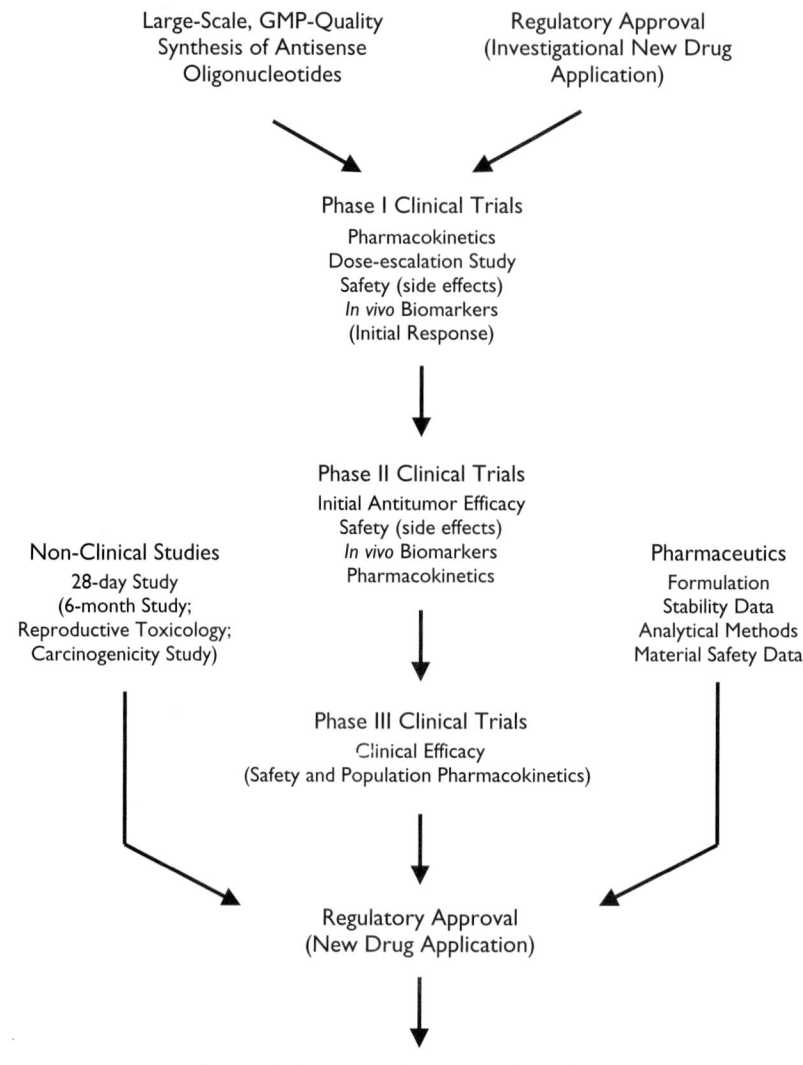

FIGURE 6.2 Outline of clinical evaluation and pharmaceutical development of anitsense oligonucleotides as therapeutic agents.

therapy is very simple: Antisense oligonucleotides specifically bind to and interact with their complimentary target RNA thereby blocking gene expression, which results in therapeutic effects in a sequence-dependent manner. It has now been realized that antisense oligonucleotides exert their biological effects on target genes through several distinct mechanisms, which include both antisense and non-antisense mechanisms in target and non-target cells or tissues [16–22].

A. Principles of Antisense Design

The biological activity of a given antisense oligonucleotide, including desired and undesired effects, may be influenced by various factors at the molecular, cellular, organ/tissue, and whole body levels (Tables 6.2 and 6.3). Many mechanisms of antisense action have been proposed [17–19]. Two major mechanisms, hybrid-arrest and RNase H activation, are generally accepted. Early studies suggested that antisense oligonucleotides bind to and interact with code region, cause blockade of ribosomal read-through of mRNA, and stop translation. Later, it was demonstrated that antisense oligonucleotides could also be targeted to initiation code and untranslated regions. In addition, antisense oligonucleotides may produce antisense effects through binding to the 5' cap region, 3' poly A, or the splicing site of the pre-mRNA [19]. RNase H activation is believed to be a major mechanism of action for several types of antisense oligonucleotides such as oligonucleotide phosphorothioates that bind to their target RNA to form RNA:DNA duplexes, which invoke the

TABLE 6.2   Factors that may Influence Experimental Results and Interpretation

Category	Factors or condition
Molecular target	Specificity of mRNA sequence chosen
	Concentration of mRNA
	Rate and synthesis of mRNA
	Degradation of mRNA
Oligonucleotides	Purity
	Sequence and structure
	Chemistry and modifications
	Impurities
In vitro study	Stability of oligonucleotides
	Test system
	Cellular uptake and distribution
	Cell type and culture conditions
	Concentrations of oligonucleotides
	Control of oligonucleotides
	Delivery approach
	Assay to determine the mRNA and protein levels of targets
In vivo study	*In vivo* stability of oligonucleotides
	Binding to protein or other macromolecules
	Pharmacokinetics: absorption, distribution, metabolism and elimination
	Toxicokinetics
	Pharmacodynamics: interaction of oligonucleotides and mRNA target
	Dose-dependent effects
	Dose-independent effects
	Pharmaceutical issues: formulations and delivery
	Test systems and disease model
	Animal use and care
	Dose, schedule, and duration of treatment
	Combination therapy
	Assay to determine the mRNA and protein levels of targets
	End points of therapeutic effects
Mechanisms of action	Antisense sequence-specific effects
	Non-antisense, sequence-dependent effects
	Non-specific effects
	RNase H activity

TABLE 6.3   Factors that may Influence Clinical Trial Results and Interpretation

Category	Factors or conditions
Subjects/patients	Expression of the target gene Disease and stage Host conditions Prior or concurrent treatment
Oligonucleotides	Purity Impurities Formulation *In vivo* stability of oligonucleotides
Pharmacology	Binding to protein or other macromolecules Pharmacokinetics: absorption, distribution, metabolism, and elimination Toxicokinetics Pharmacodynamics: interaction of oligonucleotides and mRNA target
Treatment and effects	Dose-dependent effects Dose-independent effects Dose, schedule, and duration of treatment Combination therapy Assay to determine the mRNA and protein levels of targets End points of therapeutic effects Adverse effects

RNA degradation activity of RNase. In contrast, other types of oligo-nucleotides such as methylphosphonate oligonucleotides and α-oligonucleotides do not have such a property [23].

1. Antisense Chemistry

Both antisense RNA and DNA techniques have been used in antisense research. Natural antisense RNA is involved in gene regulation in normal organisms [3], and synthetic antisense RNAs have shown antisense effects *in vitro* and *in vivo*. There are two major approaches to introduce antisense RNA into living cells: (1) nuclear expression of RNA by engineered antisense genes and (2) microinjection of artificial antisense RNA oligonucleotides. As RNAs are extremely sensitive to nuclease degradation, antisense RNA has limited potential as a therapeutic agent.

On the other hand, antisense DNAs have greater potential. They are short sequences of single-stranded DNA (~20–25 bases long) and can be produced in large quantities using automated synthetic organic chemistry. Among many chemical modifications of antisense oligonucleotides, phospho-diester oligonucleotides and their methylphosphonate and phosphorothioate analogs are considered the first generation of antisense oligonucleotides. With high affinity to their targets, phosphodiester oligonucleotides stably bind to the target mRNA and activate RNase H. The major disadvantages of phosphodiester oligonucleotides are a sensitivity to nuclease degradation and poor cellular uptake. After extensive investigation with phosphorothioate and methylphosphonate, various backbone modifications have been made to improve resistance to nucleases and the cellular uptake of antisense oligo-nucleotides. Methylphosphonate oligonucleotides, where CH_3 replaces O, were first synthesized in the late 1970s by Miller and co-workers [24]. They have been shown to be resistant to extra- and intracellular nucleases, and pass through cytoplasm membrane much better than unmodified oligonucleotides. The drawback is that they have relatively poor hybridization efficiency to target RNAs and are unable to activate RNase H [25], which limits their application as therapeutic agents.

Phosphorothioate oligonucleotides, analogs of isosteric substitution of sulfur for oxygen on the phosphorus residue, retain the negative charge and thus are more aqueously soluble than methylphosphonate analogs. They are much more resistant to nucleases and activate RNase H. Thus far, most clinically tested antisense oligonucleotides are phosphorothioate oligonucleotides. The disadvantages of phosphorothioate oligonucleotides are that they are taken up less by cells and have non-specific toxicities in some systems.

In the development of second-generation antisense oligonucleotides, major efforts have been devoted to stabilizing phosphorothioate oligonucleotides by various modifications of their structure [26–29]. One of the novel structures is that of mixed-backbone oligonucleotides (MBOs) [26, 27]. These novel oligonucleotides have segments of 2'-O-methyl oligoribonucleotide phosphorothioates at both the 3' and 5' ends. They have been shown to have an increased *in vitro* and *in vivo* stability and, therefore, increased tissue uptake and decreased total elimination [28, 29]. The MBO targeted to cAMP-dependent protein kinase (PKA) has entered clinical trials [30] (Table 6.1).

2. Target Validation and Optimization of Antisense Oligonucleotides

Although the design of antisense oligonucleotides is theoretically simple and straightforward (to identify a complementary oligonucleotide on the basis of the nucleotide sequence of the mRNA), the selection of an effective and specific antisense oligonucleotide is largely based on investigators' experience and trial-based experiments. Because certain oligonucleotide sequences such as CpG and GGGG have been shown to have sequence-dependent, non-antisense effects, these sequences should be avoided in order to identify sequence-specific antisense drugs.

a. Random "Sequence-Walking" Approach

Based on Watson-Crick base pairing rules and a known sequence of the target gene, a linear, sequence-walking method has long been used to design and select antisense oligonucleotides. Usually, a relative large number of "random" oligonucleotides (10–100, depending on the length of the gene of interest) with a certain length (15–30 mer, for example), targeted to various regions of the target mRNA, are synthesized individually and their antisense activity measured using a defined cell-free or *in vitro* screening assay. This conventional method has been used in many antisense experiments and yielded good results, although it is expensive and time- and labor-consuming. (Only less than 5% of the oligonucleotides are generally found to be effective.)

b. Computer-Aided Target Selection

It is believed that the lack of antisense efficacy of designed oligonucleotides may be largely due to targeting at inaccessible sites of the RNA. A shift in a single or a few bases has no significant change in oligonucleotide:RNA binding, but there may be large differences in antisense activity. The binding efficiency of complementary oligonucleotide to target RNA is suggested to be mainly determined by the secondary and tertiary structures of the target RNA [31]. Accessible sites in mRNAs may be predicted using computer programs through various approaches to predict the secondary structure of RNA [32]. For example, using an RNA folding program such as MFOLD (Genetics Computer Group, Madison, WI), antisense oligonucleotides may be designed to target against the regions of mRNA that are predicted to be free from intramolecular base pairing and thereby accessible to the designed oligonucleotides. However, this approach has not been successful in correctly predicting RNA structure and guiding antisense design [31].

c. Oligonucleotide Scanning Arrays

More recently, advances in DNA array technologies have led to the development of oligonucleotide scanning arrays as a novel approach to identifying active antisense oligonucleotides [31, 33]. This method allows combinatorial synthesis of a large number of oligonucleotides and parallel measurement of the binding strength of all oligonucleotides to the target mRNA. It is suggested that there be a correlation between the binding strength and the antisense activity [31, 33].

d. RNase H Digestion-Based Screening

There is convincing evidence supporting that RNase H is involved in antisense activity, especially for phosphorothioates. Therefore, one may use RNase H screening assays to identify effective antisense reagents [34, 35]. In this method, RNase H is used in combination with a random or semi-random oligonucleotide library. The target mRNA is transcribed *in vitro*, end-labeled, and mixed with the oligonucleotide library. The RNase H cleavage sites are then identified by gel electrophoresis; however, this method may not precisely define the accessible sites of the target mRNA because RNase H cleavage can occur at more than one location. Therefore it will be difficult to predict the antisense activity based on RNase mapping.

Recently, several other methods have been proposed to select optimal antisense oligonucleotides. These include DNA enzymes (deoxyribozymes) that cleave RNA in a way similar to ribozymes [36] and RNase T1 footprinting that identifies single-stranded regions of target RNA [37]. However, it is too early to determine the potential of these methods in selecting optimal antisense candidates.

B. Delivery of Antisense Oligonucleotides

In the early days of antisense research, high concentrations of oligonucleotides were frequently used due to low efficiency in cellular uptake. This practice often led to non-specific effects observed in those studies. In *in vitro* studies, lipids are now frequently used to facilitate the *in vitro* cellular uptake of oligonucleotides. Of note, the ratio of lipids/oligonucleotides will affect the results of uptake and likely the biological activity. The cytotoxicity of certain lipids alone may affect the interpretation of results from an *in vitro* cellular study. In contrast, the *in vivo* uptake of oligonucleotides seems much better than that in *in vitro* settings [38–43], which makes the use of a special carrier unnecessary. Several more detailed reviews on drug delivery of antisense oligonucleotides have been published recently as reviewed in references 44–46.

C. Pharmacological Evaluation of Antisense Oligonucleotides

In the past decade, many reports have appeared describing pharmacokinetic properties of various antisense oligonucleotides [5, 6, 8, 11, 12, 14, 22, 27–30, 38–43]. Oligonucleotides with various lengths and base compositions have been investigated in various species such as rats, mice, rabbits, monkeys, and humans and follow various routes of administration such as intravenous, intraperitoneal, subcutaneous, intradermal, oral, and inhalation. In most cases, quantification of parent oligonucleotides (and degraded products, in some cases) was reported using plasma samples. In some studies, tissue distribution of oligonucleotides was carried out [38–43].

In general, phosphorothioate oligonucleotides have a short plasma distribution half-life ($t_{1/2}\alpha$) of less than one hour and a prolonged elimination half-life ($t_{1/2}\beta$) in the range of 40–60 hours [38–43]. The plasma pharmacokinetics of oligonucleotides is not associated with the length or primary sequence, but instead associated with the backbone modification and specific segments at the 3' and/or 5' ends. Extensive and wide tissue distribution of oligonucleotides has been observed, with the highest concentrations found in the liver and kidneys. Urinary excretion is believed to be the major elimination pathway.

It has been shown that oligonucleotides bind to plasma protein extensively. Total drug concentration has been traditionally used to describe pharmacokinetics. However, for many drugs, the therapeutic and/or side effects correlate better with the concentration of diffusible, unbound drug than with the total drug concentration. Therefore, it will be helpful to determine protein binding of test oligonucleotides and related factors affecting the degree of protein binding [47]. Our studies have shown that in *in vitro* testing there is a significant species difference in plasma and serum protein binding of oligonucleotides, with the rank order of guinea pigs > rabbits > rats > humans [42]. The mechanisms for the species differences are not clear and may be associated with species differences in the total levels and compositions of plasma/serum proteins. Therefore, precautions should be undertaken when predicting drug dose for human trials based on animal data, because relatively higher free oligonucleotide levels in human plasma are expected at comparable total drug concentration.

The retention of oligonucleotides in target tissues and normal tissues is directly associated with *in vivo* stability. To increase therapeutic effects, it is desirable to increase the retention time of intact oligonucleotides in the body by means of increasing *in vivo* stability and decreasing elimination. However, due to non-specific tissue distribution and accumulation, high levels and prolonged retention of oligonucleotides in host tissue may increase the risk of toxicity. Such a risk may increase more due to individual disease status and organ function such as liver and renal. For example, significant accumulation of oligonucleotides (and metabolites) in the kidneys in patients with renal function failure may have greater impact on host toxicity than in patients with normal renal functions.

D. Evaluation of Antisense Efficacy

The concept of antisense therapy is simple and rational: to inhibit gene expression at mRNA level in a sequence-specific manner. In the last decade, there have been numerous reports that demonstrate the ability of antisense oligonucleotides, especially phosphorothioates and their analogs, to block gene expression of host genes and foreign pathogenic genes using various *in vitro* and *in vivo* disease models.

Perhaps the most important aspect of pharmacological evaluation of antisense oligonucleotides is the target effectiveness and specificity of these agents (Figure 6.1). These agents are usually tested at both *in vitro* and *in vivo* levels. In the earlier days of antisense development, biological activity of a given oligonucleotide was assayed in a cell-free, *in vitro* system using high concentrations of oligonucleotides, which resulted many false positive reports. *In vitro*, cell-based assays have been routinely employed to establish the basis for further investigation of test oligonucleotides. Although there is some variability in cellular uptake, perhaps depending on cell type, drug concentrations, cell culture conditions, and delivery system, it has been demonstrated that many oligonucleotides can cross the cell membrane and distribute to cytosol in sufficient quantities to exert the desired effect. To increase cellular uptake of oligonucleotides *in vitro*, several means of delivery, such as liposomes and phospholipids, have now been routinely used in *in vitro* experiments in order to avoid the use of extremely high concentrations of oligonucleotides that were frequently used in earlier antisense research. In the development of antisense anti-tumor agents, various assays have been used to demonstrate *in vitro* anti-tumor activity. Western and Northern blot analysis are used to demonstrate effects on protein expression and impact on mRNA metabolism of test oligonucleotides. Assays to determine cell variability, proliferation, and apoptosis are used to illustrate anti-tumor activity of test oligonucleotides. However, these assays may produce false positive and false negative results. For example, some lipids used to increase oligonucleotide uptake have cytotoxicity per se. Therefore, proper controls (e.g., negative, positive, and mismatched controls) are needed. Dose-, time-, and sequence- dependent responses are better evidence for antisense effects and desirable in order to establish a basis for further *in vivo* evaluation of the test oligonucleotides.

Evidence for *in vivo* activity of antisense oligonucleotides is critical in the development pipeline, but it is relatively harder to produce convincing, reproducible results compared to *in vitro* testing. In the development of antisense anti-tumor oligonucleotides, murine models are used most often. In fact, most anti-tumor oligonucleotides that have entered clinical trials have been tested in nude mouse xenograft models. In these models, human cancer cell lines are xenoplanted into nude mince or SCID mice. The end points for efficacy can be tumor size, survival, molecular markers, and histopathological evaluation. Three types of test models can be used, depending on the treatment schedule and time. First, the effect on tumor onset and formation of oligonucleotides can be determined using an *ex vivo* protocol in which cells are treated with oligonucleotide prior to xenoplantation, or an *in vivo* treatment protocol in which oligonucleotide treatment begins immediately after cell xenoplantation. The tumor formation rate and growth inhibition can be major end points in these models. Second, the inhibitory effects on tumor growth of oligonucleotides can be assayed using an *in vivo* treatment protocol in which oligonucleotide treatment begins in the early stage of tumor growth usually when the tumor size reaches 50–100 mg. In these models, tumor growth inhibition and molecular/pathology markers can be major end points. Third, the anti-tumor activity of oligonucleotides can also be tested in the late stage of tumors using a protocol in which oligonucleotide treatment begins usually when the tumor size reaches 500–1000 mg, depending on tumor type. In these models, tumor growth inhibition and survival can be major end points.

It is very important to establish dose-response relations in *in vivo* models. Proper controls (e.g., untreated, vehicle, oligonucleotide controls) should be included. *In vivo* evidence for a block of specific gene expression is also desirable. It should be pointed out that *in vivo* anti-tumor activity of a given antisense oligonucleotide is not necessarily the result of an antisense mechanism and can be associated with non-specific activity and/or sequence-specific, non-antisense activity.

Although most antisense oligonucleotides are tested *in vivo* as monotherapy, combination treatment of antisense oligonucleotides and conventional chemotherapeutic agents have also been widely investigated. There are a number of preclinical studies demonstrating that downregulation of specific gene products with antisense oligonucleotides sensitizes cancer cells to chemotherapeutic agents, which results in an additive or synergistic anticancer activity. These antisense targets include MDM2 [48–51], epidermal growth factor receptor [49], cAMP-dependent protein kinase [29, 53–55], c-myc [56], protein kinase Cα [57], and Bcl-2 [58]. These antisense oligonucleotides have shown to increase the therapeutic effects of chemotherapeutic agents such as paclitaxel, 5-fluorouracil, cisplatin, carboplatin, taxotere, camptothecin, irinotecan, leucovorin, gemcitabine, mafosfamide, doxorubicin, and dacarbazine. However, the mechanisms responsible for such additive or synergistic effects are not fully understood. The synergy between the two classes of agents may result from interaction on several mechanisms such as cell cycle arrest, induction of apoptosis, induction of immune responses, and production of cytokines. Although most studies showed that such additive or synergistic effects are sequence-specific, recent studies demonstrated that antisense oligonucleotides could also potentiate the anti-tumor activity of irinotecan in a sequence-independent manner [59–61], presumably through an interaction at the pharmacokinetic and/or metabolic levels to increase the conversion of the active metabolite [61].

Compared with preclinical studies, far fewer clinical studies of oligonucleotides have been reported (Table 6.1). Most clinically tested antisense anti-tumor oligonucleotides are phosphorothioates that have been shown to have an acceptable safety profile and initial anti-tumor efficacy in humans. In addition, several antisense oligonucleotides and chemotherapeutic agent combination treatments are under clinical evaluation [62].

In most published phase I trials, antisense oligonucleotides were shown to be well tolerated. Side effects include thrombocytopenia, prolongation of activated partial thromboplastin time, and slight elevation in liver enzymes. No significant liver and renal toxicity has been reported. Pharmacokinetic studies that have been carried out in patients indicate a short plasma distribution half-life and prolonged elimination half-life [38]. Urinary excretion represents the major pathway of excretion with mainly degraded products being observed. Limited phase II and III trials have been reported. Antisense oligonucleotides have now been shown to specifically inhibit expression of targeted genes and initial anti-tumor response.

E. Safety Evaluation

Thorough toxicity studies are key components of antisense drug development. A number of phosphorothioates have been studied extensively for their safety profiles in a several species such as mice, rats, monkeys, and humans. The dose-dependent side effects in experimental rats and mice included thrombocytopenia, splenomegaly, and elevation of transaminases [63, 64]. Histopathology changes included mononuclear cell infiltration in tissues such as liver, kidney, and spleen, and reticuloendothelial cell and lymphoid cell hyperplasia. The severity of side effects is dependent on the dose, frequency, and duration of the administration of oligonucleotides. In general, the toxicity profiles of phosphorothioate oligonucleotides are similar with various lengths and base compositions, with exceptions in the presence of certain sequence motifs such as CpG-dinucleotides [63, 65] and poly-G [66], which contribute to the severity of toxicity.

Preclinical toxicity studies are used to guide a starting dose and dose escalation scheme and clinical trials are expected to be conducted in accordance with current good laboratory practices (cGLP). To support clinical phase I trials, animal toxicity studies using two animal species are usually conducted in one rodent species and one non-rodent species. For antisense oligonucleotides, non-human primates have often been used. In addition, special toxicity studies have been suggested to determine cardiotoxicity, hepatotoxicity, and immunotoxicity. Interested readers are directed to a recently published review for details [67].

III. CONCLUSION

In the last decade, significant progress has been made in the development of antisense oligonucleotides as therapeutic agents. Perhaps the most important aspect of therapeutic oligonucleotides is identification of gene target and improving the targeting effectiveness of these antisense drugs. With many antisense anti-tumor oligonucleotides evaluated in the clinic, they are promising therapeutic agents used alone or in combination with other therapeutic agents. Future studies are needed not only to provide the proof of principle for antisense effects *in vitro* and *in vivo* but also to meet the full requirement for antisense therapy as a widely accepted therapeutic approach. The underlying mechanisms (antisense, sequence-dependent non-antisense, and non-sequence-specific) responsible for observed biological effects including therapeutic effects and unwanted side effects are yet to be elucidated. Therefore, more rational selection of both targets and antisense drugs, especially more and well-designed clinical studies, as well as new concepts and approaches to resolve regulatory issues related to antisense drugs are needed. With new generations of antisense drugs created and tested, therapeutic effectiveness and safety profiles of these new agents are expected to be significantly improved in the future.

ACKNOWLEDGEMENTS

This project was supported by grants from the National Institute of Health, National Cancer Institute to R. Zhang (R01 CA 80698).

REFERENCES

1. Hanahan D, Weinberg RA. The hallmarks of cancer. *Cell* 2000; 100:57–70.
2. Zamecnik PC, Stephenson ML. Inhibition of Rous sarcoma virus replication and cell transformation by a specific oligodeoxynucleotide. *Proc. Natl. Acad. Sci. U. S. A.* 1978; 75:280–284.
3. Simons RW. Naturally occurring antisense RNA control, a brief review. *Gene* 1988; 72:35–44.
4. Wickstrom E. *Clinical Trials of Genetic Therapy with Antisense DNA and DNA Vectors.* Marcel Dekker, New York, 1998.
5. Stein CA, Krieg AM. *Applied Antisense Oligonucleotide Technology.* Wiley-Liss, New York, 1998.
6. Agrawal S, Zhao Q. Antisense therapeutics. *Curr. Opin. Chem. Biol.* 1998; 2:519–528.
7. Phillips, MI. Antisense technology: Part B Applications. In *Methods in Enzymology. Vol. 314,* Academic Press, San Diego, CA, 2000.
8. Crooke ST. Antisense Drug Technology. Principles, Strategies, and Applications. Marcel Dekker, New York, 2001.
9. Wang H, Prasad G, Buolamwini JK, Zhang R. Antisense anticancer oligonucleotide therapeutics. *Curr. Cancer Drug Tar.* 2001; 1:177–196.
10. Crooke ST. Vitravene – Another piece in the mosaic. *Antisense Nucleic Acid Drug Dev.* 1998; 8:vii–viii.
11. Agrawal S. Antisense oligonucleotides: Towards clinical trial. *Trends Biotechnol.* 1996; 14:376–387.
12. Kushner DM, Silverman RH. Antisense cancer therapy: The state of the science. *Curr. Oncol. Rep.* 2000; 2:23–30.
13. Monia BP, Holmlund J, Dorr FA. Antisense approaches for the treatment of cancer. *Cancer Inv.* 2000; 18:635–650.
14. Gewirtz AM. Oligonucleotide therapeutics: A step forward. *J. Clin. Oncol.* 2000; 18:1809–1811.
15. Crooke ST. Potential roles of antisense technology in cancer chemotherapy. *Oncogene* 2000; 19:6651–6659.
16. Agrawal S. Importance of nucleotide sequence and chemical modifications of antisense oligonucleotides. *Biochim. Biophys. Acta* 1999; 1489:53–68.

17. Agrawal S, Kandimalla ER. Antisense therapeutics: Is it simple as complementary base recognition? *Mol. Med. Today* 2000; 6:72–81.
18. Lebedeva I, Stein C. Antisense oligonucleotides: Promise and reality. *Annu. Rev. Pharmacol. Toxicol.* 2001; 41:403–419.
19. Crooke ST. Molecular mechanisms of action of antisense drugs. *Biochem. Biophys. Acta* 1999; 1489:31–44.
20. Crooke ST. Comments on evaluation of antisense drugs in the clinic. *Antisense Nucleic Acid Drug Dev.* 2000; 10:225–227.
21. Crooke ST. Progress in antisense technology: The end of the beginning. *Methods Enzymol.* 2000; 313:3–45.
22. Diasio RB, Zhang R. Pharmacology of therapeutic oligonucleotides. *Antisense Nucleic Acid Drug Dev.* 1997; 7:239–243.
23. Boiziau C, Thuong NT, Toulmé JJ. Mechanisms of the inhibition of reverse transcription by antisense oligonucleotides. *Proc. Natl. Acad. Sci. U. S. A.* 1992; 89:768–772.
24. Miller PS, McParland KB, Jayaraman K, Ts'o POP. Biochemical and biological effects of nonionic nucleic acid methylphosphonates. *Biochemistry* 1981; 20:1874–1880.
25. Carter G, Lemoine NR. Antisense technology for cancer therapy: Does it make sense? *Br. J. Cancer* 1993; 67:869–876.
26. Agrawal S, Iyer RP. Modified oligonucleotides as therapeutic and diagnostic agents. *Curr. Opin. Biotechnol.* 1995; 6:112–119.
27. Agrawal S, Jiang Z, Zhao Q, Shaw D, Cai Q, Roskey A, Channavajjala L, Saxinger C, Zhang R. Mixed-backbone oligonucleotides as second-generation antisense oligonucleotides: *In vitro* and *in vivo* studies. *Proc. Natl. Acad. Sci. U. S. A.* 1997; 94:2620–2625.
28. Agrawal S, Zhang R. Pharmacokinetics and bioavailability of oligonucleotides following oral and colorectal administrations in experimental animals. In *Antisense Research and Applications*, (Crooke, S., ed.), Springer-Verlag, Heidelberg, 1998, pp. 525–543.
29. Wang H, Cai Q, Zeng X, Yu D, Agrawal S, Zhang, R. Anti-tumor activity and pharmacokinetics of a mixed-backbone antisense oligonucleotide targeted to RIα subunit of protein kinase A after oral administration. *Proc. Natl. Acad. Sci. U. S. A.* 1999; 96:13989–13994.
30. Chen HX, Marchall JL, Ness E, Martin RR, Dvorchik B, Rizi N, Marquis J, McKinlay M, Dahur W, Hawkins MJ. A safety and pharmacokinetic study of a mixed-backbone oligonucleotide (GEM231) targeting the type I protein kinase A by two-our infusion in patients with refractory solid tumors. *Clin. Cancer Res.* 2000; 6:1259–1266.
31. Milner N, Mir KU, Southern EM. Selecting effective antisense reagents on combinatorial oligonucleotide arrays. *Nat. Biotechnol.* 1997; 15:537–541.
32. Zuker M. On finding all suboptimal folding of an RNA molecule. *Science* 1989; 244:48–52.
33. Elder JK, Johnson M, Milner N, Mir KU, Sohail M, Southern EM. Antisense oligonucleotide scanning arrays. In *DNA Microarrays: A Practical Approach* (Schena, M., ed.), IRL Press, Oxford. 1999, pp. 77–99.
34. Ho SP, Bao Y, Lesher T, Malhotra R, Ma LY, Fluharty SJ, Sakai RR. Mapping of RNA accessible sites for antisense experiments with oligonucleotide libraries. *Nat. Biotechnol.* 1998; 16:59–63.
35. Lima WF, Brown-Driver V, Fox M, Hanecak R, Bruice T. Combinatorial screening and rational optimization for hybridisation to folded hepatitis C virus RNA of oligonucleotides with biological antisense activity. *J. Biol. Chem.* 1997; 272:626–638.
36. Santoro SW, Joyce GF. A general purpose of RNA-cleaving DNA enzyme. *Proc. Natl. Acad. Sci. U. S. A.* 1997; 94:4262–4266.
37. Gewirtz AM. Oligonucleotide therapeutics for human leukaemia. In *Oligonucleotides as Therapeutic Agents* (Chadwick, D.J. and Cardew, G., eds.), Ciba Foundation Symposium 209, Wiley, Chichester, England, 1997, pp. 169–194.
38. Zhang R, Yan J, Shahinian H et al. Pharmacokinetics of an oligodeoxynucleotide phosphorothioate (GEM 91) in HIV-infected subjects. *Clin. Pharmacol. Ther.* 1995; 58:44–53.
39. Zhang R, Diasio RB, Lu Z, Liu T, Jiang Z, Galbraith WM, Agrawal S. Pharmacokinetics and tissue disposition in rats of an oligodeoxynucleotide phosphorothioate (GEM 91) developed as a therapeutic agent for human immunodeficiency virus type-1. *Biochem. Pharmacol.* 1995; 49:929–939.
40. Zhang R, Lu Z, Zhao H et al. *In vivo* stability, disposition and metabolism of a "hybrid" oligonucleotide phosphorothioate in rats. *Biochem. Pharmacol.* 1995; 50:545–556.

41. Zhang R, Iyer P, Yu D, Zhang X, Lu Z, Zhao H, Agrawal S. Pharmacokinetics and tissue disposition of a chimeric oligodeoxynucleotide phosphorothioate in rats following intravenous administration. *J. Pharmacol. Exp. Ther.* 1996; 278:971–979.

42. Agrawal S, Zhang R. Pharmacokinetics of phosphorothioate oligonucleotide and its novel analogs. In *Antisense Oligodeoxynucleotides and Antisense RNA as Novel Pharmacological and Therapeutic Agents* (Weiss, B., ed.), CRC Press, Boca Raton, 1997, pp. 58–78.

43. Agrawal S, Zhang R. Pharmacokinetics of oligonucleotides. In *Oligonucleotides as Therapeutic Agents* (Chadwick, D.J. and Cardew, G., eds.), Ciba Foundation Symposium 209; Wiley, Chichester, England, 1997, pp. 60–78.

44. Akhtar S. Delivery Strategies For Antisense Oligonucleotide Therapeutics. CRC Press, Boca Raton, FL, 1995.

45. Agrawal S, Akhtar S. Advances in antisense efficacy and delivery. *TIB Tech.* 1995; 13:197–199.

46. Dokka S, Rojanasakul Y. Novel non-endocytic delivery of antisense oligonucleotides. *Adv. Drug Deliver. Rev.* 2000; 44:35–39.

47. Agrawal S, Zhang X, Cai Q et al. Effect of aspirin on protein binding and tissue disposition of oligonucleotide phosphorothioate in rats. *J. Drug Target.* 1998; 5:303–312.

48. Wang H, Zeng X, Oliver P et al. MDM2 oncogene as a target for cancer therapy: An antisense approach. *Int. J. Oncol.* 1999; 15:653–660.

49. Chen L, Agrawal S, Zhou W, Zhang R, Chen J. Synergistic activation of p53 by inhibition of MDM2 expression and DNA damage. *Proc. Natl. Acad. Sci. U. S. A.* 1998; 95:195–200.

50. Tortora G, Caputo R, Damiano V et al. Novel MDM2 anti-sense oligonucleotide Has antitumor activity and potentiates cytotoxic drugs acting by different mechanisms in human colon cancer. *Int. J. Cancer* 2000; 88:804–809.

51. Prasad G, Wang H, Agrawal S, Zhang R. Antisense anti-MDM2 oligonucleotides as a novel approach to the treatment of glioblastoma multiforme. *Anticancer Res.* 2002; 22(1A):107–116.

52. Ciardiello F, Caputo R, Troiani T et al. Antisense oligonucleotides targeting the epidermal growth factor receptor inhibit proliferation, induce apoptosis, and cooperate with cytotoxic drugs in human cancer cell lines. *Int. J. Cancer* 2001; 93:172–178.

53. Tortora G, Caputo R, Damiano V et al. Cooperative antitumor effect of mixed backbone oligonucleotides targeting protein kinase A in combination with cytotoxic drugs or biologic agents. *Antisense Nucleic Acid Drug Dev.* 1998; 8:141–145.

54. Tortora G, Caputo R, Damiano V, Bianco R, Pepe S, Bianco AR, Jiang Z, Agrawal S, Ciardiello F. Synergistic inhibition of human cancer cell growth by cytotoxic drugs and mixed backbone antisense oligonucleotide targeting protein kinase A. *Proc. Natl. Acad. Sci. U. S. A.* 1997; 94:12586–12591.

55. Tortora G, Caputo R, Pomatico G et al. Cooperative inhibitory effect of novel mixed backbone oligonucleotide targeting protein kinase A in combination with docetaxel and anti-epidermal growth factor-receptor antibody on human breast cancer cell growth. *Clin. Cancer Res.* 1999; 5:875–881.

56. Akie K, Dosaka-Akita H, Murakami A, Kawakami YA. Combination treatment of C-myc antisense DNA with all-trans-retinoic acid inhibits cell proliferation by downregulating C-myc expression in small cell lung cancer. *Antisense Nucleic Acid Drug Dev.* 2000; 10:243–249.

57. Geiger T, Muller M, Dean NM, Fabbro D. Antitumor activity of a PKC-alpha antisense oligonucleotide in combination with standard chemotherapeutic agents against various human tumors transplanted into nude mice. *Anticancer Drug Des.* 1998; 13;35–45.

58. Lopes de Menezes DE, Hudon N, McIntosh N, Mayer LD. Molecular and pharmacokinetic properties associated with the therapeutics of bcl-2 antisense oligonucleotide G3139 combined with free and liposomal doxorubicin. *Clin. Cancer Res.* 2000; 6:2891–2902.

59. Agrawal S, Kandimalla ER, Yu D et al. Potentiation of antitumor activity of irinotecan by chemically modified oligonucleotides. *Int. J. Oncol.* 2001; 18:1061–1069.

60. Wang H, Nan L, Yu D, Agrawal S, Zhang R. Antisense anti-MDM2 oligonucleotides as a novel therapeutic approach to human breast cancer: In vitro and in vivo activities and mechanisms. *Clin. Cancer Res.* 2001; 7:3613–3624.

61. Wang H, Wang S, Nan L, Yu D, Agrawal S, Zhang R. Antisense anti-MDM2 mixed backbone oligonucleotides enhance therapeutic efficacy of topoisomerase I inhibitor irinotecan in nude mice bearing human cancer xenografts: In vivo activity and mechanisms. *Int. J. Oncol.* 2002; 21:73–80.

62. Jansen B, Wacheck V, Heere-Ress E et al. Chemosensitisation of malignant melanoma by BCL2 antisense therapy. *Lancet* 2000; 356:1728–1733.

63. Agrawal S, Zhao Q, Jiang Z, Oliver C, Giles H, Heath J, Serota D. Toxicologic effects of an oligodeoxynucleotide phosphorothioate and its analogs following intravenous administration in rats. *Antisense Nucleic Acid Drug Dev.* 1997; 7:575–584.

64. Henry SP, Zuckerman JE, Rojko J, Hall WC, Harman RJ, Kitchen D, Crooke ST. Toxicological properties of several novel oligonucleotide analogs in mice. *Anticancer Drug Des.* 1997; 12:1–14.

65. Agrawal S, Zhao Q. Mixed backbone oligonucleotides: Improvement in oligonucleotide-induced toxicity in vivo. *Antisense Nucleic Acid Drug Dev.* 1998; 8:135–139.

66. Agrawal S, Iadarola PL, Temsamani J, Zhao Q, Shaw DR. Effect of G-rich sequences on the synthesis, purification, binding, cell uptake, and hemolytic activity of oligonucleotides. *Bioorg. Med. Chem. Lett.* 1996; 6:2219–2224.

67. Ahn CH, DeGeorge JJ. Preclinical development of antisense oligonucleotide therapeutics for cancer: Regulatory aspects. In *Clinical Trials of Genetic Therapy with Antisense DNA and DNA Vectors* (Wickstrom, E., ed.), Marcel Dekker, New York, 1998, pp. 39–52.

7

ANTIBODIES AND VACCINES AS NOVEL CANCER THERAPEUTICS

SVETOMIR N. MARKOVIC

Mayo Clinic
Department of Hematology
Rochester, Minnesota

ESTEBAN CELIS

Mayo Clinic
Department Immunology
Rochester, Minnesota

I. INTRODUCTION
II. ANTI-TUMOR ANTIBODIES
III. CANCER VACCINES
IV. CONCLUSIONS

I. INTRODUCTION

The past two decades have witnessed a renaissance in the field of basic and clinical immunology that has opened the doors for new approaches to treat cancer patients. Development of new methodology has allowed for an expanded understanding of the intricate mechanisms of immune cell interactions allowing for the insight into basic principles of immune defenses in general as well as anti-tumor immune responses in particular. Volumes of research in the preclinical arena have given rise to renewed enthusiasm for the use of immune-based agents as cancer therapeutics. To date, the two most significant components of cancer immunotherapeutics are anti-tumor antibodies and anti-tumor vaccines. Many of these agents have been successfully translated from preclinical studies into clinical trials. Some have already been accepted as "standards of care."

Herein we will describe the basic principles of anti-tumor antibody and vaccine development with illustrative examples of agents currently in clinical use.

II. ANTI-TUMOR ANTIBODIES

The concept of the use of antibodies for the treatment of disease dates back to Emil von Behring who was awarded the Nobel Prize in Physiology in 1901 for his work on "serum therapy and its application in diphtheria" [1]. His revolutionary concept of utilizing a normally occurring defense mechanism against disease and applying it as a medicinal agent gave rise to the theoretical framework of therapeutic antibodies. Paul Erlich who, in 1908, shared the Nobel Prize for the discovery of the concept of immunity stated: "The antibodies are therefore magic bullets which find the targets themselves . . . we must therefore concentrate all our powers and abilities on making the aim as accurate as we can contrive, so as to strike the parasites as hard and the body cells as lightly as possible." Full implementation of this principle became possible following the discovery of the methods for production of monoclonal antibodies in the mid-1970s [2]. The ability to develop antibodies capable of recognizing tumor-specific epitopes gave rise to the hope of finally specifically targeting tumor cells without injuring normal tissues and validate Erlich's "magic bullet" hypothesis.

The realm of antibody-based cancer immunotherapeutics is divided into two categories: (1) unmodified monoclonal antibodies with cytotoxic, regulatory, and immunization properties; and (2) immunoconjugates, i.e., monoclonal antibodies conjugated to toxins, chemotherapeutics, radioactive isotopes, or biologics that, in theory, should augment their effector function. In both settings, tumor target specificity is determined by the antigen-binding fragment (Fab) of the monoclonal antibody. The main distinction among the two categories is that the cytotoxic activity of these therapeutics is a function of the antibody's natural activity (via complement fixation or antibody-dependent cell cytotoxicity; ADCC) itself in the former, and the conjugate in the latter.

The most significant developments in antibody-based cancer immunotherapeutics to date has been the discovery of monoclonal antibodies demonstrating direct anti-tumor cytotoxic properties. These developments were enabled by recently described technologies for identification of tumor-specific antigens as well as techniques for "humanization" of non-human antibodies. The major drawback of conventional monoclonal antibodies, which are produced in mice, is the induction of inactivating human anti-mouse antibodies (HAMA) by the patient's own immune system. For this reason, the mouse antibodies can be genetically altered to mimic human proteins, which are not as immunogenic as their murine counterparts. The development of humanized monoclonal antibodies capable of recognizing surface antigens, highly expressed on malignant cells (her-2/neu), and normal cells (CD20, CD52 and CD33) has given rise to Herceptin, Rituxan, Campath, and gemtuzumab ozogamicin, respectively [3]. These monoclonal antibodies have completed initial clinical testing and are currently in clinical use for the treatment of breast cancer, lymphoma, chronic lymphocytic leukemia, and acute myelogenous leukemia. The exact mechanisms of anti-tumor cytotoxic activity of these antibodies in humans are not fully elucidated. Hypotheses range from induction of second messenger apoptotic signaling [4] to antibody-mediated cell cytotoxicity [5–7]. Having demonstrated clinical efficacy as single agents, most of these antibodies are currently in phase I and II clinical trials where they are used in addition to standard combination chemotherapy regimens. Preliminary reports suggest additive to synergistic effects of chemotherapy/antibody combination treatments (i.e., paclitaxel + Herceptin, Rituxan + CHOP).

A somewhat different approach in the application of therapeutic monoclonal antibodies has been with the use of antibodies directed against regulatory molecules of carcinogenesis and angiogenesis [8]. Examples of such targets include epidermal growth factor receptors (EGFR) [9], platelet-derived growth factor receptors (PDGFR) [10], vascular endothelial growth factor (VEGF), and vascular endothelial growth factor receptor (VEGFR) [11]. These molecules have been found to be upregulated in a variety of epithelial neoplasms and their inhibition/downregulation has been associated with tumor regression in preclinical models. Examples of such molecules that have successfully entered the phase II clinical trials arena are cetuximab (anti-EGFR) [12] and bevacizumab (anti-VEGF) [13]. Cetuximab has been used clinically in phase I and II studies for patients with malignancies overexpressing EGFR (breast, lung, ovary, head and neck, pancreas, and colorectal cancer) either alone or in combination with chemotherapy. Results of clinical studies reported to date are encouraging. Bevacizumab has most extensively been studied in patients with non-small cell lung cancer (NSCLC). Applied in combination with chemotherapy (carboplatin and paclitaxel), bevacizumab resulted in improved response rates, prolonged time to progression, and longer median survival times of treated NSCLC patients with non-squamous cell tumors relative to patients treated with chemotherapy alone [13]. A large number of other monoclonal antibodies directed at similar targets are currently in late stages of preclinical development entering phase I studies. One of the more encouraging new antibodies is IMC-1C11, a monoclonal antibody against VEGFR2 [14].

In a general sense, the above two applications of therapeutic monoclonal antibodies represent expansion of the basic principle of "serum therapy" utilizing state-of-the-art technology. A step away from this principle is the application of monoclonal antibodies as idiotype antigens. Namely, each antibody clone possesses an antigenically unique motif in its Fab, which represents the idiotype of the antibody. Jerne [15] theorized that each antibody idiotype is capable of generating a downregulatory anti-idiotype immune response giving rise to the "idiotype network" hypothesis of immune regulation. Considering that human B-cell malignancies (non-Hodgkin lymphomas) express surface immunoglobulins of unique idiotype as their tumor-specific antigens, the generation of anti-idiotype antibodies may be of therapeutic benefit; hence, the development of anti-idiotype vaccines. In these models, monoclonal antibodies derived from malignant B cells are used as vaccines in the hope of generating anti-idiotype immune responses that would target the parent malignant B cells. Currently, active phase I and II clinical trials utilize the patient's own malignant B cells as the source of the idiotype-specific monoclonal antibodies used as vaccines following primary "debulking" chemotherapy [16]. Preliminary reports are encouraging. Similar efforts are currently under way utilizing monoclonal antibodies specific for other tumor-associated antigens, i.e., human milk fat globule (HMFG) protein, which is expressed in >90% of breast cancer patients. The monoclonal antibody recognizing this protein is currently in phase I testing as an anti-idiotype vaccine attempting to induce anti-idiotype antibodies in the patients that would cross react with native HMFG [17].

A somewhat more innovative approach in the use of monoclonal antibodies takes advantage of a recently developed technology creating antibody molecules in which each of the two Fabs have different specificities (bispecific antibodies; BsAb). Initial work in this field utilized BsAbs in which one Fab fragment was tumor specific and the other was specific for immune effector cells surface molecules (CD3, CD16, CD64, etc.). Early, small-scale phase I studies have demonstrated encouraging results that have led to further attempts at refining the structure of the BsAbs in attempts to improve their anti-tumor efficacy [18]. This has resulted in a variety of molecules (scFv, minibodies, diabodies, and multivalent BsAbs), the clinical utility of which remains to be realized.

A somewhat different approach in the use of therapeutic monoclonal antibodies is the use of immunoconjugates. In this setting, rather than using "pure" antibodies, the antibody molecules are chemically conjugated with agents capable of inducing cell death (radioactive isotopes, toxins, chemotherapeutic agents, etc.). The rationale behind this approach stems from early observations that monoclonal antibodies are far more effective at binding to cancer cells than killing them. Therefore, "arming" the monoclonal antibody with cytotoxic agents would allow them to be delivered at high concentrations to the appropriate tumor targets, avoiding unwanted toxicity of systemic administration.

Immunotoxins represent the largest component of the immunoconjugate effort. Many different plant and bacterial toxins have been used to prepare immunotoxins. Early developments in this field utilized toxin molecules devoid of their cell binding domains/subunits coupled to whole monoclonal antibodies. These immunotoxins were chemically heterogenous, difficult to synthesize in adequate quantities, and unable to adequately penetrate solid tumors. The associated clinical trials resulted in significant toxicities with little clinical benefits. Thus, by the early 1980s endeavors in this field were nearly abandoned. By the end of the decade a renewed enthusiasm for the use of immunotoxins was brought forth following the discovery of Fv fragments [19, 20]. These fragments are genetically engineered monoclonal variable domains of the heavy and light chains of an antibody connected by a peptide linker. The decreased molecular weight of the Fv fragment relative to a whole antibody was believed to be more advantageous with respect to tumor infiltration. Some of the most exciting work in this arena was performed in patients with refractory hairy cell leukemia (HCL). A single chain Fv fragment able to recognize the IL-2 receptor (CD25) was linked to *Pseudomonas* exotoxin devoid of it's binding domain. The new molecule was designated LMB-2 and was given to four patients with refractory HCL in a phase I study. All four patients experienced major hematologic responses to therapy with limited toxicity [21]. The same group of investigators went on to a do a more expanded phase I study treating patients with multiple hematologic malignancies expressing CD25. Their results were the first to demonstrate major anti-tumor responses with the use of a recombinant immunotoxin [22]. Encouraged by these data, an increasing number of investigators are currently pursuing Fv-based immunotoxins in various phase I clinical trials targeting different tumor-associated surface molecules, thereby revitalizing the field of immunotoxin research.

Another variation to the model of immunoconjugate cancer therapy are radio-immunoconjugates. Much like the immunotoxins, the effective anti-tumor agent is the conjugated radioactive isotope, with the role of the monoclonal antibody as merely a delivery vehicle. Radio-immunoconjugates have been used for both diagnostic and therapeutic purposes. If a monoclonal antibody is conjugated to a radioisotope that could be detected by a gamma camera, the antibody could be used to visualize tumors. If the same monoclonal antibody is conjugated to an alpha- or beta-emitting radioisotope, it could be used as a therapeutic agent. The therapeutic radio-immunoconjugates would deliver the radioactive isotope to the vicinity of the tumor and allow for local radiation therapy. Because these are radioactive agents, there is no need for the isotopes to be delivered to each individual cell therefore obviating the need for high-tumor penetrance (necessary with immunotoxins). Delivery of radiation to the vicinity of tumors appeared to be sufficient. The most significant work to date in this field was performed utilizing radiolabeled monoclonal anti-CD20 antibodies for the treatment of malignant lymphoma. Malignant lymphomas are radiosensitive tumors for which a useful tumor-specific antigen (CD20) has already been recognized. Therefore, it appeared reasonable to test the principle of radio-immunotherapy in this tumor model. The two radio-immunoconjugates of greatest clinical significance to date are ^{90}Y-ibritumomab (Zevalin) and ^{131}I-tositumomab (Bexxar) [23]. Both agents have completed phase I and II studies demonstrating safety and clinical efficacy. Table 7.1 summarizes the basic characteristics of these agents. Optimal utilization of these agents is currently the subject of several ongoing clinical studies (see Table 7.1).

Immunoconjugates in which monoclonal antibodies are linked to chemotherapeutic agents have not yet made the transition to phase I clinical trials. The basic difficulties in these constructs is that chemotherapeutic agents, covalently linked to monoclonal antibodies, once delivered to the site of tumor by the antibody, need to be internalized and cleaved off the antibody in order to gain access to their intracellular targets. The obvious complexities in the synthesis and metabolism of such molecules remain a

TABLE 7.1   Basic Characteristics of Zevalin and Bexxar

	Zevalin	Bexxar
Monoclonal antibody	Murine IDEC-2B8 (parent of rituximab)	Murine IgG2a
Specificity	Anti-CD20	Anti-CD20
Radioisotope	^{90}Y beta emission	^{131}I beta emission gamma emission
Serum half-life	28 h	59.3 h
Stability of immunoconjugate	Urea-type bond	Subject to enzymatic dehalogenation
Routes of excretion	Hepatic	Urinary
Organ retention of free radioisotope	Bone marrow	Thyroid and gastrointestinal

significant obstacle to further development. In an attempt to simplify the synthesis process, several groups have attempted to coat clinically available chemotherapy-loaded liposomes with monoclonal antibodies. In principle, the chemotherapy-loaded liposomes (i.e., capecitabine) could be directed to concentrate at sites of tumor by specific monoclonal antibodies (immunoliposomes) [24]. This would in turn result in greater clinical efficacy with reduced toxicity compared to the use of the liposomal agents alone. Phase I clinical testing of several such molecules are currently nearing completion. If successful, this method would allow "packaging" of a wide array of chemotherapeutic agents into liposomes and custom "targeting" using varying tumor specific antigens. A similar attempt at utilizing the combination of monoclonal antibody tumor targeting and chemotherapy-mediated tumor killing is the antibody directed enzyme prodrug therapy (ADEPT) approach [25]. This method utilizes a two-step therapeutic approach. First, an immune conjugate consisting of a tumor-specific monoclonal antibody linked to an enzyme capable of activating a chemotherapy produg is administered. This allows the enzyme to be deployed in areas of high tumor burden. Then, a non-toxic chemotherapy prodrug is administered. The prodrug reaches the sites of its metabolizing enzyme and is converted into the active agent. Thus, active drug is produced at the site of the tumor and is capable of destroying not only tumor cells bound by the antibody, but also those in the immediate vicinity. Much like the liposomal approach, this method does not limit tumoricidal activity only to tumor cells bound by the antibody that can endocytose and translocate the conjugated chemotherapeutic agent to its intracellular target.

In summary, the use of antibodies as cancer treatment agents offers a wide variety of therapeutic possibilities based on the ability of antibodies to recognize specific tumor antigens (passive immunization). In the absence of clearly identified cell surface expressed tumor-specific antigens, antibody-based therapy is irrelevant. Therein is the most significant drawback of this mode of therapy and the source of immunologic escape of tumors recurring after initial response to antibody-based treatments. Once a cancer cell looses/alters a targeted surface antigen, it becomes invisible to the Fab of the monoclonal antibody and its anti-tumor activity is neutralized regardless of conjugates. Another important limitation in the use of antibodies for cancer immunotherapy is that this approach is limited to those tumor antigens that are expressed on the surface of the malignant cell. In contrast, immunological therapies based on tumor-specific T lymphocytes can utilize any protein that is made by the tumor cell, regardless of its localization.

III. CANCER VACCINES

As the second arm of tumor immunotherapy, cancer vaccines represent an attempt to actively immunize patients against single or multiple tumor-specific antigens. This approach takes advantage not only of the vaccine's ability to induce anti-tumor antibodies but also the ability to stimulate anti-tumor T-cell responses. The production of tumor-specific antibodies by B cells can be elicited by immunization of animals with tumor cells, and tumor-associated determinants that have been defined by their ability to stimulate an antibody response and their presence on tumor cells, but not normal cells. This is the theoretical basis for the application of anti-tumor antibodies in cancer therapy. Also, there is accumulating evidence to suggest that many tumors in experimental model systems and cancer patients express molecules that are recognized by the T-cell arm of the immune system. In contrast to antibodies, T cells recognize antigens as peptides derived from proteins, which are processed and exported to the cell surface in association with the major histocompatibility complex (MHC)-gene products. Thus, any protein made by the tumor cells can potentially function as a tumor antigen for T cells as long as it produces peptides that can bind to the MHC molecules.

Early experiments performed in the 1950s demonstrated that tumor-specific transplantation antigens were expressed by methylcholanthrene- or virus-induced tumors [26]. These antigens could provoke an immune response by the host after immunization, and rejection of antigen-expressing tumor cells was mediated by specific host cytolytic T cells [27]. The molecular cloning of a tumor-specific antigen expressed by a murine cell line that had been mutagenized has been described as well as the cloning of a naturally occurring tumor-specific antigen expressed by the murine mastocytoma P815 [28, 29]. In the mouse, cytolytic T cells that demonstrated tumor specificity could be expanded *in vitro* from splenocytes as well as from single cell enzymatic tumor digests [28, 29]. Tumor-infiltrating lymphocytes, or TIL, can mediate regression of established pulmonary tumors and cure mice with advanced tumor burdens [30, 31]. In patients bearing metastatic tumors, a number of groups have demonstrated the existence of anti-tumor cytotoxic T lymphocyte (CTL) responses. Peripheral blood mononuclear cells as well as TIL contain populations of cells and individual clones that demonstrate tumor specificity; they lyse autologous tumor cells, but not natural killer targets, allogeneic tumor cells, or autologous fibroblasts [32–35]. Tumor-specific TIL can be expanded to large numbers *ex vivo* and mediate regressions of metastatic melanoma after adoptive transfer with interleukin-2 (IL-2) [36, 37]. Therefore, tumor-specific antigens exist on metastatic human tumors, and are capable of stimulating a specific T-cell response that can be expanded to achieve objective clinical responses in tumor-bearing patients. The main goal of cancer vaccine therapy is *in vivo* expansion of tumor specific T-cell clones by boosting the already primed immune system of the host with tumor-specific antigens.

Current cancer vaccines comprise two basic elements (Figure 7.1): tumor-specific antigen and immune adjuvant. There are two basic categories of tumor-specific antigens currently in use. One utilizes clearly defined tumor-specific antigens as the vaccine immunogen (native tumor antigens, modified tumor antigens, tumor antigen specific peptides, etc). The other takes advantage of the observation that transplanted tumor cells are capable of eliciting anti-tumor immune responses and utilizes whole tumor cell (or cell components) as the vaccine immunogen (irradiated tumor cells, tumor cell lysates, fused cells, genetically engineered cells, etc.). This approach assumes that unidentified tumor-specific antigens contained in these cellular preparations could be used to upregulate anti-tumor responses when administered in conjunction with immune adjuvants.

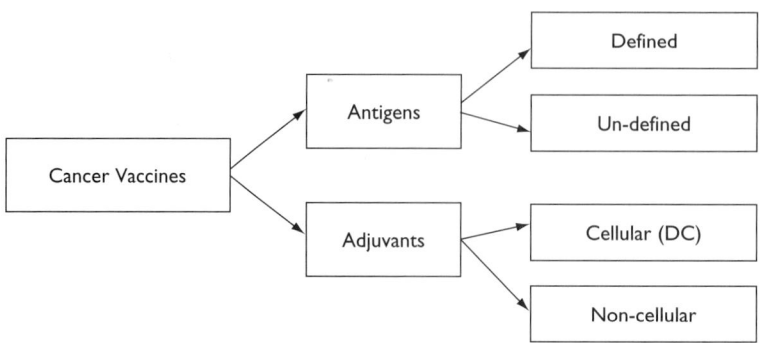

FIGURE 7.1   Current cancer vaccines comprise two basic elements.

The role of immune adjuvants in the cancer vaccine is to enhance the immunogenicity of the antigen. This can be achieved in two ways: (1) with the use of autologous dendritic cells (cellular approach) or (2) pro-inflammatory molecules able to stimulate local inflammation at the site of vaccine administration attracting immunocompetent cells to the site of antigen delivery (complete and incomplete Freund's adjuvant, cytokines, oils, etc.). In an attempt to find the optimal cancer vaccines, generations of investigators have attempted a myriad of combinations of various antigens and adjuvants. Despite decades of preclinical and clinical investigations, clinically relevant cancer vaccines remain elusive. Herein, we will describe some of the more prominent models of cancer vaccines currently in active phase II and III clinical trials.

A. Defined Tumor Antigens: Peptide Vaccines

Endogenously synthesized antigens of virtually all mammalian cells are processed in an endoplasmic reticulum compartment and converted to small epitope peptides that are subsequently displayed on the cell surface in association with class I MHC molecules. However, specialized antigen-processing cells are capable of presenting very small numbers of exogenous peptides in association with class I molecules to stimulate T-cell recognition. Tumor-specific peptides bound in association with class I molecules have been purified from the surface of melanoma cells and stimulate autologous cytotoxic T-cell recognition by cytolysis or cytokine release assay [38]. Purified epitope peptides derived from different animal viruses have been used in various preparations to immunize mice and have been shown to induce high-affinity CTL and protect mice against lethal challenges with infectious virus.

An example of a tumor-specific antigen containing immunodominant peptides capable of stimulating anti-tumor T-cell responses is MAGE-1. The MAGE-1 antigen is encoded by a gene spanning 5 kb, and the 2419 base pair sequence produces a predicted protein product of 26 kDa. The MAGE-1 antigen has been demonstrated to contain an immunodominant HLA-A1 restricted epitope (Glu-Ala-Asp-Pro-Thr-Gly-His-Ser-Tyr, or EADPTGHSY), a nonamer encoded by the third exon of the MAGE-1 gene [39]. MAGE-1 is not expressed by normal cells and tissues with the exception of testis, but it is present on approximately 40% of melanomas, 20% of breast cancers, 30% of small cell and non-small cell lung cancers, and a variety of other malignancies [40, 41]. MAGE-1 is a member of a multi-gene family of at least 15 members, of which at least two encode antigens recognized by T cells from patients with melanoma. Numerous other immunodominant peptides derived from tumor-associated and tumor-specific antigens have been described and synthesized for clinical use [42]. Several vaccines containing these peptides have already completed phase I testing and are in active phase II and III clinical trials. Most of these studies have been performed using peptides derived from malignant melanoma antigens.

One of the most significant obstacles to the development of clinically relevant peptide-based vaccines has been the poor innate immunogenicity of peptides. A number of investigators are currently engaged in attempts to overcome this problem by developing adequate immune adjuvants capable of inducing peptide-specific immune responses. Both cellular and non-cellular immune adjuvants are currently under investigation.

B. Defined Tumor Antigens: Gangliosides

Gangliosides are prominent cell surface constituents of neuroectodermal tumors, which includes melanoma. Three of them (GM2, GD2, GD3) are of particular interest in melanoma because two of the three are expressed in almost all human melanoma isolates. Initial attempts to utilize gangliosides alone as vaccines demonstrated that they were non-immunogenic. Combined with bacterial porins, they were able to induce antibody responses. Based on encouraging preclinical data, a GM2 vaccine combined with BCG was introduced into a clinical trial demonstrating an IgM response in 86% of the treated melanoma patients. In an attempt to improve the immunogenicity of GM2, the ganglioside was conjugated to keyhole limpet hemocyanin (KLH) as carrier protein and combined with QS-21 as an immune adjuvant. A preliminary report demonstrated superior immunologic antibody responses. These data gave rise to a prospective phase III clinical trial comparing vaccine versus in combination with interferon alpha for patients with resected stage III melanoma [43]. The vaccine alone group did worse compared to the vaccine plus interferon arms.

C. Undefined Tumor Antigens: Cell-Based Vaccines

Despite significant strides in our understanding of tumor-specific antigens and our ability to dissect immunodominant peptide epitopes capable of stimulating anti-tumor T-cell responses, there still exists a large number of undefined tumor antigens. Also, any tumor vaccines that immunize against single or small numbers of defined peptide antigens run the risk of selecting out peptide negative cell clones resistant to the generated immune response. Therefore, in an attempt to generate broad anti-tumor immune responses to known and unknown tumor antigens, multiple groups of investigators have used tumor-cell based vaccines. This approach is a direct outgrowth of successful vaccine strategies using killed microorganisms as immunogens. The last two decades have witnessed a multitude of various tumor cell preparations utilized as cancer vaccines. A summary of the more significant applications is presented in Table 7.2.

The most significant work in this field is attributed to Donald Morton and his introduction of CancerVax [44]. This agent is currently completing phase III testing for the treatment of stage III and stage IV melanoma. CancerVax is a whole-cell preparation of three allogeneic melanoma cell lines (M10, M24, and M101). Cells from each cell line are grown in serum-free media, harvested, pooled, and irradiated with 100–150 Gy. Irradiated cells are then cyropreserved for clinical use. Vaccine was administered intradermally every 2 weeks (×3) and then monthly (one year). After the first year of therapy, vaccine was administered every 3 months (×3) and every 6 months thereafter. The idea behind the use of such a vaccine was to introduce melanoma-specific antigens in the setting of an allogeneic MHC. The MHC mismatch would serve as a powerful stimulus to boost the immunogenicity of the putative tumor antigens. Initial reports with the use of this vaccine, administered only for one year, demonstrated an increase in median and 5-year survival times of patients with stage III and IV melanoma as compared to historic controls. The current phase III trials for both stage III and IV disease will definitively answer the questions of clinical efficacy.

Arguments that the best tumor targets for each individual patient are those of the patient's own tumor have given rise to the use of autologous tumor cells as cancer vaccines. The largest experience in this arena comes from Berd et al. [49]. In their model, patients underwent surgical excision of melanoma that was used to process an autologous cell based vaccine. The vaccine was combined with BCG as an immune adjuvant. Their initial data demonstrated five clinical responses out of 40 evaluable patients. Ongoing clinical studies utilizing this approach are attempting to improve the immunogenicity of the vaccine and improve its clinical efficacy. Other groups

TABLE 7.2 Summary of Different Applications of Cell-Based Cancer Vaccines

Tumor type (vaccine trade name)	Description	Ref:
Allogeneic melanoma (CancerVax)	A combination of three allogeneic melanoma cell lines, irradiated and administered in conjunction with incomplete Freund's adjuvant	44
Melanoma (Melacine)	A lysate derived from three allogeneic tumor cell lines administered in conjunction with immune adjuvant	45
Melanoma (Avax)	Irradiated autologous tumor cells administered with immune adjuvant	46
Renal cell carcinoma	Fused autologous tumor cells with allogeneic dendritic cells	47
Melanoma	Culture supernatants of allogeneic melanoma cell lines adsorbed to alum	48

have chosen to utilize autologous tumor cell vaccines with different immune adjuvants either administered along with the vaccine or genetically engineered and expressed by the autologous tumor cells (granulocyte macrophage colony stimulating factor; GM-CSF). Most of these approaches are still in the preclinical arena with few completing phase I trials.

Although conceptually more appealing than allogeneic tumor cell vaccines, the autologous tumor cell vaccines require significant *ex vivo* manipulations and processing, which may potentially affect expression of clinically relevant tumor-specific antigens. In an attempt to overcome this issue, several groups have embarked on the development of methods to enhance the immunogenicity of malignancies while they are still in the patients. These methods involve intra-tumor injections of various compounds (cytokines and plasmid DNA) with the hope of producing systemic anti-tumor effects following modulation of single sites of disease. Examples of such interventions include the use of intra-lesional GM-CSF therapy and intra-lesional allovectin-7 (HLA-B7 plasmid DNA). Both of these approaches have largely been applied in melanoma clinical studies. Phase I results show no significant toxicities. Phase II data are not yet available.

D. Immune Adjuvants

As is apparent from the above discussion, one of the major obstacles to the development of a potent cancer vaccine is that most tumor antigens (proteins, peptides, gangliosides, cells, and cell subunits) are poor immunogens. A large effort is currently under way attempting to define the optimal immune adjuvant for cancer vaccines. Work in this field focuses primarily on three topics: (1) modifications of oil-based immune adjuvants (incomplete Freund's adjuvant), (2) optimization of various dendritic cell-based vaccines, (3) application of cytokines as immune adjuvants (IL-2, GM-CSF, etc.).

Of the oil-based immune adjuvants, the one most widely used in peptide clinical trials is montanide ISA-51 [50]. This is a proprietary lipid preparation that has been shown to augment anti-vaccine immune responses both in preclinical and clinical models. Multiple other preparations in this category of immune adjuvants are currently in various phases of preclinical and clinical development. Due to the proprietary nature of the structure of these adjuvants, it is difficult to make adequate comparisons among the different preparations. Nevertheless, all of these agents share a few basic characteristics: (1) they do not interfere with the structure of the antigens, (2) they cause mild local inflammation at the site of injection with the purpose of attracting antigen presenting dendritic cells to the site of the antigen, and (3) they allow for slow release of the antigen allowing prolonged exposure.

Probably one of the most significant discoveries in the field of vaccine development has been the application of antigen-loaded autologous dendritic cells as cancer vaccines [51]. Dendritic cells (DCs) are the most effective antigen-presenting cells of the mammalian immune system. Therefore, if one could take DCs out of the body and "load" them with antigens, one could potentially circumvent the need to attract these cells to sites of antigen injection (skin) as is achieved with more conventional adjuvants (above). This would potentially allow for much more efficient antigen uptake and processing by the DCs and therefore much more effective presentation of these antigens to T cells once the DCs are re-infused into patients. Therein lays the principle of DC cancer vaccines in clinical trials. Initial clinical studies, despite intriguing preclinical data and phase I clinical observations, uncovered significant difficulties with reproducible production of DC cancer vaccines. There is an ongoing debate regarding the technological aspects of DC vaccine production. Optimization efforts pertaining to DC maturation conditions, antigen preparation, antigen challenge, route of administration, frequency of administration, etc., are ongoing. Unfortunately, the high cost of production of these vaccines has been a significant obstacle to a more broad-based research effort attempting to answer these questions.

One of the more interesting recent developments in cancer vaccines is the realization of the immune adjuvant potential of cytokines. The most significant work in this field deals with the application of GM-CSF as an immune adjuvant. GM-CSF is a commercially available cytokine commonly used in patients undergoing chemotherapy with the goal of shortening the duration of post-chemotherapy neutropenia. Recently published evidence also suggests that GM-CSF may play a role of an immune adjuvant [52]. Some of the demonstrated mechanisms by which GM-CSF can potentiate the immunogenicity of a given antigen stem from the following observations: (1) GM-CSF is a key mediator of DC maturation and function [53], (2) GM-CSF increases surface expression of class I and II MHC molecules as well as co-stimulatory molecules of DCs *in vitro* [53], (3) GM-CSF enhances antibody responses to known immunogens *in vivo* [54], (4) tumor cells transfected with genes encoding/expressing GM-CSF are able to induce long-lasting, specific anti-tumor immune responses *in vivo* [55], (5) GM-CSF encapsulated in biodegradable microspheres mixed with whole tumor cells resulted in systemic anti-tumor immune responses comparable to those of GM-CSF transfected tumor cells [56]. Based on these observations several ongoing clinical studies are attempting to directly ascertain the immune adjuvant potential of GM-CSF in cancer vaccines.

Despite decades of research, clinically effective cancer vaccines remain elusive. Clinical and laboratory developments in the last 5 years have provided the ability to directly quantify the immunostimulatory abilities of these vaccines beyond simple antibody titers. Having these quantitative end points (Elispot, tetramer, cytokine RT-PCR) allows us to compare the effectiveness of different vaccine preparations and learn which vaccine attributes are immunologically (clinically) relevant and which are not. This has allowed us to embark on a systematic effort and construct vaccines with increasing immunological and clinical efficacy. Only with such an effort can we hope to take the field of cancer vaccines out of the realm of clinical anecdotes.

IV. CONCLUSION

Immunotherapy of cancer remains one of the possibly most effective modes of therapy for malignant disorders, the potential of which remains unfulfilled. Recent developments in basic and clinical immunology have created tools that allow a better understanding of the mechanisms of action of these agents and gain insights into methods to improve their clinical efficacy. The first signs of the extraordinary potential of immune-based cancer therapy are evident in the development of tumor antigen-specific/associated therapeutic monoclonal antibodies. Several of these therapeutics are currently widely applied in clinical practice. Not far behind are developments in cancer vaccines. For the first time, after many decades of disappointing clinical results, cancer immunotherapeutics appear on the threshold of fulfillment of their therapeutic potential, as predicted by Erlich some 100 years ago. This chapter briefly highlights just some of the many ongoing efforts in the field of cancer immunotherapy, all of which are based on the principle of utilizing the body's own immune defenses as a blueprint and mediator of cancer therapeutics.

REFERENCES

1. Silverstein AM. *A History of Immunology*. San Diego, Academic Press, 1989.
2. Kohler G, Milstein C. Continuous cultures of fused cells secreting antibody of pre-determined specificity. *Nature* 1975; 256:495–497.
3. Johnson PW. The therapeutic use of antibodies in malignancy. *Transfus. Clin. Biol.* 2001; 8:255–259.
4. Cuello M, Ettenberg SA, Clark AS et al. Down-regulation of the erbB-2 receptor by trastuzumab (herceptin) enhances tumor necrosis factor-related apoptosis-inducing ligand-mediated apoptosis in breast and ovarian cancer cell lines that overexpress erbB-2. *Cancer Res.* 2001; 61:4892–4900.
5. Herberman RB, Morgan AC, Reisfeld R et al. Antibody-dependent cellular cytotoxicity (ADCC) against human melanoma by human effector cells in cooperation with mouse monoclonal antibodies. In UCLA Symposia on Molecular and Cellular Biology, New Series, Vol. 27: Monoclonal Antibodies and Cancer Therapy. New York, 193, 1985.
6. Herberman RB, Orew ME, Rogentine G et al. Cytolytic effects of alloantiserum in patients with lymphoproliferative disorders. *Cancer* 1971; 28:365–371.
7. Herlyn D and Koprowski H. IgG2A monoclonal antibodies inhibit human tumor growth factor through interaction with effector cells. *Proc. Natl. Acad. Sci. U. S. A.* 1982; 79:4761–4765.
8. Goustin AS, Leof EB, Shipley GD et al. Growth factors and cancer. *Cancer Res.* 1986; 46:1015–1029.
9. Herbst RS, Kim ES, Harari PM. IMC-C225, an anti-epidermal growth factor receptor monoclonal antibody, for treatment of head and neck cancer. *Expert Opin. Biol. Ther.* 2001; 1(4):719–732.
10. Plate KH, Breier G, Farrell CL, Risau W. Platelet-derived growth factor receptor-beta is induced during tumor development and upregulated during tumor progression in endothelial cells in human gliomas. *Lab. Invest.* 1992; 67(4):529–534.
11. Hasan J, Jayson GC. VEGF antagonists. *Expert Opin. Biol. Ther.* 2001; 1:703–718.
12. Baselga J. The EGFR as a target for anticancer therapy-focus on cetuximab. *Eur. J. Cancer* 2001; 37(Suppl. 4):S16–22.
13. Chen HX, Gore-Langton RE, Cheson BD. Clinical trials referral resource: Current clinical trials of the anti-VEGF monoclonal antibody bevacizumab. *Oncology (Huntingt.)* 2001; 15:1017, 1020, 1023–1026.
14. Hunt S. Technology evaluation: IMC-1C11, ImClone Systems. *Curr. Opin. Mol. Ther.* 2001; 3:418–424.
15. Jerne NK. Towards a network theory of the immune system. *Ann. Immunol.* 1974; 125C:373–389.
16. Press OW, Leonard JP, Coiffier B, Levy R, Timmerman J. Immunotherapy of Non-Hodgkin's lymphomas. *Hematology (Am. Soc. Hematol. Educ. Program)* 2001; 221–240.

17. Tripathi PK, Qin H, Bhattacharya-Chatterjee M et al. Construction and characterization of a chimeric fusion protein consisting of an anti-idiotype antibody mimicking a breast cancer-associated antigen and the cytokine GM-CSF. *Hybridoma* 1999; 18:193–202.

18. Withoff S, Helfrich W, de Leij LF, Molema G. Bi-specific antibody therapy for the treatment of cancer. *Curr. Opin. Mol. Ther.* 2001; 3:53–62.

19. Chester KA, Bhatia J, Boxer G et al. Clinical applications of phage-derived sFvs and sFv fusion proteins. *Dis. Markers* 2000; 16:53–62.

20. Todorovska A, Roovers RC, Dolezal O et al. Design and application of diabodies, triabodies and tetrabodies for cancer targeting. *J. Immunol. Methods* 2001; 248:47–66.

21. Kreitman RJ, Wilson WH, Robbins D et al. Responses in refractory hairy cell leukemia to a recombinant immunotoxin. *Blood* 1999; 94:3340–3348.

22. Kreitman RJ, Wilson WH, White DJ et al. Phase I trial of recombinant immunotoxin anti-Tac(Fv)-PE38 (LMB-2) in patients with hematologic malignancies. *J. Clin. Oncol.* 2000; 18:1622–1636.

23. Witzig TE. Radioimmunotherapy for patients with relapsed B-cell non-Hodgkin lymphoma. *Cancer Chemother. Pharmacol.* 2001; 48 (Suppl. 1):S91.

24. Bendas G. Immunoliposomes: A promising approach to targeting cancer therapy. *BioDrugs* 2001; 15:215–224.

25. Niculescu-Duvaz I, Friedlos F, Niculescu-Duvaz D et al. Prodrugs for antibody- and gene-directed enzyme prodrug therapies (ADEPT and GDEPT). *Anticancer Drug Des.* 1999; 14:517–538.

26. Prehn RT, Main JM. Immunity of methylcholanthrene-induced sarcomas. *JNCI* 1957; 18:769–778.

27. Klein G, Sjogren H, Klein E et al. Demonstration of resistance against methylcholanthrene-induced sarcomas in the primary autochthonous host. *Cancer Res.* 1960; 20:1561–1572.

28. Boon T, Van Snick J, Van Pel A et al. Immunogenic variants obtained by mutagenesis of mouse mastocytoma P815. T lymphocyte mediated cytolysis. *J. Exp. Med.* 1980; 152:1184–1193.

29. Biddison WE and Palmer JC. Development of tumor cell resistance to syngeneic cell-mediated cytotoxicity during growth of ascitic mastocytoma P815Y. *Proc. Natl. Acad. Sci. U. S. A.* 1977; 74:329–333.

30. Barth RJ Jr, Bock SN, Mule JJ et al. Unique murine tumor associated antigens identified by tumor infiltrating lymphocytes. *J. Immunol.* 1990; 144:1531–1537.

31. Boon T, Cerottini J, Van den Eynde B et al. Tumor antigens recognized by T lymphocytes. *Annu. Rev. Immunol.* 1994; 12:337–365.

32. Rosenberg S. Lymphokine activated killer cells: A new approach to the immunotherapy of cancer. *JNCI* 1985; 75:595–603.

33. Mule JJ, Shu S, Schwartz SL et al. Adoptive immunotherapy of established pulmonary metastases with LAK cells and recombinant interleukin-2. *Science* 1984; 225:1487–1489.

34. Rosenberg SA, Mule JJ, Spiess PJ et al. Regression of established pulmonary metastases and subcutaneous tumor mediated by the systemic administration of high dose recombinant interleukin-2. *J. Exp. Med.* 1985; 161:1169–1188.

35. Lafreniere R, Rosenberg SA. Successful immunotherapy of murine experimental hepatic metastases with lymphokine activated killer cells and recombinant interleukin-2. *Cancer Res.* 1985; 45:3735–3741.

36. Rosenberg SA, Spiess P, Lafreniere R. A new approach to the adoptive immunotherapy of cancer with tumor-infiltrating lymphocytes. *Science* 1986; 223:1318–1321.

37. Spiess PJ, Yan JC, Rosenberg SA. In vivo antitumor activity of tumor-infiltrating lymphocytes expanded in recombinant interleukin-2. *JNCI* 1987; 79:1067–1075.

38. Fujie T, Tanaka F, Mori M et al. Induction of antitumor cytotoxic T lymphocytes from the peripheral blood mononuclear cells of cancer patients using HLA-A2 restricted MAGE-3 peptides in vitro. *Clin. Cancer Res.* 1997; 3:2425–2430.

39. Zakut R, Topalian SL, Kawakami Y et al. Differential expression of MAGE-1, 2 and 3 messenger RNA in transformed and normal cell lines. *Cancer Res.* 1993; 53:5–8.

40. Traversari C, Van der Bruggen P, Luescher IF et al. A nonapeptide encoded by human gene MAGE-1 is recognized on HLA-A1 by cytolytic T lymphocytes directed against tumor antigen MZ2-E. *J. Exp. Med.* 1992; 176:1453–1457.

41. Van der Bruggen P, Szikora J, Boel P et al. Autologous cytolytic T lymphocytes recognize a MAGE-1 nonapeptide on melanomas expressing HLA-Cw 1601. *Eur. J. Immunol.* 1994; 24:2134–2140.

42. Rosenberg SA. Progress in human tumour immunology and immunotherapy. *Nature* 2001; 411:380–384.

43. Kirkwood JM, Ibrahim JG, Sosman JA et al. High-dose interferon alfa-2b significantly prolongs relapse-free and overall survival compared with the GM2-KLH/QS-21 vaccine in patients with resected stage IIB-III melanoma: Results of intergroup trial. *J. Clin. Oncol.* 2001; 19:2370–2380.

44. Hsueh EC, Famatiga E, Gupta RK, Qi K, Morton DL. Enhancement of complement-dependent cytotoxicity by polyvalent melanoma cell vaccine (CancerVax): Correlation with survival. *Ann. Surg. Oncol.* 1998; 5:565–602.

45. Mitchell MS. Perspective on allogeneic melanoma lysates in active specific immunotherapy. *Semin. Oncol.* 1998; 25:623–635.

46. Hsueh EC. Tumour cell-based vaccines for the treatment of melanoma. *BioDrugs* 2001; 15:713–720.

47. Kugler A, Stuhler G, Walden P et al. Regression of human metastatic renal cell carcinoma after vaccination with tumor cell-dendritic cell hybrids. *Nat. Med.* 2000; 6:332–336.

48. Mitchell MS, Kan-Mitchell J, Kempf RA, Harel W, Shau HY, Lind S. Active specific immunotherapy for melanoma: Phase I trial of allogeneic lysates and a novel adjuvant. *Cancer Res.* 1988; 48:5883–5893.

49. Berd D. Autologous, hapten-modified vaccine as a treatment for human cancers. *Vaccine* 2001; 19:2565–2570.

50. Hioe CE, Qiu H, Chend PD et al. Comparison of adjuvant formulations for cytotoxic T cell induction using synthetic peptides. *Vaccine* 1996; 14:412–418.

51. Sprinzl GM, Kacani L, Schrott-Fischer A, Romani N, Thumfart WF. Dendritic cell vaccines for cancer therapy. *Cancer Treat. Rev.* 2001; 27:247–255.

52. Jones T, Stern A, Lin R. Potential role of granulocyte macrophage colony stimulating factor as vaccine adjuvant. *Eur. J. Clin. Microbiol. Infect. Dis.* 1994; 13(Suppl. 2):s47–s53.

53. Fagerberg J. Granulocyte macrophage colony stimulating factor as an adjuvant in immunotherapy. *Med. Oncol.* 1996; 13:155–160.

54. Carlsson T, Struve J. Granulocyte macrophage colony stimulating factor given as an adjuvant to persons not responding to hepatitis B vaccine. *Infection* 1997; 25:129.

55. Pardoll DM. Paracrine cytokine adjuvants in cancer immunotherapy. *Annu. Rev. Immunol.* 1995; 13:399–415.

56. Golumbek PT, Azhari R, Jaffee EM et al. Controlled release, biodegradable cytokine depots: a new approach in cancer vaccine design. *Cancer Res.* 1993; 53:5841–5844.

8

INHIBITORS OF APOPTOSIS AS TARGETS FOR CANCER THERAPY

M. SAEED SHEIKH

YING HUANG

Department of Pharmacology
SUNY Upstate Medical University
Syracuse, New York

I. THE INHIBITORS OF APOPTOSIS
II. CONCLUDING REMARKS

It is now been well established that apoptosis is a physiological process that is essential for tissue homeostasis. A wealth of information suggests that defects in regulation of apoptosis can contribute to a number of diseases including cancer. In general, there are two major apoptotic pathways, one originates at the membrane and involves death receptors [1] and the other engages mitochondria [2]. Apoptotic signals involving either pathway engage caspases, the integral component of intracellular apoptotic machinery. Evidence suggests that the expression/function of pro-apoptotic and/or anti-apoptotic molecules is altered in cancer cells, which results in their continuous proliferation and or resistance to anticancer therapies [3, 4]. Inhibitors of apoptosis (IAPs) are anti-apoptotic molecules whose expression is generally altered in various cancer types [5–8]. This chapter deals with IAPs and will discuss the pros and cons of targeting these molecules in the development of novel anticancer agents.

I. THE INHIBITORS OF APOPTOSIS

IAPs form a growing family of proteins that inhibit apoptosis induced by a wide variety of insults [5–8]. First discovered in baculoviruses, later studies have identified IAP family members in nematodes, flies, rodents, and humans [5–8]. To date several family members have been identified in humans that include, c-IAP1, c-IAP2, NAIP, XIAP, Livin α and β (also known as ML-IAP or KIAP), Apollon, and Survivin (Figure 8.1).

Novel Anticancer Agents

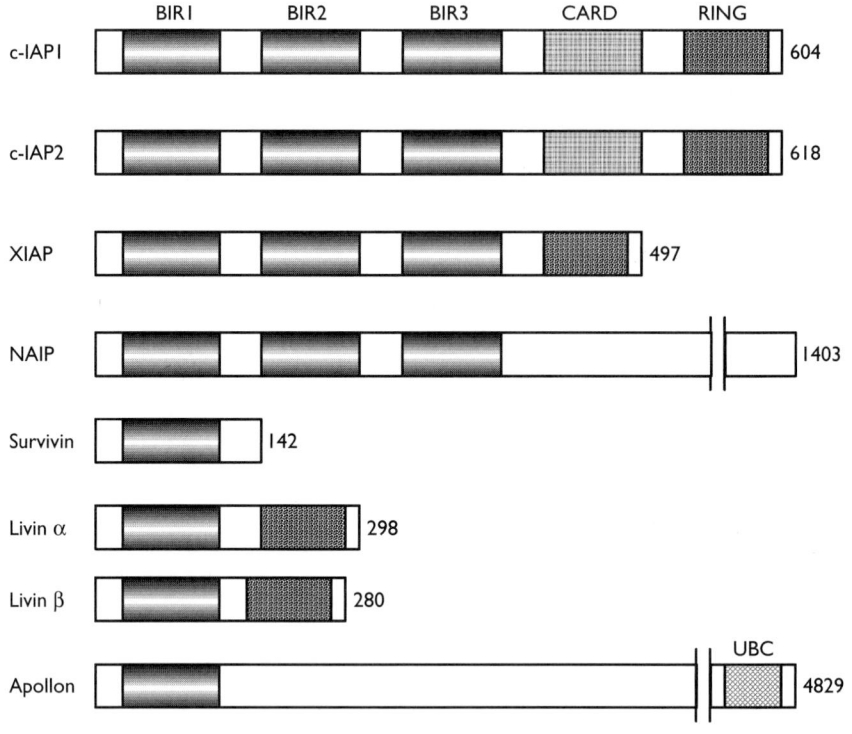

FIGURE 8.1 Structure of human IAPs. c-IAP1, c-IAP2, XIAP, and NAIP all contain three BIR domains whereas Survivin, Livin, and Apollon contain only one. Livin is also known as ML-IAP and KIAP. Two splice variants, namely Livin α and β, give rise to two different open reading frames containing 298 and 280 amino acids, respectively. Survivin is the smallest known human IAP while Apollon is the largest. Apollon also contains ubiquitin-conjugating enzyme (UBC) domain. For more information, see References 5–8.

A. Structure and Function of IAPs

Structure function analyses have revealed that all IAPs harbor varying numbers of baculoviral inhibitor of apoptosis repeat (BIR) domains. For example, Survivin, the smallest of all IAPs, contains only one BIR domain while c-IAP1, c-IAP2, XIAP, and NAIP each contains three [5, 6]. Livin (also known as ML-IAP and KIAP) and Apollon are the recent addition to this family and each contains one BIR domain [9–12]. With the exception of Survivin and NAIP, all IAPs also contain a RING zinc finger domain at the COOH terminus. In addition to these two domains, c-IAP1 and c-IAP2 contain a CARD (caspase recruitment domain) motif, and Apollon contains a ubiquitin-conjugating enzyme (UBC) domain [5, 6, 12]. A large body of evidence suggests that the BIR domain plays a central role in the IAP-mediated suppression of apoptosis [5–8]. The role of other domains in modulation of apoptosis remains unclear because removal of either RING domain or CARD domain does not affect the ability of these proteins to modulate apoptosis [5–8]. It has been proposed that the non-BIR domains may serve to diversify the function of IAPs [5].

The IAPs are believed to mediate their anti-apoptotic effects by directly inhibiting the caspases [5–8]. Caspases are cysteine proteases that are integral components of the intracellular apoptotic machinery. To date 14 caspases have been identified that are named caspase 1 through caspase 14 [13, 14]. In general, these proteases are grouped as initiator caspases and effector (executioner) caspases. Caspase 8 or 10 are the initiator caspases that are activated through apoptotic signals originating at the membrane death receptors [13, 14]. Once activated, these caspases can cleave and activate the downstream caspases such as 3, 6, and 7, and the flow of apoptotic signals moves downstream to death substrates [13, 14]. Activation of caspase 9, the other initiator caspase, involves signals originating at the mitochondria such that cytochrome c is resealed from mitochondria into cytosol, and Apaf1 is recruited into an apoptosome complex involving cytochrome c, Apaf1, pro-caspase 9, and ATP/dATP [2, 13, 14]. Assembly of apoptosome results in caspase 9 activation. Once active, caspase 9 further activates the effector caspases 3, 6, and 7 (Figure 8.2).

IAP-dependent caspase inhibition involves direct interactions between these two groups of molecules [5, 6]. For example, XIAP, c-IAP1, c-IAP2, and Survivin have been shown to bind and inhibit caspase 3, 7, and 9 [5, 6, 15–17]. These IAPs are believed to bind and inhibit the abovementioned caspases via their BIR domains at a 1:1 or 2:1 molar ratio [16, 17]. Only one BIR domain

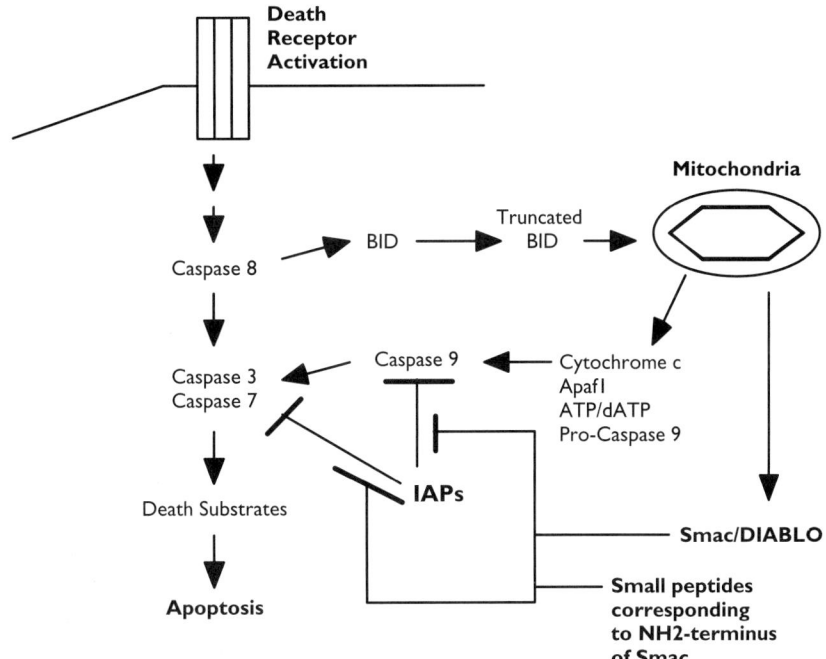

FIGURE 8.2   Death receptor and mitochondrial apoptotic pathways and the Smac/DIABLO-dependent suppression of anti-apoptotic IAPs.

has been found to be sufficient to inhibit caspase activity because Survivin, the single BIR domain-containing IAP, is capable of binding and inhibiting caspases [5–8]. Survivin, XIAP, c-IAP1, and c-IAP2 have been shown to bind to the processed and unprocessed forms of caspase 9, while only the processed forms of caspase 3 and 7 bind to these IAPs [5, 15]. Although the exact mechanisms by which these IAPs inhibit caspases remain to be elucidated, evidence points to their function as competitive inhibitors [5]. Recent structural studies have started to unravel the potential mechanism(s) of caspases and IAPs interactions (see below). The information obtained from such studies is predicted to ultimately help in elucidating the exact molecular mechanism(s) by which these IAPs inhibit caspases.

IAPs have also been implicated in the activation of anti-apoptotic nuclear factor κB (NF-κB). NF-κB is a transcription factor that is formed by the NF-κB/Rel protein family [18–20]. The members in this family include NF-κB1, NF-κB2, RelAp65, RelB, and c-Rel. All of these proteins contain a region of homology named Rel homology domain at their N terminus. The Rel homology domain is about 300 amino acids long and contains the DNA-binding and dimerization domains as well as the nuclear localization signal [18–20]. RelAp65, RelB, and c-Rel but not NF-κB1 or NF-κB2 also contain transactivation domains at their carboxyl terminal ends. These proteins are believed to form homo- and heterodimers. A possible exception is RelB, which only forms heterodimers with NF-κB1 or NF-κB2. The NF-κB transcription factor is generally referred to as the NF-κB/RelAp65 heterodimeric complex which, in its inactive state, exists in the cytoplasm in association with IκB proteins [18–20]. IκBs are inhibitory proteins and several different subunits have been identified, which include IκBα, IκBβ, IκBγ and IκBε [18–20]. Association of IκB to NF-κB/Rel complex masks the nuclear localization signal of NF-κB/Rel complex, which results in the accumulation of IκB/NF-κB/Rel complex in the cytoplasm [20].

IκB is phosphorylated, ubiquitinated, and degraded in response to NF-κB-activating signals [20, 21]. In the absence of IκB, the NF-κB dimers translocate into nucleus and transactivate their target genes. A number of anti-apoptotic genes including BclxL, A1/Bfl-1, MnSOD, A20, IEX-1L, XIAP, c-IAP, and c-IAP2 have been reported to be regulated by NF-κB [6, 20]. It is interesting that XIAP, c-IAP1, and c-IAP2 proteins have been shown to also activate NF-κB, which in turn further increases the expression of these genes and thereby forms a positive feedback loop [22, 23]. Thus, IAPs, in addition to inhibiting caspases, may also mediate the anti-apoptotic effects by activating NF-κB, which would further enhance not only the expression of IAPs but also other anti-apoptotic genes such as BclxL, A1/Bfl-1, MnSOD, A20, and IEX-1L.

There is evidence to suggest that IAPs may also mediate their anti-apoptotic effects by activation of the JNK pathway [24]. For example, XIAP has been shown to enhance pro-caspase 1 induced apoptosis. It has been speculated that XIAP might mediate such effects by its interaction with pro-caspase 1 activating protein CARDIAK/RIP-2 [5]. However, more studies are needed to explore this issue. Nevertheless, the IAPs have the demonstrated ability to mediate anti-apoptotic effects via multiple different mechanisms.

B. IAP Interactions with the Inhibitor Smac/DIABLO

Second mitochondria-derived activator of caspases (Smac) or its murine homolog direct IAP-binding protein with low PI (DIABLO) is a recently discovered protein that has been shown to mediate its apoptotic effects by binding to and neutralizing IAPs [25, 26]. Smac, itself a mitochondrial protein, is released into cytosol along with other mitochondrial proteins, which include cytochrome c and AIF (apoptosis-inducing factor) in response to apoptotic insults [25]. Smac exists in a proform and its amino-terminal sequence is believed to target Smac to the mitochondrial intermembrane space. The proform of Smac is processed into a mature form that binds to IAPs and neutralizes their ability to inhibit caspases [25]. With regard to IAPs and Smac interactions, XIAP has been more extensively studied. Evidence from structural studies suggests that Smac exists as a homodimer and binds to the BIR2 and BIR3 domains of XIAP [27]. In the case of XIAP, it is known that the BIR2 domain predominantly inhibits caspase 3 and 7 [28] while the BIR3 domain inhibits caspase 9 [29]. The mechanism of BIR3 domain-mediated caspase 9 inhibition involves BIR3 interactions with the small subunit of caspase 9 [15]. The BIR2 domain and the residues at the amino-terminal linker region promote interactions with caspase 3 and 7 [15]. Smac has been reported to interact with BIR2 and BIR3 domains of XIAP and thereby blocks XIAP-mediated inhibition of caspase 3/7 and caspase 9, respectively [15].

Evidence from structural studies suggests that the first four amino acids (Ala-Val-Pro-Ile) at the amino-terminal end of the mature Smac interact with the BIR3 domain of XIAP [15]. The tetrapeptide sequence at the amino-terminal end of Smac is critical because a single mutation involving Ala to Met has been reported to disrupt the interactions between Smac and XIAP [15 and references therein]. Smac interactions with the BIR3 domain are believed to displace the amino-terminal end of small subunit of caspase 9, which results in the release of activated enzyme from the IAP-caspase 9 complex. Once released, the active caspase 9 cleaves and activates caspase 3. Active caspase 3, in turn, cleaves the IAP binding site (15 amino-terminal residues) from the smaller subunit of caspase 9 [30]. Removal of the IAP binding site from active caspase 9 prevents XIAP from binding to and further inhibiting caspase 9. The fact that the cleaved IAP-binding residues remain bound to XIAP provides yet another level of control to further prevent XIAP from inhibiting active caspase 9 [15].

The structural interactions between BIR2 and Smac remain less well understood. It is believed that the Smac binding sites on BIR2 domain are different than those for caspase 3 and 7, and that steric hindrance prevents BIR2 domain from binding to caspase 3/7 and Smac at the same time [15].

C. IAPs as Targets for Cancer Therapy

Evidence suggests that various IAPs are not redundant but appear to exhibit distinct cell- and tissue-specific roles. For example, abrogation of XIAP but not c-IAP expression in human ovarian surface epithelial cells (hOSE) via an antisense mRNA approach has been shown to sensitize hOSE cells to cisplatin

[31]. Cisplatin also downregulates the expression of endogenous XIAP in cisplatin-sensitive but not resistant hOSE cells. Expression of exogenous XIAP in cisplatin-sensitive hOSE cells confers resistance to cisplatin-induced apoptosis [31]. These findings further implicate XIAP but not c-IAP in conferring sensitivity or resistance to chemotherapeutic drugs in hOSE cells. Cisplatin is a major chemotherapeutic agent for the treatment of hOSE; however, the development of drug resistance by hOSE cells hinders the successful use of this chemotherapeutic agent in the treatment of this malignancy. Identification of XIAP as an important determinant of cisplatin sensitivity/resistance in human ovarian cancer cells is an important finding. Further studies are needed to explore whether molecular targeting of XIAP would be a viable approach to develop novel anticancer agents against this malignancy.

ML-IAP (also known as Livin and KIAP) is a recently discovered human IAP. Expression of ML-IAP has been shown to inhibit apoptosis induced by chemotherapeutic agents or following death receptor activation [11]. ML-IAP is expressed at high levels in a majority of melanoma cell lines but not in primary melanocytes. The ML-IAP-expressing melanoma cells have been found to be more resistant to chemotherapeutic drug-induced apoptosis [11]. Although correlative, these results suggest that ML-IAP may play a role in pathogenesis of melanoma and thus could be a potentially important molecular target of cancer therapy for this malignancy.

Apollon is the largest human IAP discovered to date. It encodes a single BIR domain-containing protein of 530 kDa [12]. Apollon has been found to be expressed at high levels in human gliomas. Introduction of antisense oligonucleotides against Apollon in human glioma cells results in reduction of Apollon expression and concomitant acquisition of sensitivity to cisplatin and camptothecin-induced apoptosis [12]. Once again, these are correlative results, but they suggest that Apollon may play a role in pathogenesis and/or inherent anticancer drug resistance of human gliomas. Thus, targeting Apollon may be an important strategy to develop anticancer agents against this malignancy.

Survivin, the smallest IAP, has been found to be expressed at high levels in a wide variety of cancers compared with normal tissues [7, 8]. Survivin is expressed at high levels in fetal but not in adult tissues. Thus, constitutive overexpression of Survivin in various cancer tissues fits the onco-fetal pattern of expression [7, 8]. Survivin is a dual-function IAP that inhibits apoptosis and regulates cell division [7, 8]. The anti-apoptotic role of Survivin has been demonstrated in both *in vitro* and *in vivo* studies. *In vitro* data from a number of studies suggest that exogenous Survivin can inhibit apoptosis induced by a variety of insults [7, 8]. To study whether *in vivo* expression of Survivin would also inhibit apoptosis, investigators used the keratin 14 (K14) gene promoter to express Survivin in epidermal keratinocytes of a transgenic mouse [32]. The keratinocytes of K14-Survivin mice displayed significant resistant to UVB radiation-induced apoptosis. These findings thus demonstrate that the expression of exogenous Survivin can also inhibit apoptosis *in vivo* [32]. Because many tumors also overexpress Survivin, it is therefore likely that high levels of Survivin may mediate tumorigenic effects by suppressing apoptosis.

Although it has been proposed that Survivin inhibits caspase 3 and 9, direct evidence as to how Survivin inhibits these caspases is still absent. It has been proposed that Survivin may indirectly inhibit caspases perhaps via intermediate proteins promoting the formation of a larger complex [7]. Recent evidence suggests that Survivin appears to bind Smac [7, 8, 25]. It is, therefore, possible that Survivin may inhibit caspases indirectly by blocking Smac's ability to inhibit other IAPs, and in so doing it may promote caspase inhibition induced by other IAPs [7].

Survivin is believed to be important for cell division because defects in Survivin have been linked to aberrant mitosis involving improper chromosomal segregation [7, 8]. Consistent with this notion, Survivin has been found to be associated with microtubules and mitotic spindle apparatus. Targeted deletion of Survivin gives rise to embryonic lethality by E4.5 due to aberrant mitosis [33]. Thus, Survivin is believed to be required for normal cell division and its overexpression in cancer cells may affect the normal cell cycle controls. It is, therefore, believed that abnormal cell cycle controls due to abnormally high levels of Survivin may also account for its anti-apoptotic effects [7].

Evidence suggests that Survivin is normally phosphorylated on Thr34 by Cdc2 kinase [34]. Cdc2 is active during the G_2/M phase of the cell cycle. Mutant forms of Survivin carrying Ala34 instead of Thr34 have been shown to exhibit dominant-negative behavior and were found to inhibit the phosphorylation of endogenous Survivin that was coupled with induction of apoptosis [8]. Expression of dominant-negative Survivin is reported to also associate with pro-caspase 9 depletion and apoptosis induction. Mutant Survivin T34A-induced apoptosis is inhibited by dominant-negative caspase 9, which suggests that this mutant form of Survivin activates the mitochondrial pathway of apoptosis [8]. These results are consistent with the finding that Survivin appears to block Smac (a mitochondrial protein) and consequently suppresses Smac's ability to inhibit other IAPs such as XIAP.

Whether small peptides corresponding to the amino terminus of Smac can be used to block Survivin and Smac interactions remains to be elucidated. Information obtained form structural studies has yet to shed light on the possibility of rational drug design to target Survivin. The use of antisense methodology to target Survivin in cultured cancer cells has provided promising results with regard to affecting cell division and inducing apoptosis [35, 36]. Anti-tumor activity of T34A mutant Survivin has been demonstrated in animal models and the use of such mutants in cancer gene therapy may yield promising results [37, 38]. In view of the fact that Cdc2 kinase phosphorylates Survivin, kinase-inhibitor drugs such as falvopiridol could be tested to explore their effects in abrogating Survivin phosphorylation and thus its ability to suppress apoptosis [7, 8]. Because Survivin interacts with microtubules, antimicrotubule agents can also be tested to investigate whether Survivin's interactions with microtubules could be abrogated [7].

II. CONCLUDING REMARKS

In general, the ideal targets in molecular targeted therapy are those molecules that (1) exhibit selective expression by cancer cells and (2) are required for viability and proliferation of cancer cells. The identification of IAPs has been an important discovery in the field of cancer biology and therapy. Although further in-depth studies would be needed to explore the exact role of IAPs in carcinogenesis, available evidence suggests that the various IAPs may be important for the viability or proliferation of some tumor types. This feature, coupled with the fact that some IAPs also exhibit selective expression in cancer but not in normal cells, would suggest that the IAPs are attractive molecular targets in the development of novel anticancer agents. In this regard small peptides corresponding to the amino terminal end of Smac have been reported to relieve the XIAP-mediated inhibition of caspase 9 [15]. It has been proposed that such peptides can be used to activate caspases and to induce apoptosis [15]. Thus, the utility of small peptides corresponding to the NH2 terminal region of Smac either alone or in combination with other chemotherapeutic drugs is predicated to be a novel therapeutic strategy, particularly in IAP overexpressing tumors.

REFERENCES

1. Ashkenazi A, Dixit VM. Apoptosis control by death and decoy receptors. *Curr. Opin. Cell Biol.* 1999; 11:255–260.
2. Desagher S, Martinou JC. Mitochondria as the central control point of apoptosis. *Trends Cell Biol.* 2000; 10:369–77.
3. Strasser A, O'Connor L, Dixit VM. Apoptosis signaling. *Annu. Rev. Biochem.* 2000; 69:217–45.
4. Kaufmann SH, Grores GJ. Apoptosis in cancer: Cause and cure. *BioEssays* 2000; 22:1007–1017.
5. Deveraux QL, Reed JC. IAP family proteins-suppressors of apoptosis. *Gene Dev.* 1999; 13:239–252.
6. LaCasse EC, Baird S, Korneluk RG, MacKenzie AE. The inhibitors of apoptosis (IAPs) and their emerging role in cancer. *Oncogene* 1998; 17:3247–3260.
7. Reed JC. The Survivin saga goes in vivo. *J. Clin. Invest.* 2001; 108:965–969.
8. Altieri DC. The molecular basis and potential role of survivin in cancer diagnosis and therapy. *Trend Mol. Med.* 2001; 7:542–547.
9. Kasof GM, Gomes BC. Livin, a novel inhibitor of apoptosis protein family member. *J. Biol. Chem.* 2001; 276:3238–3246.
10. Ashhab Y, Alian A, Polliack A, Panet A, Yehuda DB. Two splicing variants of a new inhibitor of apoptosis gene with different biological properties and tissue distribution pattern. *FEBS Lett.* 2001; 495:56–60.
11. Vucic D, Sternnick HR, Pisabarro MT, Salvesen GS, Dixit VM. ML-IAP, a novel inhibitor that is preferentially expressed in human melanomas. *Curr. Biol.* 2000; 10:1359–1366.
12. Chen Z, Naito M, Hori S, Mashima T, Yamori T, Tsuruo T. A human IAP-family gene, apollon, expressed in human brain cancer cells. *Biochem. Biophys. Res. Commun.* 1999; 264:847–854.
13. Earnshaw WC, Martins LM, Kaufmann SH. Mammalian caspases: Structure, activation, substrates, and functions during apoptosis. *Annu. Rev. Biochem.* 1999; 68:383–424.
14. Nunez G, Benedict MA, Hu Y, Naohiro Inohara. Caspases: The proteases of the apoptotic pathway. *Oncogene* 1998; 17:3237–3245.
15. Fesik SW, Shi Y. Controlling the caspases. *Science* 2001; 294:1477–1478.
16. Daveraux QL, Takashashi R, Salvesen GS, Reed JC. X-linked IAP is direct inhibitor of cell death proteases. *Nature* 67; 388:300–303.
17. Roy N, Deveraux DL, Takashashi R, Salvesen GS, Reed JC. The c-IAP-1 and c-IAP-2 proteins are direct inhibitors of specific caspases *EMBO J.* 1997; 16:6914–6925.
18. Ghosh S, May MJ, Kopp EB. NF-kappa B and Rel proteins: Evolutionarily conserved mediators of immune responses. *Annu. Rev. Immunol.* 1998; 16:225–260.

19. Siebenlist U, Franzosos G, Brown K. Structure, regulation and function of NF-kappa B. *Annu. Rev. Cell Biol.* 1994; 10:405–455.

20. Schmid RM, Adler G. NF-kB/Rel/IkB: implications in gastrointestinal diseases. *Gastroenterology* 2000; 118:1208–1228.

21. Chen Z, Hagler J, Palombella VJ, Melandri F, Scherer D, Ballard D, Maniatis T. Signal-induced site-specific phosphorylation targets I kappa B alpha to the ubiquitin-proteasome pathway. *Gene Dev.* 1995; 9:1586–1597.

22. Chu ZL, McKinsey TA, Liu L, Gentry JJ, Malim MH and Ballard DW. Suppression of tumor necrosis factor-induced cell death by inhibitor of apoptosis c-IAP2 is under NF-kB control. *Proc. Natl. Acad. Sci. U. S. A.* 1997; 94:10057–10062.

23. Wang CY, Mayo MW, Korneluk RG, Goeddel DV, Baldwin Jr AS. NF-kappaB antiapoptosis: Induction of TRAF1 and TRAF2 and c-IAP1 and c-IAP2 to suppress caspase 8 activation. *Science* 1998; 1680–1683.

24. Sanna MG, Duckett CS, Richter BW, Thompson CB, Ulevitch RJ. Selective activation of JNK1 is necessary for anti-apoptotic activity of hILP. *Proc. Natl. Acad. Sci. U. S. A.* 1998; 95:6015–6020.

25. Du C, Fang M, Li Y, Li L, Wang X. Smac, a mitochondrial protein that promotes cytochrome c-dependent caspase activation by eliminating IAP inhibition. *Cell* 2000; 102:33–42.

26. Verhagen AM, Ekert PG, Pakusch M, Silke J, Connolly LM, Reid GE, Moritz RL, Simpson RJ, Vaux DL. Identification of DIABLO, a mammalian protein that promotes apoptosis by binding to and antagonizing IAP proteins. *Cell* 2000; 102:43–53.

27. Chai J, Du C, Wu JW, Kyin S, Wang X, Shi Y. Structural and biochemical basis of apoptotic activation by Smac/DIABLO. *Nature* 2000; 406:855–862.

28. Takahashi R, Deveraux Q, Tamm I, Welsh K, Assa-Munt N, Salvesen GS, Reed JC. A single BIR domain of XIAP sufficient for inhibiting caspases. *J. Biol. Chem.* 1998; 273:7787–7790.

29. Deveraux QL, Leo E, Stennicke HR, Welsh K, Salvesen GS, Reed JC. Cleavage of human inhibitor of apoptosis protein XIAP results in fragments with distinct specificities for caspases. *EMBO J.* 1999; 18:5242–5251.

30. Srinivasula SM, Hegde R, Saleh A, Datta P, Shiozaki E, Chai J, Lee RA, Robbins PD, Fernandes-Alnemri T, Shi Y, Alnemri ES. A conserved XIAP-interaction motif in caspase-9 and Smac/DIABLO regulates caspase activity and apoptosis. *Nature* 2001; 410:112–116.

31. Li J, Feng Q, Kim JM et al. Human ovarian cancer and cisplatin resistance: Possible role of inhibitor of apoptosis proteins. *Endocrinology* 2001; 142:370–380.

32. Grossman D, Kim PJ, Blanc-Brude OP, Brash DE, Tognin S, Marchisio PC, Altieri DC. Transgenic expression of survivin in keratinocytes counteracts UVB-induced apoptosis and cooperates with loss of p53. *J. Clin. Invest.* 2001; 108:991–999.

33. Uren AG, Wong L, Pakusch M, Fowler KJ, Burrows FJ, Vaux DL, Choo KH. Survivin and the inner centromere protein INCENP show similar cell-cycle localization and gene knockout phenotype. *Curr. Biol.* 2000; 10:1319–1328.

34. O'Connor DS, Grossman D, Plescia J et al. Regulation of apoptosis at cell division by p34cdc2 phosphorylation of survivin. *Proc. Natl. Acad. Sci. U. S. A.* 2000; 97:13103–13107.

35. Chen J, Wu W, Tahir SK et al. Down-regulation of survivin by antisense oligonucleotides increases apoptosis, inhibits cytokinesis and anchorage-independent growth. *Neoplasia* 2000; 2:235–241.

36. Olie RA, Simoes-Wust AP, Baumann B et al. A novel antisense oligonucleotide targeting survivin expression induces apoptosis and sensitizes lung cancer cells to chemotherapy. *Cancer Res.* 2000; 60:2805–2809.

37. Grossman D, Kim PJ, Schechner JS, Altieri DC. Inhibition of melanoma tumor growth in vivo by Survivin targeting. *Proc. Natl. Acad. Sci. U. S. A.* 2001; 98:635–640.

38. Mesri M, Wall NR, Li J, Kim RW, Altieri DC. Cancer gene therapy using a survivin mutant adenovirus. *J. Clin. Invest.* 2001; 108:981–990.

9

PRECLINICAL TESTING AND VALIDATION OF NOVEL ANTICANCER AGENTS

LLOYD R. KELLAND

St. George's Hospital Medical School
London, United Kingdom

I. INTRODUCTION
II. TARGET VALIDATION
III. A GENERIC CASCADE FOR ANTICANCER DRUG DISCOVERY
IV. HIGH-THROUGHPUT CELL-FREE SCREENS FOR ACTIVITY AGAINST THE TARGET
V. *IN VITRO* CELL LINE MODELS
VI. *IN VIVO* TESTING OF NOVEL COMPOUNDS
VII. CASSETTE-DOSING
VIII. PHARMACEUTICAL CONSIDERATIONS
IX. HIGH-THROUGHPUT *IN VIVO* ANTI-TUMOR TESTING: THE HOLLOW FIBER ASSAY
X. HUMAN TUMOR XENOGRAFTS
XI. ORTHOTOPIC, TRANSGENIC, AND OTHER ANIMAL MODELS
XII. PHARMACODYNAMICS
XIII. SUMMARY

I. INTRODUCTION

The recent revolution in genomics and programs such as the Human Genome Project and the Cancer Genome Anatomy Project (CGAP) has resulted in a marked explosion in the identification of cancer-associated genes/proteins, many of which may represent viable targets for therapeutic intervention [1]. Furthermore, the advances in generating very large numbers of molecules through combinatorial chemistry means that the efficient and effective validation of targets and preclinical testing of novel anticancer agents has become pivotal within the drug discovery process. Herein, there appears to lie a fundamental balance in the requirement to develop higher and higher throughput assays for testing but, in parallel, a need to ensure that the results are predictive of clinical utility. In the 50 years since the beginnings of cancer chemotherapy, the past paradigm of empirical-based screening of often randomly selected molecules against rapidly growing mouse leukemia cell lines has shifted. Today rational strategies are employed, often using "designer" molecules, molecularly defined testing models, and with an increased emphasis on drug pharmacokinetics (PK) and pharmacodynamics (PD). However, as always, a central theme that should not be forgotten is the requirement to progress "drug-like" molecules (i.e., those which possess good pharmaceutical properties) combined with the demonstration of a therapeutic index (i.e., selectivity for tumors over normal tissues) [2]. One consequence of targeting cancer-associated genes/proteins/pathways is that the resulting agents may be primarily cytostatic rather than cytotoxic, thus slowing tumor growth rather than leading to shrinkage. This may require a re-evaluation of the *in vivo* models developed and validated using cytotoxic drugs when testing such agents.

This chapter focuses on contemporary approaches to the preclinical testing of anticancer molecules. It describes a "generic" test cascade that has been adopted within the CRC Centre for Cancer Therapeutics, which encompasses both target validation and testing for activity in cell-free systems, against cell lines *in vitro*, and appropriate mouse models *in vivo*. Throughout, key points are illustrated by our studies using small molecules targeted against currently promising anticancer targets. These include R115777, a farnesyl protein transferase inhibitor [3]; 17-allylamino-geldanamycin (17AAG), an inhibitor of heat shock protein 90, the inhibition of which results in interference with a variety of cell signalling pathways) [4]; the cyclin dependent kinase (cdk) inhibitor roscovitine [5]; and BRACO-19 directed at telomeres/telomerase [6]. Screening strategies developed at the National Cancer Institute (NCI) are also discussed.

II. TARGET VALIDATION

Modern anticancer drug discovery is an extremely expensive and time-consuming process. Typically, from concept to the completion of phase III clinical trials and gaining regulatory approval requires in excess of 10 years and approximately 500 million dollars. Thus, at the outset before embarking on a drug-testing program, it is essential to ask and determine the answer to the question: Is the particular chosen target validated within a cancer therapeutic context? Factors to be considered include the elucidation of the function of the target gene/protein, the frequency of deregulation in cancer and whether this is linked to disease progression or prognosis, and expression in normal tissues. In recent years new possible targets have arisen from the identification of key proteins and associated pathways involved in oncogenesis or the cancer phenotype (e.g., Ras, Myc, p53, pRb, p16, HER1, HER2, Bcr-Abl, Bcl-2, PTEN, PI3K, VEGF, hTERT, etc.) [7]. However, it is generally not clear at which point in a pathway it may be best to intervene, whether cross-talk between pathways or redundancy in signaling exists or whether severe normal tissue toxicity/lack of therapeutic index may result. Another important factor concerns the relative ease by which the chosen target may be modulated.

For example, medicine is full of examples of small molecule inhibitors of enzymes, such as agonists or antagonists of receptors. In contrast, the development of drugs targeting protein-protein interactions, conformational changes in proteins, or specific sequences of genes have proven much more challenging.

One of the major components of target validation uses genetic-based studies involving creation of the malignant phenotype by mutation or a change in expression of the target gene/protein. The opposite approach is also extremely useful. Examples include the generation of knock-out mice (where the gene encoding the target of interest is deleted), the use of antisense methodologies (antisense expression vectors, application of oligonucleotides, peptide nucleic acids, ribozymes and modified RNA molecules), transfection of appropriate cells with dominant-negative forms of the target protein, the microinjection of antibodies, and the administration of inhibitory peptides. Taking telomerase as an example, such studies have proven valuable in assessing the validity of this enzyme as a cancer drug target.

Telomerase, the enzyme responsible for maintaining telomeres by the addition of TTAGGG hexanucleotide repeats, has been shown to be over-expressed in 85–90% of human tumors, while expression in normal cells is restricted to stem cells and germ cells (see reference 8 for a review). Hence, in terms of this strong association with the malignant phenotype, telomerase appears to represent a validated cancer drug target. Furthermore, a link with tumorigenesis has been established in experiments where normal human fibroblasts were transformed into fully immortalized tumor cells by the genetic addition of ras, simian virus 40 large T oncoprotein, and hTERT [9]. Nevertheless, a particular concern within a drug discovery context is that it might take a very long time for telomeres to erode upon inhibition of telomerase and for cell senescence or death to result. However, experiments with both antisense molecules directed at the RNA (hTR) component of telomerase and dominant-negative constructs of the telomerase catalytic protein (hTERT) show, that in tumors possessing relatively short telomeres, cell death may occur within 1–2 weeks *in vitro* [10, 11].

III. A GENERIC CASCADE FOR ANTICANCER DRUG DISCOVERY

Having validated the chosen target, the modern paradigm for anticancer drug discovery comprises a series of carefully constructed steps that are designed to rapidly and efficiently allow "proof of principle" pharmaceutically tractable molecules to be tested in phase I and II clinical trials. Such a cascade (Figure 9.1) may be envisaged as a large number of molecules feeding into a series of iterative stop/go tests of increasing biological complexity. The compounds may be rationally designed on the basis of structural information of the target (e.g., X-ray crystallography), a compound collection that comprises molecules of diverse structure and drug-like qualities, natural product or libraries of compounds generated using combinatorial chemistry. In broad terms, the test cascade comprises three parts. First, compounds with the desired activity against the target are identified in high-throughput screens

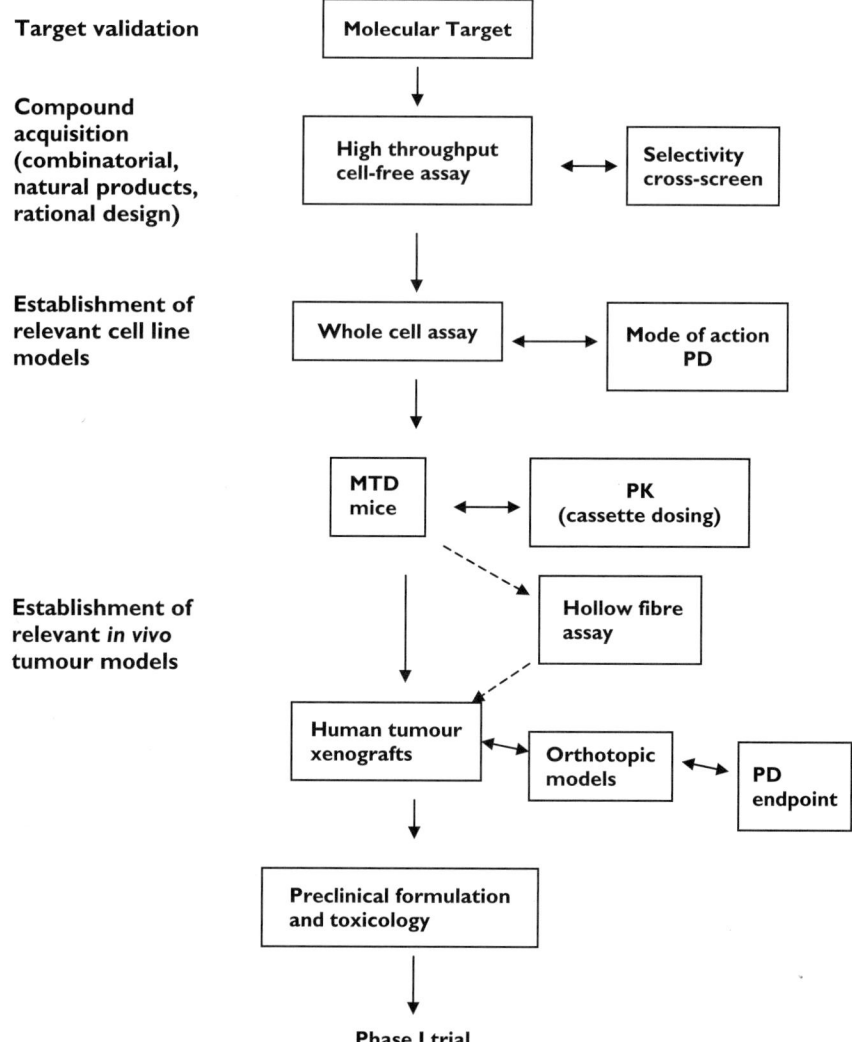

FIGURE 9.1 A generic test cascade.

(biochemical- or cell-based). Secondly, it is necessary to show inhibition of proliferation or anticancer effect against appropriate cancer cell lines by the desired mechanism, and finally anti-tumor activity *in vivo* at non-toxic doses to the host and with activity by the desired mechanism should be demonstrated. For each target evaluated, the test cascade may be customized to provide a "best-fit" with the individual target. At each step there should be feedback to allow for appropriate chemical refinement (e.g., increase potency against the target, improve oral bioavailability, decrease metabolism/improve pharmacokinetic properties, etc.). Such cascades can now be set up and run effectively in academic and small biotechnology establishments [12]. An important feature is the requirement for efficient communication between

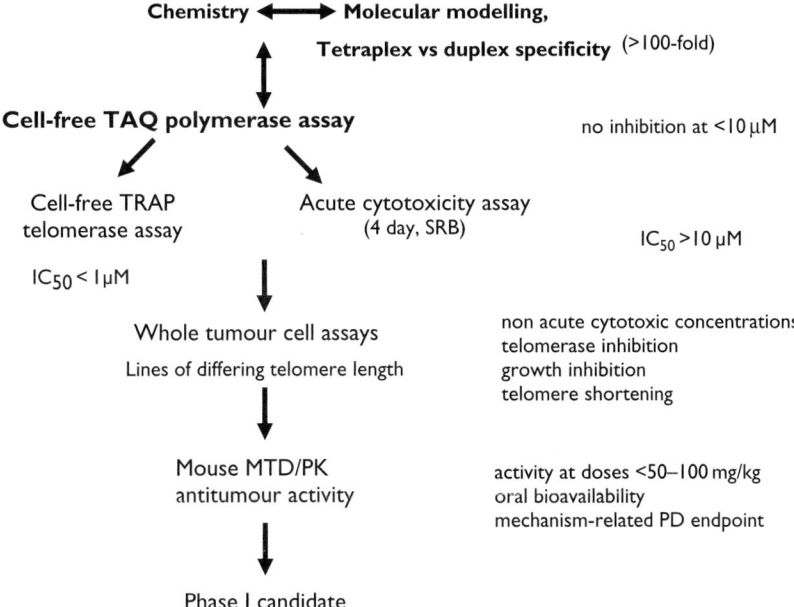

FIGURE 9.2 Evaluation cascade for G-quadruplex interactive compounds.

individuals from multiple disciplines: chemists, molecular and cell biologists, pharmacologists, pharmaceutical scientists, and medical oncologists. Today, phase I trials should involve the study of a pharmaceutically tractable drug with appropriate PK and PD assays already established and validated in the preclinical laboratory [13].

Another useful strategy is to establish an aspirational drug target profile as an adjunct to each cascade. For example, potency against the target enzyme in cell-free assays of less than 10 nM (with >10-fold selectively relative to other similar enzymes), activity in appropriate cell lines at concentrations of less than 1 μM, and anti-tumor efficacy *in vivo* in mice at doses of less than 50–100 mg/kg. Potency is an important issue, because if a dose of 100 mg/kg was found to be optimal in the mouse, at least 100 g of material would be required for formulation, toxicology, and phase I trial. An example generated for the development of G-quadruplex interactive telomerase inhibitors is shown in Figure 9.2.

IV. HIGH-THROUGHPUT CELL-FREE SCREENS FOR ACTIVITY AGAINST THE TARGET

Once a target has been identified and validated, compounds with the desired activity may be rapidly assessed in primary screens using high-throughput approaches [14]. Miniaturization of assays using microtiter plates (96, 384, or higher density formats) and automated assay procedures allow the possibility of screening many thousands of compounds on a daily basis. For cell-free screens, non-separation "mix and measure" assay technologies have been widely used for primary screening. These assay systems include scintillation proximity assays (e.g., SPA, Amersham Pharmacia and FlashPlates, PerkinElmer Life Sciences), fluorescent energy transfer assays (e.g., HTRF, Packard and LANCE, PerkinElmer Life Sciences) and chemiluminescent assays (e.g., AlphaScreen, Packard). For biochemical screens there is a requirement for relatively large quantities of active target enzyme or proteins and these are often produced by recombinant methods using a cDNA construct in *Escherichia coli*, yeast, or baculovirus infected *Spodoptera frugiperda* (Sf9) insect cells. High-throughput screens normally run at a predetermined concentration; usually 1–40 μM can be used to screen an organization's whole portfolio of tens of thousands or even millions of compounds in a matter of weeks to identify initial hits. The subsequent synthesis of lead explosion libraries then allows for structure-activity relationship (SAR) information on the target to be obtained. Typically, additional screening is carried out against other non-target but closely related enzymes, e.g., other tyrosine kinases as in the development of the bcr-abl inhibitor, STI571 [15]. Cell-based assays are also increasingly used in high-throughput screens (see below).

V. *IN VITRO* CELL LINE MODELS

Since the mid-1980s, panels of human cancer cell lines grown *in vitro* have represented the workhorse of cancer drug screening. This is largely accounted for by the empirical-based approach adopted at this time by the NCI. The NCI abandoned its use of screens involving rapidly growing mouse leukemia lines *in vivo* for a panel of 60 human tumor cell lines derived from 9 tumor types [16]. A particularly useful facilitator was the establishment of semi-automated, 96-well microtiter-plate based methods such as the microculture tetrazolium (MTT) [17] and sulforhodamine B (SRB) [18] for the rapid testing of compounds. Today, screening data for more than 30,000 compounds are available on the NCI Developmental Therapeutics Program (DTP) Web site (http://dtp.nci.nih.gov). It was hypothesized that potency within particular tumor types in the 60-cell-line screen might predict corresponding clinical activity in that tumor. The development of some drugs currently in clinical trial such as flavopiridol and UCN-01 has been assisted by evaluation through the 60-cell-line panel. However, this disease-oriented approach has not been entirely successful, especially with its use for molecularly targeted drugs where some agents could be missed. Recently, the program was modified to incorporate an *in vitro* cell line prescreen of only three cell lines (MCF-7 breast, NCI H460 non-small cell lung, and SF268 CNS), since it was found that such a prescreen could eliminate completely inactive compounds at a considerable saving in resources. [19]. Thereby only compounds showing activity in at least one of these three cell lines are forwarded to the full 60-cell-line panel.

Through the incorporation of bioinformatics, the NCI 60-cell-line panel provides a powerful resource for cancer drug screening. For each test compound, a growth inhibition "fingerprint" is produced. Thereafter, algorithms such as COMPARE developed by Dr Ken Paull and "cluster" analyses provide a means of determining whether a new agent of interest (that may possess an unknown mechanism of action) induces a pattern of growth inhibition similar or dissimilar (that is COMPARE-negative) to that of known anticancer agents [20]. Moreover, the addition of molecular profiling information from the cell line panel (e.g., enzyme or gene expression patterns; http://dtp.nci.nih.gov/mtargets/mt_index.htm) [21, 22] allows for the possibility of assigning a molecular target to a compound of hitherto unknown mechanism of action.

Further important information from specific, molecularly characterized cell lines may be attained through the incorporation of acquired drug-resistant or isogenic sublines into the test cascade. For example, we established a test cascade specifically to discover novel platinum-based drugs using a panel of human ovarian carcinoma cell lines (and companion xenografts) that possessed acquired resistance to cisplatin through defined biochemical mechanisms [23]. These cell lines were pivotal to the discovery of the sterically hindered platinum drug ZD0473 (formerly JM473, AMD473). ZD0473 was designed to circumvent acquired resistance to cisplatin due to increased inactivation by intracellular thiol-containing molecules such as glutathione, and is now undergoing phase III trials [24, 25].

Additionally, the incorporation, through gene transfection, of isogenic pairs of cell lines that differ only in the gene/protein target of interest may be particularly useful in determining whether an agent is exerting an effect in cells through the desired mechanism. For example, an isogenic human colon tumor model is currently being utilized for *NQO1* gene expression to seek prodrugs that may be selectively activated by the enzyme DT-diaphorase [26].

The use of cell-based ELISAs and appropriate cell lines may also provide a early and rapid pharmacodynamic assessment and thereby confirm that any observed anticancer effect in cells is occurring through the predicted and desired mechanism. Recently such an approach was described, which monitors the extent of phosphorylation of ERK1/2 versus total ERK1/2 expression in two human colon cancer cell lines exposed to the Hsp90 inhibitor, 17AAG [27].

As mentioned above, whole cells may also be used in high-throughput screens. Typically these might be reporter gene assays, e.g., luciferase activity as a readout and immunological or morphological assays using genetically modified cell lines. Cell-based screens have the advantage that they identify compounds that are taken up into cells. They may also identify hits for more than one target on pathways affecting the readout. Deconvolution of the assay so that the molecular target of each hit can be identified is an essential component of such cell-based screens. For example, the Mek inhibitor UO126 was identified using a COS-7 cell-based luciferase reporter assay for inhibitors of AP-1 transactivation [28].

A final important piece of information that may be easily obtained using cell lines *in vitro*, and which may guide subsequent dosing schedules *in vivo*, is a study of time of exposure versus anticancer effect. For example, with the aminopurine-based cdk inhibitor, roscovitine, it was shown that maximum growth inhibition of a human ovarian carcinoma cell line occurred after 16 hours of drug exposure (equivalent to approximately one cell cycle time)

[29]. This indicated that prolonged plasma levels would be required *in vivo* in order to achieve an anti-tumor effect.

VI. *IN VIVO* TESTING OF NOVEL COMPOUNDS

The divide between obtaining *in vitro* cytotoxic or cytostatic activity against appropriate cell lines and conferring anti-tumor activity *in vivo*, often remains the rate-limiting step in the anticancer drug discovery process. This is often attributable to poor compound PK absorption, distribution, metabolism, and excretion (ADME). In my view, from both a scientific and animal ethical standpoint, the number of anti-tumor studies conducted in mice bearing tumors should be limited only to those molecules that have successfully overcome both the above hurdles in the cascade and possess good PK properties. The random screening of molecules, especially using intraperitoneal drug administration to intraperitoneally implanted tumors, a feature of cancer drug screening prevalent in the past, is no longer acceptable. Issues of animal welfare and ethics within cancer research have recently been considered within the United Kingdom and published as a set of guidelines [30]. Therefore, a pharmacological approach should be applied whereby only molecules where plasma (or tumor) drug levels known to be required for activity against the target *in vitro* should be tested. One should also be prepared to have to compromise on potency against the target in favor of selecting an analog possessing superior PK properties.

Such a "pharmacologically guided" model has been established for some years within the European Organisation for Research and Treatment of Cancer (EORTC) for the testing of COMPARE-negative (see above) molecules arising from Europe and evaluated in the empirical NCI 60-cell-line panel [31, 32]. Herein, selected COMPARE-negative compounds are progressed for preformulation, assay development, maximum-tolerated dose (MTD), and PK studies in mice prior to beginning any anti-tumor efficacy studies. Xenograft studies, and companion mechanisms of action and PD studies, are only conducted for compounds where plasma concentrations approaching those known to be required for achieving an IC_{50} in the NCI cell screen are obtained. The NCI has recently adopted a similar approach with emphasis on PK, mechanism of action and PD post testing in the 60-cell-line screen, and prior to *in vivo* anti-tumor xenograft studies [19].

VII. CASSETTE-DOSING

A particularly useful adjunct to the pharmacologically guided approach advocated above is the development and validation of cassette- or cocktail-dosing. This allows the rapid accrual of PK information by the simultaneous administration of compound analogs to mice and measuring the different compounds in the same plasma sample by liquid chromatography mass spectrometry (LC-MS/MS). This approach has been successfully used to show that the cdk inhibitor roscovitine possesses better PK properties than either the closely chemically related olomoucine or bohemine [33]. Although one needs to validate the approach for each compound class (by comparing PK parameters when used singly or in combination) when applicable, cassette-dosing also offers another considerable advantage in using significantly fewer animals than conventional methods.

VIII. PHARMACEUTICAL CONSIDERATIONS

Having firmly established that the lead molecule possesses potent activity against the target in cell-free assays and within appropriate tumor cell lines, it is also very important to maintain a "pharmaceutical perspective" and consider at this point whether a clinically acceptable formulation of the molecule is attainable. Too many mice have been used in the past with drugs given as coarse suspensions in DMSO or detergents (e.g., Tweens), vehicles which may not be usable in man. Considerable advances in the development of biocompatible formulations for poorly water-soluble drugs have been developed in recent years (e.g., using betacyclodextrin-based systems). However, developing a vehicle is still largely empirical. For particular targets where chronic administration to patients is the likely clinical scenario based on the understanding of the target, an early evaluation of oral bioavailability may also be appropriate. This may initially be achieved using artificial permeable membranes, *in vitro* cell-line systems such as the colon cancer cell line CaCo2, or directly in rodents by determining pharmacokinetics following oral versus intravenous administration of the same dose.

IX. HIGH-THROUGHPUT *IN VIVO* ANTI-TUMOR TESTING: THE HOLLOW FIBER ASSAY

The NCI has also been instrumental in the development of a hybrid *in vitro/in vivo* assay whereby particular cell lines from the 60-cell-line panel may be grown and compounds rapidly tested *in vivo* using the hollow fiber assay [34, 35]. This assay, together with increased emphasis on PK- and PD-based molecular targeted approaches as described above, has resulted in a decreased emphasis on the use of human tumor xenografts (see below). In the hollow fiber assay, tumor cells are placed aseptically into polyvinylidine fluoride (PVDF) biocompatible hollow fibers and their ends heat-sealed at 2-cm lengths. After incubation of 1–2 days *in vitro*, fibers are then implanted into mice in two anatomically separate sites, intraperitoneally (ip) and subcutaneously (sc). The mice are then dosed ip with the test compound at two dose levels for up to 4 days. Two days later fibers are then removed and the numbers of remaining viable cells compared in treated versus control groups using the MTT assay *ex vivo*. A total of 12 cell lines is used (two each of breast, ovarian, glioma, colon, melanoma, and non-small cell lung cancer), and an overall score generated for each test compound (2 points for each fiber where a 50% or greater reduction in cell growth in comparison to vehicle controls is observed).

Although the assay is rapid (results obtained within a week), there are limitations and the assay may not be applicable to the evaluation of all novel types of agents (e.g., those affecting invasion). The use of ip implanted fibers and ip administered agents may not adequately test the PK properties of the test substance. Furthermore, it has also been shown that within the short time that fibers are implanted sc in mice, there is insufficient time for angiogenesis to the fibers to occur, thereby potentially limiting drug delivery to the cells within these fibers [36].

X. HUMAN TUMOR XENOGRAFTS

For many years, sc implanted human tumor xenografts in immunodeficient nude or SCID mice have played an important role in the cancer drug discovery process, especially at the NCI [37]. Typically, tumors are allowed to reach a diameter of around 6–8 mm prior to administering a compound (so-called advanced stage) and then effects are analyzed in control versus treated groups using caliper measurements. Xenografts are generally slower growing than previously used rodent models (such as L1210 and P388 leukemia and B16 melanoma), and because the target cells for drugs are human rather than mouse (even though the supporting stroma and blood supply is murine), they have widely been believed to represent a more dependable model of human disease and to be a reasonable predictor of clinical utility. For example, in our platinum drug development program, a good correlation was shown between the sensitivity of a panel of human ovarian carcinoma cell lines to cisplatin, their response as *in vivo* xenograft counterparts, and the response of the corresponding patient's tumor to platinum-based chemotherapy [23]. In addition, the drug-testing group at the University of Frieburg, Germany, has shown a good correlation between drug response in patients and for the same drugs when used in mice bearing xenografts [38].

An important recent analysis correlating clinical anticancer activity and preclinical responses including in human tumor xenografts has been undertaken by the NCI [39]. For 39 compounds where both xenograft and phase II data were available, activity in at least one-third of tested xenografts predicted for activity in at least some phase II trials. These data suggest that, at least for existing cytotoxic anticancer drugs, the sc xenograft model is of some predictive value. However, activity within a particular histological type of xenograft generally did not predict clinical activity in the same tumor. Interestingly, increased activity in the hollow fiber assay (especially with ip implanted fibers) also predicted increased xenograft activity (8% of all compounds tested were active in at least one-third of xenografts whereas this increased to 20% for compounds exhibiting a response in more than six ip fibers) [39]. There was also a strong correlation between potency in the 60-cell-line screen and activity in the hollow fiber assay. Although 56% of compounds with a mean 50% growth inhibition of below 0.032 μM were active in at least 6 ip fibers, only 4% of compounds with a potency of 100 μM were active to the same level.

Typical xenograft dose response curves for mice bearing an sc breast cancer tumor and treated with the FTI R115777 are shown in Figure 9.3A. A point of note in contrast to responses traditionally observed to cytotoxics (e.g., cisplatin, paclitaxel (Figure 9.3B) is that the signal transduction

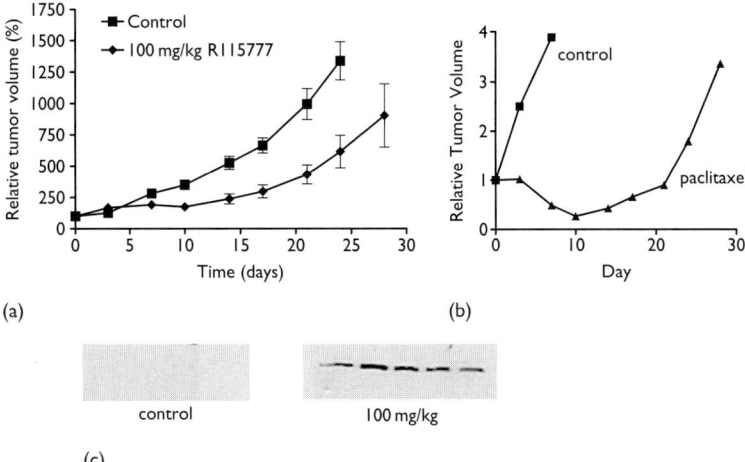

FIGURE 9.3 Comparative tumor dose—response curves for (a) the FTI R11577 (Zarnestra) and (b) paclitaxel. (c) Detection of prelamin A as a potential PD marker for R115777.

inhibitor induced a slowing (cytostatic) effect on tumor growth rather a cyto-toxic, tumor shrinkage effect. In addition, as with R115777, chronic (daily) rather than intermittent (e.g., weekly) dosing was required. Again, as emphasized above, a knowledge of both compound mechanism of action (molecular target) and PK is essential to guide xenograft experiments and to help predict what effect the compound under test might be expected to induce. Moreover, models should be selected on the basis of molecular characterization in terms of the selected target or pathway.

While the sc xenograft model is and will continue to be an important component of the test cascade, the approach does possess limitations. These include expense and foremost the fact that they generally grow relatively rapidly and do not (unlike the disease in man) metastasize. Furthermore, to date, xenografts have generally been used without characterization at the molecular level for the particular target being addressed.

XI. ORTHOTOPIC, TRANSGENIC, AND OTHER ANIMAL MODELS

The accepted limitations of the sc ectopic xenograft model for drug testing has prompted some to advocate the use of complementary tumors grown in their natural site (orthotopically) [40]. Using surgical orthotopic implantation (SOI), tumor models have been described for colon, prostate, lung, renal, bladder, and ovarian cancer and may be of particular value in studying compounds affecting metastasis and invasion (e.g., metalloproteinase inhibitors) and agents that modulate the tumor microenvironment [41]. A potentially useful recent development is the use of human and rodent tumors that stably express very high levels of the green fluorescent protein from the jellyfish, *Aequorea victoria*, thereby allowing the non-invasive, real-time whole body optical imaging of metastasis and angiogenesis [42].

In addition, transgenics (onco-mice), which spontaneously give rise to breast (e.g., ras oncogene transgenics), head and neck, or prostate cancer, and knock-out models, have also been used in drug discovery cascades for either target validation or therapy. For example, ras oncogene transgenics were used in proof of concept studies of ras farnesyltransferase inhibitors [43]. Such models that produce metastases and tumors, which are generally non-immunogenic but arise in immunocompetent mice, may also be especially applicable to the study of cancer prevention [44]. However, as with orthotopic models, these are relatively labor intensive and expensive, often requiring a long time for tumor development and large numbers of animals, in comparison to ectopic xenografts. Also there may be issues concerning the timing of potential therapies and whether the transgene products are relevant to human malignancy (e.g., knock-outs carry the targeted gene in every cell type). As used by the drug-testing group in Bradford, UK, it also remains valid to use syngeneic sc mouse tumor models such as the MAC colon adenocarcinoma series following calibration and target characterization [2]. Finally, orthotopic syngeneic tumors grown in immunocompetent mice are useful for the evaluation of agents that activate cells of the immune system and/or modulate tumor-host interactions.

XII. PHARMACODYNAMICS

As alluded to above, increased emphasis should be placed upon PD readouts, both in preclinical testing and in association with early clinical trials. As in studies of 17AAG and the farnesyl protein transferase inhibitor R115777, PD determinations using xenograft tumors in mice have proven particularly useful in guiding subsequent clinical trials. For example, it was shown that the detection of an increase heat shock protein 70 may represent a good PD marker of response in mice or patients receiving 17AAG [45]. In addition, for molecules like 17AAG that possess the potential to disrupt multiple signal transduction pathways, microarray gene expression analyses may also be useful in elucidating mechanisms of action and for identifying potential PD markers of response [46]. Another promising development, complementary to genomic approaches, is based on proteomics where large numbers of proteins may be studied simultaneously [47]. Studies with R115777 and mice bearing MCF-7 breast cancer xenografts showed that the detection of prelamin A may provide a suitable PD marker of response (Figure 9.3C) [3]. Finally, studies with the cdk inhibitor roscovitine have shown a correlation between growth inhibition of KM12 colon cancer xenografts and loss of tumor and peripheral blood lymphocyte RB phosphorylation (at serines 608 and 780) [5]. These findings are now exploited in phase I studies with roscovitine. Already in the clinic, studies with STI571 have shown a decrease in the phosphorylation of the BCR-ABL substrate CRKL in blood samples taken from patients with chronic myeloid leukemia receiving 400 mg of drug [15]. There is also considerable interest in the development of non-invasive methods for monitoring both drug PK and PD using techniques such as positron emission tomography (PET), and magnetic resonance spectroscopy (MRS) and imaging (MRI) [48].

XIII. SUMMARY

The preclinical anticancer drug discovery process has undergone a revolution in the past 10 years. Target validation is an essential component prior to initiating a drug discovery program. The amalgamation of combinatorial chemistry and robotic high-throughput screens allows for the rapid identification of "hits," which can then be converted into leads and further optimized by medicinal chemistry. There is an increased emphasis on pharmacokinetics and pharmacodynamics throughout the process. The use of mice in *in vivo* antitumor studies should be restricted to molecules possessing good pharmaceutical properties where plasma levels above those known to be required for *in vitro* anticancer effects are achievable. For some types of compounds, testing using orthotopically grown tumor models rather than sc xenografts may be more appropriate.

This more pharmacological-based approach combined with techniques to increase throughput (robotic cell-free assays, high-throughput whole cell growth inhibition and ELISA-based PD methods, cassette-dosing, hollow fiber assay) should result in the more rapid progression of carefully selected molecules for proof of principle phase I trials. The introduction of rodent-only toxicology as used successfully for many years by the Cancer Research Campaign in the UK [49] also results in a more rapid introduction of new molecules to phase I. By the time phase I trials begin, adequately sensitive and validated assays for determining drug pharmacokinetics and pharmacodynamics should be in place to allow the possibility of dosing to a biological mechanism-based PD end point rather than to the traditional dose-limiting toxicity end point used previously for cancer cytotoxics.

ACKNOWLEDGEMENTS

Studies discussed from the CRC Centre for Cancer Therapeutics were supported by grants from the UK Cancer Research Campaign. I thank Paul Workman, Wynne Aherne, and also John Double and Herbie Newell for critical appraisal of the manuscript. Thanks are also due to Ed Sausville at the NCI Developmental Therapeutics Program and to members of the EORTC Screening and Pharmacology Group (SPG) for numerous discussions.

REFERENCES

1. Workman P. Towards genomic cancer pharmacology: Innovative drugs for the new millennium. *Curr. Opin. Oncol Endometab. Invest. Drugs* 2000; 2:21–25.
2. Double JA, Bibby MC. Therapeutic index: A vital component in selection of anticancer agents for clinical trial. *J. Natl. Cancer Inst.* 1989; 81:988–994.
3. Smith V, Brunton L, Valenti M, Johnston S, Kelland L. Preclinical antitumor and pharmacodynamic studies with the farnesyl transferase inhibitor (FTI) R115777. *Proc. AACR* 2001; 42:260 (abstract).
4. Kelland LR, Sharp SY, Rogers PM, Myers TG, Workman P. DT-diaphorase expression and tumor cell sensitivity to 17-allylamino,17-demethoxygeldanamycin, an inhibitor of heat shock protein 90. *J. Natl. Cancer Inst.* 1999; 91:1940–1949.

5. Whittaker S, Walton M, Kelland L, Garrett M, Zhelev N, Workman P. RB phosphorylation as a pharmacodynamic marker of roscovitine (CYC202) activity in vitro and in vivo. *Proc. AACR* 2001; 42:926 (abstract).

6. Gowan SM, Brunton L, Valenti M, Heald R, Read MA, Harrison JR, Stevens MFG, Neidle S, Kelland LR. Preclinical antitumor properties of G-quadruplex interactive small molecule inhibitors of telomerase. *Proc. AACR* 2001; 42 (abstract).

7. Garrett MD, Workman P. Discovering novel chemotherapeutic drugs for the third millennium. *Eur. J. Cancer* 1999; 35:2010–2030.

8. Kelland LR. Telomerase: Biology and phase I trials. *Lancet Oncol.* 2001; 2:95–102.

9. Hahn WC, Counter CM, Lundberg AS, Beijersbergen RL, Brooks MW, Weinberg RA. Creation of human tumour cells with defined genetic elements. *Nature* 1999; 400:464–468.

10. Herbert BS, Pitts AE, Baker SI, Hamilton SE, Wright WE, Shay JW, Corey DR. Inhibition of human telomerase in immortal human cells leads to progressive telomere shortening and cell death. *PNAS* 1999; 96:14276–14281.

11. Hahn WC, Stewart SA, Brooks MW, York SG, Eaton E, Kurachi A, Beijersbergen RL, Knoll JHM, Meyerson M, Weinberg RA. Inhibition of telomerase limits the growth of human cancer cells. *Nat. Med.* 1999; 5:1164–1170.

12. Workman P, Garrett MD, Kelland LR, Raynaud FI, Nutley BP, Eccles SA, Jarman M, Hardcastle I, Bannister A, Kouzarides T, Aherne GW. Contemporary mechanism-based screening, combinatorial chemistry and drug development against new cancer targets in an academic research institute environment. *Clin. Cancer Res.* 2000; 6:4476s (abstract).

13. Gelmon KA, Eisenhauer EA, Harris AL, Ratain MJ, Workman P. Anticancer agents targeting signaling molecules and cancer cell environment: Challenges for drug development? *J. Natl. Cancer Inst.* 1999; 91:1281–1287.

14. Aherne W, Garrett MD, McDonald E, Workman P. Mechanism-based high throughput screening for novel anticancer drug discovery. In *Anticancer Drug Development* (Baguley, B. C., ed.), Academic Press, San Diego, 2002, pp. 249–267

15. Druker BJ, Talpaz M, Resta DJ et al. Efficacy and safety of a specific inhibitor of the BCR-ABL tyrosine kinase in chronic myeloid leukemia. *N. Engl. J. Med.* 2001; 344: 1031–1037.

16. Boyd MR, Paull KD. Some practical considerations and applications of the National Cancer Institute in vitro anticancer drug discovery screen. *Drug Dev. Res.* 1995; 34:91–109.

17. Alley MC, Scudiero DA, Monks A et al. Feasibility of drug screening with panels of human tumor cell lines using a microculture tetrazolium assay. *Cancer Res.* 1988; 48:589–601.

18. Skehan P, Storeng R, Scudiero D et al. New colorimetric cytotoxicity assay for anticancer-drug screening. *J. Natl. Cancer Inst.* 1990; 82:1107–1112.

19. Sausville EA, Feigal E. Evolving approaches to cancer drug discovery and development at the National Cancer Institute, USA. *Ann. Oncol.* 1999; 10:1287–1291.

20. Monks A, Scudiero DA, Johnson GS, Paull KD, Sausville EA. The NCI anticancer drug screen: A smart screen to identify effectors of novel targets. *Anticancer Drug Des.* 1997; 12:533–541.

21. Fitzsimmons SA, Workman P, Grever M, Paull K, Camalier R, Lewis AD. Reductase enzyme expression across the National Cancer Institute tumor cell line panel: Correlation with sensitivity to mitomycin C and EO9. *J. Natl. Cancer Inst.* 1996; 88:259–269.

22. Ross DT, Scherf U, Eisen MB, Perou CM, Rees C, Spellman P, Iyer V, Jeffrey SS, Van de Rijn M, Waltham M, Pergamenschikov A, Lee JCF, Lashkari D, Shalon D, Myers TG, Weinstein JN, Botstein D, Brown PO. Systematic variation in gene expression patterns in human cancer cell lines. *Nat. Genet.* 2000; 24:227–234.

23. Kelland LR, Jones M, Abel G, Valenti M, Gwynne JJ, Harrap KR. Human ovarian carcinoma cell lines and companion xenografts: A disease oriented approach to new platinum anticancer drug development. *Cancer Chemother. Pharmacol.* 1992; 30:43–50.

24. Raynaud FI, Boxall FE, Goddard PM, Valenti M, Jones M, Murrer BA, Abrams M, Kelland LR. Cis-amminedichloro(2-methylpyridine) platinum(II) (AMD473), a novel sterically hindered platinum complex: In vivo activity, toxicology and pharmacokinetics in mice. *Clin. Cancer Res.* 1997; 3:2063–2074.

25. Holford J, Sharp SY, Murrer BA, Abrams M, Kelland LR. In vitro circumvention of cisplatin-resistance by the novel sterically hindered platinum complex AMD473. *Br. J. Cancer* 1998; 77:366–373.

26. Sharp SY, Kelland LR, Valenti MR, Brunton LA, Hobbs S, Workman P. Establishment of an isogenic human colon tumor model for *NQO1* gene expression: Application to investigate the role of DT-diaphorase in bioreductive drug activation in vitro and in vivo. *Mol. Pharmacol.* 2000; 58:1146–1155.

27. Aherne W, Hardcastle A, Newbatt Y, Boxall K, Clarke P, Di Stefano F, Maloney A, Workman P. Mechanism-based cell ELISAs for lead optimization in drug discovery. *Proc. AACR* 2001; 42:485 (abstract).

28. Favata MF, Horiuchi KY, Manos EJ et al. Identification of a novel inhibitor of mitogen-activated protein kinase kinase. *J. Biol. Chem.* 1998; 273:18623–18632.

29. Kelland LR, Rogers PM, Pestell KE et al. Preclinical antitumor evaluation of cyclin-dependent kinase (cdk) inhibitors. *Proc. AACR* 1999; 40:125.

30. Workman P, Twentyman P, Balkwill F et al. United Kingdom Co-ordinating Committee on Cancer Research (UKCCCR) guidelines for the welfare of animals in experimental neoplasia (second edition). *Br. J. Cancer* 1999; 77:1–10.

31. Hendriks HR, Burtles S, Radke S et al. Cell-based screening and pharmacological strategies for the selection of new anticancer agents: A collaboration between the National Cancer Institute (NCI), Cancer Research Campaign (CRC) and EORTC. NCI-EORTC Symposium New Drugs In Cancer Therapy 1998; 10:40 (abstract).

32. Burger AM, McGown AM, Kelland L, Fiebig HH, Harter M, Sausville EA. Antivascular effects and antitumor activity of NSC 643314 in vitro and in vivo. Proceedings of AACR/NCI/EORTC 1999; 82 (abstract).

33. Raynaud FI, Nutley BP, Fischer P et al. Cassette dosing does not affect the individual pharmacokinetics of the cell cycle inhibitors olomoucine, roscovitine and bohemine in Balb C mice. *Proc. AACR* 2000; 41:816 (abstract).

34. Casciari JJ, Hollingshead MG, Alley MC et al. Growth and chemotherapeutic response of cells in a hollow-fiber in vitro solid tumor model. *J. Natl. Cancer Inst.* 1994; 86:1846–1852.

35. Hollingshead MG, Alley MC, Camalier RF et al. In vivo cultivation of tumor cells in hollow fibers. *Life Sci.* 1995; 57:131–141.

36. Phillips RM, Pearce J, Loadman PM et al. Angiogenesis in the hollow fiber tumor model influences drug delivery to tumor cells: Implications for anticancer drug screening programs. *Cancer Res.* 1998; 58:5263–5266.

37. Plowman J, Dykes DJ, Hollingshead M, Simpson-Herren L, Alley MC. Human tumor xenograft models in NCI drug development. Teicher B. 101–125, 1997, Totowa NJ, Humana Press. Anticancer Drug Development Guide. Ref Type: Serial (book monograph).

38. Scholz CC, Berger DP, Winterhalter BR, Henz H, Fiebig HH. Correlation of drug response in patients and in the clonogenic assay with solid human tumour xenografts. *Eur. J. Cancer* 1990; 26:901–905.

39. Johnson JI, Decker S, Zaharevitz D et al. Relationships between drug activity in NCI preclinical in vitro and in vivo models and early clinical trials. *Br. J. Cancer* 2001; 84(10):1424–1431.

40. Killion JJ, Radinsky R, Fidler IJ. Orthotopic models are necessary to predict therapy of transplantable tumors in mice. *Cancer Metast. Rev.* 1999; 17:279–284.

41. Hoffman RM. Orthotopic metastatic mouse models for anticancer drug discovery and evaluation: A bridge to the clinic. *Invest. New Drugs* 1999; 17:343–359.

42. Yang M, Baranov E, Jiang P et al. Whole-body optical imaging of green fluorescent protein-expressing tumors and metastases. *Proc. Natl. Acad. Sci. U. S. A.* 2000; 97:1206–1211.

43. Kohl NE, Omer CA, Conner MW et al. Inhibition of farnesyltransferase induces regression of mammary and salivary carcinomas in *ras* transgenic mice. *Nat. Med.* 1995; 1:792–797.

44. Rosenberg MP, Bortner D. Why transgenic and knockout animal models should be used (for drug efficacy studies in cancer). *Cancer Metast. Rev.* 1999; 17:295–299.

45. Banerji U, Walton M, Raynaud F, Kelland L, Judson I, Workman P. Validation of pharmacodynamic endpoints for the HSP90 molecular chaperone inhibitor 17-allylamino 17-demethoxygeldanamycin (17AAG) in a human tumor xenograft model. *Proc. AACR* 2001; 42 (abstract).

46. Clarke PA, Hostein I, Banerji U et al. Gene expression profiling of human colon cancer cells following inhibition of signal transduction by 17-allylamino-17-demethoxygeldanamycin, an inhibitor of the hsp90 molecular chaperone. *Oncogene* 2000; 19:4125–4133.

47. Page MJ, Amess B, Rohlff C, Stubberfield C, Parekh R. Proteomics: A major new technology for the drug discovery process. *Drug Discov. Today* 1999; 4:55–62.
48. Price P. Changes in ^{18}F-FDG uptake measured by PET as a pharmacodynamic end-point in anticancer therapy. How far have we got? *Br. J. Cancer* 2000; 83:281–283.
49. Newell DR, Burtles SS, Fox BW, Jodrell DI, Connors TA. Evaluation of rodent-only toxicology for early clinical trials with novel cancer therapeutics. *Br. J. Cancer* 1999; 81:760–768.

II

METHODS FOR CLINICAL TESTING OF NOVEL AGENTS

10
SURROGATE END POINTS AND BIOMARKERS FOR EARLY TRIALS OF NOVEL ANTICANCER AGENTS

ALEX A. ADJEI

Mayo Clinic and Foundation
Rochester, Minnesota

I. INTRODUCTION
II. WHAT ARE TARGET AGENTS?
III. SURROGATE MARKERS OR BIOMARKERS?
IV. BIOMARKERS AS INDICATORS OF DRUG EFFECT *IN VIVO*
V. BIOMARKERS AS PREDICTIVE FACTORS
VI. BIOMARKERS AS PROGNOSTIC FACTORS
VII. TECHNICAL ISSUES IN THE EVALUATION OF DRUG EFFECTS *IN VIVO*
VIII. LESSONS FOR THE FUTURE

I. INTRODUCTION

Traditional anticancer drug development has focused on testing large numbers of chemicals on rapidly growing transplantable rodent tumors, and more recently, human tumor xenografts. This approach identified DNA-directed drugs, which have been considerably toxic and have limited efficacy. In recent years, advances in genetics and tumor biology have elucidated the molecular pathways implicated in the pathogenesis and progression of cancers and resulted in the discovery of a variety of novel molecular targets for therapeutic intervention. These targets are components of signal transduction pathways, cell cycle regulation, apoptosis, angiogenesis, and the tumor stroma. Because a number of current anticancer compounds have been designed to selectively inhibit these targets, there is considerable interest in assessing their cellular and subcellular effects in the clinical setting. Conceptually, assays of drug action *in vivo* can serve two purposes. In early clinical trials, these assays can determine whether the drug target has been inhibited at drug concentrations that are achievable in the clinical setting. In later clinical trials, these assays could potentially provide an early marker of drug efficacy if a strong correlation between assay results and clinical outcome can be established. More important, assays could improve the efficacy of a given compound by selecting the patient population that is likely to respond to therapy. This chapter will discuss conceptual and technical issues involved in the incorporation of biomarker evaluation in phase I and II clinical trials of targeted anticancer agents. The focus will be on biochemical markers. The reader is referred to Chapter 13 for a discussion of imaging modalities in the determination of drug effects *in vivo*.

II. WHAT ARE TARGETED AGENTS?

As discussed in the introductory section, a number of novel agents have been developed to selectively target aberrant molecular pathways in cancer cells. Because of this selective targeting, these agents tend to be less toxic when compared to standard cytotoxic chemotherapy agents. In addition, their toxicity profile tends to be different from that of cytotoxic agents. Thus alopecia is not seen, and myelosuppression, mucositis, and severe nausea and vomiting are uncommon. These agents have been referred to by multiple terms: "targeted agents," "novel agents," and "molecularly-targeted agents." All of these terms have created some confusion. A number of novel agents, including cytotoxic agents such as oxaliplatin, have been introduced into the clinic. There are interesting standard cytotoxic agents such as pemetrexed (Alimta), whose molecular targets are known, and thus can be called targeted agents. Regardless of which term is used, it is important to establish criteria to be met for agents to be considered targeted, and by implication, intrinsically different from cytotoxic agents. Targeted agents of interest, which could potentially be successful in the clinic, should be directed against a target that is biologically relevant to human cancer. The target must have a causal, rather than a simply correlative role in cancer development. Specifically, if the target is an antigen for immunotherapy, it must be expressed only on cancer cells and not on any normal cells. If it is an enzyme or protein, it must be present in cancer cells but not normal cells, and its continued normal functioning must be essential to the continued survival of the cancer cells. The presence of the target must correlate with clinical benefit when the drug is employed — blocking the target should impair tumor growth. Tumors that are devoid of a target should not respond to agents directly solely against that target. If an agent meets these criteria, designing valid *in vivo* correlative studies should be relatively simple.

III. SURROGATE MARKERS OR BIOMARKERS?

The terms "surrogate markers" and "biomarkers" have been sometimes used interchangeably, but may not have the same meaning. A recently organized workshop by the U. S. National Institutes of Health in Bethesda, MD, defined a biomarker (also called biological marker) as "a characteristic that is objectively measured and evaluated as an indicator of biologic processes, pathogenetic processes, or pharmacologic responses to therapeutic intervention" [1]. The term surrogate marker should probably be reserved for a marker that may be an accurate measure of drug effect, but may not directly measure the drug target. Thus, if one utilizes an inhibitor of the epidermal growth factor receptor tyrosine kinase in a clinical study and evaluates the induction of a non-specific effect such as apoptosis in tumor samples, this will be the utilization of a surrogate marker [1]. In general the term "surrogate marker" can be imprecise, creates confusion, and should probably not be used.

A biomarker is generally accepted as a measure of drug effect on its target. Thus, the evaluation of the inhibition of ERK phosphorylation after utilization of a MEK inhibitor represents the use of a biomarker [2]. A biomarker can, of course, be evaluated in surrogate tissue such as skin, lymphocytes, or buccal mucosa cells [3–5].

In addition, a surrogate end point could be defined as a biomarker response intended to substitute for a clinical end point, where a clinical end point is a characteristic or variable that reflects how a patient feels or functions, the extent of tumor shrinkage, or how long a patient survives [1].

A. Why are Surrogate End-Points Needed?

If surrogate endpoints might only measure drug effects but may not measure the drug target, why are they needed? There are several reasons why a surrogate end-point may be of considerable importance. The most important reason is the drug target may not be known with any certainty at the time the agent is introduced into the clinic. For example, there may be drugs with ubiquitous targets such as proteasome inhibitors [6], where the basis of cytotoxicity may not be known. In such circumstances, evaluation of a non-specific marker of drug effect such as inhibition of proliferation or induction of apoptosis may be very useful. Second, as a pharmacodynamic marker, a surrogate end-point may help to reliably establish a dosing schedule in phase I studies. If an *in vivo* effect persists for up to 24 hours after a single dose, investigators will be much more comfortable with administering the agent once daily, rather than relying on traditional pharmacokinetic measures to pick a schedule. Thirdly, as mentioned above, surrogate endpoints can provide proof of *in vivo* effects that complement traditional pharmacokinetic studies.

B. The Ideal Biomarker

If biomarkers are used, there are clearly properties that would make such markers ideal for use in conjunction with clinical trials. First, as is the case of any measures of biologic activity, the ideal bio marker should be sensitive and specific. Second, the marker should be present in easily accessible tissue in order to make it simple for patients to consent to sample collection. The commonly accessible tissues that have been utilized in current clinical trials are peripheral blood mononuclear cells (PBMCs), skin biopsies, and buccal mucosa cells [4, 7, 8]. Third, assays for the bio marker should be simple and adaptable to clinical use. In this regard, even though immunohistochemistry has been assailed as a very subjective and unreliable method for biomarker studies, it remains a simple, widely available method that can be utilized in virtually all hospitals world-wide. This explains, in part, why the measurement of estrogen and progesterone receptor status in breast cancer evolved from quantitative measures of protein content to an immunohistochemistry method. Finally, results in surrogate tissue of an ideal biomarker should correlate with results in tumor tissue, thus obviating the need of invasive tumor biopsies to document drug effects. Unfortunately, no such biomarker exists at present.

IV. BIOMARKERS AS INDICATORS OF DRUG EFFECT *IN VIVO*

When biomarkers are evaluated in surrogate tissues, this use represents the utilization of the marker as a pharmacodynamic marker. In this instance, one can categorically state that the drug is inhibiting its target in human tissues *in vivo*. In first-in-man phase I studies, this represents an important proof-of-principle (see Chapter 11). These studies are important in the phase I setting, because they provide information that complements traditional pharmacokinetic data. It is important to show that steady-state drug levels are consistent with the drug concentrations needed to inhibit the target enzyme *in vitro*, but it is much more compelling to show that the target is inhibited in patient tissues.

One of the problems facing drug development is that investigators continue evaluating biomarkers in surrogate tissue in phase II clinical trials. The utility of this approach is difficult to discern, since after proof-of-concept phase I studies, demonstrating that the drug target is inhibited in surrogate tissue provides no additional useful information.

V. BIOMARKERS AS PREDICTIVE FACTORS

Biomarkers can be used as predictive factors to identify patients likely to respond to a particular therapeutic agent. Examples in current oncology practice indicate that this approach is feasible. The expression of estrogen and progesterone receptors on breast cancer cells is a predictive marker for response to tamoxifen [9] and aromatase inhibitors [10]. The expression of HER-2/neu protein in breast cancer cells predicts for response to trastuzumab [11]. Clearly, the expression of ER/PR or HER-2/neu protein on breast cancer cells is necessary, but not sufficient for these tumors to respond to therapy with the above agents. Therefore, response rates in expressors of these proteins are approximately 20–50%, rather than close to 100%. In contrast, patients with tumors that are devoid of these proteins almost never respond to agents that target them [9, 12]. These biomarkers therefore allow for the enrichment of the treatment population in order to maximize responses. In designing trials to evaluate predictive markers, the end point of the study should be objective response rates, because the hypothesis tested is the ability of the marker to predict for a response to therapy. Theoretically, a marker that is only predictive of response could select patient populations that would yield high response rates in clinical trials without an effect on survival.

A. Why is the Positive Predictive Value of Biomarkers not 100%?

Reasons why a large proportion of human tumors that express a specific drug target do not respond to therapy that selectively and specifically inhibits the particular target are not exactly known; however, several contributing factors can be identified.

1. Tumors Possess Multiple Molecular Abnormalities

Most common epithelial tumors possess multiple molecular abnormalities. In addition, signal transduction pathways in tumors form a complex network with redundancies and cross-talk, rather than the parallel linear pathways that are often illustrated in manuscripts for simplicity (see Table 10.2) [13, 14]. Thus, inhibiting only one protein or pathway is not likely to kill the vast majority of tumors. There are examples in oncology in this regard. The most successful targeted agent to date, imatinib, is much more active in chronic phase chronic myelogenous leukemia (CML; complete cytogenic response rates of 20%) [15]. In this phase the tumor is driven predominantly by the bcr-abl oncogene, and is much less active in accelerated phase CML (complete cytogenetic response rates of 7% or less) [16], where multiple molecular abnormalities begin to appear, akin to the situation in a number of epithelial tumors. These considerations suggest that the limitation is not in the biomarkers, but the narrowly effective agents themselves.

2. Pharmacology is Important

In assessing biochemical targets with cell and molecular biology approaches, it can be forgotten that the drug has to get to its target. Most of the current targeted agents are orally administered, and are substrates for the CYP450 enzyme system. Polymorphisms in these enzymes combined with the concomitant ingestion of inhibitors and inducers of these enzymes [17] lead to highly variable systemic exposures to the drug. This problem is compounded by flat dosing of most of these agents in all patients. It is probably unreasonable to give 250 mg of gefitinib to the 45-kg, non-smoking lady and the 100-kg weightlifter who smokes, ingests alcohol regularly, and consumes anabolic steroids.

A number of these agents are further inactivated by phase II enzymes such as the sulfotransferases, which are known to possess functionally relevant polymorphisms [18]. Finally, there may be polymorphisms in the target, as has been recently described for epidermal growth factor receptor (EGFR) [19].

VI. BIOMARKERS AS PROGNOSTIC FACTORS

Biomarkers may also be used as prognostic factors. In these situations, the presence of a biomarker would correlate with the clinical outcome of a patient. The end point of a clinical trial to evaluate a prognostic factor should be survival, or some other clinical parameter such as time to progression. Part of the current confusion regarding the relevance and utility of biomarkers is related to the use of inappropriate end points for studies. Overexpression of the

TABLE 10.1 Biomarkers in Standard and Experimental Clinical Practice

Marker	Clinical use	Anticancer agent	Specific disease	Methodology
AFP	Predictive and prognostic marker	Non-specific	Hepatoma/germ cell tumor	ELISA
BCR-ABL	Predictive and prognostic marker	Non-specific	CML	Polymerase chain reaction
c-kit	Predictive and prognostic marker	Non-specific	GIST, AML	IHC
CA-125	Predictive and prognostic marker	Non-specific	Ovarian cancer	ELISA
CEA	Predictive and prognostic marker	Non-specific	Colon cancer liver metastasis	ELISA
ER	Predictive and prognostic marker	Non-specific	Breast cancer	IHC
Her2/Neu	Predictive and prognostic marker	Non-specific	Breast cancer Ovarian cancer	FISH IHC
β-HCG	Predictive and prognostic marker	Non-specific	Germ cell tumor	ELISA
p-ERK	PD marker	MEK, Raf kinase inhibitors	Multiple tumors	IHC Western blotting
PSA	Predictive and prognostic marker	Non-specific	Prostate cancer	ELISA
P70S6K	PD marker	mTOR inhibitors	No	IHC, Western blotting
Prelamin A/HDJ-2	PD Marker	FTIs	Multiple tumors	IHC, Western blotting

Abbreviations: AFP, alpha fetoprotein; BCR-ABL, break point cluster region of the ABELSON oncogene; c-kit, stem cell factor receptor (CD117); CA-125, cancer antigen 125; CEA, carcinoembryonic antigen; AML, acute myelogenous leukemia; β-HCG; beta subunit of human chorionic gonadotropic hormone.

HER-2/neu protein correlates with a poor outcome, and thus, successful inhibition of HER-2/neu with trastuzumab leads to improvements in survival [20].

Part of the reason why investigators have confused the predictive end points of response and prognostic end points of survival in clinical trials is because all the successful paradigms in clinical practice today involve biomarkers that are both predictive and prognostic (Table 10.1).

VII. TECHNICAL ISSUES IN THE EVALUATION OF DRUG EFFECTS *IN VIVO*

Evaluation of biomarkers in patient samples can be radically different from what occurs with pre-clinical samples for a variety of reasons. First, in the laboratory, significant manipulation of cell lines by transfections or gene knock-outs can occur in an effort to maximize the reproducibility of a particular assay. Secondly, experiments can be repeated as many times as necessary, with the same cell populations until reproducible results are obtained. Third, there is biological homogeneity in the cell lines and animal models used to test hypotheses. Thus, individual experiments can be pooled to increase statistical certainty of results.

In clinical translational work, limited amounts of tissue samples are obtained at a particular time point, experiments in individual patients cannot be repeated to test reproducibility and generate confidence intervals. Even more frustrating is the fact that it is impossible to repeat an assay, if technical difficulties render the one experiment uninterpretable. This means that strict attention to detail and extensive preliminary laboratory studies are needed to work out specific assays before their introduction into a clinical trial. Specific examples will be highlighted in this section.

A. Choice of Tissue for Biomarker Assays

In all correlative studies in drug development, the ideal tissue to be sampled is tumor. However, this is always difficult, because of cost, patient safety, and technical difficulties. In a number of tumor types such as lung cancer, prostate cancer, and brain tumors, tissue cannot be accessed in a safe, consistent manner because of the anatomic location. Because these biopsy procedures are utilized for investigational purposes with no possibility of a therapeutic benefit in most instances, obtaining consent becomes ethically difficult. As a compromise, most initial correlative studies are performed with surrogate tissue.

Two approaches have been utilized in an attempt to incorporate the successful utilization of tumor tissue in early phase studies. The first approach involves the use of surrogate tissue for biomarkers in the dose-escalation phase, with accrual of a relatively large (by phase I standards) cohort of 10–20 patients at the maximum tolerated dose (MTD) in whom tumor biopsies are obtained. Special efforts are made to accrue patients with readily accessible tumors for biopsies (melanoma, lymph node, and cutaneous metastases from various tumors) [2].

In the second approach, a phase IB study is performed in a tumor that is easily sampled (hematologic malignancies, melanoma, head and neck tumors) to specifically test the biomarker after assays are refined in surrogate tissue in the initial phase I study [8, 21]. The most common tissue surrogates utilized to date are skin, PBMCs, and buccal mucosa [3–5].

1. Skin as Surrogate Tissue

Clinical studies of the EGFR tyrosine kinase inhibitors, particularly gefitinib, have pioneered the use of skin as surrogate tissue for measuring drug effects. These assays are typically pharmacodynamic assays, which indicate that the drug has affected the target. They are important in phase I testing as proof-of-principle, but they may not have any predictive or prognostic value.

The utilization of skin has several advantages. The sampling is relatively non-invasive and can be performed by oncologists in the office. In some institutions, biopsies are obtained by dermatologists. Multiple serial biopsies can be performed with minimal morbidity.

The disadvantage relates to the types of assays that can be performed on this tissue. Because of small amounts of tissue normally obtained, immunohistochemistry and PCR-based studies can be performed, but not Western blotting. Tissue procurement and analysis has been previously described [3]. Briefly, skin specimens are obtained from an area of normal skin by an approximately 8 × 4 mm punch biopsy to the level of subcutaneous tissue or by an incisional biopsy of at least a 0.5 × 0.5 cm tissue. Specimens can be frozen, batched, and thawed for analysis at a later date. For immunohisto-chemistry, specimens are embedded in paraffin after thawing.

2. Peripheral Blood Mononuclear Cells as Surrogate Tissue

PBMCs are the most widely utilized surrogate tissue. Blood sampling is such an integral part of modern medical care, especially in phase I clinical trials where repetitive samples are drawn for pharmacokinetic analysis, that obtaining an extra tube of blood for correlative studies is never seen as a burdensome exercise. For this reason, this is the most convenient and practical surrogate tissue for clinical trials. The advantages are the ready availability of multiple samples, the large number of health-care workers (physicians, nurses, phlebotomists) who can safely procure samples, and typically, the ability of adequate material for a variety of assays.

The main disadvantage was the time-intensive procedure involved in isolation of PBMCs from whole blood by Ficoll gradients and the preparation of samples for Western blotting. With the advent of pre-prepared PBMC separation kits such as the Vacutainer CPT tubes, this process has been greatly simplified. These assays have been previously described [4, 8]. In brief, about 10 mL of blood is collected in Vacutainer CPT tubes (Beckton Dickinson) and centrifuged at room temperature for 15 minutes at 2500 rpm. After centrifugation, the mononuclear cell layer is diluted to 50 mL with 1X PBS and sedimented at 1200 rpm × 10 minutes Cells are re-suspended in 10.5 mL RPMI-HEPES pH 7.4) and counted. A 10-mL aliquot is solubilized in alkylation buffer consisting of 6 M guanidine hydrochloride, 250 mM Tris-HCl (pH 8.5 at 21°C), 10 mM EDTA, 1% (v/v) β-mercaptoethanol, and 1 mM 2-phenylmethylsulfonyl fluoride (freshly added from a 100-mM stock in anhydrous isopropanol). After the cell lysates are dialyzed and lyophilized as previously described [8], aliquots containing approximately 50 μg of protein (assayed by the bicinchoninic acid method) are subjected to electrophoresis on SDS-polyacrylamide gels, transferred to nitrocellulose, and probed with the relevant primary and secondary antibodies.

3. Buccal Mucosa Cells as Surrogate Tissue

The use of buccal mucosa cells as surrogate markers of drug activity was recently highlighted by Adjei and colleagues in their work with farnesyl transferase inhibitors (see Figure 10.1) [8].

Buccal mucosa cells are probably the easiest surrogate tissue to obtain. The collection procedure is painless, and any health-care worker can be trained to obtain samples. Their easy accessibility and the rapid turnover of these cells make them ideal for the study of agents that may interfere with proliferation. They share the same disadvantages of a restrictive assay choice with skin. Because small amounts of cells are obtained, IHC- and PCR-based techniques are the only approaches that can be used.

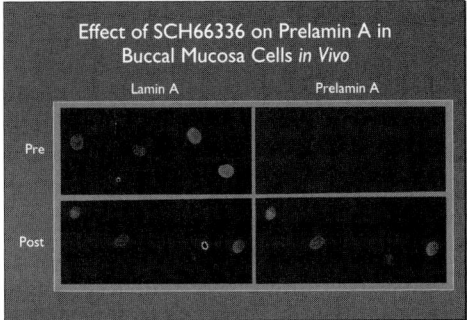

FIGURE 10.1   Detection of prelamin A in buccal mucosa cells from SCH66336-treated patients. Buccal smears were double labeled with mouse anti-lamin A (left) and rabbit anti-prelamin A (right) followed by fluorochrome-labeled secondary antibodies. Corresponding fields were photographed. Bottom panel: samples harvested on day 8 from patients treated with 300 mg b.i.d. of SCH66336. Upper panel: pretreatment sample from same patient. See Color Plate 16.

The procedure for sample collection and preparation for double-label IHC is described briefly here. The samples are best obtained prior to breakfast to minimize the presence of proteolytic enzymes that can digest the buccal mucosa cells and interfere with results. The patient should have no food for approximately 15 minutes prior to this procedure. Patients gently swish and spit approximately 100 mL of saline. This is repeated twice. The inside of the mouth is firmly scraped with a clean wooden tongue depressor. The scraped cells are spread on a clean charged microscope slide (Superfrost$^+$, Fischer Scientific). Using a fresh tongue depressor each time, the scraping and deposition are repeated until a total of four slides are obtained. These slides are air-dried and fixed in acetone within 3 hours of harvest. Samples can be stored in buffer A consisting of 10% (w/v) powdered milk in 150 mM NaCl, 10 mM Tris-HCl (pH 7.4 at 21°C), 100 U/mL penicillin G, 100 μg/ml streptomycin, and 1 mM sodium azide and subjected to immunohistochemical assay in batches [8, 22].

4. Rational Use of Biomarker Assays in Surrogate Tissue

A major problem in the use of correlative markers in clinical trials is the failure of investigators to evaluate assays in the relevant tissue before incorporating them into clinical trials. Surrogate tissue should be selected based on its expression of the biomarker of interest. Thus, skin is an appropriate surrogate tissue for the evaluation of the effect of EGFR inhibitors, because EGFR is widely expressed in skin [7]. However, skin was found not to be an appropriate surrogate tissue for the evaluation of the effect of MEK inhibitors, because phosphorylated ERK is not expressed in skin. In a completed phase I trial of the MEK inhibitor, CI-1040 PBMCs were used as surrogate tissue. However, preliminary studies in PBMCs isolated from volunteers demonstrated the lack of expression of p-ERK. Thus assays were developed that involved the *ex vivo* stimulation of isolated PBMCs with phorbol esters to activate p-ERK [2]. Similarly, in a study of the FTI lonafarnib (SCH 66336) our group identified prelamin A, a protein that is farnesylated and cleaved to form lamin A, which is a good biomarker of FT inhibition. Preliminary laboratory studies indicated that PBMCs do not express lamin A. Further investigation identified buccal mucosa as an ideal surrogate tissue for evaluating the effects of lonafarnib on the target enzyme, FT (see Figure 10.1) [23].

5. Shortcomings of Surrogate Tissue

The major advantage of utilizing normal tissue surrogates is that these are easily accessible and amenable to multiple sampling. The disadvantages have been discussed in recent publications [4, 24]. A clear disadvantage is that events in surrogate tissue may not reflect intra-tumoral events. Thus assays in surrogate tissue are useful in the phase I setting, where an attempt is made to show that a known target can be inhibited *in vivo*. In the phase II setting, these assays are of limited use. Demonstrating that EGFR phosphorylation may be inhibited in skin does not address events in the tumor. There are no convincing data that biomarkers in any surrogate tissue correlate with events in tumor. However, it needs to be stated that there are few studies that have attempted to correlate changes in markers in surrogate tissue with changes in tumor.

B. Evaluation of Biomarkers in Tumor Tissue

Evaluating biomarkers in tumor tissue is the gold standard for correlative studies evaluating drug effects. Predictive markers, prognostic markers, or a combination can be tested in tumor tissue. Current equivocal results from tumor-based studies are partly due to the testing of faulty hypotheses and poor assay development.

1. Sampling of Tumor Tissue

Tumor samples are obtained by two main procedures. The more common approach is to obtain biopsies, either at the time of surgery, by incision into a superficial lesion, or with a needle in deep lesions. Needle biopsies are usually aided by imaging modalities such as an ultrasound or computed axial tomography (CT scans).

2. Tumor Biopsies

Procedures that yield adequate tissue for multiple analyses include samples taken at surgery and biopsies of superficial tissues by incision or with a large-bore (14–16 gauge) needle. An example of how our group handles biopsy specimens is given below. For studies where multiple assays (Western blotting, PCR, and IHC) are performed on tissue, fresh biopsies are immediately split into four aliquots constituting approximately 15, 35, 35, and 15%, respectively. Each of the 35% aliquots can be snap frozen on liquid nitrogen in preparation for Western blotting and PCR. One 15% aliquot can be frozen at $-20°C$ in OCT compound in preparation for immunohistochemistry, and the other aliquot is processed for normal H&E stains to confirm the tissue diagnosis by pathology.

3. Collection of Circulating Tumor Cells

An approach that is being developed, which holds promise for easy access to tumor tissue for correlative assays, is the isolation of circulating tumor DNA in patients' plasma. It has long been demonstrated that small quantities of DNA circulate in the plasma of healthy subjects [25, 26]. A number of recent studies have shown that tumor DNA is shed in the plasma of cancer patients in much greater quantities — up to four- and five-fold higher concentrations than in the normal population [27].

Specific mutations found in genes in the primary tumors but not present in the patient's genomic DNA can be identified in the DNA from plasma, which demonstrates that the source of the DNA in plasma is the tumor. Abnormalities that have been detected in a number of pilot studies include microsatellite alterations, immunoglobulin rearrangements, mutant DNA (K-ras, APC), and hypermethylation of several genes [27]. As an example, Sozzi and colleagues [28] have quantified free circulating DNA in patients with lung cancer. They utilized real-time quantitative polymerase chain reaction (RT-PCR) and human telomerase catalytic component (hTERT) primers. Median concentration of circulating plasma DNA in patients was almost eight times the value detected in age-, sex-, and smoking-matched controls (24.3 vs. 3.1 ng/mL) [28]. In other studies, methylation-specific PCR techniques have been used to quantitate the methylation of the promoter regions of a number of oncogenes [29–31]. This approach holds promise for easy access to tumor material for correlative, predictive, and prognostic studies, once methodologic issues and inconsistent results from different studies are sorted out [32].

4. Shortcomings of Assays in Tumor Tissue

A number of drawbacks in the assessment of biomarkers using tumor tissue exist. A common criticism is that only parts of the tumor is sampled, and because of tumor cell heterogeneity, the sampled tumor may not represent the total tumor population. This is a valid criticism; however, the advantages of performing assays on tumor rather than normal surrogate tissue far outweigh this disadvantage. Nevertheless, investigators have attempted to resolve this by sampling multiple sites in a single tumor, when feasible. The other criticism of assays utilizing tumor samples relates to the fact that biopsy samples contain tumor as well as vascular and connective tissue. A biomarker may therefore be identified that may not be present in tumor tissue, but rather in the normal supporting structures. Laser capture microdissection to isolate tumor cells has been used to overcome this problem [33].

The most common problem encountered in the use of tumor samples for biomarker assays is the limited samples available for performing assays. Occasionally, biopsy samples are made up entirely of adipose and connective tissue with no tumor cells present. Most often, there is only a limited amount of tumor available. Strategies to overcome this include taking multiple samples of adequate size. This approach requires investigators to identify patients with superficial lesions that lend themselves to multiple sampling. It is difficult to obtain multiple 0.5-cm samples from metastatic liver or lung lesions under ultrasound or CT guidance, because of the high risk of serious complications. More refined PCR assays in the future requiring a minimal amount of tumor tissue will also help circumvent this problem.

a. Prediction of Response versus Patient Enrichment

The most successful use of biomarkers in oncology involve the selection of patients who are likely to respond to particular therapies (Table 10.1). A number of researchers have invested considerable effort in trying to demonstrate that the inhibition of a target in tumor tissue correlates with clinical outcome, with disappointing results. There are many potential reasons for these negative results. A major reason is that the hypothesis tested in these situations is inherently flawed. Unless a tumor depends solely on one protein or pathway without any cross-talk with parallel pathways, it is difficult to imagine how inhibiting that protein may be tightly correlated with clinical response. Many epithelial tumors such as lung cancer contain multiple genetic abnormalities (see Table 10.2). It may be necessary to inhibit multiple proteins or pathways in order to achieve significant tumor shrinkage and prolong the survival of patients with current targeted therapy. Secondly, there are multiple factors that contribute to tumor response, apart from biochemical inhibition of a target. As a reminder, the only examples in clinical practice where changes in a "marker" may correlate with clinical response are those of a select few tumor markers: prostate specific antigen (PSA) in prostate cancer, cancer antigen 125 (CA-125) in ovarian cancer, human chorionic gonadotropin (HCG) and alpha fetoprotein (AFP) in germ cell tumors.

TABLE 10.2   Molecular Abnormalities in Non-Small Cell Lung Cancer

Molecular abnormality	Incidence in NSCLC (%)	Agent(s) targeting aberrant pathway
Ras mutation	40	Farnesyltransferase inhibitors, antisense oligonucleotides, raf inhibitors, MEK inhibitors, 17AAG
Myc amplification	10	None
EGFR expression	40–80	EGFR tyrosine kinase inhibitors; EGFR antibodies
c-erb B-2 overexpression	30	Trastuzumab, EGFRTK inhibitors, 17AAG
c-kit/SCFR co-expression	15	STI-571, SU11248
bcl-2 expression	35	PS-341, G3139
p53 mutation	50	PS-341, flavopiridol
RB deletion (protein)	20	CCI-779, flavopiridol
p16 inactivation	70	CCI-779
COX-2 expression	70	COX-2 inhibitors
3p deletion	50	None
VEGF expression	50–90	Monoclonal antibodies, RTK inhibitors, FTI
Matrix metalloproteinase (gelatinase)	65	Matrix metalloproteinase inhibitors

VIII. LESSONS FOR THE FUTURE

Clearly, with the introduction of novel drugs whose targets are known, there is considerable interest in assessing the cellular and subcellular effects of these drugs in the clinical setting. Conceptually, assays of drug action could serve two purposes. In early clinical trials, these assays will be required to determine whether the target has been inhibited at drug concentrations that are achievable in the clinical setting. In later clinical trials, these assays could potentially provide an early marker of drug efficacy if a strong correlation between assay results and clinical outcome can be established. Investigators may be more successful if they try to use baseline biochemical tumor characteristics such as the expression of a protein to select those patients most likely to respond to therapy. As bioinformatics becomes established as a discipline and vast amounts of data from microarray and mass spectroscopy experiments are analyzed consistently, proteomics and genomics might improve the accuracy of predicting tumors that are more likely to respond to specific therapeutic agents. This approach, by evaluating a large array of proteins and genes, can pick up patterns of overexpression.

ACKNOWLEDGMENTS

The author wishes to thank Mrs. Raquel Ostby for excellent secretarial support.

REFERENCES

1. De Gruttola VG, Clax P, DeMets DL et al. Considerations in the evaluation of surrogate endpoints in clinical trials. summary of a National Institutes of Health workshop. *Control Clin. Trials* 2001; 22:485–502.
2. LoRusso PM AA, Meyer MB et al. A phase I clinical and pharmacokinetic evaluation of oral CI-1040 administered for 21 consecutive days, repeated every 4 weeks in patients with advanced cancer. *Proc. ASCO* 2002; 21.
3. Albanell J, Rojo F, Averbuch S et al. Pharmacodynamic studies of the epidermal growth factor receptor inhibitor ZD1839 in skin from cancer patients: Histopathologic and molecular consequences of receptor inhibition. *J Clin. Oncol.* 2002; 20:110–124.
4. Peralba JM, DeGraffenried L, Friedrichs W et al. Pharmacodynamic Evaluation of CCI-779, an Inhibitor of mTOR, in Cancer Patients. *Clin. Cancer Res.* 2003; 9:2887–2892.
5. Adjei AA. Immunohistochemical assays of farnesyltransferase inhibition in patient samples. In *Novel Anticancer Drug Protocols* (Buolamwinin J and Adjei AA, eds.), Humana Press, Totowa, NJ, 2003, pp. 141–145.
6. Williams S, Pettaway C, Song R et al. Differential effects of the proteasome inhibitor bortezomib on apoptosis and angiogenesis in human prostate tumor xenografts. *Mol. Cancer Ther.* 2003; 2:835–843.
7. Malik SN, Siu LL, Rowinsky EK et al. Pharmacodynamic evaluation of the epidermal growth factor receptor inhibitor OSI-774 in human epidermis of cancer patients. *Clin. Cancer Res.* 2003; 9:2478–2486.
8. Adjei AA, Erlichman C, Davis JN et al. A Phase I trial of the farnesyl transferase inhibitor SCH66336: evidence for biological and clinical activity. *Cancer Res.* 2000; 60: 1871–1877.
9. Anonymous. Tamoxifen for early breast cancer. Early Breast Cancer Trialists' Collaborative Group. *Cochrane Database Syst. Rev.* 2001; 1:CD000486.

10. Smith IE, Dowsett M. Aromatase inhibitors in breast cancer. *N. Engl. J. Med.* 2003; 348:2431–2442.

11. Takahashi M, Inoue K, Goto R et al. Metastatic breast cancer of HER2 scored 2+ by IHC and HER2 gene amplification assayed by FISH has a good response to single agent therapy with trastuzumab: A case report. *Breast Cancer* 2003; 10:170–174.

12. Leyland-Jones B. Maximizing the response to Herceptin therapy through optimal use and patient selection. *Anticancer Drugs* 2001; 12:S11–17.

13. Dy GK, Adjei AA. Novel targets for lung cancer therapy: Part I. *J. Clin. Oncol.* 2002; 20:2881–2894.

14. Dy GK, Adjei AA. Novel targets for lung cancer therapy: Part II. *J. Clin. Oncol.* 2002; 20:3016–3028.

15. Druker BJ, Talpaz M, Resta DJ et al. Efficacy and safety of a specific inhibitor of the BCR-ABL tyrosine kinase in chronic myeloid leukemia. *N. Engl. J. Med.* 2001; 344:1031–1037.

16. Sawyers CL, Hochhaus A, Feldman E et al. Imatinib induces hematologic and cytogenetic responses in patients with chronic myelogenous leukemia in myeloid blast crisis: results of a phase II study. *Blood* 2002; 99:3530–3539.

17. McLeod HL, Yu J. Cancer pharmacogenomics: SNPs, chips, and the individual patient. *Cancer Invest.* 2003; 21:630–640.

18. Weinshilboum R. Inheritance and drug response. *N. Engl. J. Med.* 2003; 348:529–537.

19. Liu W, Innocenti F, Chen P et al. Interethnic difference in the allelic distribution of human epidermal growth factor receptor intron 1 polymorphism. *Clin. Cancer Res.* 2003; 9:1009–1012.

20. Ross JS, Fletcher JA, Linette GP et al. The Her-2/neu gene and protein in breast cancer 2003: Biomarker and target of therapy. *Oncologist* 2003; 8:307–325.

21. Karp JE, Lancet JE, Kaufmann SH et al. Clinical and biologic activity of the farnesyltransferase inhibitor R115777 in adults with refractory and relapsed acute leukemias: A phase 1 clinical-laboratory correlative trial. *Blood* 2001; 97:3361–3369.

22. Adjei AA, Mauer A, Bruzek L et al. Phase II study of the farnesyl transferase inhibitor R115777 in patients with advanced non-small-cell lung cancer. *J. Clin. Oncol.* 2003; 21:1760–1766.

23. Adjei AA, Davis JN, Erlichman C, Svingen PA, Kaufmann SH. Comparison of potential markers of farnesyltransferase inhibition. *Clin. Cancer Res.* 2000; 6:2318–2325.

24. Arteaga CL, Baselga J. Clinical trial design and end points for epidermal growth factor receptor-targeted therapies: Implications for drug development and practice. *Clin. Cancer Res.* 2003; 9:1579–1589.

25. Steinman CR. Free DNA in serum and plasma from normal adults. *J. Clin. Invest.* 1975; 56:512–515.

26. Raptis L, Menard HA. Quantitation and characterization of plasma DNA in normals and patients with systemic lupus erythematosus. *J. Clin. Invest.* 1980; 66:1391–1399.

27. Kawaguchi T, Holland WS, Gumerlock PH. Methods for isolation and genetic analysis of circulating tumor DNA in patient plasma. *Methods Mol. Med.* 2003; 85:257–262.

28. Sozzi G, Conte D, Leon M et al. Quantification of free circulating DNA as a diagnostic marker in lung cancer. *J. Clin. Oncol.* 2003; 21:3902–3908.

29. Usadel H, Brabender J, Danenberg KD et al. Quantitative adenomatous polyposis coli promoter methylation analysis in tumor tissue, serum, and plasma DNA of patients with lung cancer. *Cancer Res.* 2002; 62:371–375.

30. Ramirez JL, Sarries C, de Castro PL et al. Methylation patterns and K-ras mutations in tumor and paired serum of resected non-small-cell lung cancer patients. *Cancer Lett.* 2003; 193:207–216.

31. Bearzatto A, Conte D, Frattini M et al. p16(INK4A) Hypermethylation detected by fluorescent methylation-specific PCR in plasmas from non-small cell lung cancer. *Clin. Cancer Res.* 2002; 8:3782–3787.

32. Bunn PA, Jr. Early detection of lung cancer using serum RNA or DNA markers: ready for "prime time" or for validation? *J. Clin. Oncol.* 2003; 21:3891–3893.

33. Barisoni L, Star RA. Laser-capture microdissection. *Methods Mol. Med.* 2003; 86:237–255.

11

REGULATORY CONSIDERATIONS IN CLINICAL TRIALS OF NOVEL ANTICANCER DRUGS

GRANT WILLIAMS
RICHARD PAZDUR

Division of Oncology Drug Products
Center for Drug Evaluation and Research
Food and Drug Administration
Rockville, Maryland

I. INTRODUCTION
II. OVERVIEW OF CANCER DRUG REGULATION
III. REGULATORY CONSIDERATIONS IN EARLY CANCER
   DRUG DEVELOPMENT
IV. REGULATORY CONSIDERATIONS IN LATE DRUG
   DEVELOPMENT
V. CONCLUSION

I. INTRODUCTION

This chapter discusses regulatory considerations in clinical trials for "novel" anticancer drugs. Novel anticancer drugs are often designed to be more specific and less cytotoxic than conventional anticancer drugs. Although no special regulations exist for these agents, the implications of existing regulations may differ. This chapter addresses general regulatory principles for cancer drug approval and comments on issues specific for novel agents where appropriate (see Table 11.1).

The examples given in this chapter are from regulatory experience in the Division of Oncology Drug Products (DODP) in the United States Food and Drug Administration (FDA)'s Center for Drug Evaluation and Research (CDER). This chapter was not written to address cancer biological products and does not address some of the special considerations in biologic drug development.

The chapter is divided into three parts: overview of cancer drug regulation, regulatory considerations in early trials, and regulatory considerations in late trials.

The overview of cancer drug regulation discusses the FDA's role in cancer drug development. The section on early trials discusses the Investigational

TABLE 11.1   Differences Between Novel Drugs and Conventional Cytotoxic Drugs

Expected difference from conventional drug	Trial phase most affected	Considerations for trial design
Less toxicity	I	MTD not goal of phase I
	III	Affects benefit to risk ratio. Less benefit may be acceptable if toxicity is less
Different toxicity profile	I, II, III	Clinical trials should evaluate new toxicities
Chronic treatment with drug	I, II, III	Evaluate whether preclinical chronic testing is needed
	III	Design clinical trials to evaluate chronic toxicities
Early use in combination	I, II	Evaluate whether preclinical tests of drug combinations are required
		Design phase I trials of combinations
	III	Demonstrate the contribution of each drug to efficacy of the combination
Different clinical benefits	II, III	Design endpoints to measure new clinical benefit (e.g., measuring bone morbidity of biphosphonate drugs)
Blinding of trials possible	III	May use more subjective end points (e.g., pain or symptoms)

New Drug Application (IND) (the initial application to the FDA for evaluating a drug in humans) and the design of phase I and phase II trials. The section on later trials discusses the FDA's role in evaluating end points and trial designs for phase III marketing trials. It presents a comprehensive table of study end points used in cancer drug approvals.

II. OVERVIEW OF CANCER DRUG REGULATION

A. IND Regulations

The responsibilities of the FDA and of sponsors of INDs are outlined in the Code of Federal Regulations (CFR) 21 part 312. Any use of a drug that is not marketed in the United States must be carried out under an IND. The IND provides permission to use an investigational drug according to a protocol filed with the FDA. The regulatory definitions of two parties involved with INDs are presented below:

- The *sponsor* initiates and assumes responsibility for the clinical investigation. The sponsor is usually a pharmaceutical company, but individuals or academic institutions may also serve as sponsors.
- The *investigator* performs the trial. The regulations stipulate that a sponsor shall "select only investigators qualified by training and experience as appropriate experts to investigate the drug." The FDA expects the investigator to be a licensed physician with training and experience in treating cancer.

The FDA role varies with the stage of drug development and includes: (1) experimental subject protection, (2) guidance on clinical trial design, and (3) verification of clinical trial results and of supporting data in marketing applications such as new drug applications (NDAs) for drugs or biologics license applications (BLAs) for biologic products.

A clinical study of a marketed drug product is exempt from the requirement to file an IND if it meets all of five criteria [21 CFR 312.2(b) (1)]: The study (1) is not intended to support approval of a new indication or a significant change in the product labeling, (2) is not intended to support a significant change in advertising, (3) does not involve a route of administration or dosage level or use in a patient population or other factor that significantly increases the risks (or decreases the acceptability of the risks) associated with the use of the drug product, (4) is conducted in compliance with Institutional Review Board (IRB) and informed consent regulations, and (5) will not be used to promote unapproved indications. Although an IND is not needed for such studies, requirements for informed consent and IRB approval are unchanged. The practice of oncology frequently involves treatment of cancer patients for indications not yet included in the drug label. An FDA guidance document assists investigators to determine whether an IND is required for oncology drug studies. Literature data from phase 1 or phase 2 trials can often supply sufficient information to support an IND exemption [1].

B. IND Process

The IND process is initiated by submission of an IND application and continues throughout the period a drug is under investigation. For conventional cancer drugs, the first study is usually a dose-escalating phase I trial to identify dose-limiting toxicities and the maximally tolerated dose. Phase II trials are usually single-arm studies that screen for anti-tumor activity in selected tumors. If the drug is active, the sponsor conducts larger randomized phase III registration trials that usually evaluate the drug's effect compared to (or added to) standard therapy. The objective is to demonstrate whether the drug produces clinical benefit, such as improvement in survival or disease-related symptoms.

C. NDA Process

If the sponsor concludes that the drug is safe and effective, it submits detailed study results and supporting data in an NDA. The FDA is committed under the Prescription Drug User Fee Act (PDUFA) to review most NDAs in 6 or 10 months (depending on the importance of the drug). NDAs contain all data from IND investigations. The NDA includes chemistry and manufacturing data, animal data, and human clinical trial data. The application is reviewed by a team of FDA reviewers, which includes oncologists, chemists, toxicologists, clinical pharmacologists, and statisticians. A field team evaluates selected clinical sites to validate clinical data and to inspect manufacturing facilities. The FDA often presents results of the review to the Oncology Drugs Advisory Committee (ODAC) for advice.

The FDA subsequently takes an action, which is communicated to the company by one of three types of letters: (1) an Approval Letter that allows the sponsor to market the drug, (2) an Approvable Letter that states the deficiencies that must be corrected prior to marketing, and (3) a Not Approvable Letter that indicates that the drug is not approved.

D. Review by CDER or CBER

A new agent will be reviewed by either the FDA's CDER or the Center for Biologics Evaluation and Research (CBER). Several recent and anticipated changes affect the assignment of FDA review authority for cancer drug applications. Prior to 2003, all biologic drug products were reviewed in CBER. In 2003, review responsibility for biotechnology derived biologics was transferred to CDER. FDA has announced that in 2005 review of these cancer biologics, most other cancer drugs, chemoprevention agents, and imaging drug products will be assigned to one office of cancer drug review in CDER. Cancer vaccines and cell-derived biologic products will continue to be reviewed in CBER.

E. The FDA Regulatory Approach to Cancer Drugs

Compared to patients with less serious medical conditions, cancer patients and physicians accept greater risks in exchange for the potential of life prolongation [2]. Risks and potential benefits of treatment vary with cancer type and stage. The FDA incorporates the oncology community perspective into the review process. IND and NDA review teams are led by FDA oncologists and include outside oncology experts during the planning and review of clinical trials. Patient and consumer representatives are present on the ODAC.

The intensity of FDA involvement in the design and analysis of cancer clinical trials varies with the stage of drug development. The FDA frequently offers input to sponsors during planning of early trials and late trials (i.e., during early phase I and during phase III development). During late phase I and during phase II development, the challenges are more scientific than regulatory. In late phase I, a dose is selected for further testing and in phase II preliminary evidence is collected regarding drug activity — neither of these tasks pose regulatory concerns regarding safety or efficacy.

The FDA review of phase I trials emphasizes safety. The sponsor submits an IND application containing the phase I clinical protocol and data on chemistry, manufacturing, and preclinical testing. The FDA must evaluate the safety of the IND plan within 30 days to determine whether the trial may proceed. FDA reviewers evaluate these data and the clinical protocol to ensure that the proposed dose, schedule, and monitoring plan are safe. Thirty days after the FDA receives the IND, the study may proceed unless the FDA notifies the sponsor otherwise. (Irrespective of the FDA findings, sponsors should expect notification of the FDA's findings and recommendations within 30 days.) If the FDA determines the plan is unsafe, the sponsor is notified by telephone that the study should not proceed (the study is on *clinical hold*) and receives a letter detailing the deficiencies. The clinical hold is removed after FDA verifies that the sponsor has addressed the deficiencies.

After the initial protocol submission, new protocols submitted to the IND may proceed without any waiting period. The FDA can place subsequent trials on clinical hold if safety concerns arise.

Prior to conducting phase III trials, sponsors are encouraged to meet with the FDA to discuss trial design in *end-of-phase 2 meetings*. At these meetings, the sponsor and the FDA agree on end points and trial designs that would support a marketing claim. When phase III trials are complete, the sponsor submits the trial results in an NDA. The FDA performs an in-depth multidisciplinary review to verify that results demonstrate that the drug is effective and safe for the labeled use, thus meeting the statutory standard for NDA approval. Guidances, suggesting approaches to evaluating particular tumors or providing general advice, and transcripts from meetings of the ODAC, which "update" the guidances by indicating recent agency and advisory committee deliberations, are available from FDA Web sites [3, 4].

III. REGULATORY CONSIDERATIONS IN EARLY CANCER DRUG DEVELOPMENT

Early cancer drug development is described in three subsections: (1) preclinical studies supporting the IND submission, phase I trial design, and phase II trial design.

A. Preclinical Studies Supporting the IND Submission

During pre-IND meetings, the FDA indicates the toxicology testing required to support initial clinical trials. Although the preclinical tests for cytotoxic drugs have been discussed [5] requirements for novel drugs may need clarification.

An early challenge with novel anticancer agents is the selection of agents for human studies. Although the selection of cytotoxic drugs is often based on human tumor xenograft models in nude mice, these models may not be useful with novel agents. First, the models are most sensitive to drugs that cause tumor necrosis, and this may not be the mechanism of action for selected novel agents. Second, some molecular targets of novel agents are unique to humans (e.g., complementary strands of some antisense drugs).

Animal studies should support the safety of the starting dose of phase I clinical trials. For oncology drugs, at least two studies are needed, one in a rodent and another in a non-rodent species. Animal studies should use the same schedule and route of administration proposed for the phase I clinical study. The starting dose for human studies is usually one-tenth of the mouse STD_{10} (dose where 10% of animals have severe toxicity) calculated on a milligrams per meter squared basis provided this dose does not result in irreversible toxicity in non-rodents. If this dose causes irreversible toxicity, one-sixth of the highest dose that does not produce irreversible toxicity is selected for the starting dose [5].

The above preclinical testing procedure may also be adequate for most novel drugs, with two possible exceptions. First, if a drug's molecular target is unique to humans, routine animal models may not predict mechanism-specific toxicity likely to occur in humans. Mechanism-specific toxicities might be predicted by special tests, such as knock-out mouse models for antisense products or human tissue binding patterns for monoclonal antibodies. Second, with novel agents, chronic testing in animals should be considered earlier in development. The FDA does not usually require chronic animal studies prior to phase I clinical testing of cytotoxic drugs because these drugs are administered periodically (usually every 21 to 28 days). The FDA assumes full recovery from toxic effects between doses. However, selected novel anticancer agents may be given daily, on prolonged, continuous schedules, and recovery from toxicities between doses would not be expected. If the starting dose has been identified but chronic studies have not yet been performed, consultation with toxicologists in the FDA Oncology Group may identify a mechanism for proceeding with human studies prior to completing chronic studies.

B. Phase I Trial Design

In contrast to other therapeutic areas, phase I oncology trials are infrequently performed in healthy volunteers, because oncology drugs are usually toxic (often genotoxic) and oncology studies usually escalate until some patients experience severe toxicities. Limited phase I or pharmacokinetic studies are sometimes performed in healthy volunteers for oncology drugs that are relatively nontoxic.

1. Traditional Phase I Trial Design

In recent years investigators have used several different phase I dose-escalation methods. In the 1980s and early 1990s, the modified Fibonacci scheme was commonly used. This scheme used large initial dose-escalation steps that become progressively smaller. This scheme is seldom used today. Pharmacologically guided dosing was evaluated in the early 1990s with limited success, but was difficult logistically [6].

2. Accelerated Dose Escalation Designs

During the early and mid-1990s, the FDA permitted investigators to use several new methods for accelerating dose escalation. With very careful monitoring, 100% dose-escalation steps were used until investigators observed the first sign of biologic activity, when more modest escalation steps of 25–50% were used. Several accelerated phase I designs were formalized by Simon et al., in 1997 [7]. In these designs, the occurrence of grade 2 toxicity is the harbinger of early drug toxicity. The occurrence of two instances of grade 2 toxicity ends the accelerated phase of dose escalation. The occurrence of a single grade 2 toxicity in a cohort of three patients is attributed to chance, and the accelerated escalation phase continues. If these designs are used and grade 2 toxicity is encountered in one patient, escalation should not continue until additional patients are evaluated at that dose.

In standard phase I designs, multiple patients are included at each dose level to detect differences in toxicities due to inter-patient differences in drug metabolism. However, single-patient cohorts may be used in accelerated dose-escalation designs. In these accelerated escalation trials, differences in blood levels and toxicities between dose groups are likely to exceed inter-patient differences. If no toxicity is observed in the first patient, additional patients at the same dose are unlikely to be helpful. A disadvantage to single-patients cohorts in accelerated escalation trials is that when grade 2 toxicity occurs in one patient, the study must be delayed for evaluation of additional patients at the same dose.

In the 1990s many phase I studies used accelerated dose-escalation designs with few problems [8]. While the apparent safety of using accelerated dose-escalation schemes is encouraging, concern has been expressed in several circumstances as listed below:

1. Animal dose-toxicity curve is steep
2. Preclinical dose-limiting toxicities are unusual
3. Drugs are intended for continuous chronic dosing

Accelerated-escalation designs assume that the dose of investigational drug can be doubled without lethal or irreversible toxicity. Although there is no proven association between dose-toxicity curves in animals and humans, when animal studies show a steep dose-toxicity curve (e.g., when no animals in a cohort treated at one dose die and all of the animals at the next dose die), caution may be advised in using accelerated dose-escalation designs.

Accelerated dose-escalation schemes rely on detection of mild toxicities to terminate the rapid escalation phase. Experience with accelerated dose escalation designs is predominantly from trials using cytotoxic drugs that have predictable, reversible, and easily-monitored toxicities (e.g., bone marrow suppression). Reservations have been expressed about using accelerated designs when lethal toxicities observed in animals are poorly characterized or when the predicted human toxicity may be irreversible (e.g., CNS toxicity).

A third concern involves continuous administration schedules. Most oncology drugs have been administered over a short time, which allows for recovery from toxicities between courses. Selected novel drugs will be given daily and chronically, and dose-limiting toxicity may sometimes be delayed, which reflects chronic drug accumulation. Rapid escalation schedules, especially those including intra-patient escalation, may lead to confusion regarding the relationships among duration, dose, and toxicity.

3. Other Phase I Trial Designs

Other phase I designs have been used including the modified Continual Reassessment Method (mCRM) [9]. A goal of this method is to better estimate the optimal phase II dose. This approach seems acceptable provided the maximum size of dose-escalation steps is limited.

C. Phase II Trial Design

Phase II cancer trials are used to select promising drugs for further testing. Historically, there has been comparatively little regulatory attention to the design of these trials because efficacy results were seldom submitted to support marketing claims. However, in recent years phase II studies in refractory patients have supported accelerated approvals in specific settings (see Section IV.B.2).

Evaluating novel anticancer drugs in phase II studies presents scientific challenges. The traditional phase II trial design, which requires limited patient numbers, is based on objective response rates (RR) that can be measured in single-arm studies. This single-arm trial design is inappropriate for novel cytostatic drugs, which may delay tumor progression rather than causing tumor size reduction.

New phase II trial designs have been proposed [10]. One design uses single-arm trials and compares results to historical experience. Trial results may be questioned, however, because historical controls are often unreliable. Variation in prognoses between populations is often larger than the treatment effects attributed to anticancer drugs.

A second approach is to use a randomized control group and measure time to progression (TTP), but require a less definitive p value for claiming success, ($p = 0.10$ or 0.20, rather than 0.05). This design may provide a high rate of false positive trials. Even if the trial were positive, considerable doubt would exist regarding drug activity.

Another approach is to evaluate the rate of progression of a surrogate marker over a selected time period prior to treatment and determine whether this rate of change is altered after treatment. This assumes that the tumor possesses a relatively constant growth rate over time and that the surrogate accurately reflects tumor growth.

A randomized discontinuation design has been proposed for phase II evaluations [11]. All patients are given the investigational drug during a "run-in period." Patients with stable disease during the run-in period are randomized to continue drug or switch to placebo. The numbers of patients demonstrating progressive disease are compared after a pre-specified time. If a statistically significant difference is demonstrated, the randomized discontinuation design provides strong evidence of drug activity. Relative to other randomized study designs, accrual may be improved because all patients will receive the investigational drug initially. In addition, patients who receive placebo during the discontinuation phase can again receive investigational drug upon progression. There are, however, weaknesses of the randomized discontinuation design. The rate of anti-tumor activity is not measured in the overall study population, so it is difficult to estimate the size of the observed treatment effect for designing subsequent studies. In addition, this design only detects activity that continues after the initial 2 months of treatment. Drugs that impart benefit only during the first treatment months may be missed.

Because the maximum tolerated dose is routinely given, sponsors seldom design phase II trials that compare different doses of cancer drugs. However, the multiple-dose randomized phase II design, frequently used for non-cancer drugs, may be useful for evaluating novel anticancer drugs. This design can detect anticancer activity by demonstrating a dose-response relationship and allows selection of the optimal dose by assessing comparative safety.

IV. REGULATORY CONSIDERATIONS IN LATE DRUG DEVELOPMENT

Late drug development involves the design, conduct, and analysis of trials to support marketing. This section discusses meetings, regulatory requirements, end points, and trial designs.

A. End-of-Phase II Meetings

When phase II studies near completion, sponsors should meet with the FDA DODP at end-of-phase II meetings to establish the design of phase III trials. This ensures that trial designs will be considered adequate to support initial marketing of a drug (submitted in an NDA) or additional efficacy claims for already marketed drugs (submitted in an efficacy supplement to the NDA). Meeting agreements are part of the administrative record.

B. Requirements for Drug Approval

This section describes the requirements for regular new drug approval and for accelerated approval.

1. Requirements for Regular Approval

Drug approval usually requires two adequate and well-controlled studies demonstrating that the drug is effective and studies that show it is safe for its intended use. The requirement to demonstrate safety and efficacy prior to approval results from two laws promulgated in 1938 and 1962. The safety requirement is derived from the Federal Food Drug and Cosmetic Act of 1938 (FD&C Act). The efficacy requirement is from a 1962 amendment to that Act requiring "substantial evidence that the drug will have the effect it purports or is represented to have under the conditions of use prescribed, recommended, or suggested in the proposed labeling . . . ." This amendment required "evidence consisting of adequate and well-controlled investigations."

Subsequent legislative and judicial history clarified the legislative intent to require a minimum of two trials [12]. Exceptions exist and include where a "single multicenter study of excellent design provided highly reliable and statistically strong evidence of an important clinical benefit, such as an effect on survival, and a confirmatory study would have been difficult to conduct on ethical grounds" [13]. An amendment to the FD&C Act in 1997 specifically allows reliance on a single study in selected cases [14]. In many situations, a single study may be required for approval of new *efficacy supplements* (applications to the FDA for new indications for treatment with already marketed drugs). See Table 11.2 and FDA guidance [15].

Although the 1962 efficacy amendment did not directly address whether the drug effect must be clinically meaningful, the risk-benefit assessment needed to determine that a drug is "safe for its intended use" implies some value of the effect be shown. A critical court decision (*Warner Lambert v Heckler*, 1986) established that the effect shown must be of clinical value (i.e., provide clinical benefit) [12].

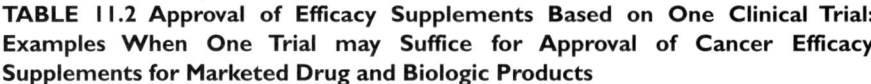

TABLE 11.2 Approval of Efficacy Supplements Based on One Clinical Trial: Examples When One Trial may Suffice for Approval of Cancer Efficacy Supplements for Marketed Drug and Biologic Products

- For treating a second type of cancer similar to that in the approved indication
- For treating a pediatric cancer similar to that in the adult indication
- For use of a chemoprotectant for a new type of tumor
- For a new dosing regimen for the same tumor
- For treating an earlier stage of the same disease
- For use in a new combination regimen when previously approved for use alone or in a different combination regimen

2. Requirements for Accelerated Approval

In 1992, Subpart H was added to the NDA regulations to allow *accelerated approval* of drugs for diseases that are serious or life-threatening, where the new drug appears to provide benefit over available therapy. Accelerated approval may be based on the effect of a drug on a *surrogate end point* that is reasonably likely to predict clinical benefit. After accelerated approval, the sponsor is required to perform a post-marketing study to demonstrate that treatment with the drug is indeed associated with clinical benefit. If the studies fail to demonstrate clinical benefit or if the sponsor does not show "due diligence" in performing the studies, the regulations describe a rapid process for removing the drug from the market [16]. Surrogate end points and clinical design related to accelerated approval are discussed in Section IV.D.

3. Other Regulatory Mechanisms for Important Drugs

In addition to accelerated approval, Fast Track Designation and Priority NDA Review are two other regulatory mechanisms designed to expedite drug development of important drugs[17, 18] (see Table 11.3).

C. Efficacy End Points for Regular Approval of Cancer Drugs

Sponsors must first select the primary clinical end point. The end point must reliably measure clinical benefit, and trial design should minimize bias. Blinding of randomized trials is the most reliable method to prevent bias. The common stance that oncology trials cannot be blinded should be carefully evaluated because blinding allows additional end points to be used, such as tumor-related symptoms, and enhances the credibility of end points like TTP.

The law requires demonstration of clinical benefit for drug approval. Clinical benefit can be defined as treatment effects judged to be clinically meaningful and suitable as the primary efficacy endpoint for regular drug approval. In oncology, the most reliable end point is survival. However, the FDA also considers other end points to represent clinical benefit in cancer patients. In the following subsections, several non-survival end points are described which have supported cancer drug approval.

TABLE 11.3 Regulatory Procedures for Important Drugs: Accelerated Approval, Fast Track Designation, and Priority Review Status

	Accelerated approval	Fast track designation	Priority review status
Description	Approval based on a surrogate end point reasonably likely to predict clinical benefit (but not as convincing as fully accepted surrogates)	Designation of a drug development plan allowing early FDA review of "rolling NDA" (NDA submitted in parts)	Status conferring FDA commitment to a six-month NDA review goal
Requirements	• Drug treats serious or life-threatening disease • Drug provides benefit over available therapy • After approval, sponsor must perform phase 4 IV study to prove clinical benefit	• Drug treats serious or life-threatening disease • Drug has potential to address unmet medical need	• Drug treats any disease[a] • Drug would be a significant improvement compared to marketed products
Timing	At NDA submission (although endpoints are also considered during protocol design).	At any time during drug development	At NDA submission
Policy source	1992 accelerated approval regulations (21 CFR 314.500) Also incorporated into the Food and Drug Modernization Act of 1997 (FDAMA)	The Food and Drug Administration Modernization Act of 1997 [16]	Definition of a priority application is given in CDER Manual of Policy and Procedures. The six-month review goal is from the Prescription Drug User Fee Act of 1992 [17].

[a]The CBER definition of a priority review is stricter than the definition that CDER uses. The biological drug, if approved, must be a significant improvement in the safety or effectiveness of the treatment diagnosis or prevention of a serious or life-threatening disease.

Additional information on trial designs and results from trials supporting approval of cancer drugs can be found in the Clinical Trials Section of approved package inserts, in transcripts from meetings of the ODAC [4], and in FDA guidance documents [3].

1. Regular Approval, RR, and TTP

In the early 1980s FDA approved cancer drugs based on RR. In the mid-1980s, upon the advice of the ODAC, the FDA determined that RR should not generally be the sole basis for approval. The possible benefit associated with partial responses did not necessarily outweigh the substantial toxicity of cancer drugs, and RR was not established as a surrogate for survival. The new FDA position subsequently required an improvement in survival or patient symptoms for approval [19].

However, the FDA has, in selected indications, based approval on other end points; their acceptability was determined on a case-by-case basis with advice from the ODAC. The FDA stated that under selected circumstances, impressive tumor-related outcomes could be considered clinical benefits [20]:

- An improvement in disease-free survival can be an end point for an adjuvant clinical trial if a large proportion of recurrences are symptomatic.
- Complete responses of reasonable duration may represent clinical benefit.
- The appropriateness of RR as an end point depends on duration of response and the toxicity of the treatment.
- Quality of life could be an efficacy end point if validated measures of disease-related symptoms were included and bias was minimized.

indications. End points supporting regular approval of cancer drugs by the FDA's Division of Oncology Drugs from 1990–2002 are summarized in Table 11.4 [21]. Non-survival end points were the primary end points in 68% (39/57) of the trials supporting regular approval, and tumor related end points (RR or TTP) were the basis of 27 approvals. RR alone supported 10 of these 27 approvals; nine were based on both tumor response and tumor-specific symptoms; seven were based on both RR and TTP; and one approval was based on TTP alone. Treatment indications approved using RR and/or TTP included hormonal treatment of breast cancer, treatment of hematologic malignancies, and treatment of cutaneous lesions from Kaposi's sarcoma or cutaneous T-cell lymphoma.

Whether FDA judges objective tumor response to be clinical benefit depends on the toxicity of treatment, the type of tumor, the efficacy of available therapy, the rate of response, the type of response (CR vs. PR), and the duration of response. Further information can be found in the package inserts of approved drugs. Below is a discussion of reasons for approval in different tumor settings:

- Hormonal agents for breast cancer: Approved in 1995, anastrozole was the first hormonal agent for breast cancer to be approved in the 1990s.

TABLE 11.4　End Points for Regular Approval of Cancer Drugs[21]*

Total	57
Survival	18
RR	26
-RRalone	10
-RR + ↓ Tumor Specific Symptoms	9
-RR + TTP	7
↓ Tumor Specific Symptoms	4
DFS	2
TTP	1
Recurrence Malignant Pleural Effusion	2
Occurrence Breast Cancer	2
Decreased Impairment Creatinine Clearence	1
Decreased Xerostomia	1

*Based on applications approved by CDER's DODP from 1990–2002.

The NDA trials compared the RR and TTP of anastrozole and tamoxifen. Other hormonal agents subsequently approved were exemestane, letrozole, toremifene. Because of the minimal toxicity, the well-accepted beneficial role of tamoxifen in this indication, and the lack of a demonstrated survival effect, RR was deemed a satisfactory end point for evaluating the clinical benefit for breast cancer hormone treatment [22]. NDAs of hormonal drugs for breast cancer have always included randomized trials comparing the new drug to a standard hormonal agent, usually with RR as the primary end point and TTP and survival as secondary end points.

- Hematologic malignancies: Drugs approvals for treatment of hematologic malignancies were based on complete responses (pentostatin, cladribine, tretinoin, arsenic trioxide) or partial responses associated with improvements in blood counts from levels likely to be symptomatic (fludarabine).
- Kaposi's sarcoma: Cutaneous responses of Kaposi's sarcoma (altretinoin, DaunoXome) and cutaneous T-cell lymphoma (altretinoin, bexarotene, DaunoXome) were considered clinical benefit in part because lesions are visible to patients and responses were thought to be of palliative benefit based on cosmesis.
- Other solid tumors: Partial responses in solid tumors were judged to be clinical benefit in several approvals. Prior to the advent of the accelerated approval regulations, altretamine and paclitaxel were approved for durable partial responses in refractory ovarian cancer. Topotecan approval in refractory small cell carcinoma was based on RR and symptom benefit. During deliberations, the ODAC indicated that RR alone (with adequate response duration) represents clinical benefit in the treatment of refractory small cell carcinoma because of the disease's rapidly progressive course [23].

2. Regular Approval, Quality of Life (QOL), and Patient Reported Outcomes

Until methods for evaluating and quantifying the overall quality of a patient's life are widely accepted, global QOL is not likely to be a useful primary end point. For a subjective measure to support approval, the end point should be clinically relevant, collected in ways that minimize bias, statistically robust, and clearly understood by practitioners and cancer patients [24]. The term patient-reported outcomes (PRO) has been recently adopted to describe a variety of tests that depend on patient input. Use of the term PRO rather than QOL avoids confusion as to whether the end point is measuring the overall quality of a patient's life or other important patient-derived outcomes [25].

Over the past 15 years, FDA has encouraged development of primary and secondary end points to evaluate patient symptoms. In 1985, the FDA position was that "a favorable effect on survival and/or quality of life is generally required for approval." The author's definition of QOL, however, was described as an assessment of performance status or pain [19]. Since that time, cancer drugs have been approved based on improvement in pain or morbidity, but no drugs have been approved based on a scale purporting to capture a patient's global QOL [26]. The following are examples of drug approvals utilizing PROs as primary or co-primary:

- In 1995, porfirmer sodium (Photofrin) was approved for photodynamic therapy (PDT) in completely obstructing esophageal cancer. In 1998, approval was extended to completely or partially obstructing endo-bronchial non-small cell lung cancer. FDA reviewers relied on patient-reported improvements in obstructive symptoms to determine that luminal responses were clinically meaningful [27].
- In 1996, mitoxantrone (Novantrone) was approved for treatment of advanced prostate cancer based primarily on improvement in pain demonstrated in randomized (but not blinded) controlled trials [28].
- In 1996, gemcitabine (Gemzar) was approved for treatment of pancre-atic cancer in part on the basis of *clinical benefit response*, an composite end point of pain, performance status, and weight gain; a survival benefit was also shown [29].
- In 1998 topotecan (Hycamtin) was approved for treatment of small cell lung cancer. An improvement in pulmonary symptoms was supportive for this application [30].
- In 1999, amifostine (Ethyol), a radiation therapy protectant, was approved to decrease xerostomia after radiation therapy for head and neck cancer. Approval was based primarily on xerostomia scores with support from measurements of salivary production from randomized trials [31].

3. Composite Clinical Benefit End Points

a. Composite End Points in Biphosphonate Trials

An composite end point may be appropriate when the drug's benefit is multifaceted. Pamidronate (Aredia) was the first biphosphonate drug approved for the treatment of skeletal metastases, initially for myeloma, and subsequently for breast cancer. The goal of treatment was to decrease the morbidity of bone metastases. The sponsor developed an composite end point (skeletal-related events; SRE) that included any of the following: pathologic fractures, radiation therapy for local pain, surgery to stabilize pending fractures, or spinal cord compression. Hypercalcemia was origi-nally proposed as an element in this composite end point, but was deemed to be qualitatively different than the other elements. Pamidronate was already marketed for the treatment of hypercalcemia. In the sponsor's myeloma and breast cancer trials, treatment with pamidronate resulted in both a decrease in the proportion of patients with at least one SRE and an increase in time to first SRE [32].

Two aspects of the pamidronate trials are notable. First, even though the trials evaluated intravenous drugs, placebo controls were used. The use of a placebo control was acceptable because all patients continued to receive stan-dard anticancer therapy in addition to study drug. The placebo control increased the credibility of the composite end point that could have been affected by bias. Second, patients did not discontinue study drug at the time of tumor progression. Pamidronate was continued after the first SRE and even after anticancer therapy was changed for tumor progression.

b. Other Composite End Points

Composite end points can also be constructed from symptoms, such as the *clinical benefit response* used in the approval of gemcitabine. A similar end point, perhaps more useful for novel cytostatic agents, is *time to symptomatic progression*. For trials using this end point, asymptomatic patients are entered and remain in the study until they experience a symptom related to tumor progression. Careful definition of symptomatic progression in the protocol and case report form is essential for this design. Blinding of the trial is important to minimize bias. A significant problem with this end point is that patients are often discontinued from the study when there are preliminary indications of progression, such as increased levels of a tumor marker, which leads to missing data and crossover to other treatments. One solution, for drugs that are relatively nontoxic, is to continue monitoring patients for symptomatic progression even after anticancer therapy changes. This solution decreases the missing data, but requires consideration of the impact of the additional therapy on the end point of symptomatic progression.

Another approach is to enroll symptomatic patients, identifying each patient's primary symptom. Each primary symptom is assessed on a suitable scale. The final analysis is a comparison of the number of patients on each study arm with an improvement in their pre-specified symptom. The credibility of this end point is reinforced if a correlation between improvement in the patients' symptoms and objective tumor response is observed. This approach has not yet supported a new drug approval.

c. Time To Treatment Failure

Time to treatment failure (TTF) is often defined as the time from randomization to discontinuation of treatment for any reason, including progression of disease, treatment toxicity, and death. TTF is an end point that combines efficacy and measures of safety and tolerability; it is seldom useful for regulatory purposes. The agency must determine that approved drugs are effective, and TTF does not provide evidence of efficacy. Separate analyses of the components of TTF (TTP, survival, and toxicity) are preferred end points.

4. Conclusions on End Points for Regular Approval of Cancer Drugs

Clinical end points for regular approval of cancer drugs measure clinical benefit. Although survival is the "gold standard" for measuring clinical benefit, in appropriate clinical settings, tumor response or an improvement in patient symptoms has supported approval. Innovative drug developers should consider what benefits their drug may provide and consider whether new end points need to be developed.

D. Surrogate End Points for Accelerated Approval

Under accelerated approval regulations, the FDA may approve a drug for serious or life-threatening disease based on a surrogate end point that is *reasonably likely to predict clinical benefit*. The drug must also represent an improvement over *available therapy*. Twenty two anticancer drugs and biologics received accelerated approval based on surrogate end points celerated approval from 1992 to 2004 [33]. Fifteen of these approvals were based on study designs that did not involve a randomized comparison (single arm designs or dose-comparison designs), and in each case, a response endpoint (tumor response, hematologic response, cytologic response, or cytogenetic response) was the surrogate end point supporting accelerated approval.

Drug-development strategies should not focus only on single-arm trials (intended for accelerated approval) to the exclusion of more reliable phase III trials (intended for regular approval) for several reasons:

- The use of RR as the surrogate end point may allow accelerated approval based on relatively small single-arm trials. For cytostatic agents, however, tumor size reduction may not be observed. Delays in tumor progression must be assessed in randomized trials to be credible.
- Under accelerated approval regulations, the new drug must have a "meaningful therapeutic benefit" over available therapy. Alternative drugs are increasingly available for second-line and subsequent therapy. Only randomized trials can demonstrate benefit of investigational therapy over available therapy.
- Even if there is no available therapy when a study is begun, therapy may become available prior to NDA submission, and randomized trials would then be required. Relying on single-arm trials and accelerated approval could be risky. A recent FDA guidance on "available therapy" has clarified that accelerated approval of a drug would not necessarily prevent FDA from granting a second accelerated approval for the same indication [34].
- If new data become available about the predictive value of the surrogate end point, a judgment that a surrogate is reasonably likely to predict clinical benefit could change.
- Small single-arm trials do not provide comprehensive evaluations of toxicity and do not allow comparisons to other therapies.
- Reliance on accelerated approval leads to evaluation of new drugs only in the most refractory populations. The demonstration of the drug's activity may not be observed in a heavily treated population.

After a drug is granted accelerated approval for treating a refractory cancer, it may be difficult to perform randomized trials to assess clinical benefit in the approved indication.

A better strategy is to include randomized comparative studies that evaluate both clinical benefit end points (that would support regular approval) and also the oncology surrogates, RR, and TTP (that might support accelerated approval).

E. Surrogate End Points for Regular Approval

For accelerated approval, the FDA relies upon surrogate end points that are not completely validated, but are reasonably likely to predict clinical benefit. This reasonable likelihood is then verified by post-marketing trials evaluating clinical benefit. Many end points have been proposed as appropriate surrogates for clinical benefit that could be used for regular drug approval. There are relatively few surrogate end points that have been adequately validated. Even what constitutes a valid surrogate is debatable. Prentice has argued that a valid surrogate should not only correlate with the outcome (clinical benefit), but should fully capture the net effect of treatment on the clinical outcome [35]. Others have suggested less stringent requirements. In any event, in order to validate a surrogate, one needs multiple clinical trials with each demonstrating the predictive value of the surrogate for the effect of treatment on the clinical outcome of interest [36]. Some surrogates are accepted as representing clinical benefit even if there are no formal survival benefit data; examples are prolonged complete responses in acute leukemia and testicular cancer.

Figure 11.1 displays the ideal surrogate end point [36]. The surrogate lies on the only causal pathway for the clinical end point and fully reflects the intervention's effect on the clinical outcome.

Figure 11.2 illustrates the problems that can arise with surrogate end points. Although the surrogate end point does lie on one causal pathway and does measure some of the treatment effect, clinical outcome is also affected by

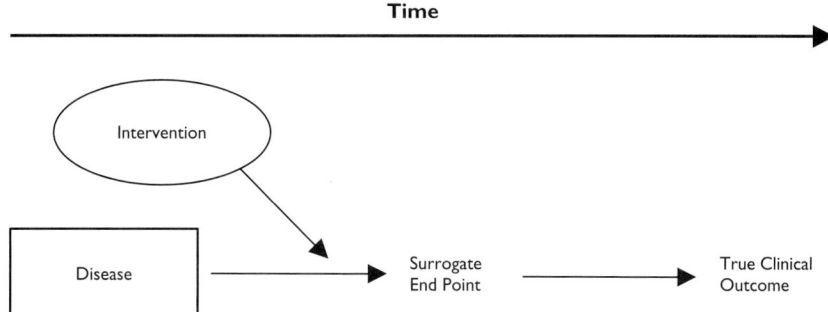

FIGURE 11.1   Ideal setting for surrogate end point. (From Fleming T, DeMets D. *Ann. Intern. Med.* 1996; 125:605–613. With permission.)

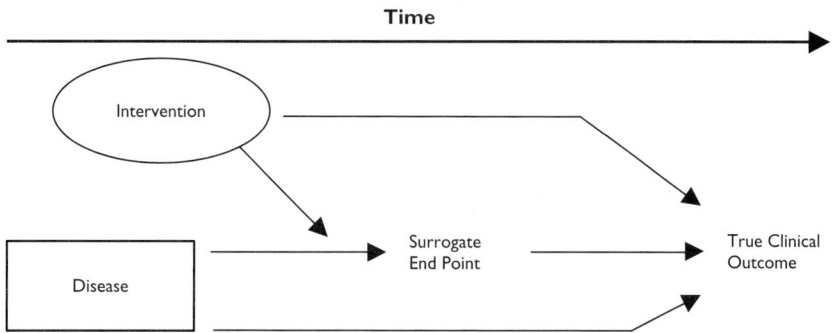

FIGURE 11.2   Unfavorable setting for surrogate end point. (From Fleming T, DeMets D. *Ann. Intern. Med.* 1996; 125:605–613. With permission.)

an independent pathway unrelated to treatment, and treatment also directly affects outcome [36]. An example in oncology is the use of a low RR as a surrogate to assess treatment with a toxic chemotherapy regimen. The RR might accurately predict benefit in the few patients who respond (middle pathway in Figure 11.2), but the surrogate does not reflect the direct negative effects of chemotherapy toxicity (upper pathway) and does not reflect progression of disease occurring in the large majority of patients (lower pathway).

F. Tumor Markers as Clinical End Points

The FDA has not accepted changes in tumor markers alone as primary end points for NDA studies, but these could become accepted surrogates if future data show that changes in tumor markers are reasonably likely to predict clinical benefit (accelerated approval) or that they have been validated for measuring clinical benefit (regular approval).

Although tumor markers have not been used alone as primary end points, the FDA has accepted them in protocol designs as elements in composite end points. For instance, women with ovarian cancer often show clinical deterioration from progression of unmeasured tumor. In blinded trials in advanced refractory ovarian cancer, the FDA has allowed use of a composite end point that included CA-125. The occurrence of certain clinical events (a significant decrease in performance status or bowel obstruction) coupled with marked increases in CA-125 was considered progression in these patients.

G. Clinical Trial Designs for the Approval of Cancer Drugs

The number of study arms, the type of control arm, and superiority or noninferiority to a control are discussed below. This section ends with a discussion of clinical trial design for chemotherapy protectants and radiotherapy protectants.

1. Single-Arm Trials

Single-arm, historically controlled trials have occasionally provided support for regular approval of new cancer drugs. A requirement for approval is proof of efficacy. Time-to-event end points (survival or TTP) are not well assessed in historical comparisons. Randomized trials are needed to adequately assess these end points. When standard therapy produces cures or substantial improvement in survival, a concurrent comparison to standard therapy is critical. Single-arm studies also do not optimally characterize toxicities.

Sponsors have sometimes demonstrated the clinical benefit of anticancer drugs in single-arm studies when there were convincing clinical findings, such as durable complete remissions in acute leukemia or restoration of the ability to swallow in esophageal cancer. Most examples of regular approvals based on single-arm trials were cytotoxic drugs causing tumor shrinkage.

2. Placebo Control

Placebo control increases the reliability of end points subject to bias, such as tumor-related symptoms and time-to-tumor progression. Placebo controls may be more acceptable in studies of novel agents than in studies of conventional cytotoxic drugs; many novel agents are given by the oral route and their favorable toxicity profile will help maintain the study blind. As discussed below, the comparison to placebo may be done either with treatment and placebo each added to standard therapy, or with treatment and placebo alone.

a. Comparison to Placebo Alone

Placebo-only controls are often considered inappropriate in cancer trials where effective therapy exists but may be appropriate in some other settings. For instance, in early stage cancers when standard practice is not to administer treatment, comparing a relatively non-toxic treatment to a placebo would be acceptable. This might be an optimal setting for detecting anti-tumor activity, because such patients usually have a good performance status and because tumor volume is low. This design could be useful in early myeloma, where a treatment-induced delay in the need for toxic chemotherapy may be a clinical benefit. Similarly, in patients with prostate cancer who have only PSA elevation, time to bone-scan- evident disease may be a reasonable end point for a phase 3 study.

b. Comparison to Placebo in Combination with Other Therapy

A randomized trial comparing an investigational drug to placebo, each in combination with standard therapy, is the optimal design for evaluating novel therapies. This design can demonstrate patient benefit and may establish a new standard of care. The placebo control allows credible analysis of subjective end points. Pilot phase I/II studies of the combination regimen would be needed prior to undertaking a phase III study.

3. Active Control Trials, Superiority Design

Most phase III cancer trials randomize patients to an investigational treatment versus an active control regimen, usually a standard therapy, or compare new drug plus standard drug to standard drug alone (add-on design). The latter design is expected to be more sensitive for detecting activity because there is no head-to-head comparison to an active agent. The add-on design was employed in the trials supporting the approval of three drugs for lung cancer (vinorelbine [37], paclitaxel [38], gemcitabine [29]). Each used cisplatin as the control arm.

4. Active Control Trials, Non-Inferiority Design with Single-Drug Regimens

Non-inferiority is the proper statistical term for what many investigators call *equivalence*. (This term is no longer used because, from a statistical stand point, it is impossible to prove equivalence.) Such trials seek to demonstrate that the new drug is not meaningfully less than the standard drug's efficacy of the standard drug by ruling out statistically a degree of inferiority of the new treatment to the standard. Non-inferiority designs pose formidable methodological difficulties, notably the need for reliable historical data to establish the active control treatment effect. Furthermore, whereas sloppiness in trial conduct decreases the likelihood that a superiority trial will be positive, it increases the likelihood that a non-inferiority trial will be "positive," i.e., show no difference [39]. Designing these trials requires a comprehensive meta-analysis of prior studies that reproducibly demonstrate that the control agent is effective and define the magnitude of the effect. The new trial must rule out that degree of difference between treatment and control (or some fraction of that difference) statistically. Given the complexity of the statistical approach needed to evaluate non-inferiority trials, early consultation with FDA is advisable.

5. Trial Designs for Radiotherapy Protectants and Chemotherapy Protectants

Radiotherapy protectants and chemotherapy protectants are drugs designed to ameliorate radiotherapy or chemotherapy toxicities. The first objective is to assess whether the new drug decreases the toxicity of the anticancer agent. Unless the mechanism of chemotherapy protection is clearly unrelated to the anti-tumor activity of anticancer drugs (e.g., anti-nausea agents), a second objective should be to demonstrate that the new agent does not compromise anti-tumor efficacy.

The need to demonstrate that anti-tumor efficacy is not compromised by chemotherapy protectants has been an important issue in several recent regulatory decisions:

- Dexrazoxane is a chelating agent intended to retain the benefits of doxorubicin while decreasing the associated cardiotoxicity. Approval of dexrazoxane was delayed for several years because the RR in the largest study submitted in the NDA showed a significantly lower RR when dexrazoxane was added to doxorubicin (63% vs. 48%, $p = 0.007$). Based on additional data, dexrazoxane was subsequently approved for delayed use after a cumulative doxorubicin dose of 300 mg/m^2 [40].
- Liposome-encapsulated doxorubicin (Myocet, The Liposome Company, Elan Corporation, Princeton, NJ), a liposomal formulation of doxorubicin also designed to decrease cardiac toxicity, was evaluated by the ODAC in 1998. The committee voted not to approve the NDA because one of the studies comparing doxorubicin to Myocet had inadequate statistical power to assess tumor protection and showed an adverse trend in survival [41].
- In 1999, amifostine (Ethyol, Alza, Mountain View, CA) was approved to decrease the incidence of moderate to severe xerostomia in patients receiving postoperative radiotherapy for head and neck cancer. The approved indication was limited to use with postoperative radiotherapy after an ODAC deliberation suggested that the studies had insufficient statistical power to rule out tumor protection by amifostine in the setting of definitive radiation [42].

In summary, trials to evaluate chemotherapy or radiotherapy protectants should be powered to rule out a reduction in anticancer efficacy from tumor protection.

V. CONCLUSION

The FDA regulation of anticancer drugs is fundamentally the same for novel and conventional (cytotoxic) drugs. Preclinical testing is similar for both classes of drugs. The design of phase I and phase II trials for novel drugs may present unique challenges. These challenges include identifying the optimal dose and selecting from several novel therapies for phase III development. In phase III trials, a variety of end points and trial designs should be considered. The most useful design is to compare standard therapy plus new therapy to standard therapy plus placebo. The add-on nature of this design optimizes the detection of activity or benefit from the new drug and the placebo control reduces bias, which allows subjective end points to be used for evaluating clinical benefit. Sponsors are encouraged to meet with review teams in the DODP in the FDA's Center for Drug Evaluation and Research.

ACKNOWLEDGEMENTS

We thank Robert Temple, M.D., for his critical reading of this chapter. The opinions expressed in this chapter are solely those of the authors and do not necessarily reflect those of any government agency.

REFERENCES

1. Guidance for Industry: IND exemptions for studies of lawfully marketed drug or biological products for the treatment of cancer, September, 2003. Available at: http://www.fda.gov/cder/guidance/545.htm
2. U.S. Food and Drug Administration. Reinventing the regulation of cancer drugs: Accelerating approval and expanding access. National Performance Review, Washington (DC), March 1996.
3. FDA Guidances may be found on the internet guidance page at http://www.fda.gov/cder/guidance.
4. Transcripts from meetings of the Oncologic Drugs Advisory Committee are available on the CDER Freedom of Information Home Page, http://www.fda.gov/cder/foi.
5. DeGeorge J, Ahn C, Andrews P. Regulatory considerations for preclinical development of anticancer drugs. *Cancer Chemother. Pharmacol.* 1998; 41:173–185.
6. Collins JM, Grieshaber CK, Chabner BA. Pharmacologically guided phase I trials based upon preclinical development. *J. Natl. Cancer Inst.* 1990; 82:1321–3126.
7. Simon R, Freidlin B, Rubinstein L, Arbuck S, Collins J, Christian M. Accelerated titration designs for phase I clinical trials in oncology. *J. Natl. Cancer Inst.* 1997; 89:1138–1147.
8. Eisenhauer P, O'Dwyer P, Christian M, Humphrey J. Phase I clinical trial design in cancer drug development. *J. Clin. Oncol.* 1997; 18:684–692.
9. Goodman SN, Zahurak ML, Piantadosi S. Some practical improvements in the continual reassessment method for phase I studies. *Stat. Med.* 1995; 14:911–922.
10. Korn E, Arbuck S, Pluda M, Simon R, Kaplan R, Christian M. Clinical trial designs for cytostatic agents: Are new approaches needed? *J. Clin. Oncol.* 2001; 19:265–272.
11. Kopec J, Abrahamowicz M, Esdaile J. Randomized discontinuation trials: Utility and efficiency. *J. Clin. Epidemiol.* 1993; 46:959–971.
12. Temple R. Development of drug law, regulations, and guidance in the United States. In *Principles of Pharmacology: Basis Concepts and Clinical Application* (Munson PL, Mueller RA and Breese GR, eds.), (NY:Chapman and Hall, 1996; 1643).

13. Guidance for industry: Providing clinical evidence of effectiveness for human drug and biological products. *Food and Drug Administration* 1998; 1–20. (FDA Guidances may be found on the FDA internet guidance page at http://www.fda.gov/cder/guidance.)

14. Food and Drug Administration Modernization Act of 1997, Sec. 115. Available on CDER guidance home page at the following address: http://www.fda.gov/cder/regulatory.

15. Guidance for industry: FDA approval of new cancer treatment uses for marketed drug and biological products. 1998; 1–10. (FDA Guidances may be found on the FDA CDER internet guidance page at http://www.fda.gov/cder/guidance.

16. 21 Code of Federal Regulations, Part 314.530.

17. Guidance for Industry, Fast Track Drug Development Programs — Designation, Development, and Application Review, 1998. (FDA Guidances may be found on the FDA internet guidance page at http://www.fda.gov/cder/guidance.)

18. Priority Review Policy, FDA Center for Drug Evaluation and Research Manual for Policies and Procedures, MAPP #6020.3, 1996. CDER MAPPs are available at www.fda.gov/cder/mapp.htm.

19. Johnson JR, Temple R. Food and Drug Administration requirements for approval of anticancer drugs. *Cancer Treat. Rep.* 1985; 69:1155–1159.

20. O'Shaughnessy J, Wittes R, Burke G et al. Commentary concerning demonstration of safety and efficacy of investigational anticancer agents in clinical trials. *J. Clin. Oncol.* 1991; 9:2225–2232.

21. Johnson JR, Williams G and Pazdur R. End points and United States Food and Drug Administration approval of oncology drugs. *J. Clin. Oncol.* 21:1404–1411, 2003.

22. Arimidex® package insert, AstraZeneca, Wilmington, DE.

23. Transcript of the 57th Meeting of the Oncologic Drugs Advisory Committee. Rockville MD. June 8, 1998. Transcripts available at the CDER Freedom of Information Home Page, http://www.fda.go.

24. Beitz J, Gnecco C, Justice R. Quality-of-life end points in cancer clinical trials: The U.S. Food and Drug Administration perspective. *Monogr. Natl. Cancer Inst.* 1996; 20:7–9.

25. Draft guidance for industry *Patient-Reported Outcome Measures: Use in Medical Product Development to Support Claim, 2004.* Most recent version of CDER guidance are at http://www.fda.gov/cder/guidance/index.htm.

26. Williams G, Pazdur R, Temple R. Assessing tumor-related signs and symptoms to support cancer drug approval. J Biopharm Stat., Feb 2004; 14:5.

27. Photofrin® package insert, Sanofi Pharmaceuticals, Inc., New York, NY.

28. Novantrone® package insert, Immunex Corporation, Seattle, WA.

29. Gemzar® package insert, Eli Lilly, Indianapolis, IN.

30. Hycamtin® package insert, Smithkline Beecham, Pittsburgh, PA.

31. Ethyol® package insert, Alza, Mountain View, CA.

32. Aredia® package insert, Novartis Pharmaceuticals, East Hanover, NJ.

33. Dagher R, Johnson J, Williams G et al- Accelerated Approval of Oncology Products: A Decade of Experience. J Natl Cancer Inst 2004; 96:1500–9.

34. Guidance for industry: Available therapy. July 2004. FDA guidances are available at http://www.fda.gov/cder/guidance/index.htm.

35. Prentice RL. Surrogate endpoints in clinical trials: definition and operational criteria. Stat Med. 1989; 3:1065–73.

36. Fleming T, DeMets D. Surrogate end points in clinical trials: Are we being misled? *Ann. Intern. Med.* 1996; 125:605–613.

37. Navelbine®, Glaxo Wellcome, Research Triangle Park, NC.

38. Taxol® package insert, Bristol-Myers Squibb Co., New York, NY.

39. ICH E10 Guideline: E-10 Choice of control group and related design issues in clinical trials. July 2000; 1–ICH guidelines may be found at http://www.fda.gov/cder/guidance/index.htm.

40. Swain SM, Whaley FS, Gerber MC et al. Delayed administration of dexrazoxane provides cardioprotection for patients with advanced breast cancer treated with doxorubicin-containing therapy. *J. Clin. Oncol.* 1997; 15:1333–1340.

41. Cortazar P. Presentation to Oncologic Drugs Advisory Committee. Rockville MD. September 16, 1999. Transcript available at the CDER Freedom of Information Home Page, http://www.fda.gov/cder/foi.

42. Chico G. Presentation to Oncologic Drugs Advisory Committee. Rockville MD. June 8, 1999. Transcript available at the CDER Freedom of Information Home Page, http://www.fda.gov/cder/foi.

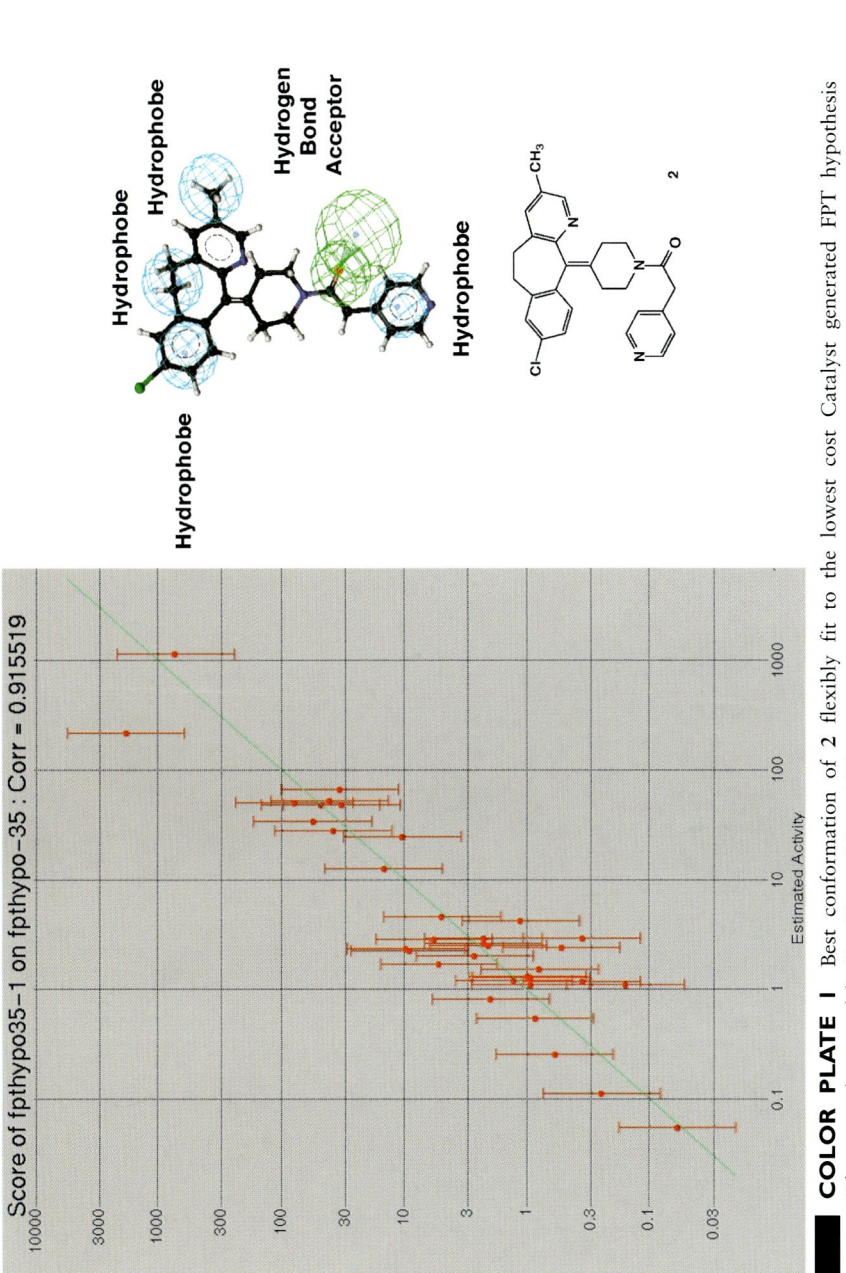

COLOR PLATE I Best conformation of 2 flexibly fit to the lowest cost Catalyst generated FPT hypothesis (Pharmacophore model). (See Figure 4.2, p. 100)

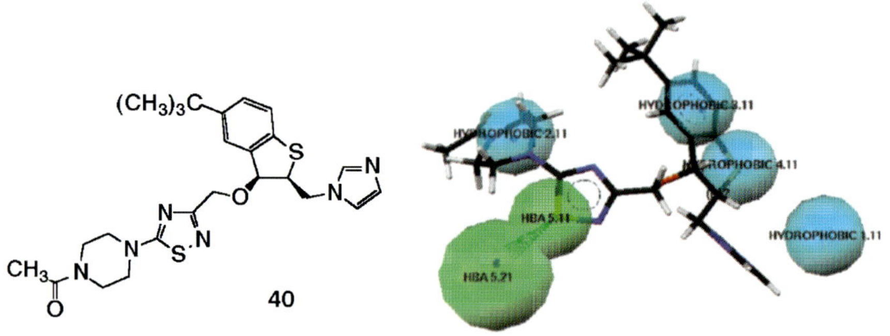

COLOR PLATE 2 Best conformation of **40**, *cis*-isomer, flexibly fit to the lowest cost Catalyst generated FPT hypothesis. (See Figure 4.5, p. 103)

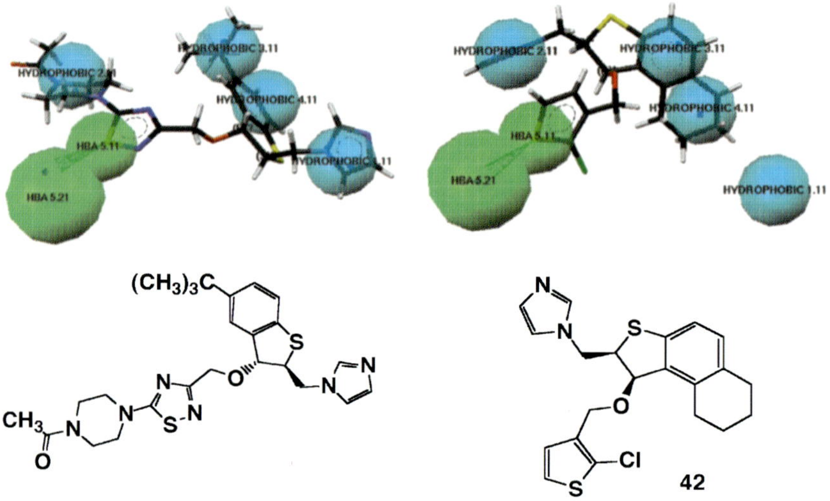

COLOR PLATE 3 A conformation of the *trans*-isomer of **40** and the best conformation of **42** flexibly fit to the lowest cost Catalyst generated FPT hypothesis. (See Figure 4.6, p. 103)

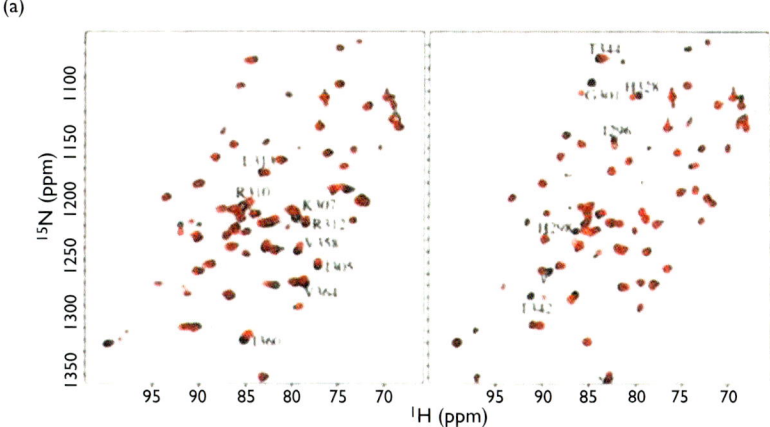

(a)

^{15}N (ppm)

^{1}H (ppm)

(b)

1. IC$_{50}$ > 1000 μm

2. IC$_{50}$ > 1000 μm

21. IC$_{50}$ = 150 μm

30. IC$_{50}$ = 75 μm

40. IC$_{50}$ = 10 μm

COLOR PLATE 4   Examples of the application of the SAR by NMR screening approach with human papillomaviruses (HPV) DNA binding protein E2 and stromelysin. (a) Two examples of ^{1}H-^{15}N HSQC spectra of E2 in the absence of added ligand (black) and the presence of added ligand (red). Some residues that exhibit chemical shift changes upon binding are labeled. (b) Summary of the discovery of a 10-μM inhibitor of E2 starting from mM leads identified using SAR by NMR. (c) Ribbons depiction of (left) stromelysin complexed with acetohydroxamic acid and a biphenyl compound; (right) the stromelysin linked compound complex (green) superimposed with a collagenase:inhibitor complex (cyan). (d) A summary of the SAR by NMR approach applied to the discovery of stromelysin inhibitors. (Reprinted with permission from references [79, 80]. Copyright 1997 by American Chemical Society.) (See Figure 5.1, p. 112)

(c)

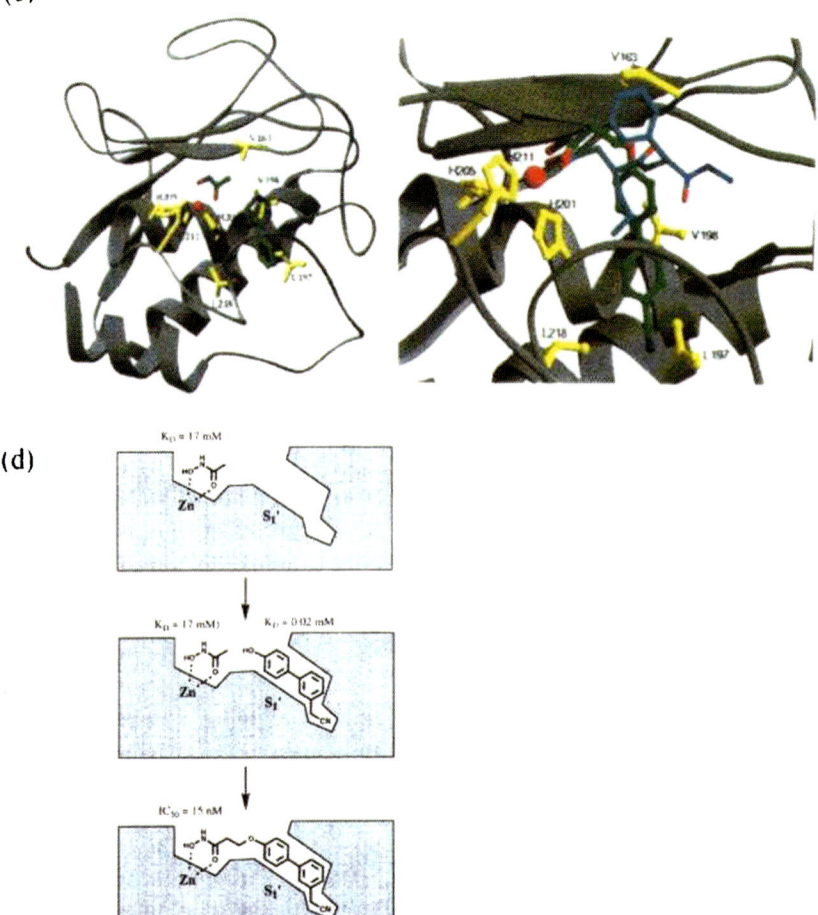

(d)

COLOR PLATE 4 (Continued)

a)

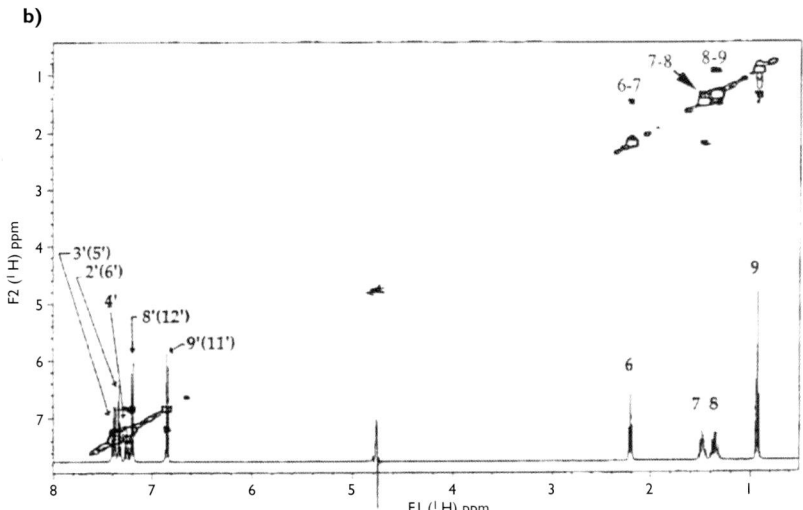

b)

c)

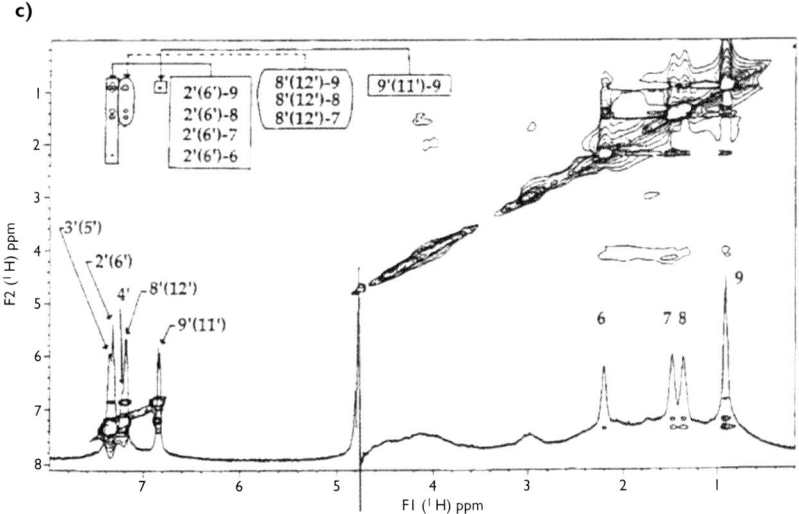

COLOR PLATE 5 Example of the 2D-trNOE experiment to identify binders to a protein target. (a) Chemical structure of OXY. (b) 2D ^{1}H NOESY spectra of OXY (5 mM) and a corresponding 1D ^{1}H trace. (c) spectra of OXY (5 mM) in the presence of 0.083 mM of human serum albumin. The observed trNOEs for OXY upon binding human serum albumin are boxed and labeled. (Reprinted with permission from reference [91]. Copyright 1998 by John Wiley & Sons, Inc.) (See Figure 5.2, p. 117)

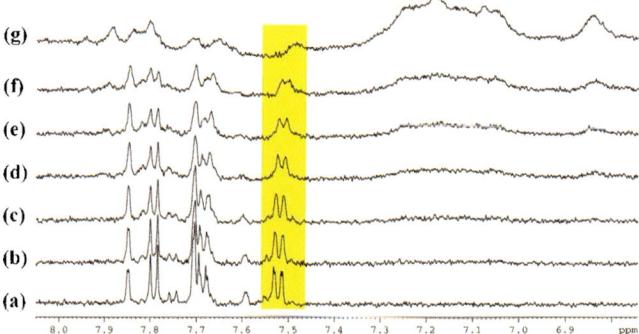

COLOR PLATE 6 Illustration of the application of 1D line-broadening to identify binders [423]. (a) The 1D-NMR spectrum of the free compound (50 μM). (b–g) Addition of 2 μM to 50 μM of ER-α to the compound in (a). The observed line-broadening indicates the compound binds ER-α. The resonances centered around 7.52 ppm are outlined in yellow to highlight the observed line-broadening and chemical shift changes upon the addition of ER-α. (See Figure 5.3, p. 118)

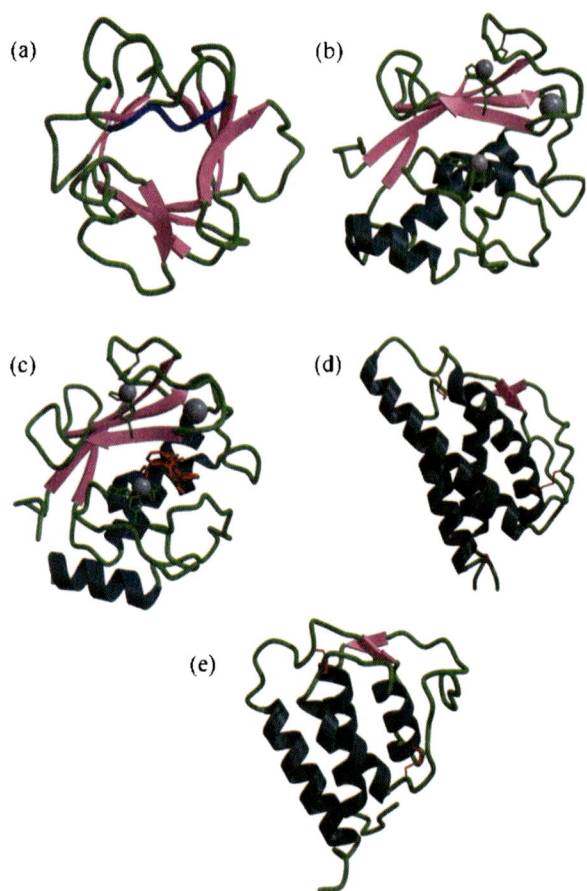

COLOR PLATE 7 Ribbon diagrams of the NMR solution structures of (a) FGF-2, (b) MMP-1, (c) MMP-13:CPD-693, (d) IL-4, and (e) IL-13 (from [113, 150, 151, 161]). (Reprinted with permission from references [154, 167]. Copyright 2001 and 2000 by Elsevier Science.) (See Figure 5.6, p. 128)

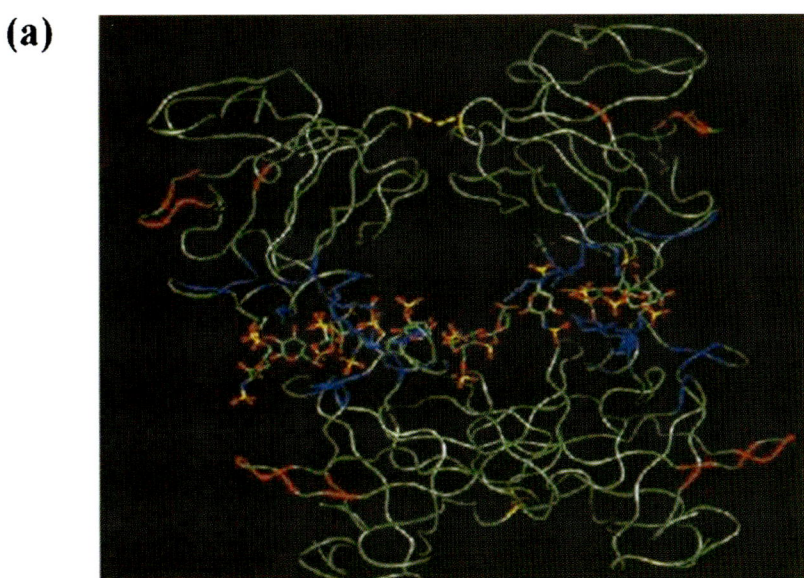

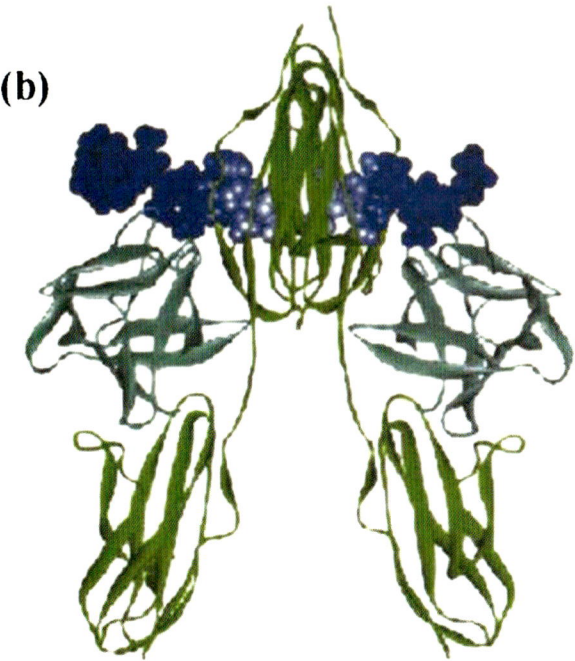

COLOR PLATE 8 (a) NMR model of the heparin-induced oligomerization of FGF-2 as a prerequisite to receptor binding. FGF-2 is shown as a ribbon where side chains for residues involved in heparin binding are illustrated. Heparin is shown as a licorice bond representation colored by atom type. The putative receptor binding site is colored red and residues that incur chemical shift changes in the heparin-binding site from heparin-binding site are colored blue. (Reprinted with permission from reference [114], Copyright 1997 by American Chemical Society.) (b) X-ray model of an FGF2-FGFR1-heparin complex with 2:2:2 stoichiometry. FGFR (green) and FGF (cyan) are in ribbon representation and heparin is in a spacefill representation. (Reprinted with permission from reference [118]. Copyright 2001 by Elsevier Science.) (See Figure 5.7, p. 129)

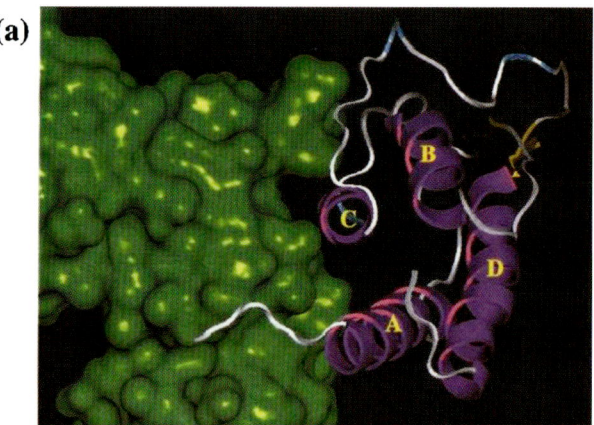

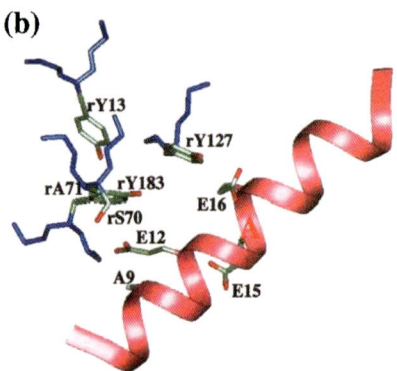

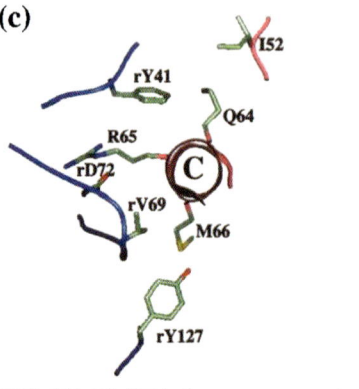

COLOR PLATE 9 Interaction of IL-13 with its receptor. (a) IL-13/IL-4Rα model based on the IL-4/IL-4Rα X-ray structure (PDB ID:1IRA) [422]. IL-13 replaced IL-4 in the IL-4/IL-4Rα X-ray structure by overlaying IL-13 onto IL-4 based on the common secondary structure elements and cysteines. IL-4Rα is shown as a molecular surface (green) and IL-13 as a ribbon diagram colored by secondary structure, where the helices are colored purple and the β-sheets are colored yellow. Only the IL-13/IL-4Rα interface is illustrated. The secondary structure elements are labeled. (b) Expanded view of the IL-13/IL-4Rα binding site indicating the interaction with helix αA from IL-13. (c) Expanded view of the IL-13/IL-4Rα binding site illustrating the interaction with helix αC from IL-13. The side chains for critical residues based on the IL-4/IL-4Rα X-ray structure and mutational data are shown and labeled. Residues from IL-4Rα are labeled with the prefix "r." The side chains are colored by element type; the backbone atoms for IL-13 and IL-4Rα are colored magenta and blue, respectively. (Reprinted with permission from reference [154]. Copyright 2001 by Elsevier Science.) (See Figure 5.8, p. 131)

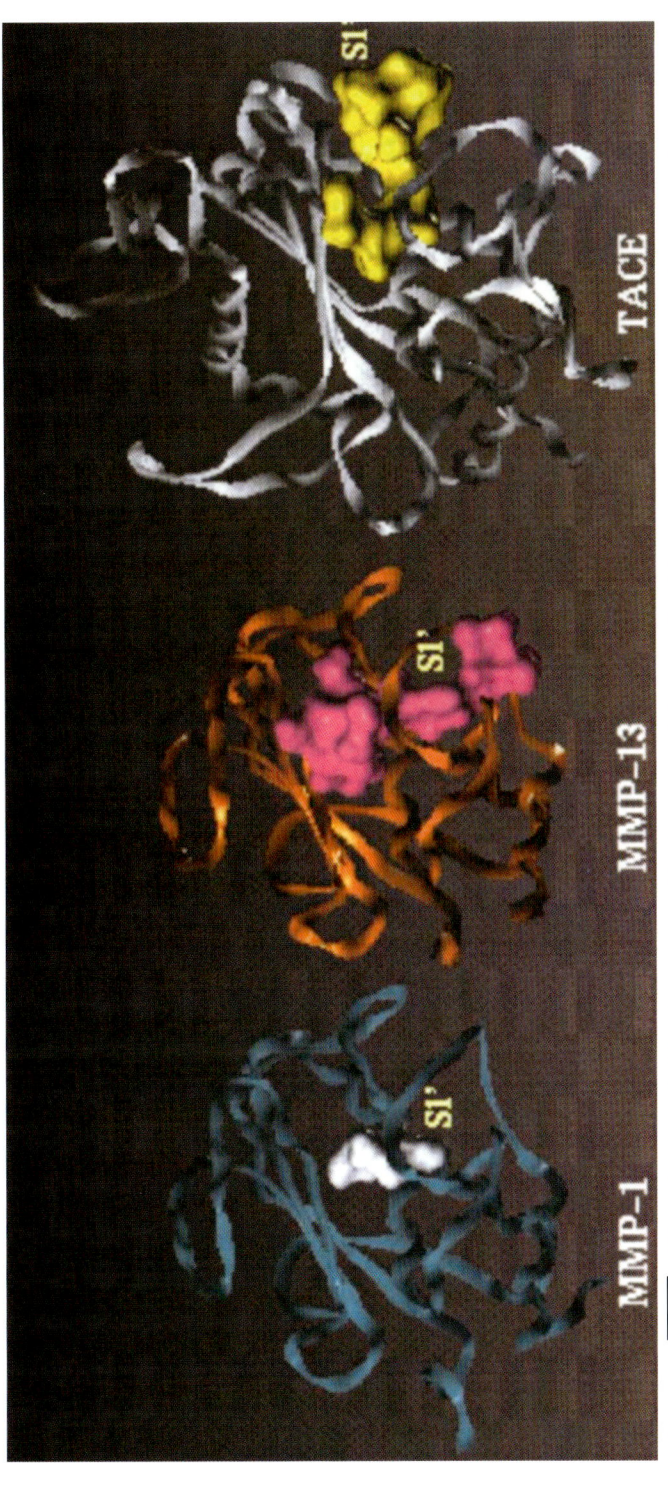

COLOR PLATE 10 Illustration of the differences in the size and shape of the S1' pocket for MMPs and related proteins. Ribbon diagrams and S1' pockets for MMP-1, MMP-13, and TACE. (See Figure 5.9, p. 135)

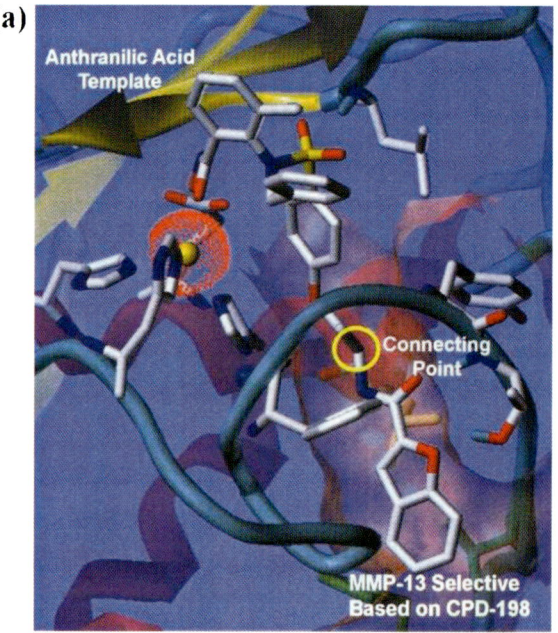

(a)

Anthranilic Acid
Template

Connecting
Point

MMP-13 Selective
Based on CPD-198

(b)

CPD-177   +   CPD-198

CPD-523

MMP-13	MMP-1	MMP-9	TACE
17nM	16%(10μM)	945 nM	19% (1μM)
selectivity	>5800x	56x	>500x

COLOR PLATE II Application of the MMP NMR structures for the design of a novel, potent, and selective inhibitor for MMP-13. (a) Expanded view of the NMR MMP-13:CPD-198 complex overlaid with the MMP-13:CPD-177 model. This demonstrates the approach to forming the hybrid inhibitor CPD-523 where the MMP-13 active site is shown as a grid surface with CPD-198 and CPD-177 are shown with licorice bonds. (b) Design scheme showing the flow from CPD-198 and CPD-062 to CPD-523. The observed IC_{50} and selectivity against MMPs and TACE for inhibitor CPD-523 are listed below the design scheme. (Reprinted with permission from reference [191]. Copyright 2000 by American Chemical Society.) (See Figure 5.10, p. 136)

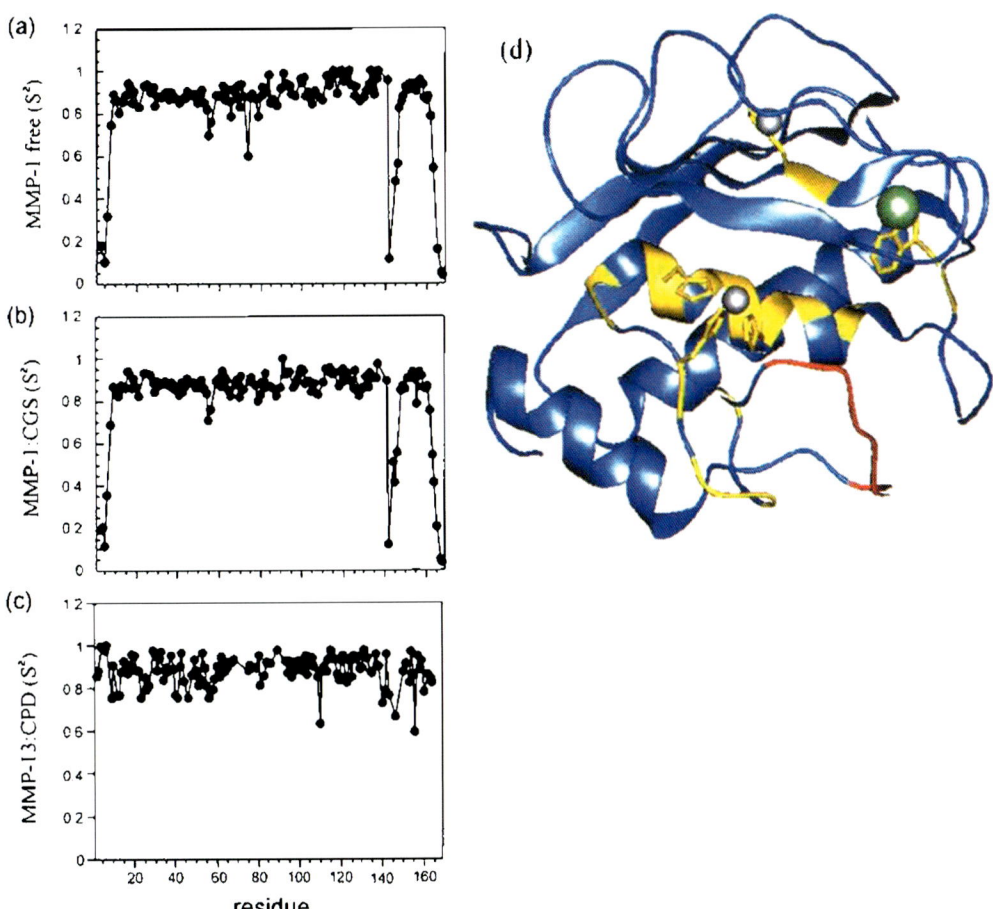

COLOR PLATE 12 Residue plot of the order parameters (S^2) for (a) MMP-1 free, (b) MMP-1 complexed with CGS-27023A, and (c) MMP-13 complexed with CPD-693, which illustrates the mobility of the MMP active site and the effect of inhibitors on the mobility (from [167, 197]). (d) Ribbon diagram of MMP-1 with residues exhibiting doubling of peaks in the ^{1}H-^{15}NHSQC colored yellow, which indicates slow exchange, and the mobile active site loop is colored red. (Reprinted with permission from reference [167]. Copyright 2000 by Elsevier Science. Also reprinted with permission from reference [197]. Copyright 1997 by Kluwer Academic Publishers.) (See Figure 5.11, p. 139)

Chromatogram

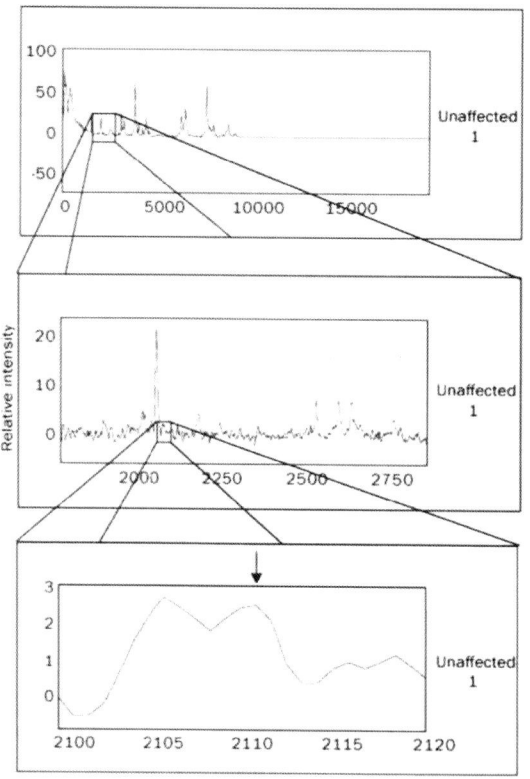

Density plot

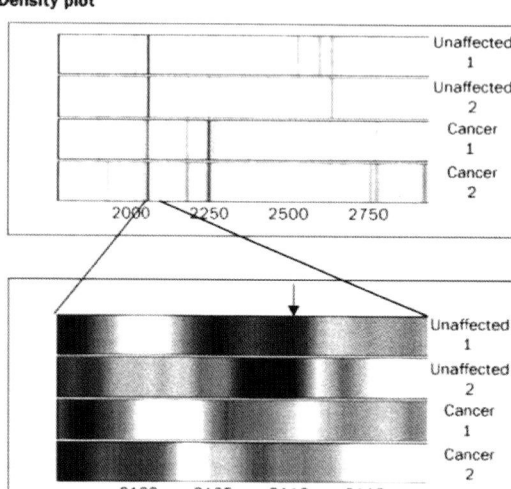

M/Z values

COLOR PLATE 13 SELDI mass spectra of sera obtained from patients without (Unaffected) and diagnosed with ovarian cancer (Cancer). The top three panels illustrate the exploded regions in a SELDI mass spectrum where a protein biomarker was identified using statistical methods at m/z 2111 to be present in patients free of ovarian cancer. Similar exploded views are illustrated in the bottom two panels indicating the presence of the m/z 2111 protein in patients without ovarian cancer but absent in patients with ovarian cancer. Statistical analyses of similar SELDI mass spectral data were instrumental in identifying spectral patterns for diagnosing ovarian cancer. (Reprinted with permission from reference [361]. Copyright 2002 by the Lancet Publishing Group.) (See Figure 5.20, p. 159)

Compound mixtures + protein passed through gel-filtration column

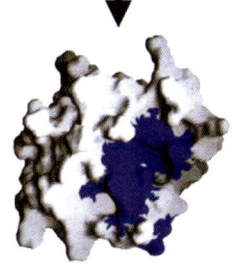

Mass Spectroscopy

NMR chemical shift perturbations (2D ^{1}H-^{15}N HSQC)

Mapping of chemical shift perturbations on protein surface

High-resolution NMR structure of protein-ligand complex

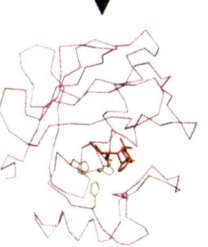

COLOR PLATE 14 Pictorial flow diagram of MS/NMR assay using data from the MMP-1 binding assay. (Reprinted with permission from reference [393]. Copyright 2001 by American Chemical Society.) (See Figure 5.21, p. 163)

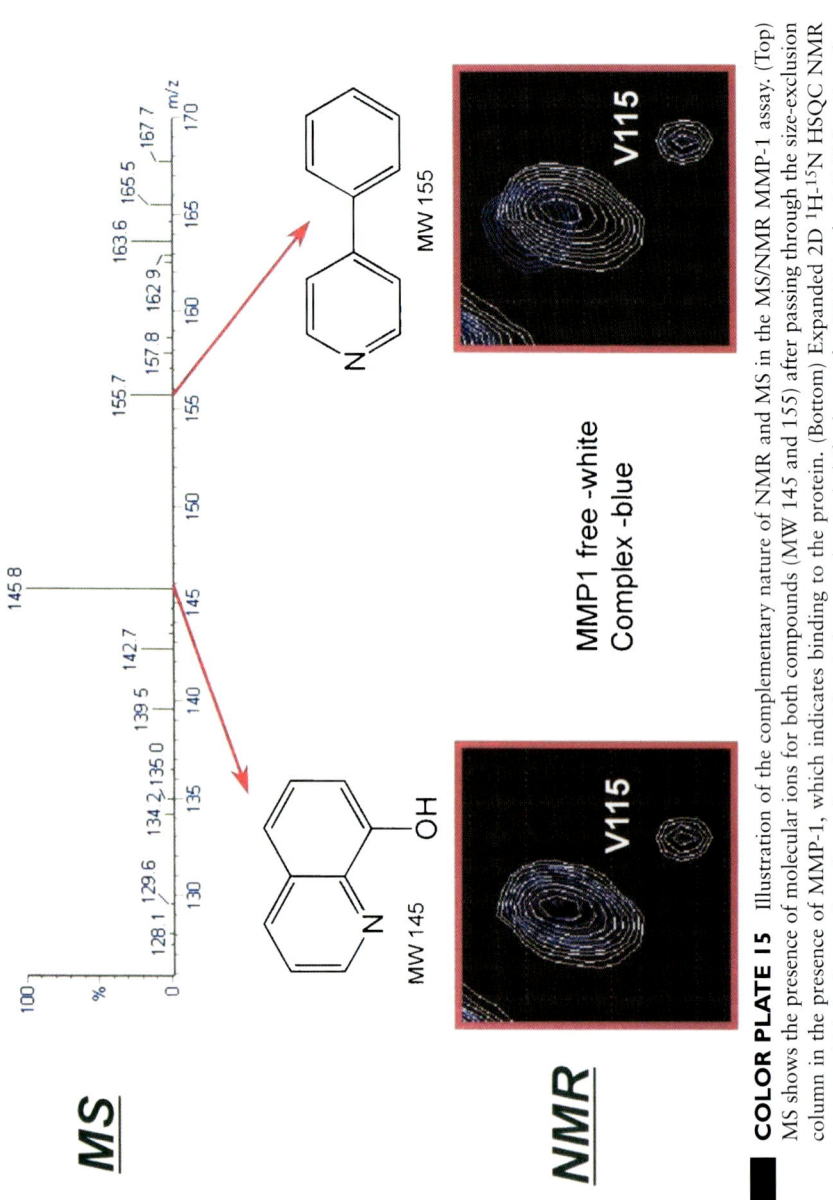

COLOR PLATE 15 Illustration of the complementary nature of NMR and MS in the MS/NMR MMP-1 assay. (Top) MS shows the presence of molecular ions for both compounds (MW 145 and 155) after passing through the size-exclusion column in the presence of MMP-1, which indicates binding to the protein. (Bottom) Expanded 2D ^1H-^{15}N HSQC NMR spectra which indicates that the *p*-phenyl pyridine induces a chemical shift change for V115 in the MMP-1 active site. (See Figure 5.27, p. 171)

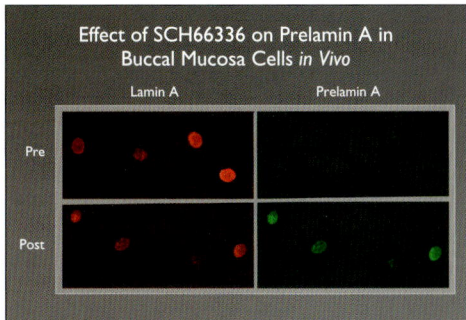

COLOR PLATE 16 Detection of prelamin A in buccal mucosa cells from SCH66336-treated patients. Buccal smears were double labeled with mouse anti-lamin A (left) and rabbit anti-prelamin A (right) followed by fluorochrome-labeled secondary antibodies. Corresponding fields were photographed. Bottom panel: samples harvested on day 8 from patients treated with 300 mg b.i.d. of SCH66336. Upper panel: pretreatment sample from same patient. (See Figure 10.1, p. 257)

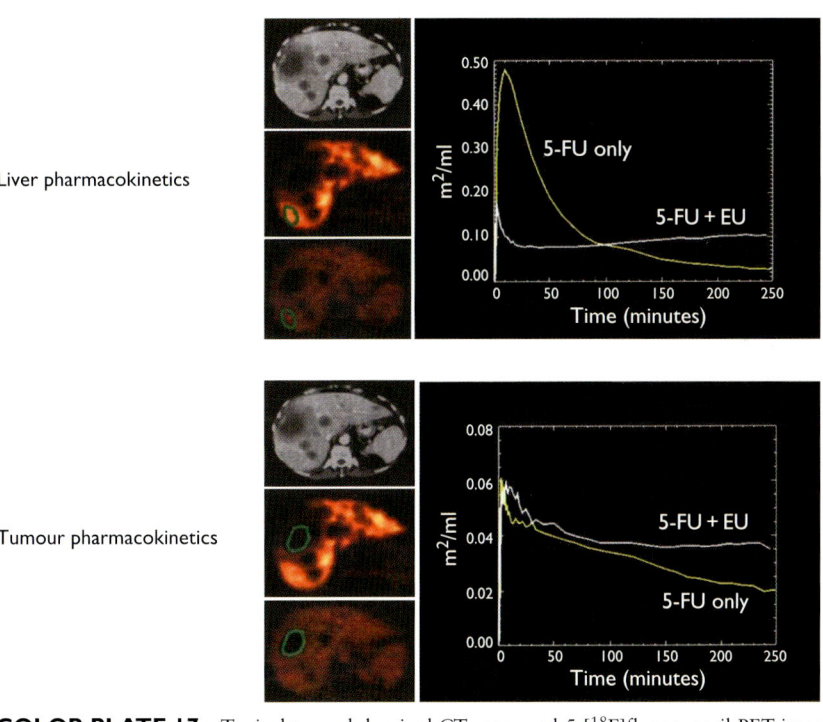

COLOR PLATE 17 Typical transabdominal CT-scans and 5-[^{18}F]fluorouracil-PET images of a patient before and after treatment with eniluracil. There was a substantial decrease in liver radioactivity (top panel) after eniluracil treatment due to the inactivation dihydropyrimidine dehydrogenase, and hence, absence of [^{18}F]fluoro-β-alanine. Such studies of enzyme activity are useful in providing proof of principle of mechanism in humans. The half-life of tumor 5-[^{18}F]fluorouracil-derived radioactivity increased after eniluracil treatment. (See Figure 13.3, p. 305)

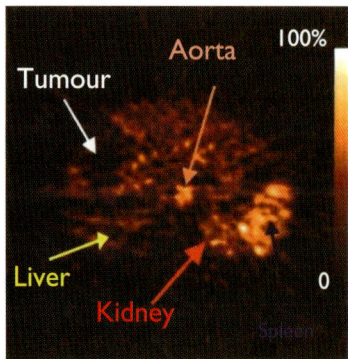
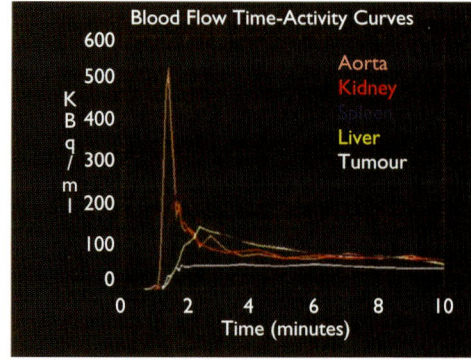

Blood flow model: $\quad C_t(t) = F.C_a(t) \otimes \ell^{-(\frac{F}{V_d} + \lambda).t}$

COLOR PLATE 18 Measurement of tissue perfusion and volume of distribution of water (exchanging water space) using $H_2{}^{15}O$-PET. Cumulative tissue localisation of $H_2{}^{15}O$ and its time-course in tissues are shown. The model for deriving parameters of flow and volume of distribution is also shown, where $C_t(t)$ is the regional tissue concentration of $H_2{}^{15}O$ [$Bq.ml^{-1}$ (tissue)] as a function of time t, $C_a(t)$ is the arterial whole blood concentration of $H_2{}^{15}O$ [$Bq.ml^{-1}$ (blood)] as a function of time, F is the regional flow in ml (blood)$.ml^{-1}$ (tissue)$.min^{-1}$, Vd is the volume of distribution of water [ml (blood)$.ml^{-1}$ (tissue)], and λ is the decay constant of ^{15}O (0.338 min^{-1}). (See Figure 13.4, p. 306)

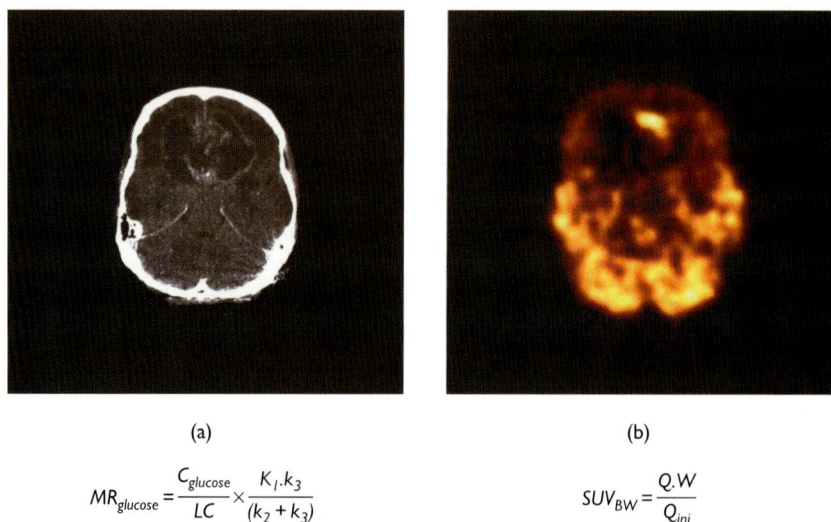

(a)   (b)

$$MR_{glucose} = \frac{C_{glucose}}{LC} \times \frac{K_1.k_3}{(k_2 + k_3)} \qquad\qquad SUV_{BW} = \frac{Q.W}{Q_{inj}}$$

COLOR PLATE 19 (a) A CT-scan of the brain showing a tumour mass, and (b) [^{18}F]FDG-PET scan showing hypermetabolic regions within the tumour and in normal brain. Such images when acquired dynamically may be analysed to provide measures of the metabolic rate of glucose utilisation ($MR_{glucose}$, $\mu mol.min^{-1}.ml^{-1}$) or the standardised uptake value normalised to body weight (SUV_{BW}, Kg (body weight)$.l^{-1}$ (tissue)), where $C_{glucose}$, LC are the plasma glucose concentration and lumped constants, respectively and K_1, k_2 and k_3 are as previously defined in figure 2. Q, W, and Q_{inj} represent the tumour radiotracer concentration (units = $MBq.l^{-1}$), body weight (units = Kg) and injected activity (units = MBq), respectively. (See Figure 13.6, p. 311)

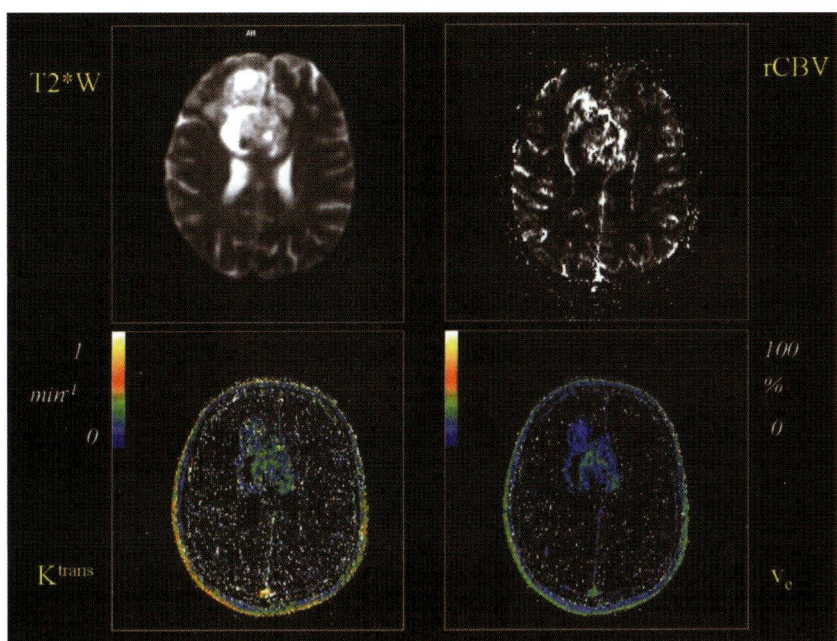

COLOR PLATE 20 Multifunctional vascular characterisation of brain oligodendroglioma. (a) Top left. Axial T2-weighted MR image of a transformed malignant cerebral oligodendroglioma. A large necrotic mass is seen in the frontal lobe. Tumour extends across the midline. High signal areas within the mass are presumed to represent necrosis. (b) Top right. Relative cerebral blood volume (rCBV) map at the same slice location. The tumour is noted to be markedly hypervascular with a blood volume equal to or greater than normal cortical grey matter. Note that the areas of highest blood volume are not immediately adjacent to the areas of necrosis. (c) Bottom left. Transfer constant (K^{trans}) map (maximum transfer constant displayed = 1 minute^{-1}). The areas of highest permeability surface area product (transfer constant) are noted in the centre of the tumour. In particular, there are areas of high transfer constant immediately adjacent to the areas of necrosis seen in the axial T2-weighted image. The distribution of transfer constant values does not match the distribution of relative cerebral blood volume spatially. (d) Leakage space (v_e) map. Maximum leakage space demonstrated 100%. There is a good spatial match of leakage space with transfer constant values.(See Figure 13.7, p. 315)

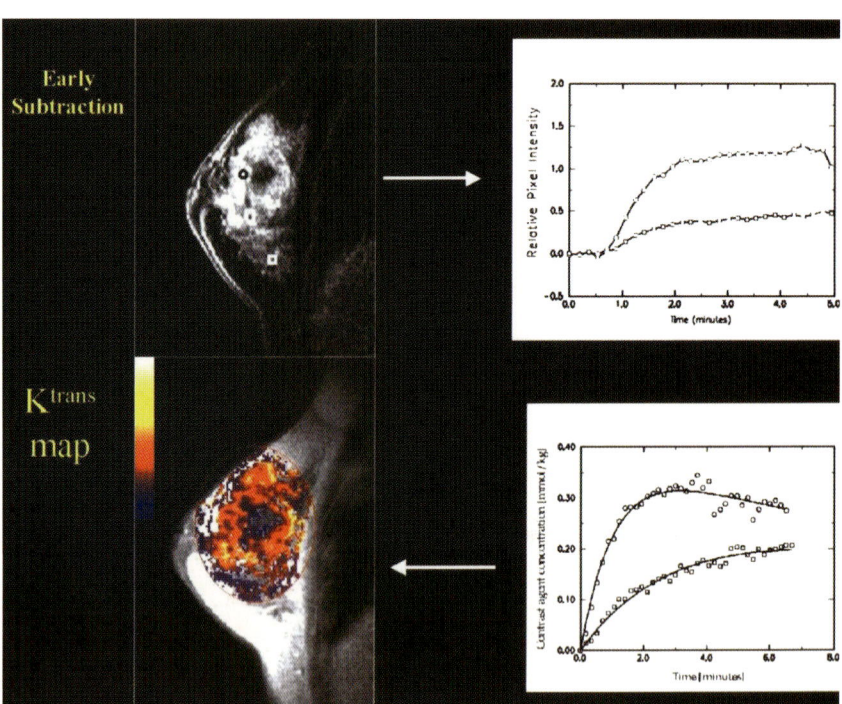

COLOR PLATE 21 Converting signal intensity into contrast concentration and model fitting; data obtained from a patient with invasive ductal cancer. (a) Top-right. This early subtraction image (90 second image following contrast medium minus pre-contrast image) demonstrates a large heterogeneously enhancing mass characteristic for malignancy. This mass is applied to the anterior chest wall. There is a central area of non-enhancement presumably representing an area of necrosis. (b) Top-left. Signal-intensity time curves for the two regions of interest shown in the early subtraction image. Regions of interest are taken from the edge of the enhancing tumour (O) normal tissue ( ). (c) Bottom-right. Conversion of signal intensity information into contrast agent concentration is performed according to the method described by Parker *et al*. The model fitting (continuous line) is done using the Tofts' model. Model fitting is performed after calculation of time of onset of enhancement. (d) Bottom-left. Model fitting is done on each pixel and colour parametric maps (K^{trans}) are displayed. (See Figure 13.8, p. 316)

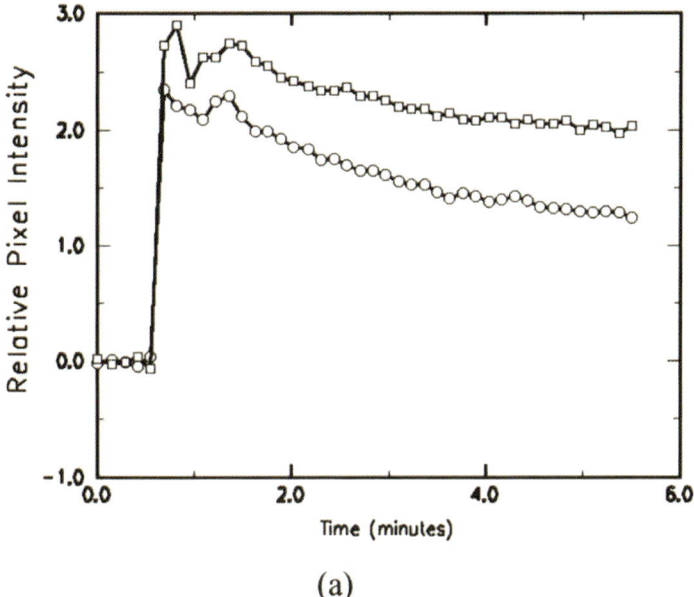

(a)

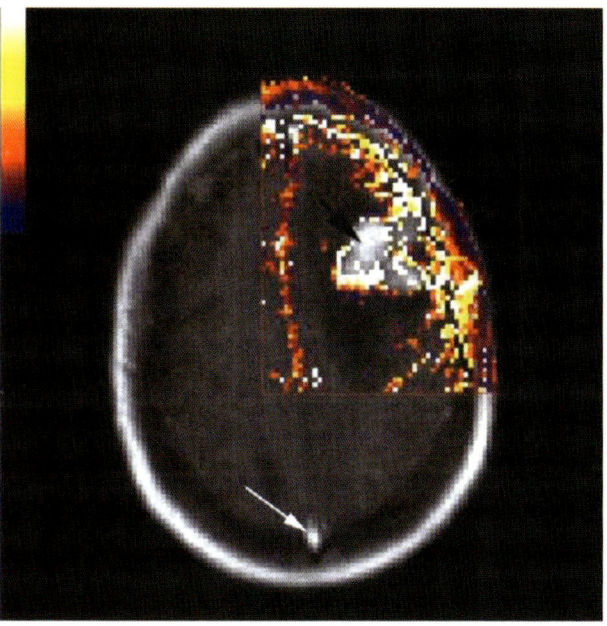

(b)

COLOR PLATE 22 Significant vascular contribution leading to modelling failure. (a) Time signal intensity curve from the centre of metastatic tumour (-black arrow in b) and superior sagittal sinus (O – white arrow in b). The shape of the signal intensity time curves are very similar suggesting that there is a large vascular contribution to the signal obtained from the tumour. Such curves cannot be fitted to the Tofts' model, which results in a large number of modelling pixel failures as shown on the transfer constant map (b). (See Figure 13.10, p. 322)

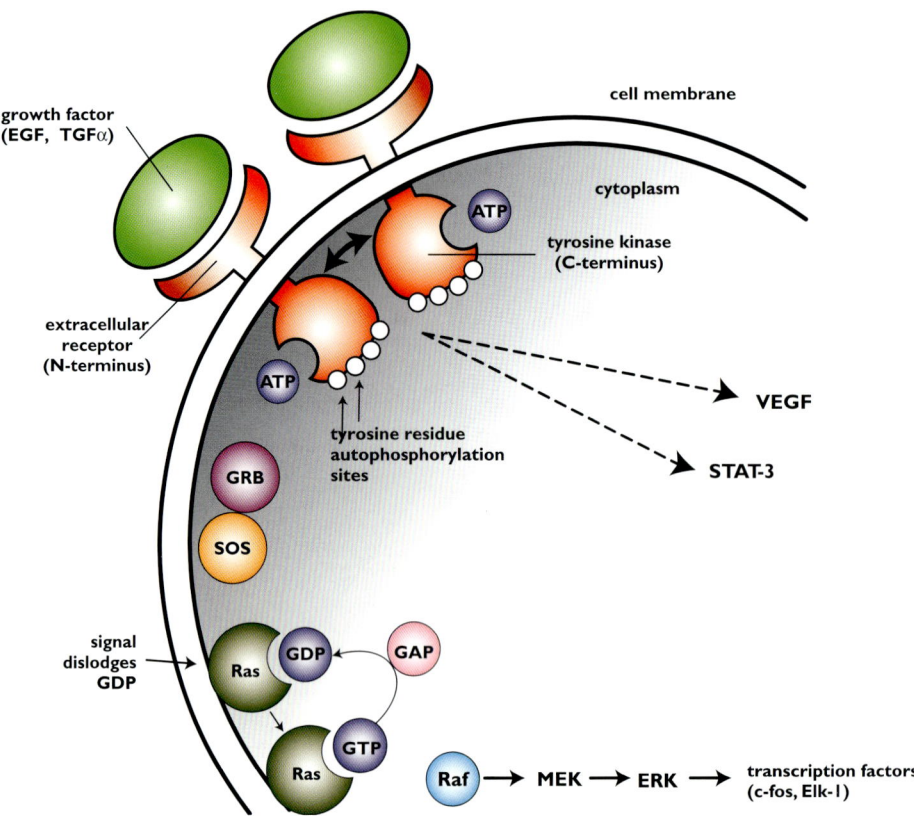

COLOR PLATE 23   Schematic of EGFr signal transduction. EGFr is a class I transmembrane tyrosine kinase receptor with each receptor interacting with a separate ligand (EGF). Interaction induces dimerization and autophosphorylation of the intracellular C terminus portion, which leads to conformational changes enhancing tyrosine kinase activity and allowing interaction with substrates. The growth stimulus is transmitted via the growth factor receptor binding protein (GRB) and son of sevenless (SOS), which leads to dissociation of GDP from membrane bound Ras. Ras then binds with GTP, which is more prevalent than GDP in the cytoplasm. This leads to interaction with Raf and stimulation of the MAP kinase pathway. Ras is returned to the rest state by GAP, which dephosphorylates GTP. EGFr also leads to increased VEGF production, and in addition has anti-apoptotic effects by decreasing levels of phophorylated STAT-3. (See Figure 17.1, p. 393)

12
IMPROVING THE EFFICACY AND SAFETY OF ANTICANCER AGENTS — THE ROLE OF PHARMACOGENETICS

MARGARET-MARY AMEYAW
HOWARD L. McLEOD

Departments of Medicine, Molecular Biology and Pharmacology, and Genetics
Washington University School of Medicine
The Siteman Cancer Center
St. Louis, Missouri

I. INTRODUCTION
II. THIOPURINE METHYLTRANSFERASE
III. DIHYDROPYRIMIDINE DEHYDROGENASE
IV. THYMIDYLATE SYNTHASE
V. ATP-BINDING CASSETTE FAMILY OF DRUG TRANSPORTERS
VI. UDP-GLUCURONOSYLTRANSFERASE 1A1 PHARMACOGENETICS AND IRINOTECAN
VII. METHYLENETETRAHYDROFOLATE REDUCTASE PHARMACOGENETICS
VIII. CYTOCHROME P4503A PHARMACOGENETICS
IX. CONCLUSION

The response to chemotherapeutic drug treatment is a complex process involving multiple factors. Many proteins for example, carrier proteins, drug transporters, metabolizing enzymes, and receptors and their transduction components take part in the response to a drug. Many genes coding for such proteins contain polymorphisms that alter the activity or the level of expression of the encoded proteins. Therefore, the response of a given anticancer agent reflects the interaction of multiple genetic factors that cause important variations in drug metabolism, distribution, and action on its drug target. Pharmacogenetic applications are most relevant for drugs with a narrow therapeutic range between desired effectiveness and toxicity or for drugs with severe side effects or substantial toxicity. Anticancer drugs fall into this category. Some of these pharmacogenetic polymorphisms, for example thiopurine methyltransferase (TPMT), have been studied in detail and are being applied to patient treatment. For patients it will be important to distinguish patient populations based on their expected response and toxicity to target therapy accordingly. Preventing toxicity and improving efficacy will not only help patients but may also help save health-care dollars.

This chapter uses the examples of TPMT, dihydropyrimidine dehydrogenase (DPD), thymidylate synthase (TS), ATP-binding cassette (ABC) group of transporters, UDP-glucuronosyltransferase (UGT), methylenetetrahydrofolate reductase (MTHFR), and CYP3A to illustrate the role of pharmacogenetics in improving the efficacy and safety of anticancer agents.

I. INTRODUCTION

Pharmacogenetics is the study of how genetic variations affect an individual's response to drugs. These variations can affect a patient's toxic response to anticancer agents. Various studies have demonstrated that, not only toxicity, but also response to chemotherapy and patient outcome could be influenced by pharmacogenetic polymorphisms in several genes. Through the study of pharmacogenetics, genetic variations that affect drug efficacy and toxicity will eventually enable physicians to individualize the selection of optimal medications and specific dose for patients, which results in fewer adverse reactions. Currently in oncology, the administration of anticancer agents uses fixed doses normalized by body surface area and does not take into account existing differences between individuals in pharmacokinetics and pharmacodynamics as a result of genetic polymorphisms. Pharmacogenetic screening before cancer therapy may enable the prospective identification of patients at increased risk of toxicity and improve the efficacy of these chemotherapeutic agents.

The role of pharmacogenetics in the optimization of the efficacy and safety of cancer chemotherapy is important in oncology, because cancer chemotherapeutic agents generally have a narrow margin of safety and exhibit significant inter-patient variability in pharmacokinetics and toxicity. Many of these agents are prodrugs that are converted to the active drug by polymorphic enzymes and certain anticancer agents are detoxified by polymorphic enzyme systems.

This chapter will focus on the role of genetic polymorphisms of well-known classes of enzymes involved in cancer chemotherapy. These include TPMT, DPD, TS, ABC group of transporters, UGT, MTHFR, and cytochrome P450 3A (CYP3A).

II. THIOPURINE METHYLTRANSFERASE

TPMT catalyzes the S-methylation of thiopurine drugs such as 6-mercaptopurine (6-MP), 6-thioguanine, and azathioprine to inactive metabolites [1–3]. Thiopurines form part of the routine treatment for patients with acute lymphoblastic leukemia, rheumatoid arthritis, autoimmune diseases such as systemic lupus erythematosus (SLE) and Crohn's disease, and are used as an immunosuppressant following organ transplantation.

TPMT enzyme activity and immunoreactive protein levels in human tissues are controlled by a common genetic polymorphism [1, 4]. Variation in TPMT activity regulates thiopurine toxicity and therapeutic efficacy of thiopurine drugs. Approximately 1 in 300 white subjects have low activity, 6–11% have intermediate activity, and 89–94% have high activity [1, 3, 5]. Patients with low or undetectable levels of TPMT activity develop severe myelosuppression when treated with "standard" doses of thiopurines, while patients with very high TPMT are more likely to have a reduced clinical response to these agents [6–11]. 6-MP and the other thiopurines, azathioprine and thioguanine, are all inactive prodrugs that require metabolism to thioguanine nucleotides (TGNs) in order to exert cytotoxicity [3]. The principal mechanism by which these drugs exert cytotoxicity is considered to be as a result of incorporation of TGNs into DNA and RNA. 6-MP is converted to TGNs by a multistep pathway that is initiated by hypoxanthine phosphoribosyl transferase [3]. Alternatively, these agents can undergo S-methylation catalyzed by TPMT to methylmercaptopurine or oxidation to thiouric acid via xanthine oxidase. TPMT can also S-methylate 6-thioinosine 5′ monophosphate (TIMP) to form the S-methylated derivative methylTIMP. MethylTIMP is a potent inhibitor of de novo purine synthesis and represents an alternative mechanism for cytotoxicity [3, 12]. TPMT shunts more drug down the methylation pathway, therefore making less drug available for activation to TGNs. TPMT is the main enzyme in hematopoietic cells as there is very little xanthine oxidase in these cells. Several studies have documented that TPMT-deficient patients accumulate very high TGN concentrations in erythrocytes (RBC), about 10- to 20-fold higher than controls when given standard doses of thiopurines [7, 8]. This results in severe hematopoietic toxicity in TPMT-deficient patients, unless the thiopurine dosage is reduced 10- to 15-fold [7, 8]. The use of azathioprine in a patient with complete TPMT deficiency resulted in death from neutropenic sepsis [10].

The association between low TPMT activity and excessive hematological toxicity is now well recognized [6, 8, 13]. Molecular analysis of TPMT genotype is able to identify patients at risk for acute toxicity from thiopurines. A recent study in 180 children also identified an important role for TPMT genotype on tolerance to 6-MP therapy [14]. Two of the patients were TPMT deficient and tolerated full-dose 6-MP for only 7% of weeks of therapy. Heterozygous and homozygous wild-type patients tolerated full doses for 65 and 84% of weeks of therapy over 2.5 years of treatment, respectively [14]. The percentage of weeks in which 6-MP dosage had to be decreased to prevent toxicity was 2, 16, and 76% in wild-type, heterozygous and homozygous mutant individuals, respectively (Figure 12.1).

The relationship between *TPMT* genotype and phenotype has been most clearly defined for *TPMT*2, *TPMT*3A, and *TPMT*3C in patients with leukemia and normal volunteers and has been shown to be clinically important [15–16]. The presence of *TPMT*2, *TPMT*3A, or *TPMT*3C predicts phenotype with heterozygous subjects all having intermediate activity and homozygous subjects being TPMT deficient [15]. Coulthard et al., established that *TPMT* genotype not only predicts RBC TPMT activity but also influences TPMT activity in blast cells from leukemia patients [16].

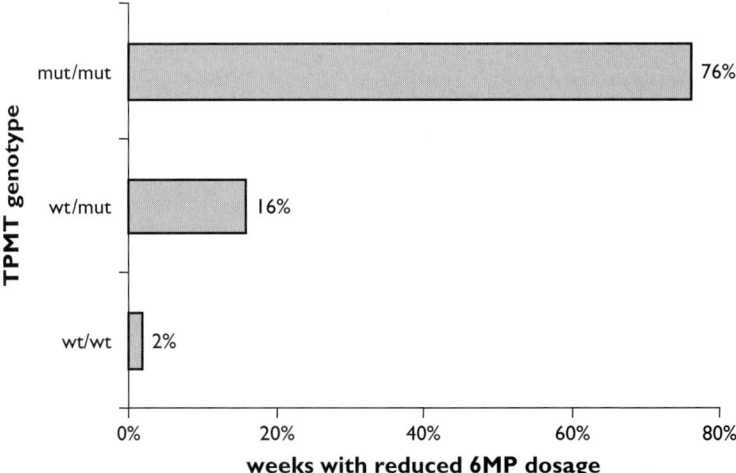

FIGURE 12.1   Percentage of weeks in which (6-MP) dosage reductions were required due to toxicity. Data derived from reference 14.

Knowledge of *TPMT* genotype has been shown to be important in the clinical management of patients receiving thiopurine therapy. A child with acute lymphocytic leukemia (ALL) who was homozygous mutant for TPMT was unable to receive therapy for 53% of the maintenance period and tolerated full 6-MP dosage for only 2% of the maintenance period [17]. 6-MP had to be decreased to prevent toxicity after 2 and 16% of weeks of treatment in children with ALL who were homozygous mutant and heterozygous, respectively, compared with 76% in wild-type TPMT patients. Overall these studies demonstrate that the influence of TPMT genotype is most dramatic for homozygous mutant patients, but is also of clinical relevance for heterozygous individuals.

III. DPD

DPD catalyzes the rate-limiting step in the catabolism of pyrimidines such as thymine and uracil and the fluoropyrimidine, 5-fluorouracil (5-FU). 5-FU is used in the treatment of breast, head, neck, and colorectal cancers [18]. Significant inter-individual variations in 5-FU clearance, tumor response, and host toxicity have been reported after 5-FU therapy [19–20]. In cancer patients with defective DPD, 5-FU toxicity occurs with standard doses of 5-FU and may be severe and life-threatening due to grade 4 myelosuppression and grade 3–4 neurological and gastrointestinal toxicities. DPD activity is completely or partially deficient in about 0.1 and 3–5% of individuals, respectively [21]. The occurrence of severe toxicity usually requires 5-FU discontinuation and dose reduction in the following cycles of therapy, hospitalization, and sometimes change of therapy. A few cases of death from 5-FU toxicity with documented DPD defects have been reported [22–24].

Over 30 variant *DPYD* alleles in the coding and promoter region of the gene have been reported in pediatric patients with total or near-total deficiency of DPD activity and on cancer patients with low activity [25–30]. Eight of these are rare polymorphisms and do not result in decreased DPD activity. Potential mutations with clinical relevance are DPYD*2A and DPYD*9A. DPYD*2A is a splice site mutation (IVS14 + 1G>A) resulting in the production of a truncated mRNA. The molecular basis for DPD deficiency in cancer patients has not been clearly defined; however, analysis of the prevalence of the various mutations among pediatric patients with complete DPD deficiency has shown that the splice-site mutation IVS14 + 1G>A was the most common (52%) [27]. Several studies have shown the frequency of this allele to be low and seen only in some patients with severe toxicity [25, 30–33]. In other studies, discordance was demonstrated between DPYD*2A and DPD activity [26].

The high prevalence of the DPYD*2A polymorphism may warrant screening for the DPYD*2A mutation in cancer patients prior to 5-FU administration. The clinical relevance of DPD deficiency may diminish due to the availability of potent inhibitors of DPD. The use of such inhibitors may result in an improved therapeutic index of 5-FU by enabling the administration of smaller doses of 5-FU [34]. Further studies of DPD pharmacogenetics may help clarify the role of DPD as a marker to identify patients prone to 5-FU toxicity, which may provide a more individualized approach in the administration of 5-FU-based therapies.

IV. THYMIDYLATE SYNTHASE

Thymidylate synthase (TS, TYMS) catalyzes the intracellular transfer of a methyl group to deoxyuridine-5-monophosphate (dUMP) to form deoxythymidine-5-monophosphate (dTMP), which is anabolized in cells to the triphosphate (dTTP). This pathway is the only de novo source of thymidine, an essential precursor for DNA synthesis and repair. The methyl donor for this reaction is the folate co-factor 5,10-methylenetetrahydrofolate (CH2-THF).

TS has been of considerable interest as a target for cancer chemotherapeutic agents such as 5-FU and raltitrexed [35–36]. Fluoropyrimidine resistance in several tumors, including colorectal cancer, has been shown to be mediated through increased mRNA and TS protein levels [37]. High levels of TS expression have been correlated with poor prognosis in breast, gastric, and colorectal cancer [38–41]. This may be due to increased tumor cell proliferation as a result of increased TS levels [42]. The human TS promoter has recently been characterized, which identifies several important mechanisms for gene regulation. In 1995, Horie et al., described a polymorphic tandem repeat found in the 5′-untranslated region of the thymidylate synthase gene [43].

The essential promoter sequence is located –242 to –148 nucleotides upstream of the initiation start site [43]. Polymorphic tandem repeat sequences containing either two (TSER*2) or three (TSER*3) 28 bp repeat units per allele were identified in this region in a Japanese population [44]. In vitro studies have shown that increasing the number of repeats leads to stepwise increases of TS gene expression with the presence of a triple repeat resulting in a 2.6-fold greater TS expression than a double repeat [44–45]. In vivo studies in human gastrointestinal cancer have shown a significant increase in TS protein levels and functional activity in patients with *TSER*3* compared to individuals with *TSER*2* [46]. As TS tumor levels are important for resistance and survival prediction, this may have important implications for TS-based chemotherapy.

There have been many studies from different laboratories on different continents that all suggest that patients homozygous for *TSER*3* have a higher TS activity and a poorer response to 5-FU therapy than patients homozygous for *TSER*2*. In one study involving 65 rectal cancer patients, the probability of achieving tumor downstaging after radiation and 5-FU treatment was dependent on *TSER* genotype. *TSER*2* carriers exhibited a 3.7-fold higher probability of achieving downstaging (a measure of therapeutic success) when compared to *TSER*3* homozygotes [47]. Marsh et al., also showed that *TSER* genotypes correlated with tumor response after 5-FU treatment in 24 metastatic colorectal cancer patients [48]. This study showed that the *TSER*2/TSER*2* genotype was nearly twice as common in the responders to chemotherapy, compared to non-responders (40% *vs.* 22%, respectively). In addition, the study also showed a decrease in median survival with increasing numbers of TSER repeats (median survival 16 months for *TSER*2/TSER*2*, 14 months for *TSER*2/TSER*3*, 12 months for *TSER*3/TSER*3*) [48]. These data were confirmed by Pullarkat et al., who showed that in 50 patients receiving 5-FU for metastatic colorectal cancer, there was a higher response rate in patients with lower numbers of TSER repeats (50% for *TSER*2/TSER*2*,15% for *TSER*2/TSER*3*, and 9% for *TSER*3/TSER*3*; Figure 12.2) [49].

The TS enhancer region polymorphism may be one mechanism responsible for increasing TS gene expression. Two, three, four, and nine copies of 28-bp

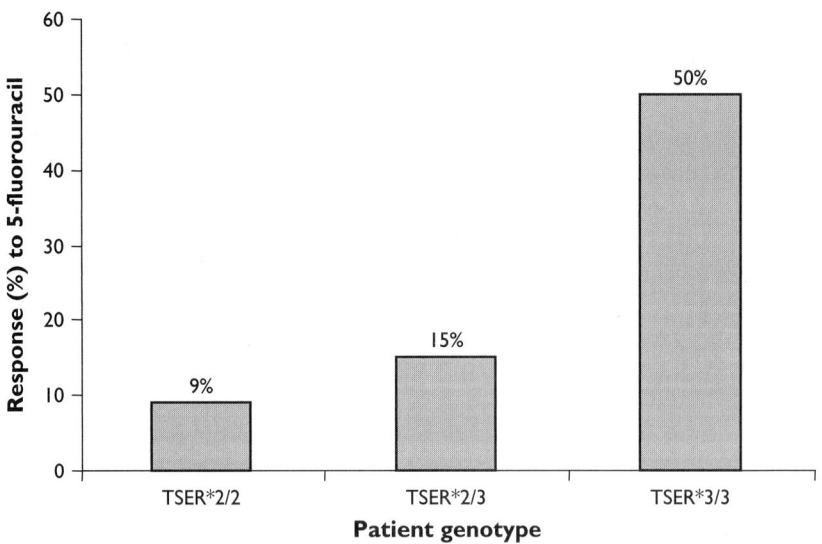

FIGURE 12.2 The relationship between TSER genetic status and response to 5-FU chemotherapy for colorectal cancer. Data derived from reference 49.

tandem repeated sequences have been described in the enhancer region of the TS promoter [44, 50, 51]. A translational regulatory element within the coding region and a 6-bp deletion in the 3′-untranslated region of TS mRNA stability and translation have also been found [52, 53]. Genotyping for tandem repeat promoter polymorphisms, as well as other mutations, that maybe distributed throughout the linear sequence and three-dimensional structure of the human TS gene [54] could be used to select other chemotherapeutic agents that have a different mechanism of action.

V. ABC FAMILY OF DRUG TRANSPORTERS

The ABC transporter family comprises several drug transport proteins. The best characterized ABC drug pump is the *ABCB1* gene, formerly known as *MDR1* or *PGY1*. The *ABCB1* (*MDR1*) gene encodes an integral membrane protein, P-glycoprotein (PGP), a member of the ABC family of membrane transporters [55, 56]. PGP was originally identified by its ability to confer multidrug resistance on tumor cells against a variety of structurally unrelated anticancer agents. The main function of PGP is the energy-dependent efflux of substrates, which include bilirubin, cancer drugs (such as vinca alkaloids, anthracyclines, colchicine, epipodophyllotoxins, actinomycin D, taxanes), cardiac glycosides, immunosuppressive agents, glucocorticoids, HIV-1 protease inhibitors, and many other drugs [57–61].

PGP protein level is highly variable between subjects [62]. However, the molecular basis for inter-patient variation in PGP is not clear. Recently, fifteen different single nucleotide polymorphisms (SNPs) were detected in the *ABCB1* gene. One of these SNPs, resulting in a C to T transition in exon 26 (C3435T), showed a correlation with PGP protein levels and function where the homozygous T allele was associated with more than two-fold lower duodenal PGP protein levels compared with C3435 homozygotes [62]. Homozygosity of the T3435 variant was observed in 24% of 188 German Caucasians. Heterozygous individuals displayed an intermediate phenotype. Evaluation of *ABCB1* genotype status may be a valuable tool in identifying individuals who may have altered drug absorption or be at higher risk for clinically significant drug interactions.

In addition to the PGP transported neutral organic compounds, *ABCC1* (MRP1), *ABCC2* (MRP2), and *ABCC3* (MRP3) also transport drugs conjugated to GSH, glucuronate, or sulfate and other organic anions such as methotrexate. The newer family members, *ABCC4* (MRP4) and *ABCC5* (MRP5), are able to cause resistance to nucleotide analogs, such as PMEA and purine base analogs, such as 6-MP and thioguanine. Transport by the other members of the ABC family, therefore, affects a wide range of anticancer drugs. The *ABCC1* pump confers resistance to doxorubicin, daunorubicin, vincristine, colchicines, and several other compounds; this is a similar profile to that of *ABCB1* [63]. *ABCG2* confers resistance to anthracycline anticancer drugs and is amplified or involved in chromosomal translocations in cell lines selected with topotecan, mitoxantrone, or doxorubicin treatment [64–66].

Pharmacogenetic research involving characterization of drug transporter polymorphisms will enhance our insights into the molecular mechanisms involved in transporter function, especially for anticancer agents. Such findings will become important components of individualized drug therapy in the future.

VI. UDP-GLUCURONOSYLTRANSFERASE 1A1 PHARMACOGENETICS AND IRINOTECAN

Irinotecan is a prodrug, and hydrolysis of irinotecan by the carboxyesterase-2 enzyme in many normal tissues is responsible for activation of irinotecan to SN-38, a potent topoisomerase I inhibitor [67–69]. Glucuronidation of SN-38 is the major elimination pathway of SN-38 and protects patients from irinotecan toxicity. The pharmacogenetics of irinotecan is mainly focused on the polymorphic glucuronidation of SN-38 to SN-38G. Inter-patient variability in SN-38 glucuronidation is considerably high in cancer patients [70]. A recent prospective trial of UGT1A1 pharmacogenetics in cancer patients receiving irinotecan found that the presence of the UGT1A1*28 allele (characterized by a TA insertion in the promoter region of UGT1A1 gene) markedly altered SN-38 disposition [71]. The presence of UGT1A1*28 allele has been shown to be a significant risk factor for severe toxicity from irinotecan in several studies where patients homozygous for 7 repeats experiencing approximately four-fold greater neutropenia (Figure 12.3) [71, 72]. These studies propose UGT1A1 genotyping as a reliable test to predict the risk of severe toxicity after irinotecan.

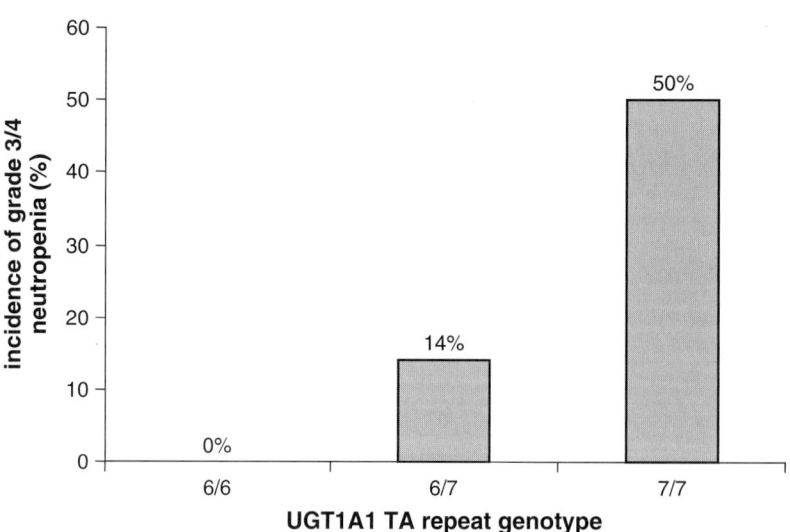

FIGURE 12.3 A higher incidence of severe neutropenia (grade 3–4) from irinotecan is observed in patients homozygous for 7 TA repeats in UGT1A1 (UGT1A1*28). Data derived from reference 71

VII. MTHFR REDUCTASE PHARMACOGENETICS

MTHFR regulates the pool of intracellular folates for nucleic acid and protein synthesis. *MTHFR* converts 5,10-methylene tretrahydrofolate (CH_2THF) to 5-methyltetrahydrofolate (CH_3THF), a methyl donor in the conversion of homocysteine to methionine during protein synthesis [73]. A recent study has reported an association between the occurrence of severe myelotoxicity after CMF and a single nucleotide polymorphism (C677T mutation in exon 4) in *MTHFR* [74]. This SNP is common with approximately 10% of homozygous variant individuals (TT) in Caucasian populations and ranges between 5–54% in other populations [75]. The C677T mutation in the *MTHFR* gene results in an enzyme variant with *in vitro* thermolability and 35% reduction in activity compared to wild type [76]. When TS converts dUMP into dTMP, CH_2THF is required as a donor of monocarbon groups. *MTHFR* deficiency as a result of TT genotype results in reduced activity of MTHFR enzyme, which implies increased levels of CH_2THF that probably increase 5-FdUMP inhibition of TS and lead to severe myelosuppression [77]. Five of six patients with grade 4 leukopenia after CMF were TT homozygotes [74]. The clinical relevance of the C677T mutation was also highlighted in a phase I trial of CPT11/raltitrexed combination [78]. Patients with a TT genotype showed no toxicity compared with CC/CT patients. These findings highlight a possible role of *MTHFR* polymorphism in selecting cancer patients at higher risk of toxicity after receiving the CMF regimen.

VIII. CYTOCHROME P4503A PHARMACOGENETICS

Cytochrome P450 enzymes are responsible for activation of anticancer drugs or might be involved in forming metabolites that are toxic to host tissues. The CYP3A enzymes account for approximately half of the metabolism carried out by cytochrome P450 enzymes. Two main forms are expressed in humans, CYP3A4 and CYP3A5. Genetic polymorphisms in both genes have been described [79–83]. Polymorphisms in CYP3A4 have not been consistently associated with altered catalytic activity. There are at least two distinct single nucleotide polymorphisms in CYP3A5 that demonstrate significant ethnic differences in allele frequency and altered enzyme activity.

CYP3A enzymes are involved in the metabolism of teniposide and etoposide [84], ifosfamide [85], vindesine [86], vinblastine [87, 88], vincristine [87], cyclosphosphamide [85], paclitaxel [89], and docetaxel [90]. The contribution of the SNPs to the effect of anticancer drugs has not yet been elucidated, but because almost half of all anticancer drugs are CYP3A substrates, polymorphisms in CYP3A are likely to affect the pharmacodynamics of anticancer drugs.

IX. CONCLUSION

Clinical trials that individualize therapy based on each patient's individual genetic constitution need to be undertaken to test whether such individualization benefits patients. Once the functional significance of a drug disposition pathway has been established, anticancer agents can be optimized and individualized by pharmacogenetic approaches into the routine care of patients receiving anticancer drugs.

The availability of reliable genotyping techniques for functional polymorphisms can change the way patients will receive chemotherapy in the near future.

ACKNOWLEDGEMENTS

The authors are supported by NIH grants U01 GM63340 and P30 CA091842.

REFERENCES

1. The number is off by 1, as the 'weinshilboum/sladek' reference below should be reference 1. Weinshilboum RM, Sladek SL. Mercaptopurine pharmacogenetics: Monogenic inheritance of erythrocyte thiopurine methyltransferase activity. *Am. J. Hum. Genet.* 1980; 32:651–662.
2. McLeod HL, Krynetski EY, Willimas JA, Evans WE. Higher activity of polymorphic thiopurine S-methyltransferase in erythrocytes from neonates compared to adults. *Pharmacogenetics* 1995; 5:281–286.
3. Krynetski EY, Tai H-L, Yates CR et al. Genetic polymorphism of thiopurine methyltransferase: Clinical importance and molecular mechanisms. *Pharmacogenetics* 1996; 6:279–290.
4. Tai HI, Krynetski EY, Schuetz EG, Yashinevski Y, Evans WE. Enhanced proteolysis of thiopurine S-methyltransferase (TPMT) encoded by mutant alleles in human (*TPMT*3A, TPMT*2): Mechanism for the genetic polymorphism of TPMT activity. *Proc. Natl. Acad. Sci. U. S. A.* 1997; 94:6444–6449.
5. McLeod HL, Lin J-S, Scott EP, Pui C-H, Evans WE. Thiopurine methyltransferase activity in American white subjects and black subjects. *Clin. Pharmacol. Ther.* 1994; 55:15–20.
6. Lennard L, Lilleyman JS, Van Loon JA, Weinshilboum RM. Genetic variation in response to 6-mercaptopurine for childhood acute lymphoblastic leukaemia. *Lancet* 1990; 1336:225–229.
7. Evans WE, Horner M, Chu YO, Kalwinsky D, Roberts WM. Altered mercaptopurine metabolism, toxic effects and dosage requirement in a thiopurine methyltranferase-deficient child with acute lymphoblastic leukaemia. *J. Paediatr.* 1991; 119:985–989.
8. McLeod HL, Miller DR, Evans WE. Azathioprine-induced myelosuppression in thiopurine methyltransferase deficient heart transplant recipient. *Lancet* 1993; 1341:1151.
9. Lennard L, Gibson BES, Nicole T, Lilleyman JS. Congenital thiopurine methyltransferase deficiency and 6-mercaptopurine toxicity during treatment for acute lymphoblastic leukaemia. *Arch. Dis. Child.* 1993; 69:577–579.
10. Schutz E, Gummert J, Mohr F, Oellerich M. Azathioprine induced myelosuppression in thiopurine methyltransferase deficient heart transplant recipient. *Lancet* 1993: 341:436.
11. Lilleyman JS, Lennard L. Mercaptopurine metabolism and risk of relapse in childhood lymphoblastic leukaemia. *Lancet* 1994; 343:1188–1190.
12. Krynetski EY, Evans WE. Pharmacogenetics as a molecular basis for individualised drug therapy: The thiopurine S-methyltransferase paradigm. *Pharmaceut. Res.* 1999; 16:342–349.
13. McLeod HL, Relling MV, Liu Q, Pui CH, Evans WE. Polymorphic thiopurine methyltransferase in erythrocytes is indicative of activity in leukaemic blasts from children with acute lymphoblastic leukaemia. *Blood* 1995; 85:1897–1902.
14. Relling MV, Hancock HL, Rivera GK et al. Intolerance to mercaptopurine therapy related to heterozygosity at the thiopurine methyltransferase gene locus. *J. Natl. Cancer Inst.* 1999; 91:2001–2008.

15. Tai HL, Krynetski EY, Yates CR et al. Thiopurine S-methyltransferase deficiency: Two nucleotide transitions define the most prevalent mutant allele associated with loss of catalytic activity in Caucasians. *Am. J. Hum. Genet.* 1996; 58:694–702.

16. Coulthard SA, Howell C, Robson J, Hall AG. The relationship between thiopurine methyltransferase activity and genotype in blasts from patients with acute leukemia. *Blood* 1998; 92:2856–2862.

17. McLeod HL, Coulthard S, Thomas AE et al. Analysis of thiopurine methyltransferase variant alleles in childhood acute lymphoblastic leukaemia. *Br. J. Haematol.* 1999; 105:696–700.

18. Diasio RB, Harris BE. Clinical pharmacology of 5-fluorouracil. *Clin. Pharmacokinet.* 1989; 16:215–37.

19. Milano G, Etienne MC, Cassuto-Viguier E et al. Influence of sex and age on fluorouracil clearance. *J. Clin. Oncol.* 1992; 10:1171–1175.

20. Diasio RB, Van Kuilenburg AB, Lu Z et al. Determination of dihydropyrimidine dehydrogenase (DPD) in fibroblasts of a DPD deficient pediatric patient and family members using a polyclonal antibody to human DPD. *Adv. Exp. Med. Biol.* 1994; 370:7–10.

21. Lu Z, Zhang R, Diasio RB. Dihydropyrimidine dehydrogenase activity in human peripheral blood mononuclear cells and liver: Population characteristics, newly identified deficient patients, and clinical implication in 5-fluorouracil chemotherapy. *Cancer Res.* 1993; 53:5433–5438

22. Stephan F, Etienne MC, Wallays C, Milano G, Clergue F. Depressed hepatic dihydropyrimidine dehydrogenase activity and fluorouracil-related toxicities. *Am. J. Med.* 1995; 99:685–688.

23. Milano G, Etienne MC, Pierrefite V, Barberi-Heyob M, Deporte-Fety R, Renee N. Dihydropyrimidine dehydrogenase deficiency and fluorouracil-related toxicity. *Br. J. Cancer* 1999; 79:627–630.

24. Fleming RA, Milano GA, Gaspard MH et al. Dihydropyrimidine dehydrogenase activity in cancer patients. *Eur. J. Cancer* 1993; 29A:740–744.

25. van Kuilenburg AB, Haasjes J, Richel DJ et al. Clinical implications of dihydropyrimidine dehydrogenase (DPD) deficiency in patients with severe 5-fluorouracil-associated toxicity: Identification of new mutations in the DPD gene. *Clin. Cancer Res.* 2000; 6:4705–4712.

26. Collie-Duguid ES, Etienne MC, Milano G, McLeod HL. Known variant DPYD alleles do not explain DPD deficiency in cancer patients. *Pharmacogenetics* 2000; 10:217–223.

27. van Kuilenburg AB, Vreken P, Abeling NG et al. Genotype and phenotype in patients with dihydropyrimidine dehydrogenase deficiency. *Hum. Genet.* 1999; 104:1–9.

28. Ridge SA, Sludden J, Brown O et al. Dihydropyrimidine dehydrogenase pharmacogenetics in Caucasian subjects. *Br. J. Clin. Pharmacol.* 1998; 46:151–156.

29. Ridge SA, Sludden J, Wei X et al. Dihydropyrimidine dehydrogenase pharmacogenetics in patients with colorectal cancer. *Br. J. Cancer* 1998; 77:497–500.

30. van Kuilenburg AB, Dobritzsch D, Meinsma R et al. Novel disease-causing mutations in the dihydropyrimidine dehydrogenase gene interpreted by analysis of the three-dimensional protein structure. *Biochem. J.* 2002; 364:157–163.

31. Wei X, McLeod HL, McMurrough J, Gonzalez FJ, Fernandez-Salguero P. Molecular basis of the human dihydropyrimidine dehydrogenase deficiency and 5-fluorouracil toxicity. *J. Clin. Invest.* 1996; 98:610–615.

32. van Kuilenburg AB, Vreken P, Beex LV, De Abreu RA, van Gennip AH. Severe 5-fluorouracil toxicity caused by reduced dihydropyrimidine dehydrogenase activity due to heterozygosity for a G→A point mutation. *J. Inherit. Metab. Dis.* 1998; 21:280–284.

33. Johnson MR, Hageboutros A, Wang K, High L, Smith JB, Diasio RB. Life-threatening toxicity in a dihydropyrimidine dehydrogenase-deficient patient after treatment with topical 5-fluorouracil. *Clin. Cancer Res.* 1999; 5:2006–2011.

34. Adjei AA, Reid JM, Diasio RB et al. Comparative pharmacokinetic study of continuous venous infusion fluorouracil and oral fluorouracil with eniluracil in patients with advanced solid tumors. *J. Clin. Oncol.* 2002; 20:1683–1691.

35. Rustum YM, Harstrick A, Cao S, Vanhoefer U, Yin MB, Wilke H, Seeber S. Thymidylate synthase inhibitors in cancer therapy: Direct and indirect inhibitors. *J. Clin. Oncol.* 1997; 15:389–400.

36. Leichman CG, Lenz HJ, Leichman L et al. Quantitation of intratumoral thymidylate synthase expression predicts for disseminated colorectal cancer response and resistance to protracted-infusion fluorouracil and weekly leucovorin. *J. Clin. Oncol.* 1997; 15:3223–3229.

37. Berger SH, Jenh CH, Johnson LF, Berger FG. Thymidylate synthase overproduction and gene amplification in fluorodeoxyuridine-resistant human cells. *Mol. Pharmacol.* 1985; 28:461–467.

38. Pestalozzi BC, Peterson RD, Gelber A et al. Prognostic importance of thymidylate synthase expression in early breast cancer. *J. Clin. Oncol.* 1997; 15:1921–1931.

39. Lenz H-J, Leichman CG, Danenberg KD et al. Thymidylate synthase mRNA level in adenocarcinoma of the stomach: A predictor for primary tumour response and overall survival. *J. Clin. Oncol.* 1995; 14:176–182.

40. Johnston PG, Fisher ER, Rockette HE et al. The role of thymidylate synthase expression in prognosis and outcome of adjuvant chemotherapy in patients with rectal cancer. *J. Clin. Oncol.* 1994; 12:2640–2647.

41. Kornmann M, Link KH, Lenz H-J et al. Thymidylate synthase is a predictor for response and resistance in hepatic artery infusion chemotherapy. *Cancer Lett.* 1997; 118:29–35.

42. Kaye SB. New antimetabolites in cancer chemotherapy and their clinical impact. *Br. J. Cancer* 1998; 78:1–7.

43. Horie N, Takeishi K. Identification of functional elements in the promoter region of the human gene for thymidylate synthase and nuclear factors that regulate the expression of the gene. *J. Biol. Chem.* 1997; 272:18375–18381.

44. Horie N, Aiba H, Oguro K, Hojo H, Takeishi K. Functional analysis and DNA polymorphism of the tandemly repeated sequences in the 5′-terminal regulatory region of the human gene for thymidylate synthase. *Cell Struct. Funct.* 1995; 20:191–197.

45. Kawakami K, Salonga D, Omura K et al. Effects of polymorphic tandem repeat sequence on the in vitro translation of messenger RNA. *Proc. Am. Assoc. Cancer Res.* 1999; 40:436–437.

46. Kawakami K, Omura K, Kanehhira E, Morishita M, Watanabe Y. Polymorphic tandem repeats in the thymidylate synthase gene is associated with its protein expression in human gastrointestinal cancers. *Anticancer Res.* 1999; 19:3249–3252.

47. Villafranca E, Okruzhnov Y, Dominguez MA et al. Polymorphisms of the repeated sequences in the enhancer region of the thymidylate synthase gene promoter may predict downstaging after preoperative chemoradiation in rectal cancer. *J. Clin. Oncol.* 2001; 19:1779–1786.

48. Marsh S, McKay JA, Cassidy J, McLeod HL. Polymorphism in the thymidylate synthase promoter enhancer region in colorectal cancer. *Int. J. Oncol.* 2001; 19:383–386.

49. Pullarkat ST, Stoehlmacher J, Ghaderi V et al. Thymidylate synthase gene polymorphism determines response and toxicity of 5-FU chemotherapy, *Pharmacogenomics J.* 2001; 1:65–70.

50. Kaneda S, Horie N, Takeishi K, Takayanagi A, Seno T, Ayusawa D. Regulatory sequences clustered at the 5′ end of the first intron of the human thymidylate synthase gene function in cooperation with the promoter region. *Somat. Cell Molec. Gen.* 1992; 18:409–415.

51. Marsh S, Ameyaw M-M, Githang'a J, Indalo A, Ofori-Adjei D, McLeod HL. Novel thymidylate synthase enhancer region alleles in African populations. *Hum. Mutat.* 2000; 16:528.

52. Lin X, Parsels LA, Voeller DM et al. Characterization of a cis-acting regulatory element in the protein coding region of thymidylate synthase mRNA. *Nucleic Acids Res.* 2000; 28:1381–1389.

53. Ulrich CM, Bigler J, Velicer CM, Greene EA, Farin FM, Potter JD. Searching expressed sequence tag databases: discovery and confirmation of a common polymorphism in the thymidylate synthase gene. *Cancer Epidemiol. Biomarkers Prev.* 2000; 9:1381–1385.

54. Kawate H, Landis DM, Loeb LA. Distribution of mutations in human thymidylate synthase yielding resistance to 5-fluorodeoxyuridine. *J. Biol. Chem.* 2002; 1277:36304–36311.

55. Ueda K, Cornwell MM, Gottesman MM et al. The *MDR1* gene, responsible for multidrug resistance, codes for P-glycoprotein. *Biochem. Biophys. Res. Commun.* 1986; 141:956–962.

56. Borst P, Evers R, Kool M, Wijnholds J. A family of drug transporters: The multidrug resistance-associated proteins. *J. Natl. Cancer Inst.* 2000; 92:1295–1302.

57. Gottesman MM, Hrycyna CA, Schoenlein PV, Germann UA, Pastan I. Genetic analysis of the multidrug transporter. *Ann. Rev. Genet.* 1995; 29:607–649.

58. de Lannoy IAM, Silverman M. The *MDR1* gene product P-glycoprotein, mediates the transport of the cardiac glycoside, digoxin. *Biochem. Biophys. Res. Commun.* 1992; 189:551–557.

59. Saeki T, Ueda K, Tanigawara Y, Hori R, Komano T. Human P-glycoprotein transports cyclosporin a and FK 506. *J. Biol. Chem.* 1993; 1268:6007–6080.

60. Ueda K, Okamura N, Hirai M et al. Human P-glycoprotein transports cortisol, aldosterone, and dexamethasone but not progesterone. *J. Biol. Chem.* 1992; 267:24248–24252.

61. Kim RB, Fromm MF, Christoph W, Leake B, Wood AJJ, Roden D. The drug transporter P-glycoprotein limits oral absorption and brain entry of HIV-1 protease inhibitors. *J. Clin. Invest.* 1998; 101:289–294.

62. Hoffmeyer S, Burk O, von Richter O et al. Functional polymorphisms of the human multidrug-resistance gene: Multiple sequence variations and correlation of one allele with P-glycoprotein expression and activity in vivo. *Proc. Natl. Acad. Sci. U. S. A.* 2000; 97:3473–3478.

63. Cole SP, Bhardwaj G, Gerlach JH et al. Overexpression of a transporter gene in a multidrug-resistant human lung cancer cell line. *Science* 1992; 258:1650–1654.

64. Doyle LA, Yang W, Abruzzo LV, Krogmann T, Gao Y, Rishi AK, Ross DD. A multidrug resistance transporter from human MCF-7 breast cancer cells. *Proc. Natl. Acad. Sci. U. S. A.* 1998; 95:15665–15670.

65. Miyake K, Mickley L, Litman T et al. Molecular cloning of cDNAs which are highly over-expressed in mitoxantrone-resistant cells: Demonstration of homology to ABC transport genes. *Cancer Res.* 1999; 59:8–13.

66. Allikmets R, Schriml LM, Hutchinson A, Romano-Spica V, Dean M. A human placenta-specific ATP-binding cassette gene (ABCP) on chromosome 4q22 that is involved in multidrug resistance. *Cancer Res.* 1998; 58:5337–5339.

67. Kawato Y, Furuta T, Aonuma M, Yasuoka M, Yokokura T, Matsumoto K. Antitumor activity of a camptothecin derivative, CPT-11, against human tumor xenografts in nude mice. *Cancer Chemother. Pharmacol.* 1991; 28:192–198.

68. Humerickhouse R, Lohrbach K, Li L, Bosron WF, Dolan ME. Characterization of CPT-11 hydrolysis by human liver carboxylesterase isoforms hCE-1 and hCE-2. *Cancer Res.* 2000; 60:1189–1192.

69. Rivory LP, Bowles MR, Robert J, Pond SM. Conversion of irinotecan (CPT-11) to its active metabolite, 7-ethyl-10-hydroxycamptothecin (SN-38), by human liver carboxylesterase. *Biochem. Pharmacol.* 1996; 52:1103–1111.

70. Gupta E, Lestingi TM, Mick R, Ramirez J, Vokes EE, Ratain MJ. Metabolic fate of irinotecan in humans: Correlation of glucuronidation with diarrhea. *Cancer Res.* 1994; 54:3723–3725.

71. Iyer L, Hall D, Das S, Mortell MA, Ramirez J, Kim S, Di Rienzo A, Ratain MJ. Phenotype-genotype correlation of in vitro SN-38 (active metabolite of irinotecan) and bilirubin glucuronidation in human liver tissue with UGT1A1 promoter polymorphism. *Clin. Pharmacol. Ther.* 1999; 65:576–582.

72. Innocenti F, Undevia SD, Iyer L et al. Genetic variants in the UDP-glucuronosyltransferase 1A1 gene predict the risk of severe neutropenia of irinotecan. *J. Clin. Oncol.* 2004; 22:1382–8.

73. Toffoli G, Veronesi A, Boiocchi M, Crivellari D. MTHFR gene polymorphism and severe toxicity during adjuvant treatment of early breast cancer with cyclophosphamide, methotrexate, and fluorouracil (CMF). *Ann. Oncol.* 2000; 11:373–374.

74. Brattstrom L, Zhang Y, Hurtig M et al. A common methylenetetrahydrofolate reductase gene mutation and longevity. *Atherosclerosis* 1998; 141:315–319.

75. Ueland PM, Hustad S, Schneede J, Refsum H, Vollset SE. Biological and clinical implications of the MTHFR C677T polymorphism. *Trends Pharmacol. Sci.* 2001; 22:195–201.

76. Frosst P, Blom HJ, Milos R et al. A candidate genetic risk factor for vascular disease: A common mutation in methylenetetrahydrofolate reductase. *Nat. Genet.* 1995; 10:111–113.

77. Innocenti F, Ratain MJ. Update on pharmacogenetics in cancer chemotherapy. *Eur. J. Cancer* 2002; 38:639–644.

78. Stevenson JP, Redlinger M, Kluijtmans LA et al. Phase I clinical and pharmacogenetic trial of irinotecan and raltitrexed administered every 21 days to patients with cancer. *J. Clin. Oncol.* 2001; 19:4081–4087.

79. Kuehl P, Zhang J, Lin Y et al. Sequence diversity in CYP3A promoters and characterization of the genetic basis of polymorphic CYP3A5 expression. *Nat. Genet.* 2001; 27:383–391.

80. Paulussen A, Lavrijsen K, Bohets H et al. Two linked mutations in transcriptional regulatory elements of the CYP3A5 gene constitute the major genetic determinant of polymorphic activity in humans. *Pharmacogenetics* 2000; 10:415–424.

81. Sata F, Sapone A, Elizondo G et al. CYP3A4 allelic variants with amino acid substitutions in exons 7 and 12: Evidence for an allelic variant with altered catalytic activity. *Clin. Pharmacol. Ther.* 2000; 67:48–56.

82. Ball SE, Scatina J, Kao J et al. Population distribution and effects on drug metabolism of a genetic variant in the 5′-promoter region of CYP3A4. *Clin. Pharmacol. Ther.* 1999; 66:288–294.

83. Rebbeck TR, Jaffe JM, Walker AH, Wein AJ, Malkowicz SB. Modification of clinical presentation of prostate tumours by a novel genetic variant in CYP3A4. *J. Natl. Cancer Inst.* 1998; 90:1225–1229.

84. Relling MV, Evans R, Dass C, Desiderio DM, Nemec J. Human cytochrome P450 metabolism of teniposide and etoposide. *J. Pharmacol. Exp. Ther.* 1992; 261:491–496.

85. Chang TK, Weber GF, Crespi CL, Waxman DJ. Differential activation of cyclophosphamide and ifosphamide by cytochromes P-450 2B and 3A in human liver microsomes. *Cancer Res.* 1993; 53:5629–37.

86. Zhou XJ, Zhou-Pan XR, Gauthier T, Placidi M, Maurel P, Rahmani R. Human liver microsomal cytochrome P450 3A isozymes mediated vindesine biotransformation. Metabolic drug interactions. *Biochem. Pharmacol.* 1993; 45:853–861.

87. Wacher VJ, Wu CY, Benet LZ. Overlapping substrate specificities and tissue distribution of cytochrome P4503A and P-glycoprotein: implications for drug delivery and activity in cancer chemotherapy. *Mol. Carcinogen.* 1995; 13:129–134.

88. Zhou-Pan XR, Seree E, Zhou XJ et al. Involvement of human liver cytochrome P450 3A in vinblastine metabolism: drug interactions. *Cancer Res.* 1993; 53:5121–5126.

89. Harris JW, Rahman A, Kim BR, Guengerich FP, Collins JM. Metabolism of taxol by human hepatic microsomes and liver slices: Participation of cytochrome P450 3A4 and an unknown P450 enzyme. *Cancer Res.* 1994; 54:4026–4035.

90. Royer I, Monsarrat B, Sonnier M, Wright M, Cresteil T. Metabolism of docetaxel by human cytochromes P450: Interactions with paclitaxel and other antineoplastic drugs. *Cancer Res.* 1996; 56:58–65.

13
IMAGING OF PHARMACODYNAMIC END POINTS IN CLINICAL TRIALS

ERIC O. ABOAGYE

PET Oncology Group
Department of Cancer Medicine
Imperial College School of Medicine
London, United Kingdom

A. R. PADHANI

Paul Strickland Scanner Centre
Mount Vernon Hospital
Middlesex, United Kingdom

PATRICIA M. PRICE

PET Oncology Group
Department of Cancer Medicine
Imperial College School of Medicine
London, United Kingdom

I. INTRODUCTION
II. PET
III. EVALUATION OF CANCER THERAPEUTICS WITH PET
IV. MRI ASSESSMENT OF MICROVESSEL FUNCTION
V. CONCLUSIONS

Anticancer drug discovery and development are experiencing a paradigm shift from cytotoxic therapies to more selective therapies that target underlying oncogenic abnormalities. To a large extent, these newer therapies are cytostatic and, thus, difficult to evaluate by current methods such as maximum tolerated dose and radiologic tumor shrinkage. Furthermore, there is an increasing need to include selection of patients possessing particular oncogenic abnormalities in clinical trial designs. In this chapter the application of non-invasive imaging methods (positron emission tomography; PET) and dynamic contrast-enhanced magnetic resonance imaging; DCE-MRI) for the pharmacodynamic evaluation of existing and new cancer therapeutics will be described. These imaging modalities have potential application in the evaluation of novel agents including cell cycle inhibitors, anti-angiogenic and anti-vascular agents, thymidylate synthase inhibitors, inhibitors of ras farnesylation, apoptosis-inducing agents, gene therapies, multidrug resistance modulators, receptor antagonists, and inhibitors of drug metabolism. The success of incorporating these new technologies into drug development programs will depend on close collaboration and risk sharing in technology development between academia and industry.

I. INTRODUCTION

There is a lot of enthusiasm about the development of molecular target-directed anticancer agents. These agents, discovered through our increased understanding of tumor biology, target specific alterations that drive malignant transformation including genes and pathways involved in angiogenesis, cell cycle, signal transduction, cell death, drug resistance, cell invasion, and metastasis. With these advances, the need to revise the way new drugs are tested has become apparent. The conventional way of testing drugs including studies aimed at defining the maximum tolerated dose (phase I), and those aimed at evaluating the efficacy of a particular dose and schedule in a number of disease types (phase II) may be inadequate. Although safety studies are still needed, phase I studies also need to incorporate an evaluation of mechanism of action. Such hypothesis-testing studies could also be used to establish appropriate dosing schedules for phase II studies. Two key issues that need to be addressed in early clinical trial design for new agents are (1) pathophysiology-based (based on specific molecular abnormalities) selection of patients for clinical trials, and (2) pharmacodynamic evaluation of mechanism of action or of response to therapy. Evaluation of drugs in a more homogeneous population of patients expressing the molecular abnormality of interest is ethically debatable but is likely to provide answers in fewer patients and in less time. In addition, patients unlikely to respond to a specific therapy would be excluded.

The ability to include new ideas in clinical trial design presupposes that one can measure the molecular abnormality of interest. Assays of protein levels, for instance, have been reported in Chapters _____ for monitoring the pharmacodynamics of farnesyl transferase inhibitors. In this chapter the use of imaging to measure pathophysiology and pharmacodynamics for existing and newer cancer therapeutics will be described. The imaging methods have the advantage that the same patients can be studied over time avoiding multiple biopsies, which can be problematic in recruiting patients for proof-of-principle studies. Furthermore, the imaging studies allow the "effect" compartment (e.g., tumor) to be examined *in situ*. In some cases this may be superior to pharmacodynamic assessment using non-tumor cells such as peripheral blood mononuclear cells (PBMC). This is particularly the case when the response in PBMCs is more sensitive than in tumors as was the case for the inactivation of alkyltransferase by benzylguanine [1]. Imaging modalities are not, however, straightforward. There are specific methodological challenges: technologies are not as widely available and they may be expensive. In this chapter the scientific basis underlying PET and DCE-MRI will also be described, potential for quantification and validation studies performed to date will be reviewed, and their potential application for testing cancer therapeutics will be explored. Specific challenges will also be discussed.

II. PET

PET is a sensitive technique that involves the administration of a compound labeled with a short-lived positron emitting isotope, followed by data acquisition to obtain the *in vivo* three-dimensional (3D) distribution and kinetics of the compound. The radiopharmaceuticals used are administered in very small quantities so as not to modify underlying tissue biological and biochemical properties. As such they are known as radiotracers.

A. Radiotracers

PET employs proton-rich radionuclides, which decay by positron emission. Positron-emitting radionuclides frequently used in medicine including oxygen-15 (physical half-life, $t_{1/2}$ = 2.03 min), nitrogen-13 ($t_{1/2}$ = 10 min), carbon-11 ($t_{1/2}$ = 20.4 min), fluorine-18 ($t_{1/2}$ = 109.8 min), and iodine-124 ($t_{1/2}$ = 4.2 days) are produced by a cyclotron. One limitation of PET is related to the short half-life of some of these positron-emitting radionuclides. This presents difficulties in the time available for radiochemical synthesis and the need for an on-site cyclotron. This problem is illustrated for the radiosynthesis of carbon-11 radiolabeled thymidine (Figure 13.1). For PET to play a major role in drug development, extensive resources will need to be invested to support radiochemistry. Currently, not all ligands and tracers can be radiolabeled with sufficient radioactivity to make them useful for investigational studies. The ability to radiolabel a compound depends on the availability of suitable functional groups. For instance, compounds with N-, S-, or O-methyl (or -ethyl) groups, as well as proteins and antibodies can be radiolabeled fairly easily. In some cases the multistep chemistry required to produce a radiotracer precludes radiolabeling and purification of molecules rapidly enough to avoid substantial decay of radioactivity. Constraints in the availability of suitable labeling reagents including precursors can also limit the ability to synthesis a radiotracer. The position of labeling should be resistant to metabolic degradation, which further limits the number of compounds that can be radiolabeled.

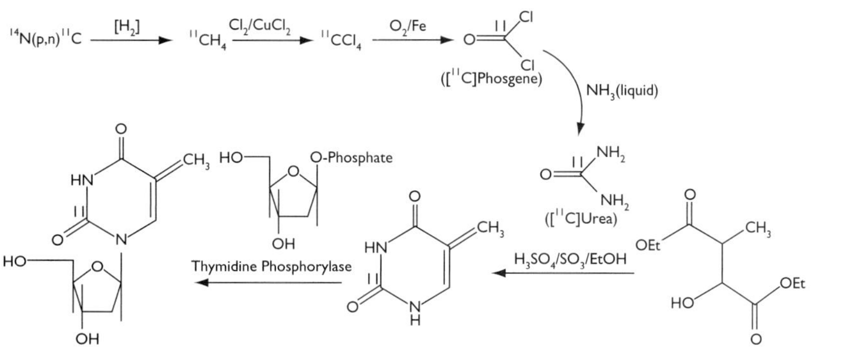

FIGURE 13.1   Synthesis of 2-[^{11}C]thymidine from [^{11}C]methane via [^{11}C]phosgene and anhydrous [^{11}C]urea. Using a fully automated system, Steel and co-workers reliably prepared 2-[^{11}C]thymidine by this method within 45–50 min from [^{11}C]methane with an average yield of 1.5–3.3 GBq (40–90 mCi) which corresponds to ~14% radiochemical yield (Steel, C.J. *et al.*, *Appl. Radiat. Isot.*, 51, 1999, 377–388). The specific radioactivity was typically 29.6–51.8 GBq μmol^{-1} (0.8–1.4 Ci μmol^{-1}) corresponding to 6–12 μg of stable thymidine.

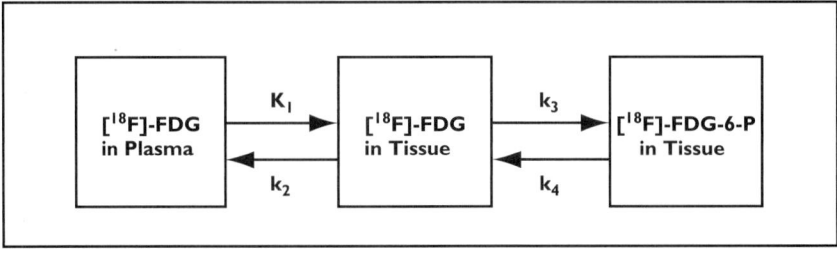

FIGURE 13.2 Compartmental model for glucose metabolism using [^{18}F]fluorodeoxyglucose. The rate constants K_1, k_2, k_3, and k_4 are defined as delivery, washout, phosphorylation and dephosphorylation, respectively. In most tumours, dephosphorylation of [^{18}F]FDG is insignificant. [^{18}F]FDG-6-P, [^{18}F]FDG-6-phosphate

B. Acquisition and Processing of PET Images

The signal used to create the 3D image in PET comes from the simultaneous detection of two 511-keV gamma rays emitted at approximately 180° from each other following the decay of positron-emitting radionuclides. The emitted photons are recorded by opposing coincidence detectors [2]. Data are obtained as sinograms that are corrected for detector efficiency and attenuation of photons and reconstructed into image data using mathematical algorithms. The data depict the spatial and temporal distribution of total radioactivity within a number of tomographic image planes. Most currently available commercial clinical PET scanners have intrinsic resolution of 4–8 mm (1–2 mm on animal scanners). PET images are usually analyzed by defining regions of interest and extracting radioactivity versus time curves for the region. In more advanced situations, functional parametric images are generated on a voxel-to-voxel basis using generic kinetic analysis.

Mathematical kinetic modeling is employed to enhance data interpretation within a framework of important kinetic behaviors and to obtain quantitative parameters of relevance and universal comprehension. This is necessary if the effect of a drug needs to be quantified. In practice, this involves comparing the concentrations of radioactivity in tissue with that in arterial plasma and calculating plasma/tissue exchange rate constants [3]. A tracer kinetic model for [^{18}F] fluorodeoxyglucose is illustrated in Figure 13.2. The usual approach in deriving such a mathematical description is to assign the possible distribution of the tracer to a limited number of discrete compartments, within which it could be free, specifically, or non-specifically bound. Special mathematical approaches such as spectral analysis [4] and graphical analysis [5] have been explored as alternatives to compartmental modeling.

III. EVALUATION OF CANCER THERAPEUTICS WITH PET

Ligands and tracers are being developed for measuring pathophysiology and for pharmacodynamic imaging. Some of these are in preclinical development and are not ready for use in early clinical trials. A list of existing and potential

PET ligands and tracers are presented in Table 13.1. These tracers can be used to select patients possessing specific oncogenic abnormalities, provide proof-of-mechanism, and quantify response or efficacy.

A. Evaluation of Pathophysiology to Enable Patient Selection or Prediction of Response

Some of the ligands and tracers listed in Table 13.1 could be used to measure baseline pathophysiology. The use of PET to assess pathophysiology and to enable prediction of response is reviewed below with specific examples.

I. Receptor Occupancy

Several growth factors produce therapeutic effects by interacting with specific receptors or binding to cell surface molecules. It is possible to study such drug-receptor interactions with ligands or antibodies radiolabeled with a positron emitter, and measure the regional uptake of radioligands to enable derivation of values for receptor number (Bmax), affinity (K_d), and binding potential (Bmax/K_d). Drug receptor studies are helpful in predicting response and optimal dose and for selecting patients likely to respond to specific therapies. Receptor occupancy studies involving the estrogen receptor (ER), for instance, have been used to predict response. The majority of breast cancers are hormone-dependent as indicated by an increase in ER and progesterone receptor content of breast tumors. The clinical course of disease in patients with ER-positive tumors is less aggressive and characterized by a longer disease-free interval and greater overall survival. Moreover, ER-positive tumors are likely to respond to hormonal manipulation. 16α-[^{18}F]fluoro-17β-estradiol (FES), a radioligand for ERs has been used to assess the ER status of breast tumors. McGuire et al. [6] found a decrease in FES uptake in metastatic breast cancers after the administration of tamoxifen. This demonstrated the presence of functional ERs in the tumors. Furthermore, the decrease in FES uptake after tamoxifen was significantly greater in patients who responded to hormonal therapy [7]. Thus, the ER occupancy status can be used to predict response to hormonal therapy.

2. Multidrug Resistance

The multidrug resistance (MDR) phenotype plays a major role in the treatment of cancer with anthracyclines, vinca alkaloids, and podophyllotoxins [8, 9]. Modulators of P-glycoprotein (PGP)-mediated efflux including verapamil, cyclosporin A, and PSC 833, which are also PGP substrates, have been used to circumvent MDR. However, their effect thus far in the treatment of solid cancers has been disappointing [10–12]. ^{99m}Tc-sestamibi [hexakis(2-methoxy-isobutyl-isonitrile)technetium(I)]-SPECT is the most common non-invasive method used for assessing MDR with decreased accumulation in MDR-proficient tumors. Kostakoglu et al. [13] demonstrated accumulation of ^{99m}Tc-sestamibi in breast and lung tumors expressing lower amounts of PGP. A 2.7-fold higher efflux rate [14] and a more rapid tumor clearance ($t_{1/2} < 204$ min) of ^{99m}Tc-sestamibi have been demonstrated in breast cancers with high PGP expression [15]. PGP modulation by PSC 833 was associated with an increase in the accumulation of ^{99m}Tc-sestamibi in tumors and liver of treated patients [16].

PET tracers for studying MDR status are only in preclinical development, with [11C] daunorubicin and [11C] verapamil the most promising. *In vitro* studies with [11C] daunorubicin has shown a 16-fold accumulation of [11C]daunorubicin in drug sensitive compared to PGP expressing human ovarian carcinoma cells [17]. The addition of verapamil resulted in increased accumulation of [11C]daunorubicin in the resistant cells, which confirms the modulatory nature of verapamil on PGP [17]. Similarly, *in vivo* rat studies have shown a lesser accumulation of [11C]verapamil in PGP overexpressing tumors compared to PGP negative ones. Modulation of PGP has also been demonstrated by an 18-fold increase in [11C]verapamil accumulation after pretreatment with cyclosporin A [18].

3. Tumor Hypoxia

Hypoxia in tumors results from an inadequate supply of oxygen to cells due to the inefficient and aberrant vasculature within tumors. These hypoxic cells are resistant to conventional radiotherapy and certain chemotherapeutic agents. [18F]fluoromisonidazole has been used as a PET marker to quantify hypoxia in tumors [19–21]. Other hypoxia markers such as SR 4554 and ^{64}Cu-ATSM are being developed for similar *in vivo* assessment [22, 23]. Using [18F]fluoromisonidazole as a marker, Rasey and co-workers found that hypoxia was present in 97% of 37 tumors studied [21]. The extent of hypoxia varied markedly between tumors in the same site or of the same histology. They also found that there was a heterogeneous distribution of hypoxia between regions within a single tumor. Such knowledge gained about tumor hypoxia non-invasively could find utility in the selection of patients for treatment with radiation, bioreductive agents, anti-angiogenic agents, anti-vascular agents, and hypoxia-targeted gene therapy.

B. Proof-of-Principle of Mechanism of Action

There is an increasing need to obtain information on the mechanism of action of drugs in patients to ensure that new drugs behave in a predictable manner. Examples of such studies are described below.

1. Modulation of Dihydropyrimidine Dehydrogenase Activity

The synthetic pyrimidine, 5-FU, is the most commonly used anticancer agent for the treatment of gastrointestinal malignancies. Up to 80% of systemically administered 5-FU is degraded through catabolism to α-fluoro-β-alanine (FBAL) [24], which decreases the amount of drug available for formation of cytotoxic anabolites. One aspect of current research with 5-FU has been to provide proof-of-principle of the mechanism of action of eniluracil, an inactivator of the proximal and rate-limiting catabolic enzyme, dihydropyrimidine dehydrogenase (Figure 13.3). Using PET, it was demonstrated that in eniluracil-naïve patients, 5-[18F]FU-derived radioactivity localized strongly in normal liver (0.0234% of the injected activity per milliliter at 11 min) due to the rapid formation and retention of [18F]FBAL [25]. Furthermore, there was a distinct localization of radioactivity in the gallbladder consistent with hepatobiliary clearance of [18F]FBAL [25]. In eniluracil-treated patients, there was a

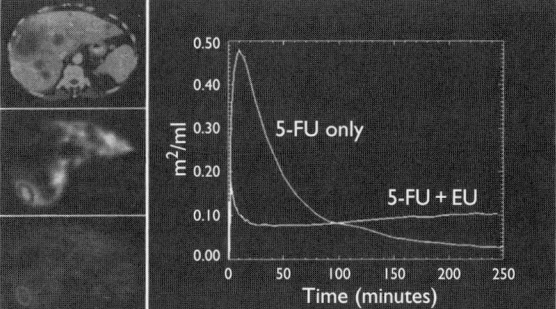

Liver pharmacokinetics

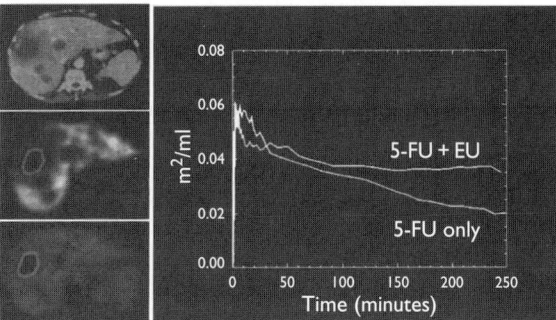

Tumour pharmacokinetics

FIGURE 13.3 Typical transabdominal CT-scans and 5-[^{18}F]fluorouracil-PET images of a patient before and after treatment with eniluracil. There was a substantial decrease in liver radioactivity (top panel) after eniluracil treatment due to the inactivation dihydropyrimidine dehydrogenase, and hence, absence of [^{18}F]fluoro-β-alanine. Such studies of enzyme activity are useful in providing proof of principle of mechanism in humans. The half-life of tumor 5-[^{18}F]fluorouracil-derived radioactivity increased after eniluracil treatment. See Color Plate 17.

substantial reduction in radiotracer disposition in normal liver and kidneys. Other effects observed were the absence of hepatobiliary clearance and an increase in plasma uracil and unmetabolized 5-[^{18}F]FU [25]. The half-life of 5-[^{18}F]FU-derived radioactivity in tumors increased from 2.3 to >4 hours following eniluracil administration. This is a large increase given that tumor radioactivity in eniluracil-naïve patients is comprised mainly of [^{18}F]FBAL.

2. Anti-Angiogenic and Anti-Vascular Therapies

Angiogenesis, the sprouting of capillaries from pre-existing vasculature, represents an important target and a challenge for drug development. Two main therapeutic approaches that researchers are pursuing include (1) inhibition of new vessel formation (anti-angiogenic agents), and (2) inhibition of blood flow (anti-vascular agents). Vascular properties, which describe the angiogenic phenotype, can be estimated by PET making the technique suitable for monitoring the pharmacodynamics of anti-angiogenic and anti-vascular therapies. Perfusion (blood flow per unit volume) and volume of distribution of water in tissues can be measured in most human tissues by i.v. injection of $H_2{}^{15}O$ and PET scanning. Typical $H_2{}^{15}O$-PET image and time activity curves are illustrated in Figure 13.4. The equation used to derive perfusion and volume of distribution is also shown.

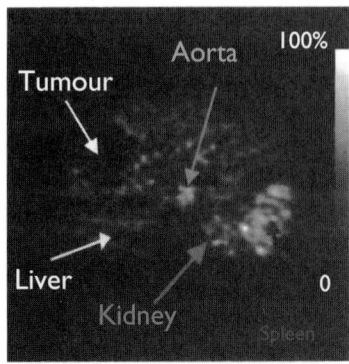
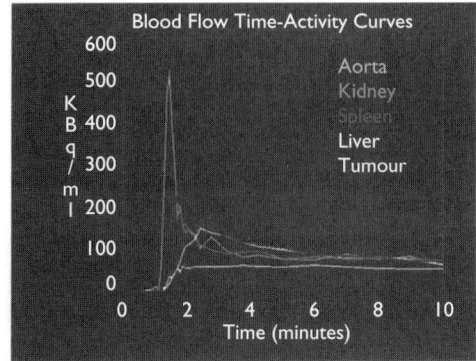

Blood flow model: $\qquad C_t(t) = F.C_a(t) \otimes \ell^{-(\frac{F}{V_d} + \lambda).t}$

FIGURE 13.4 Measurement of tissue perfusion and volume of distribution of water (exchanging water space) using $H_2{}^{15}O$-PET. Cumulative tissue localisation of $H_2{}^{15}O$ and its time-course in tissues are shown. The model for deriving parameters of flow and volume of distribution is also shown, where $C_t(t)$ is the regional tissue concentration of $H_2{}^{15}O$ [Bq.ml^{-1} (tissue)] as a function of time t, $C_a(t)$ is the arterial whole blood concentration of $H_2{}^{15}O$ [Bq.ml^{-1} (blood)] as a function of time, F is the regional flow in ml (blood).ml^{-1} (tissue).min^{-1}, Vd is the volume of distribution of water [ml (blood).ml^{-1} (tissue)], and λ is the decay constant of ^{15}O (0.338 min^{-1}). See Color Plate 18.

Blood volume is measured with $C^{15}O$-PET. Following inhalation of $C^{15}O$, time is allowed for steady state to be achieved. The relative tumor blood volume (rTBV), which is essentially the volume of distribution of carboxyhemoglobin (units = mL blood/mL of tissue) can be calculated using the following equation:

$$rTBV = \frac{\int_{t1}^{t2} C_{tissue}}{\int_{t1}^{t2} C_{blood}}$$

where t1 and t2 are the start and end of scan, respectively, and the concentrations (C) of blood and tissues are corrected activities in kBq/mL. These data may be corrected for the ratio of tumor small-vessel hematocrit to large-vessel hematocrit if this is known. The repeatability of such perfusion, volume of distribution, and blood volume measurements has been established (Anderson et al., unpublished). It has been hypothesized that vascular shutdown, for instance, will be characterized by a decrease in all three parameters, whereas hypoperfusion will only show up as a decrease in perfusion without any change in volume of distribution or blood volume. To assess the pharmacodynamics of the anti-vascular agent combretastatin A4 [26] as part of a UK Cancer Research Campaign (CRC) phase I trial, Anderson et al. [26] performed paired PET scans with $H_2{}^{15}O$ and $C^{15}O$. Perfusion and blood volume parameters were unchanged in untreated patients and at low doses of the drug. At higher doses ($\geq$40 mg/m^2), a 30–60% decrease in tumor perfusion was seen in 4 out of 5 patients at 30 min resolving in 3 out of 4 patients by 24 hours after injection of combretastatin A4 [26]. These studies demonstrated the combretastatin A4 effects a vascular shutdown in human tumors [26]. The non-selective effect of the drug on other tissues (kidney and spleen), as well as on cardiac output, were also noted [26, 27]. Of interest, reduction in perfusion for tumors and spleen were similar to that seen in tumor-bearing rodents [28]. It should be emphasized that the success of this trial was based on the ability to predict the time course of vascular shutdown in patients from rodent data [28].

3. Gene Expression

It is anticipated that post-genome drug discovery and development will have several strategies aimed at correcting oncogenic abnormalities. This has prompted the need to develop assays for demonstrating expression. Traditional gene expression assays at the gene, mRNA, or protein levels are impractical for providing proof-of-mechanism in clinical trials. Molecular imaging approaches using "*in vivo* reporter strategies" are more suited to experimental and clinical pharmacodynamic evaluation of the location, magnitude, and time course of gene expression [29]. Several PET reporter strategies are being developed to monitor gene therapy (Table 13.1). The principle underlying the approach is illustrated in Figure 13.5. When HSV1-tk is the reporter gene, the reporter substrate may be a radiolabeled pyrimidine or purine tracer such as FIAU (Table 13.1) and the gene delivery vector, e.g., adenovirus may contain the reporter gene under the control of a tumor-selective promotor, or the reporter gene and a therapeutic gene in a bicistronic construct [30]. If gene expression occurs in tumors, then following i.v. administration of the radiolabeled substrate, "trapping" of the substrate occurs through phosphorylation catalyzed by the protein product of the reporter gene (HSV1-tk). The retention of the radiolabeled substrate is proportional to the degree of gene expression. Although such PET methodologies are ready for the clinic, no clinical studies have as yet been reported.

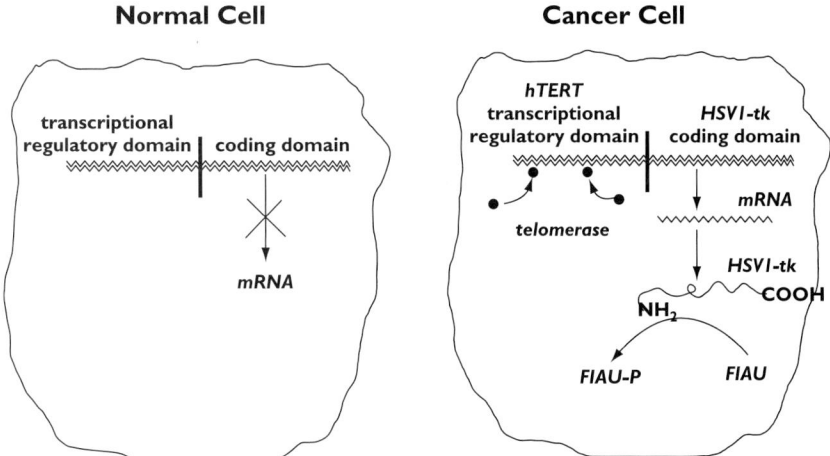

FIGURE 13.5 Measurement of gene expression with the PET using a notional binary vector system involving the human telomerase reverse transcriptase (hTERT) promoter linked to the HSV1-tk gene. Telomerase is highly expressed in tumour cells but repressed in somatic cells. Hence activation of the promoter in tumour cells will result in transcription, and consequently translation of the message into the HSV1-tk enzyme. Thus, tumour cells but not normal cells will phosphorylate FIAU to FIAU-phosphate (FIAU-P) which is trapped and can be quantified by PET.

4. Assessment of Intermediate Cascades in Mitogenic Signal Transduction

There are efforts to develop agents that inhibit mitogenic signal transduction. This is because signaling mechanisms that drive cell proliferation tend to be associated with malignant transformation and progression. For instance, Gibbs [31, 32] has recently described a variety of new compounds targeted against components of mitogenic signal transduction, which include monoclonal antibodies to erbB2, kinase inhibitors of Raf-1, inhibitors of molecular chaperone HSP 90, Raf-1 antisense oligonucleotides, and farnesyl transferase inhibitors [31, 32]. Imaging methods are in development for monitoring the pharmacodynamics of these promising agents. With respect to receptor imaging, an antibody for c-erbB2 is in development for monitoring erbB2 levels [33]. This could find utility as a pharmacodynamic probe for new therapies aimed at erbB2 such as herceptin [31, 32]. Developing end points for intermediate cascades in signal transduction, however, represents a significant challenge. This is because molecular events such as changes in phosphorylation and protein-protein interactions, are difficult to measure in intact animals or humans. One approach for investigating the effect of Ras protein inhibitors has been developed [34]. This involved iodination of a farnesyl transferase inhibitor for assessing farnesyl transferase enzyme occupancy. The labeling strategy employed by Hamill and co-workers permitted incorporation of other radioisotopes such as carbon-11 and fluorine-18 [34]. Studies in dogs have already demonstrated enzyme-specific binding of the iodinated radiotracer.

5. Thymidylate Synthase Inhibition

Thymidylate synthase (TS) is still an attractive target for drug development. The first TS inhibitor to be clinically used was 5-FU. Over the years, knowledge of TS has increased, which resulted in more efficacious and selective TS inhibitors that are now in development. For instance, the crystal structure of TS protein in its native form and in the ternary complex is now known and the molecular basis of properties such as substrate binding, catalytic activity, and transport via reduced folate carrier proteins have been well described [35–37]. In addition, prodrugs, which are activated by TS overexpression, which could result from treatment with fluoropyrimidines, are in development. All of these advances require an ability to measure TS inhibition or TS levels. One emerging area of research is the use of thymidine analogs to monitor thymidine salvage kinetics following TS inhibition. Using PET, Wells et al. [38] demonstrated increased fractional retention of 2-[^{11}C]thymidine in tumors at 1 hour after patients were treated with the non-classical TS inhibitor, AG337. Related to this, Collins et al. [39] are investigating the utility of 2'-[^{18}F]fluoro-ara-deoxyuridine-PET for imaging TS activity.

C. Evaluation of Efficacy and Response to Therapy

1. Evaluation of Cellular Proliferation

Most cancer therapeutics such as cell cycle inhibitors, inhibitors of mitogenic signal transduction, and differentiating agents inhibit cellular proliferation. PET methodology is available for measuring thymidine incorporation into DNA and thus for providing an index of proliferation rate. The PET methods may be superior to current methods for monitoring tumor response such as tumor shrinkage and time to progression, because cytostatic effects may be incorrectly assessed and response assessment with anatomical images may be confounded by inflammatory or fibrotic masses. The optimal probe for measuring proliferation is, however, an issue of current debate. 2-[^{11}C]thymidine is the gold standard for measuring proliferation. It has the advantage of being a natural compound, is readily taken up by cells and incorporated into DNA, and has been used extensively in *in vitro* studies (in the form of ^{3}H-thymidine). The main limitation of using 2-[^{11}C]thymidine-PET is its rapid catabolism *in vivo* ultimately to [^{11}C]CO$_2$. A dual-scan approach comprised of an initial scan with [^{11}C]HCO$_3$ followed after a brief period by a 2-[^{11}C]thymidine scan permits metabolite correction, and hence determination of fractional retention of thymidine or incorporation rate constants for thymidine [40–43]. The deconvolution approach for metabolite correction is based on the derivation of a unit impulse response function (IRF) as described below [42]:

In the [^{11}C]HCO$_3$ scan,

$$[\text{tissue activity}](t) = [\text{blood HCO}_3](t) \; \text{IRF, HCO}_3(t) \tag{1}$$

The IRF, HCO$_3$ obtained can then be used in a 2-[^{11}C]thymidine scan to derived the tissue component of HCO$_3$.

$$[\text{tissue HCO}_3 \text{ activity}](t) = [\text{blood HCO}_3](t) \; \text{IRF, HCO}_3(t) \tag{2}$$

Subtraction of the tissue HCO$_3$ activity from the total tissue activity in the 2-[^{11}C]thymidine scan gives leaves thymidine (and intermediate catabolites).

$$[\text{tissue thymidine activity}](t) =$$
$$[\text{total tissue activity}](t) - [\text{tissue HCO}_3 \text{ activity}](t) \tag{3}$$

In practice IRF is defined as a sum of exponentials using spectral analysis [4].

$$IRF(t) = \sum_{i=1}^{n} \alpha_i l^{-\beta_i t} \tag{4}$$

where n is the number of identifiable kinetic components, β is constant such that $\lambda < \beta_i < 1$ (λ = decay constant of carbon-11), and α is the intensity of the kinetic component at β_i.

Wells et al., have demonstrated that fractional uptake of 2-[^{11}C]thymidine-derived radioactivity correlates with a well-known index of cell proliferation, the MIB-1 index [43], thus, making it a suitable radiotracer for monitoring response to antiproliferative therapy. 2-[^{11}C]thymidine has been used in a number of pilot studies to measure response to therapy. For example, in patients with metastatic small cell lung cancer and abdominal sarcoma, with 2-[^{11}C]thymidine flux constant, measured at 1 week following chemotherapy (compared to baseline), declined by 100% in complete responders and 35% in a partial responder compared to a much smaller decline (15%) in a patient with progressive disease [44]. One of the biggest challenges in such studies is to determine when to make the measurements (length of time after chemotherapy to obtain a snapshot of the dynamics of an antiproliferative effect). Preclinical studies in tumor-bearing animals may aid in defining such time points. [^{124}I]iododeoxyuridine has also been used to measure proliferation [45]. The rapid metabolic de-iodination of the radiotracer, however, limited the usefulness of this probe *in vivo* [45]. One of the more promising probes for measuring proliferation is 3′-deoxy-3′-[^{18}F]fluorothymidine (FLT) [46]. This radiotracer is metabolized to a lesser extent than 2-[^{11}C]thymidine. The retention of FLT is determined not only by the degree of proliferation but also by levels of cell-cycle-regulated thymidine kinase-1 protein. Studies are ongoing to evaluate the role of this tracer in clinical imaging of proliferation. Thus far, 2-[^{11}C]thymidine appears to be the radiotracer widely used for imaging tumor proliferation.

2. Evaluation of Tumor Energy Metabolism

[^{18}F]fluorodeoxyglucose ([^{18}F]FDG) is one of the commonly used radiotracers in PET studies. [^{18}F]FDG follows the same route as glucose into cells where it is phosphorylated by hexokinase to [^{18}F]FDG-6-phosphate. Unlike glucose, there is little further metabolism and [^{18}F]FDG-6-phosphate remains essentially trapped within cells, with the rate of accumulation proportional to the rate of glucose utilization. [^{18}F]FDG-6-phosphate has low membrane permeability and although dephosphorylation does occur, it is very slow in brain, heart, and tumors, which have very low levels of glucose-6-phosphatase. The increased levels of the key enzyme hexokinase and corresponding decreased levels of glucose-6-phosphatase characterizes de-differentiation of cancer cells and has been attributed to transformation- and progression-linked reprogramming of gene expression [47–49]. FDG uptake in tumors probably reflects a combination of factors, which include phosphorylating activity of mitochondria, degree of hypoxia, and levels of glucose transporters [50, 51].

[^{18}F]FDG is used in oncology to grade tumors, to determine tumor extent, as a prognostic indicator, and as a measure of tumor response [52]. [^{18}F]FDG kinetics follow a three-compartment model (Figure 13.2). The retention of the radiotracer may be calculated as the standardized uptake value (SUV) or metabolic rate of glucose uptake. As a pharmacodynamic end point, [^{18}F]FDG has been used in several relatively small studies to monitor response to treatment. For instance, single-agent (tumor type in parenthesis) evaluation has been performed for temozolomide (glioma) [53] and hormone therapy (breast) [54]. Evaluation of combination therapies has also been performed, e.g., 5-FU + mitomycin-C (pancreatic cancers) [55], 5-FU ± interferon (colorectal liver metastases) [56], and radiotherapy + combination chemotherapy (glioma) [57].

Pharmacodynamic studies with [^{18}F]FDG are usually carried out at baseline and soon after the first or second cycle of therapy. A typical example of an [^{18}F]FDG image in a brain tumor is shown in Figure 13.6. The European organization for research and treatment of cancer-PET (EORTC-PET) group has recently published guidelines for common measurement criteria and reported alterations in FDG-PET studies to enable much needed comparison of smaller clinical studies and larger scale multicenter trials [58]. Tumor-response assessment as defined by the group (progressive, stable, partial, or complete metabolic response) is based on the observation that, on average, a 15–30% reduction in SUV or metabolic rate of glucose utilization can predict response and that this precedes tumor shrinkage and clinical response [58].

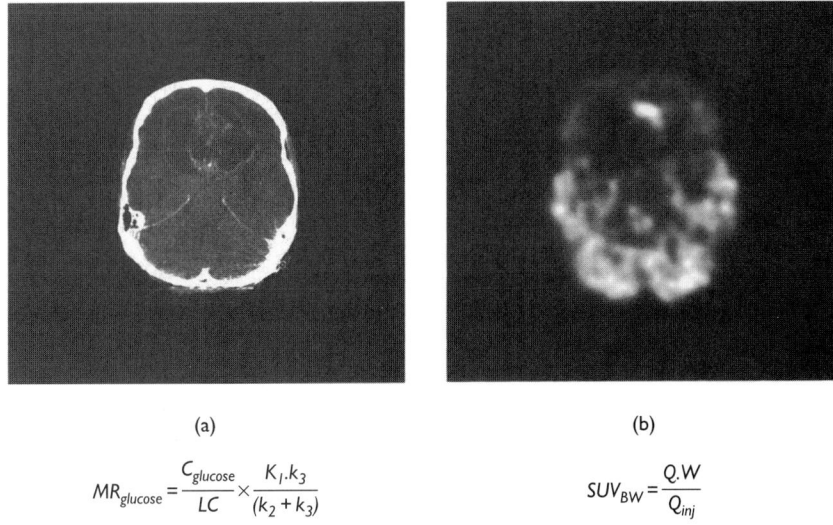

$$MR_{glucose} = \frac{C_{glucose}}{LC} \times \frac{K_1 . k_3}{(k_2 + k_3)} \qquad\qquad SUV_{BW} = \frac{Q.W}{Q_{inj}}$$

FIGURE 13.6 (a) A CT-scan of the brain showing a tumour mass, and (b) [18F]FDG-PET scan showing hypermetabolic regions within the tumour and in normal brain. Such images when acquired dynamically may be analysed to provide measures of the metabolic rate of glucose utilisation ($MR_{glucose}$, μmol.min^{-1}.ml^{-1}) or the standardised uptake value normalised to body weight (SUV_{BW}, Kg (body weight). l^{-1} (tissue)), where $C_{glucose}$, LC are the plasma glucose concentration and lumped constants, respectively and K_1, k_2 and k_3 are as previously defined in figure 2. Q, W, and Q_{inj} represent the tumour radiotracer concentration (units = MBq.l^{-1}), body weight (units = Kg) and injected activity (units = MBq), respectively. See Color Plate 19.

3. Assessment of Programmed Cell Death (Apoptosis)

Cell death by apoptosis is a pharmacodynamic end point for several anti-cancer therapies. Current methods for monitoring apoptosis are based on excision of tumors followed by immunohistochemical or flow cytometric analysis. PET methodology for measuring apoptosis holds promise for detecting apoptosis within patient tumors over time. The probe most amenable to PET studies is annexin V, an endogenous protein that has high affinity for membrane-bound phosphatidylserine. An early event in apoptosis is the rapid exposure of phosphatidylserine groups, which are normally confined to the inside of the cell. Binding of radiolabeled annexin V to such phosphatidylserine groups allows dying cells to be detected. Annexin V has been labeled with ^{99m}Tc for imaging with single photon computed tomography [59]. Annexin V has also been labeled with iodine-124 for PET studies (Glaser M et al., unpublished). These radiotracers are currently being validated in preclinical models and will soon be available for clinical imaging.

IV. MRI ASSESSMENT OF MICROVESSEL FUNCTION

MRI can be used experimentally and clinically to characterize tumor microvessel structure and function [60]. MRI techniques can be divided into non-enhanced and contrast media enhanced methods [61]. The latter can be further divided by the type of contrast medium utilized: (1) non-specific techniques that utilize small-molecular agents that distribute rapidly in the extracellular space (ECF agents), (2) techniques that use large-molecular agents designed for prolonged intravascular retention (macromolecular contrast media or blood pool agents), and (3) methods that use agents intended to accumulate at sites of concentrated angiogenesis mediator molecules. ECF contrast agents are available commercially, and in this section the pathophysiological basis, validation, quantification, and clinical applications of DCE-MRI will be discussed. Macromolecular contrast media are being investigated in clinical trials, but are not currently approved for human use. Molecular targeted contrast media are in preclinical development. Deoxyhemoglobin can also be used as an intrinsic contrast agent for tumor vascular characterization and this technique will also be discussed briefly.

MRI methods of evaluating microvessel function have the advantage of good spatial resolution often equal to that of corresponding morphologic images. MRI techniques are minimally invasive and involve little patient risk. As such they can be incorporated into routine patient studies. Limitations of MRI techniques are discussed below. Other imaging techniques that assess microvasculature have a number of drawbacks [62–64]. For example, ultrasound examinations are limited by poor depth of penetration and organs such as the brain and lungs remain inaccessible. Ultrasound is also highly operator dependent. Radiation exposure considerations and the small volume of tissue that can be examined limits CT assessments. PET is limited by high cost and limited availability of equipment. Furthermore, the short lives of radioisotopes used require that a cyclotron and onsite radiochemistry be present (see above).

A. Contrast Agent Kinetics Using Extracellular Contrast Agents

DCE-MRI is able to distinguish malignant from benign tissues by exploiting differences in their contrast agent kinetics [65, 66]. When a bolus of paramagnetic contrast agent passes through a capillary bed it is initially confined in the intravascular space. Within this space, it produces magnetic field (Bo) inhomogeneities that result in a decrease in the signal intensity of surrounding tissues. In most extracranial tissues and in some brain tumors, the contrast agent then passes into the extravascular-extracellular space (EES) at a rate determined by the permeability of the capillaries and their surface area. The early phase of contrast enhancement (often referred to as the first pass) includes the arrival of contrast medium and lasts many cardiac cycles. In this phase, the contrast medium gains access to the extracellular space via diffusion and causes shortening of tissue T1-relaxation times. The early signal increase observed on T1-weighted images arises from the both the vascular and interstitial compartments. Contrast medium also begins to diffuse into tissue compartments further removed from the vasculature including areas of necrosis and fibrosis. Over a period typically lasting several minutes to half an hour, the contrast agent diffuses back into the vasculature from which it is excreted (usually by the kidneys). Contrast medium elimination from very slow-exchange tissues such as fibrosis and necrosis occurs more slowly, which explains the persistent delayed enhancement characteristic of some tumors, e.g., cholangiocarcinoma and breast cancer [67].

MR sequences can be designed to be sensitive to the vascular phase of contrast medium delivery (so-called T2* methods, which reflect on tissue perfusion and blood volume). Similarly, sequences sensitive to the presence of contrast medium in the EES reflect microvessel permeability and extracellular leakage space (so-called T1 methods). The analytical methods for evaluating these techniques have their foundations in basic physiology and pharmacology [68–70]. These two methods are compared in Table 13.2.

B. T2*-Weighted Imaging

1. Pathophysiological Basis

Perfusion-weighted images can be obtained with "bolus-tracking techniques" that monitor the passage of contrast material through a capillary bed [71, 72]. The decrease in signal intensity of tissues can be observed with susceptibility-weighted T1- or T2*-weighted sequences, the latter providing greater sensitivity and contrast to perfusion effects. The degree of signal loss seen is dependent on the vascular concentration of the contrast agent and microvessel size [73] and volume. The signal–to-noise ratio (SNR) of such images can be improved by using higher doses of contrast medium (i.e., ≥ 0.2 mmol/kg body weight) [74]. High specification, echo-planar-capable MRI systems capable of rapid image acquisition are required to adequately characterize these effects. However, such studies are possible with conventional MRI systems using standard gradient-echo sequences (with long repetition and echo times employing low flip angles) but are limited to a few slices.

2. Quantification

Tracer kinetic principles can be used to provide estimates of relative blood volume (rBV), relative blood flow (rBF), and mean transit time (MTT) derived from the first pass of contrast agent through the microcirculation [75]. These variables are related by the central volume theorem equation BF = BV/MTT. BV measurements are obtained from the integral of the time-susceptibility curve, but a number of conditions of the central volume theorem are not met. For example, injection time is not instantaneous (in general, not obtainable in biological tissues) and as the arterial input function is not typically measured, these parameter estimates are qualitative or "relative." Recently, quantification of these parameters has been undertaken by simultaneous monitoring of the concentration of contrast agent in a large neck or brain vessel [76], and quantified perfusion parameters in normal brain and low-grade gliomas have been obtained [76, 77].

3. Limitations of T2* Methods

Limitations specific to T2* MRI methods are discussed here and those related to T1W methods and DCE-MRI techniques in general are discussed below. Recirculation of contrast medium can impair the calculation of T2*-weighted parameter estimates. Other physiological characteristics that hinder accurate measurements include non-laminar flow, which arises from the presence of irregular caliber vessels and non-dichotomous branching and high vascular permeability, which leads to increased blood viscosity (from hemoconcentration). In addition, factors such as machine stability, patient motion, and intrinsic patient variables, particularly cardiac output and upstream stenoses, can affect the computations. The quantification techniques described above also cannot readily be applied to areas of marked blood-brain barrier breakdown or to extracranial tumors with very leaky blood vessels. This is because the T1-enhancing effects of gadolinium chelates can counteract T2* signal lowering effects, which results in falsely low blood volume values in very leaky vessels. Quantitative imaging is thus most reliably used for normal brain and non-enhancing brain lesions, because the contrast medium is retained within the intravascular space. One solution to overcoming these problems is to use non-gadolinium susceptibility contrast agents based on dysprosium, which has a strong T2* effect but a weak T1 effect [78, 79].

4. Clinical Experience with T2* Techniques

The signal loss observed with T2*-weighted sequences has been used qualitatively in clinical studies to characterize liver, breast, and brain tumors [80–82]. Relative cerebral blood volume (rCBV) mapping can be used to detect areas of increased vascularity in brain gliomas (Figure 13.7) [83, 84]. Areas of high tumor rCBV appear to correlate with tumor grade and vascularity but not with cellular atypia, endothelial proliferation, necrosis, or cellularity [83]. CBV maps appear to have a high negative predictive value when excluding the presence of high-grade tumor in untreated patients regardless of their enhancement characteristics on T1-weighted MRI. In low-grade gliomas, homogeneous low rCBV is found whereas higher grade tumors display both low and high rCBV components [85]. CBV maps can therefore be used to direct stereotactic biopsy to areas where the highest tumor grade may be found [86, 87]. Other potential uses of T2*W imaging in patients with brain tumors include distinguishing radiation necrosis from recurrent disease, determining prognosis, and monitoring response to radiotherapy [77]. T2*W imaging techniques have not as yet been used to evaluate anti-angiogenic/anti-vascular treatments.

C. T1-Weighted Imaging

1. Pathophysiological Basis

Extracellular contrast media readily diffuse from the blood into the EES of tissues at a rate determined by the permeability of the capillaries and their surface area. T1 relaxation time shortening caused by contrast medium is the mechanism of tissue enhancement seen. Most DCE-MRI studies employ gradient-echo sequences (short repetition and echo times employing large flip angles) to monitor the tissue-enhancing effects of contrast media. This is because gradient-echo sequences have good contrast medium sensitivity, good SNR, and data acquisition can be performed rapidly. The degree of signal enhancement seen on T1-weighted images is dependent on a number of physiological and physical factors. These include tissue perfusion, capillary permeability to contrast agent, volume of the extracellular leakage space, native T1-relaxation time of the tissue, contrast agent dose, imaging sequence used, parameters utilized, and machine scaling factors [88, 89].

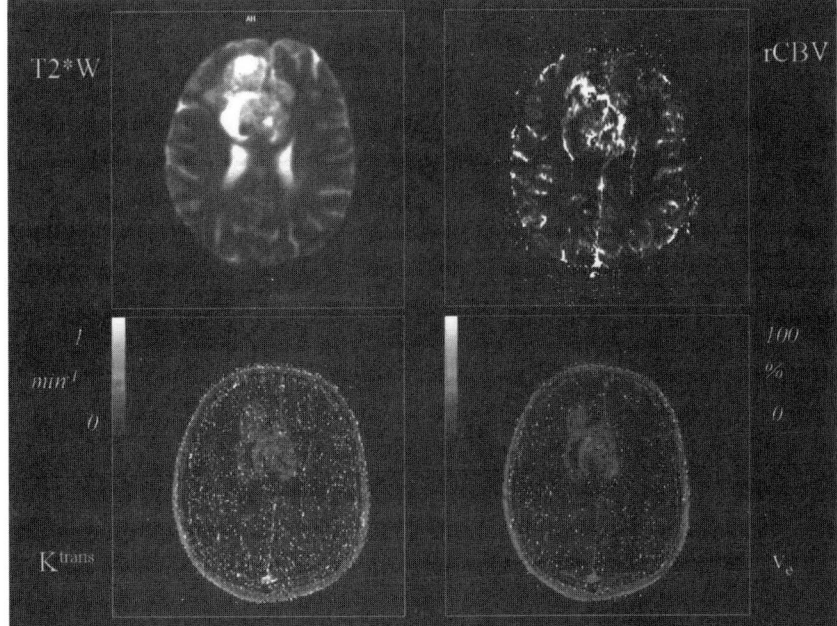

FIGURE 13.7 Multifunctional vascular characterisation of brain oligodendroglioma. (a) Top left. Axial T2-weighted MR image of a transformed malignant cerebral oligodendroglioma. A large necrotic mass is seen in the frontal lobe. Tumour extends across the midline. High signal areas within the mass are presumed to represent necrosis. (b) Top right. Relative cerebral blood volume (rCBV) map at the same slice location. The tumour is noted to be markedly hypervascular with a blood volume equal to or greater than normal cortical grey matter. Note that the areas of highest blood volume are not immediately adjacent to the areas of necrosis. (c) Bottom left. Transfer constant (K^{trans}) map (maximum transfer constant displayed = 1 minute^{-1}). The areas of highest permeability surface area product (transfer constant) are noted in the centre of the tumour. In particular, there are areas of high transfer constant immediately adjacent to the areas of necrosis seen in the axial T2-weighted image. The distribution of transfer constant values does not match the distribution of relative cerebral blood volume spatially. (d) Leakage space (v_e) map. Maximum leakage space demonstrated 100%. There is a good spatial match of leakage space with transfer constant values. See Color Plate 20.

2. Quantification

Signal enhancement seen on a dynamic acquisition of T1-weighted images can be assessed in two ways: by the analysis of signal intensity changes (semiquantitative) and/or by quantifying contrast agent concentration change using pharmacokinetic modeling techniques [90]. Semiquantitative parameters describe tissue signal intensity enhancement by using a number of descriptors. These parameters include onset time (time from injection to the arrival of contrast medium in the tissue), initial and mean gradient of the upsweep of enhancement curves, maximum signal intensity, and washout gradient. As the rate of enhancement is important for improving the specificity of examinations, parameters that include an additional time element have been introduced (e.g., maximum intensity time ratio; MITR [91] and maximum focal enhancement at one minute [92, 93]). The shape of time signal intensity curves has also been correlated with breast lesion histology [94]. Semiquantitative parameters are advantageous because they are straightforward to calculate but have a number of limitations. These include the fact that they do not accurately reflect tissue contrast medium concentration or the vascular end point of interest (tissue perfusion). Semiquantitative estimates are also subject to the variabilities of scanner manufacture and examination settings (including gain and scaling factors). These limitations can and do make between-patient and system comparisons difficult.

Quantitative techniques use pharmacokinetic modeling algorithms that are applied to tissue contrast agent concentration changes. The signal intensity changes observed during a dynamic enhancement acquisition can be used to estimate contrast agent concentration *in vivo* (Figure 13.8) [90, 95, 96]. Concentration-time curves are then mathematically fitted using one of a number of recognized pharmacokinetic models (Figure 13.9) [97]. Examples of modeling parameters include the volume transfer constant of the contrast agent

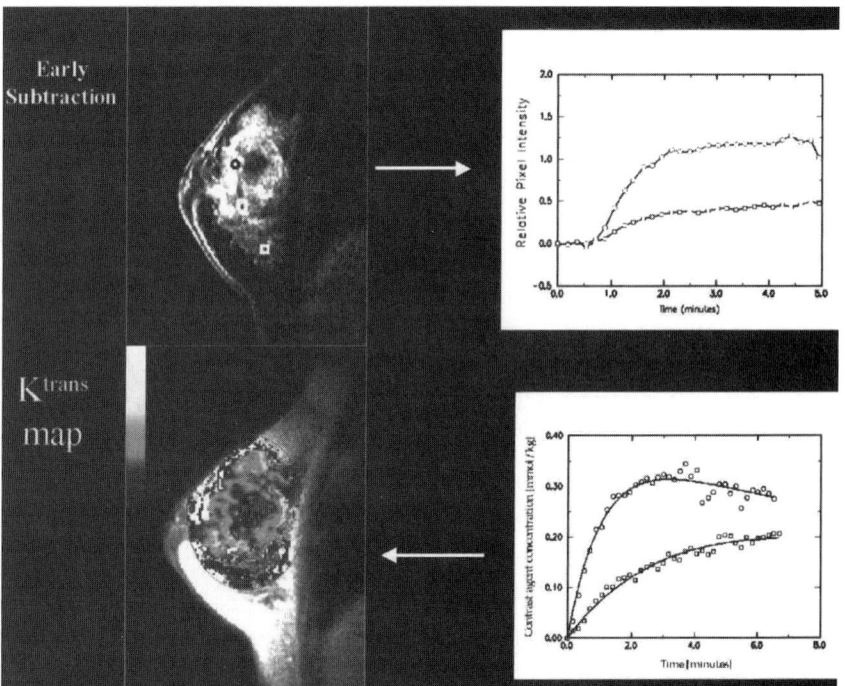

FIGURE 13.8 Converting signal intensity into contrast concentration and model fitting; data obtained from a patient with invasive ductal cancer. (a) Top-right. This early subtraction image (90 second image following contrast medium minus pre-contrast image) demonstrates a large heterogeneously enhancing mass characteristic for malignancy. This mass is applied to the anterior chest wall. There is a central area of non-enhancement presumably representing an area of necrosis. (b) Top-left. Signal-intensity time curves for the two regions of interest shown in the early subtraction image. Regions of interest are taken from the edge of the enhancing tumour (O) normal tissue ( ). (c) Bottom-right. Conversion of signal intensity information into contrast agent concentration is performed according to the method described by Parker *et al.* The model fitting (continuous line) is done using the Tofts' model. Model fitting is performed after calculation of time of onset of enhancement. (d) Bottom-left. Model fitting is done on each pixel and colour parametric maps (K^{trans}) are displayed. See Color Plate 21.

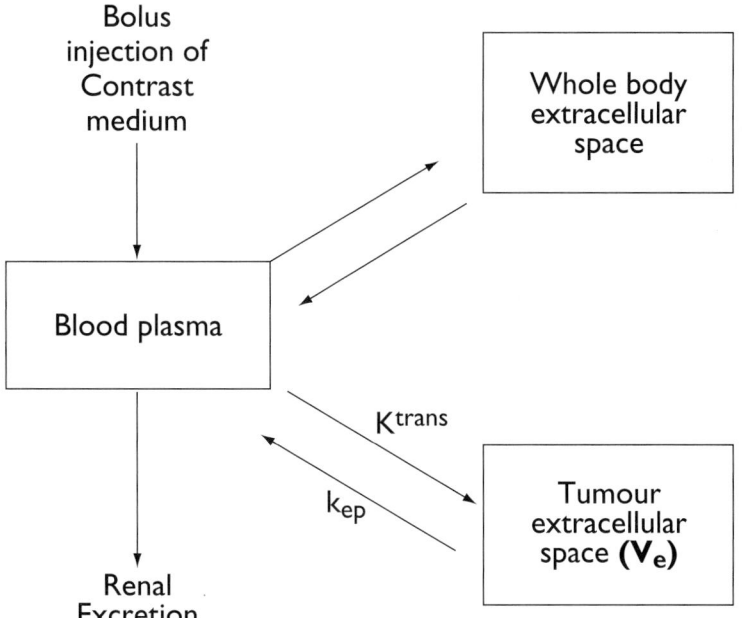

Modified from Tofts 1991 and 1995

FIGURE 13.9 Compartments assumed for the Tofts' model and parameters obtained. K^{trans} = transfer constant, k_{ep} = rate constant, v_e = extravascular, extracellular leakage space.

(K^{trans-} formally called permeability-surface area product per unit volume of tissue), leakage space as a percentage of unit volume of tissue (v_e), and the rate constant (k_{ep} also called K_{21}). These parameters are related mathematically ($k_{ep} = K^{trans}/v_e$) and recently have been reconciled with others that appear in the literature [98]. It is important to note that in tissues with highly permeable vessels, the rate at which the contrast medium enters the EES is limited by perfusion and in this situation the transfer constant (K^{trans}) is equivalent to the plasma flow per unit volume of tissue [98]. In a tissue such as the brain where an intact blood-brain barrier is present, the rate at which the contrast medium enters the EES is limited by vessel permeability and in this situation, K^{trans} is equivalent to permeability surface area product. In malignant tumors, vessels in general are more permeable than normal tissues but are heterogeneously distributed, therefore, K^{trans} reflects a combination of permeability surface area product and perfusion. Quantitative parameters are more complicated to derive compared to those derived semiquantitatively. The model chosen may not fit the data obtained, and each model makes a number of assumptions that may not be valid for every tissue or tumor type [97, 98]. Nonetheless, if contrast agent concentration can be measured accurately and the type, volume, and method of administration are consistent, then it may be possible to directly compare pharmacokinetic parameters acquired serially in a given patient and in different patients imaged at the same or different scanning sites [99].

3. Analysis Methods and Display

Analysis methods and presentation of DCE-MRI data vary in the literature. Most dynamic MRI studies apply user-defined regions of interest (ROI) (Figure 13.8). ROI methods yield enhancement curves with good SNR, but lack spatial resolution and are prone to partial volume averaging errors. It should be recognized that the placement of ROIs can have profound effects on the outcome of the analysis. In its simplest form, an ROI encompassing the whole tumor is drawn from which an average enhancement curve is extracted. This method ignores heterogeneity of tumor enhancement by assuming that the averaged kinetic parameter estimate equates to those that would be obtained from individual pixels. This method is acknowledged to be inappropriate [73, 80, 84] because many malignant tumors show markedly heterogeneous areas of enhancement (an important diagnostic feature). This regional variability of enhancement probably reflects variations in microvessel density [100–102] such as vascular endothelial growth factor (VEGF) expression, areas of fibrosis, avascularity, and necrosis [67, 103]. Therefore, selective sampling of regions within a tumor is used by most researchers based on the premise that the discrimination of lesions is improved [104].

Another approach of displaying dynamic data is by pixel mapping (Figures 13.7 and 13.8). This method depicts quantitative enhancement information as color maps exactly co-registered with anatomic images on a pixel-by pixel basis. This type of display has a number of advantages, which include an appreciation of heterogeneity of enhancement and removal of the need for selective placement of user-defined ROIs. The risk of missing important diagnostic information and of creating ROIs that contain more than one tissue type is thus reduced. Pixel mapping techniques have the disadvantages of having poorer SNR and require specialist software for their generation [95, 105]. Although visual appreciation of heterogeneity is improved by pixel displays, quantification of the same is more difficult. Recently, histogram analysis has been used to quantify the heterogeneity of tumors for comparative and longitudinal studies and for monitoring the effects of treatment. It can also show the regression or development of angiogenic hotspots [106, 107]. Simple frequency distributions are plotted and numerical descriptive statistics quantify the variability therein.

4. Validation

Many studies have attempted to correlated tissue MR enhancement with immunohistochemical microvessel density (MVD) measurements (Table 13.3) [61]. Many studies have found that vascular density in malignant tissue is higher than normal in the parenchyma, but there is an overlap with benign lesions including inflammatory and proliferative processes [108, 109]. Some studies have shown a broad correlation between MR enhancement and MVD [109–112], whereas others have found no correlation [113, 114]. Experience shows that factors other than MVD must be important in determining the degree of tissue enhancement. For example, in the brain, retina, and testis high vascular density and capillary permeability estimates do not correlate because of an intact capillary-interstitial space barrier. Recently VEGF, a potent vascular permeability and angiogenic factor, has been implicated as an additional explanatory factor that determines MR signal enhancement. Knopp et al. [115] reported that vascular permeability to contrast media closely correlated with tissue VEGF expression in breast tumors. In tumors without significant VEGF expression, a linear correlation of K_{21} (now called rate constant or k_{ep} and MVD) was seen. Once tissue VEGF staining became prominent, then K_{21} increased rapidly, independently of MVD. The importance of the role of VEGF in determining microvascular permeability is supported by the spatial association of hyperpermeable capillaries and VEGF expression on histological specimens [116, 117]. A correlation between serum VEGF levels and rectal tumor transfer constant values has recently been reported [118]. Furthermore, the observation that MR kinetic measurements can detect suppression of vascular permeability after anti-VEGF antibody [119] and after the administration of inhibitors of VEGF signaling [120] lends weight to the important role played by VEGF in determining MR enhancement. Other characteristics that have been correlated with enhancement patterns include the degree of stromal cellularity and fibrosis [67, 103] and tissue oxygenation [114].

5. Clinical Experience

Analysis of enhancement seen on dynamic T1-weighted images has been found to be a valuable diagnostic tool in a number of clinical situations. The most established role is in lesion characterization where it has found a role in distinguishing benign from malignant breast and musculoskeletal lesions [92, 121]. Simple observations from time signal-intensity curves have shown that malignant tissues generally enhance early, with a rapid and large increase in signal intensity compared with benign tissues, which in general show a slower increase in signal intensity. In the breast, a clear overlap of enhancement rates of benign and malignant breast lesions is seen [91, 92, 122–126]. Breast fibroadenomas in particular demonstrate enhancement patterns similar to that of invasive cancer [127]. Non-malignant tissues such as benign prostatic hyperplasia also enhance avidly with an enhancement pattern similar to prostate cancer [128, 129]. Dynamic T1-weighted MRI studies have also been found to be of value in staging gynecological malignancies and bladder and prostate cancers [130–132].

DCE-MRI is also able to predict response or monitor the effects of a variety of treatments. These include neoadjuvant chemotherapy in bladder and breast cancers and bone sarcomas [133–136]. In breast cancer, for example, it has recently been shown that a decrease in transendothelial permeability accompanies tumor shrinkage, and that an early (1–2 cycles of chemotherapy) increase or no change in permeability can predict non-responsiveness [137]. Other treatments that can be monitored include radiotherapy of rectal and cervix cancers [106, 138], androgen deprivation in prostate cancer [139], and vascular embolization of uterine fibroids [140–142]. All of these studies show that successful treatment results in a decrease in the rate of enhancement, and that poor response results in persistent abnormal enhancement however judged (semiquantitatively or quantitatively). Most recently, enhancement parameters have been shown to predict survival in patients with cervix cancers; that is, tumors with fast initial rate of enhancement or vascular permeability were more likely to have a poorer prognosis [143] despite having a higher radiotherapy response rate [144]. DCE-MRI studies have also been found to be of value in detecting tumor relapse within treated tissues of the breast and pelvis [123, 145–151]. For example, in the breast, early rapid enhancement is reliable at discriminating between scar tissue and recurrent tumor. Many studies now suggest that recent surgery and prior radiotherapy can result in false positive results when evaluating the activity of residual disease [149, 150].

6. Clinical Experience in Anti-Angiogenesis/Anti-Vascular Studies

About 50 patients at two UK institutions (Royal Marsden Hospital and Mount Vernon Cancer Treatment Centre, London) have been evaluated by DCE-MRI in phase I clinical trials of anti-angiogenic/anti-vascular agents. The aim of both studies was to seek biological evidence of drug action in early clinical trials. These studies have evaluated the dose-related effects of two compounds on blood vessel permeability in metastatic solid tumors using DCE-MRI. The Royal Marsden study evaluated the anti-angiogenic compound SU-5416, a small molecule inhibitor of the VEGF receptor FLK-1/KDR [152, 153]. Recently, SU-5416 has been to shown to induce endothelial and tumor apoptosis in a xenograft model of colon cancer liver metastases [154]. The Mount Vernon Cancer Treatment Centre study is part of a CRC trial to evaluate the drug combretastatin phosphate (CA4P). CA4P is a tubulin binding agent that has been shown to have vascular targeting activity in preclinical models, which causes rapid tumor vascular occlusion [28]. It has also been shown to increase permeability in endothelial cell monolayers *in vitro*, and in the first few minutes after treatment in tumors *in vivo* [155] the mechanism of which appears to be changes in endothelial shape [156].

Patients were chosen on the basis of evaluable disease at anatomic sites with little physiological motion. As a result, many patients with lung and liver lesions were excluded as potential candidates unless the volume of disease was large (leading to fixity of these organs). Patients evaluated included those with brain masses, head and neck tumors, bony disease, or large pelvic masses. Despite these precautions, a number of patients were subsequently excluded from final analysis because of significant physiological motion. The CA4P trial incorporated a reproducibility study as part of the study protocol. To date there has been little published material on the reproducibility of DCE-MRI examinations between sessions on different days. This important aspect is considered further in Section IV.D.3. Both trials evaluated morphological and functional responses to the treatments. The CA4P study used a manual i.v. contrast injection procedure whereas the SU-5416 study used a mechanical power injector. The importance of consistent and reproducible delivery of contrast medium is also discussed in Section IV.D.3. The Mount Vernon reproducibility study recently reported three unreliable injections of the contrast medium due to fracturing of glass syringes, and leakage of contrast medium at the site of the i.v. cannula [157]. Similarly, the SU-5416 study reported unreliable mechanical injections in a number of patients and extravasations of contrast medium were also noted [158]. The data acquisition protocols for the two studies were similar; 5-slice saturation recovery Turbo-FLASH (fast low-angle shot) sequence for SU-5416 study [96] and, spoiled gradient echo sequence (FLASH) sequence [90] for the CA4P trail. Analysis methods for both studies were similar with the Tofts' model applied to the change in contrast medium concentration (Section IV.C.2). ROIs were drawn to include the whole tumor edge where possible excluding pulsatility artifacts from blood vessels and susceptibility artifacts from bowel. ROIs were also drawn in areas of skeletal muscle, which served as a normal tissue control. Some patients had a large number of pixels with modeling failures that resulted in unreliable parameter estimates, and this aspect is discussed in Section IV.D.2. An assessment of the shape of the contrast medium concentration time curves for these pixels suggests a significant vascular contribution (Figure 13.10). The estimation of kinetic parameters was therefore inaccurate, as the Tofts' model assumes no contribution of the intravascular compartment. Significant reductions in kinetic parameter estimates were observed in both trials (Figure 13.11) [158, 159].

D. Challenges for DCE-MRI Examinations

1. Imaging Protocol Standardization

No standardized, generally accepted technique has emerged for DCE-MRI examinations. This has resulted in difficulties in making meaningful comparisons between different cancer types and between data from different imaging centers. It is recognized that high-resolution and short imaging time represent competing examination strategies on current equipment and software. Higher temporal resolution imaging necessitates reduced spatial resolution, decreased anatomic coverage, or a combination thereof. Higher temporal resolution techniques appear to improve specificity of T1-weighted examinations because of better characterization of signal intensity time curves; one study has suggested that characterization of breast lesions is optimal using 1- to 2-second image acquisition times [122]. Even though data collection procedures for quantitative examinations differ from those used in routine clinical practice, there is debate on which technique(s) is best [95, 160, 161]. A standardized method for T1-weighted data collection has recently been published [61]. Currently, DCE-MRI studies are performed in body parts where there is little physiological movement, but motion compensation techniques based on navigator technologies may overcome these restrictions and allow application of these techniques to organs such as the liver and lungs.

2. Methods of Quantification and Modeling

As previously discussed, simple morphologic and semiquantitative analyses work well in a number of clinical situations. However, it is important to realize these semiquantitative diagnostic criteria cannot be simply applied from one center to another, particularly when different equipment and sequences are used. For example, it is known that the baseline signal intensity for any given tissue will differ by the choice of machine type even if identical sequences are used. Thus, the calculation of the degree of enhancement (e.g., percentage increase in signal intensity from baseline) can be profoundly

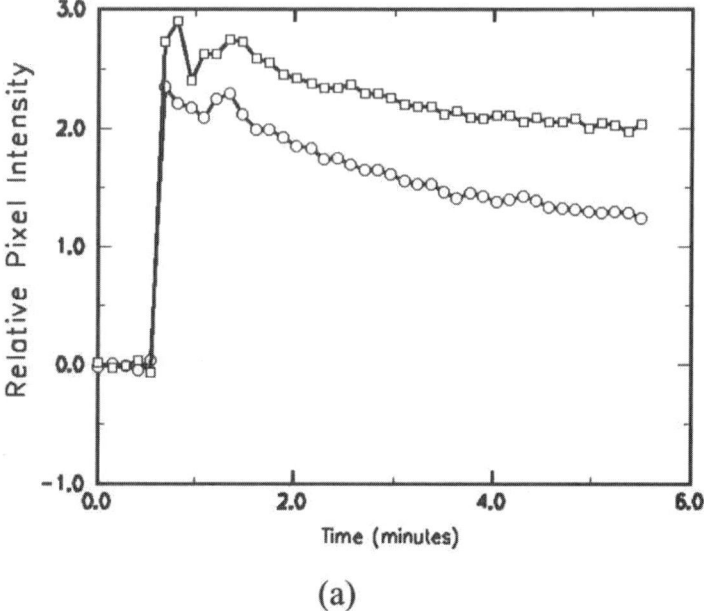

(a)

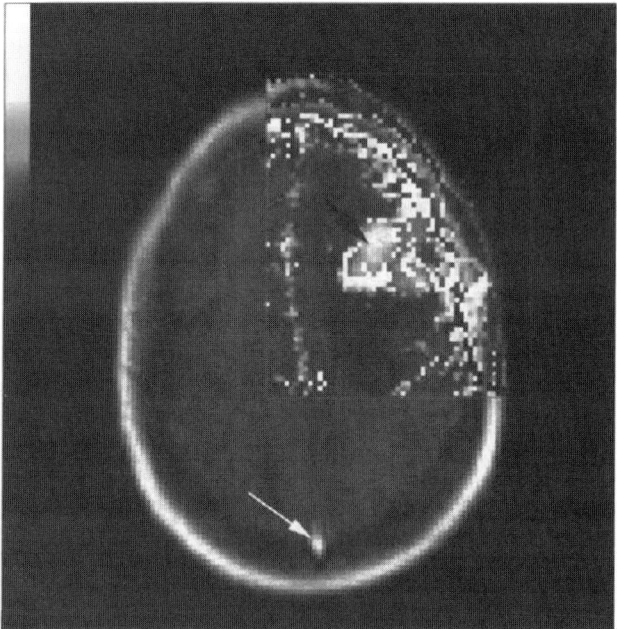

(b)

FIGURE 13.10 Significant vascular contribution leading to modelling failure. (a) Time signal intensity curve from the centre of metastatic tumour (-black arrow in b) and superior sagittal sinus (O – white arrow in b). The shape of the signal intensity time curves are very similar suggesting that there is a large vascular contribution to the signal obtained from the tumour. Such curves cannot be fitted to the Tofts' model, which results in a large number of modelling pixel failures as shown on the transfer constant map (b). See Color Plate 22.

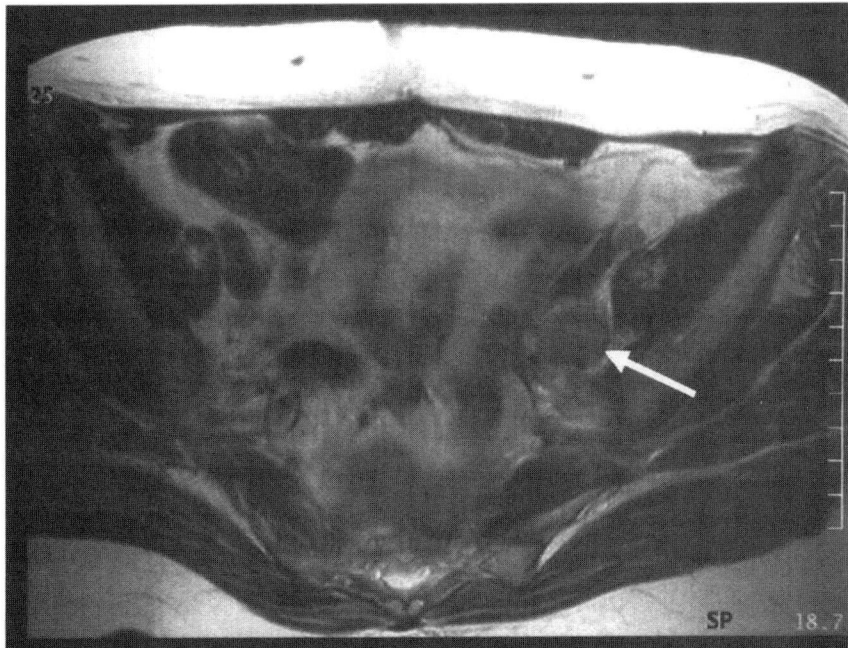

(a)

FIGURE 13.11 Significant reductions in tumour blood flow following combretastatin treatment. (a) An axial T2-weighted MR image through the middle of the pelvis shows a large malignant lymph node in the left inferior hypogastric group (arrow) in a patient with malignant peritoneal carcinoma. (b) Early subtraction images from four studies at the same level as the anatomical image (a). These subtraction images are obtained by subtracting a ninety-second image from a pre-contrast image. Arrows demonstrate the site of the malignant lymph node. Two studies were obtained before treatment as part of a reproducibility study (-3 days and -1 day). The bottom left hand image shows marked reduction in the delivery of the contrast medium to the lymph node particularly in the centre with the relative sparing of the periphery, four hours after administration of Combretastatin (52 mg.m^{-2}). The bottom right hand image shows some recovery in enhancement 24 hours after the administration of Combretastatin. (c) Time signal density curves from the tumour ROI on the days indicated in (b). The x-axis displays the time in seconds before and after the administration of contrast medium (arrow). The y-axis displays the enhancement above baseline values as a percentage. Note that at four hours, there is a significant reduction in the initial gradient and maximal amplitude of enhancement visible (yellow line). Some recovery of curve shape is seen at 24 hours.

affected. Consequently, the degree of enhancement that distinguishes one tissue from another on a particular machine type may give erroneous results on another. Quantification techniques aim to minimize these variabilities and thus allow comparisons between and within patients and between different imaging centers. Furthermore, quantification techniques enable the derivation of kinetic parameters that are based on some understanding of physiological processes and thus can provide insights into tumor biology. Quantitative techniques are therefore the preferred method of evaluating anti-angiogenic and anti-vascular treatments.

Experience shows that the model chosen may not fit the data acquired (modeling failures) (Figure 13.10) and that apparently sensible kinetic values

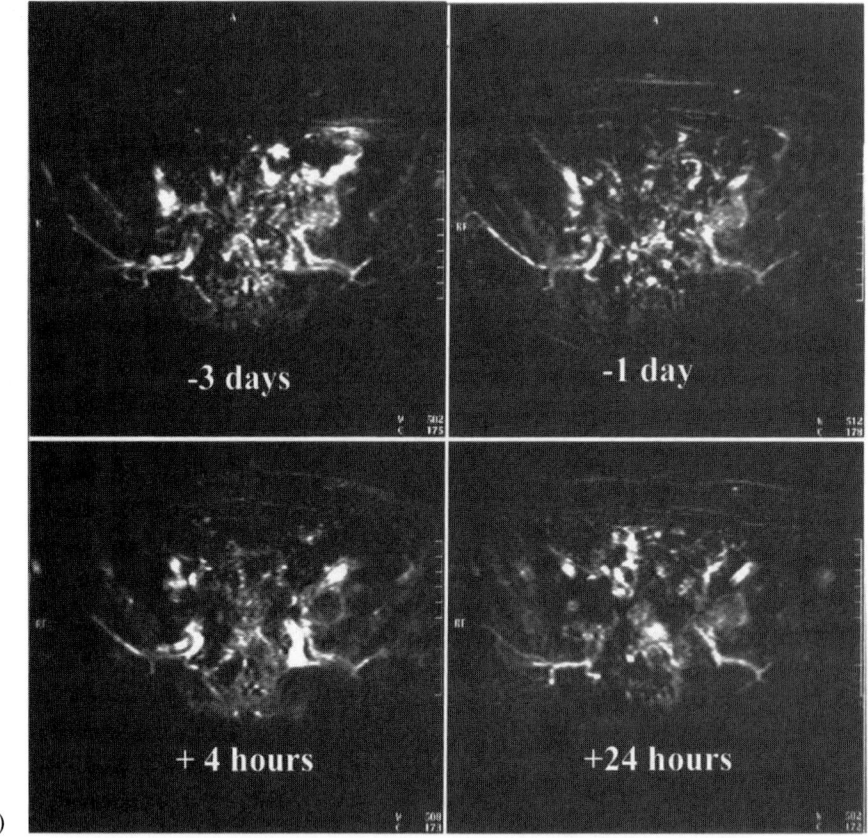

(b)

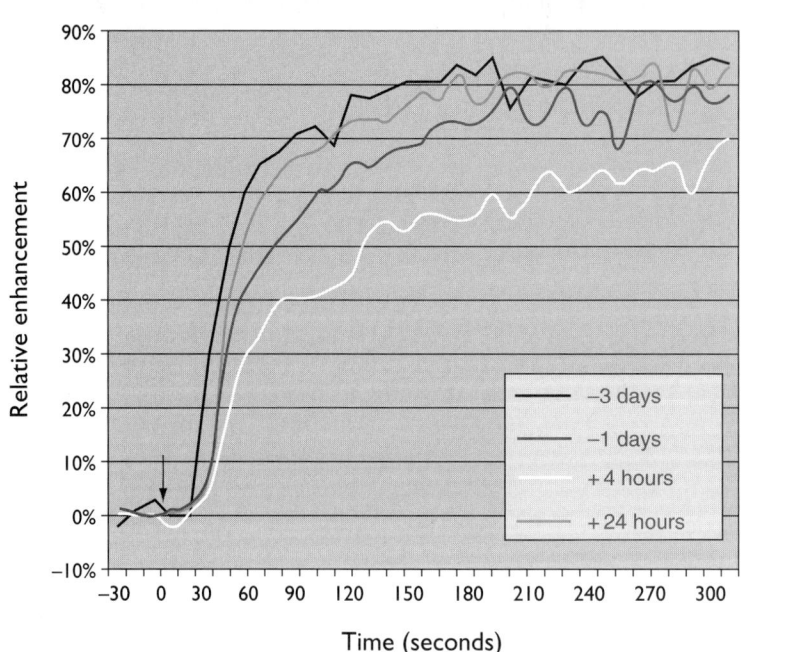

(c)

FIGURE 13.11 (*Continued*)

may be obtained even from noisy data. The causes for modeling failures are complex and often not well understood and include high permeability situations (i.e., when the intravascular contrast medium concentration cannot be maintained due to marked leaky vessels in the setting of limited blood flow), high tissue blood volume, multiple tissue compartments, and an incorrect arterial input function. We do not have models that fit all acquired data and more sophisticated, multicompartment models that provide insights into tissue compartment behavior are needed [162].

3. Precision of Measurements

Measurement error is the variation between measurements of the same quantity on the same individual. An estimate of measurement error enables us to decide whether a change in an observation represents a real change. An important question that needs addressing is the precision and measurement variability of DCE-MRI parameter estimates. These data are urgently needed and should be an integral part of any new prospective study that uses DCE-MRI data to evaluate new anti-angiogenic/anti-vascular drugs. We have recently reported that tumor leakage space and maximum enhancement are highly reproducible variables and that quantitative parameters such as K^{trans} and gradient of enhancement are more variable [157]. The factors that determine measurement error need to be defined for a given quantitative modeling technique. An example is the input function, which is an estimate of the delivery of the contrast medium to the tissue in question. The precision of perfusion and permeability estimates is dependent on the compactness of the contrast medium bolus injection and in this regard, the recent availability of MR-compatible automated injection devices is particularly welcome. The effect of the measured arterial input function on the precision of kinetic parameter estimates can be quantified using mathematical simulations. However, a reliable method for measuring and incorporating input function into DCE-MRI studies has not yet emerged.

4. Validation of DCE-MRI Techniques

Any imaging assay of tumor microvascular characteristics that seeks to define the state of tumor angiogenesis must be rigorously compared to accepted surrogates of angiogenesis, even if they are imperfect. Unfortunately no single imaging assay or surrogate may be adequate to reflect the whole spectrum of events involved in angiogenesis. Nonetheless, to keep the evaluation of new techniques as reasonable as possible, only positive significant correlations with accepted surrogates on angiogenesis should be accepted as supporting evidence for an imaging assay. Commonly used and appropriate surrogates include histologic MVD as counted on factor VIII- or CD34-stained tumor specimens. Also quantitative measures of VEGF, or other known mediators of angiogenesis, in the tumor tissue itself or in the plasma can be compared to MRI assay results [61]. Similarly, DCE-MRI techniques should also be tested against other imaging techniques that measure vascular function including ultrasound, PET, and computed tomography [62–64].

E. Promising New MR Approaches

1. Simultaneous Perfusion and Permeability Imaging Using ECF Agents

Technical developments in MRI hardware and software are continuing and more rapid, high-spatial resolution and simultaneous T1 and T2* data acquisition techniques have been described [163–165]. The ability to simultaneously acquire spatially registered perfusion and permeability data will enable the interrelationship between diverse parameters to be appreciated and correlated with morphological appearances (Figure 13.7).

2. Macromolecular MR Assays of Microvascular Function

MRI assays of tumor angiogenesis using macromolecular contrast agents (MMCM) should be feasible soon. MMCM-enhanced MRI assays of tumor microvessel characteristics include vascular permeability (kPS) and the fractional plasma volume (fPV) [166]. As noted above, high permeability of ECF contrast media is observed both in normal and in tumor microvessels. This accounts, at least in part, for the variability of the clinical results described. Physiologists have observed that the microvessels of cancer are hyperpermeable to macromolecules, a feature largely absent in normal vessels [167, 168]. Hyperpermeability to macromolecules is considered important, even essential, to angiogenesis because it allows plasma proteins to seep into the tumor interstitium forming the matrix for the subsequent in-growth of new capillaries. Data analyses in animal models have shown good correlation between MRI-derived assays of tumor kPS and fPV with histologic MVD [169, 170]. Preclinical studies have also demonstrated that MMCM-enhanced MRI could identify and measure the effect of an anti-VEGF antibody [119]. This study showed that MMCM estimates of permeability were highly sensitive to angiogenesis modulation as early as 24 hours after a single dose of anti-VEGF antibody (kPS declined a dramatic 98%). The fractional plasma volume did not change significantly, which suggests that this characteristic, dependent on vessel morphology (MVD and surface area), is less sensitive than permeability to inhibition of VEGF. As yet, however, the ideal macromolecular MRI contrast media for use in clinical studies of anti-angiogenesis/anti-vascular drugs has not been identified. A major research goal is to identify one or more MMCM agents that are suitable for development as clinical pharmaceuticals.

3. Imaging Vascular Function Using Hemoglobin as a Contrast Agent

Analysis of vascular function can be accomplished by using deoxyhemoglobin as an intrinsic, paramagnetic contrast agent (blood oxygenation level dependent or BOLD contrast) [171]. Gradient-echo T_2*-weighted images that are sensitive to changes in blood volume, blood oxygenation, and blood flow are used (Figure 13.12). BOLD contrast can be used for mapping changes in blood volume fraction, and vascular functionality associated with angiogenesis [172, 173]. Vascular function can be evaluated by analysis of BOLD contrast changes in response to hyperoxia and hypercapnia [172, 174]. Clinical application of this method revealed high signal enhancements in

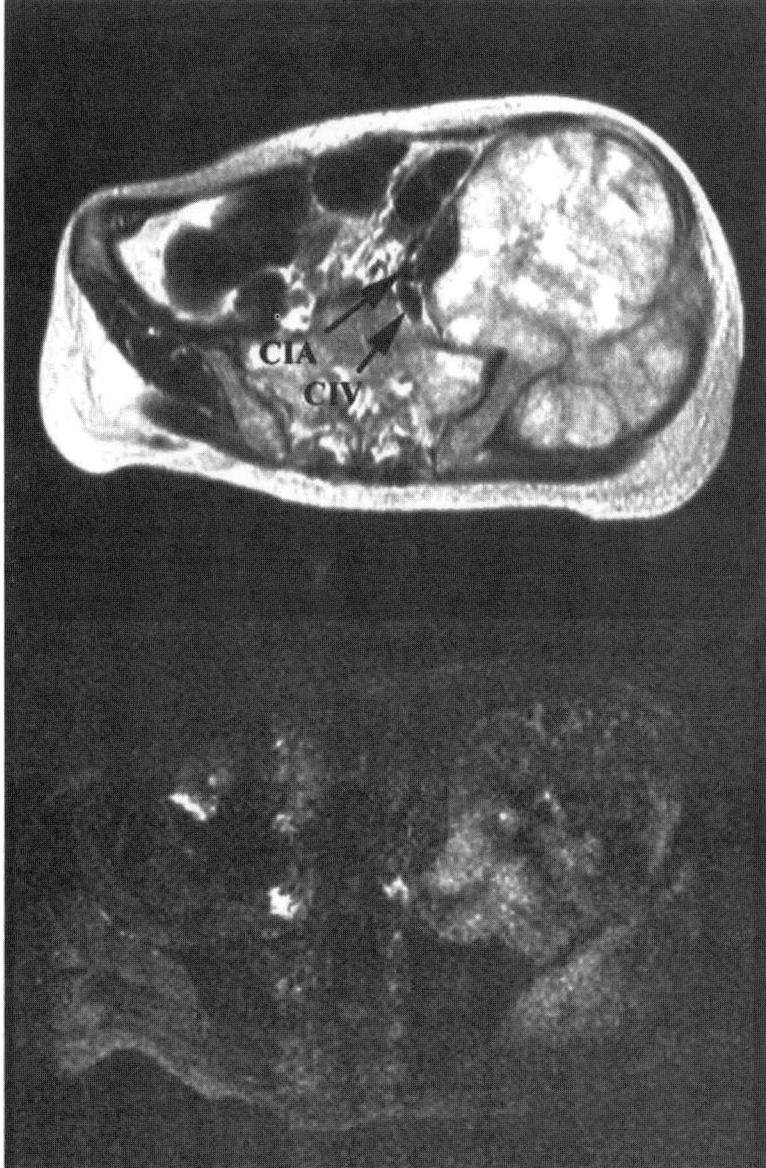

FIGURE 13.12 BOLD contrast for mapping tissue oxygenation and blood flow. (a) Top image. Axial T2-weighted image of the pelvis in a patient with a large metastatic leiomyosarcoma in the left iliac bone. Bony destruction is visible with displacement of muscles from the bones. (b) Bottom image. BOLD (Blood oxygenation Level Dependent) image at the same level shows marked heterogeneity in signal intensity within the tumour that is not readily appreciable on the anatomical image (a). High signal areas are seen adjacent to the bone and is also visible close to the iliac vessels (labelled as CIA = common iliac artery and CIV = common iliac vein in a). High signal probably relates to the delivery of oxygenated blood via vessels from the bone and iliac vessels.

response to carbogen inhalation in human tumors [175, 176]. Taylor et al., also reported that human studies are technically challenging [176]. The primary advantage of the intrinsic contrast is that there is no need to administer contrast material. Measurements can be repeated as needed with almost no limitation. BOLD contrast is not sensitive to fluctuation in permeability. A major reservation for intrinsic contrast imaging is the reduced contrast to noise ratio in the images obtained.

V. CONCLUSIONS

PET methodology is being developed to enable evaluation of pathophysiology and pharmacodynamics in oncology. The high sensitivity and specificity of PET assays allow the mechanism of drug action to be assessed in patients. There are, however, difficult methodological challenges in ligand/tracer discovery, radiochemistry, data processing, and modeling. These challenges need to be overcome to fully realize the potential of PET in clinical trials of novel cancer therapeutics.

There are definite clinical needs to develop non-invasive, imaging assays of tumor angiogenesis. Such imaging techniques will have a central role in the evaluation of novel anti-angiogenesis therapies [177]. DCE-MRI is one of a number of MRI techniques that evaluates tumors with respect to their state of angiogenesis. There are a number of requirements that need to be met before DCE-MRI techniques can become mainstream diagnostic tools. Requirements include agreed protocols for data acquisition, analysis, and presentation methods. Appropriate imaging processing and visualization tools will be needed to achieve this. New image acquisition techniques able to sample the whole tumor volume will also be needed, particularly if the technique is to be extended to organs with significant physiological motion. In time, macromolecular contrast enhanced MRI may become the preferred choice for these evaluations. Given the lead-time between the development of a new therapeutic approach or drug in the laboratory and its evaluation in the clinic, radiologists need to fully evaluate currently available and new imaging methods for evaluating tumor microvascular function.

REFERENCES

1. Spiro TP, Gerson SL, Liu L et al. O6-benzylguanine: A clinical trial establishing the biochemical modulatory dose in tumor tissue for alkyltransferase-directed DNA repair. *Cancer Res.* 1999; 59:2402–2410.

2. Cho ZH, Chan JK, Ericksson L et al. Positron ranges obtained from biomedically important positron-emitting radionuclides. *J. Nucl. Med.* 1975; 16(12):1174–1176.

3. Huang SC, Phelps ME. Principles of tracer kinetic modeling in positron tomography and autoradiography. In *Positron Emission Tomography and Autoradiography: Principles and Applications for the Brain and Heart* (Phelps ME, Mazziota JC, Schelbert HR, eds.), Raven Press, New York, 1986; 287–346.

4. Cunningham VJ, Jones T. Spectral analysis of dynamic PET studies. *J. Cereb. Blood Flow Metab.* 1993; 13(1):15–23.

5. Patlak CS, Blasberg RG, Fenstermacher JD. Graphical evaluation of blood-to-brain transfer constants from multiple-time uptake data. *J. Cereb. Blood Flow Metab.* 1983; 3(1):1–7.

6. McGuire AH, Dehdashti F, Siegel BA et al. Positron tomographic assessment of 16 alpha-[18F] fluoro-17 beta-estradiol uptake in metastatic breast carcinoma. *J. Nucl. Med.* 1991; 32(8):1526–1231.

7. Dehdashti F, Flanagan FL, Mortimer JE, Katzenellenbogen JA, Welch MJ, Siegel BA. Positron emission tomographic assessment of "metabolic flare" to predict response of metastatic breast cancer to antiestrogen therapy. *Eur. J. Nucl. Med.* 1999; 26(1):51–56.

8. Bellamy WT, Dalton WS, Dorr RT. The clinical relevance of multidrug resistance. *Cancer Invest.* 1990; 8(5):547–562.

9. Gottesman MM, Pastan I. Biochemistry of multidrug resistance mediated by the multidrug transporter. *Annu. Rev. Biochem.* 1993; 62:385–427.

10. Hendrick AM, Harris AL, Cantwell BM. Verapamil with mitoxantrone for advanced ovarian cancer: A negative phase II trial. *Ann. Oncol.* 1991; 2(1):71–72.

11. Rodenburg CJ, Nooter K, Herweijer H et al. Phase II study of combining vinblastine and cyclosporin-A to circumvent multidrug resistance in renal cell cancer. *Ann. Oncol.* 1991; 2(4):305–356.

12. Wood L, Palmer M, Hewitt J et al. Results of a phase III, double-blind, placebo-controlled trial of megestrol acetate modulation of P-glycoprotein-mediated drug resistance in the first-line management of small-cell lung carcinoma. *Br. J. Cancer* 1998; 77(4):627–631.

13. Kostakoglu L, Elahi N, Kiratli P et al. Clinical validation of the influence of P-glycoprotein on technetium-99m-sestamibi uptake in malignant tumors. *J. Nucl. Med.* 1997; 38(7):1003–1008.

14. Vecchio SD, Ciarmiello A, Potena MI et al. In vivo detection of multidrug-resistant (MDR1) phenotype by technetium- 99m sestamibi scan in untreated breast cancer patients [see comments]. *Eur. J. Nucl. Med.* 1997; 24(2):150–159.

15. Ciarmiello A, Del Vecchio S, Silvestro P et al. Tumor clearance of technetium 99m-sestamibi as a predictor of response to neoadjuvant chemotherapy for locally advanced breast cancer. *J. Clin. Oncol.* 1998; 16(5):1677–1683.

16. Chen CC, Meadows B, Regis J et al. Detection of in vivo P-glycoprotein inhibition by PSC 833 using Tc-99m sestamibi. *Clin. Cancer Res.* 1997; 3(4):545–552.

17. Elsinga PH, Franssen EJ, Hendrikse NH et al. Carbon-11-labeled daunorubicin and verapamil for probing P-glycoprotein in tumors with PET. *J. Nucl. Med.* 1996; 37(9):1571–1575.

18. Hendrikse NH, de Vries EG, Eriks-Fluks L et al. A new in vivo method to study P-glycoprotein transport in tumors and the blood-brain barrier. *Cancer Res.* 1999; 59(10):2411–2416.

19. Casciari JJ, Graham MM, Rasey JS. A modeling approach for quantifying tumor hypoxia with [F-18]fluoromisonidazole PET time-activity data. *Med. Phys.* 1995; 22(7):1127–1139.

20. Koh WJ, Bergman KS, Rasey JS et al. Evaluation of oxygenation status during fractionated radiotherapy in human non-small cell lung cancers using [F-18]fluoromisonidazole positron emission tomography. *Int. J. Radiat. Oncol. Biol. Phys.* 1995; 33(2):391–398.

21. Rasey JS, Koh WJ, Evans ML et al. Quantifying regional hypoxia in human tumors with positron emission tomography of [18F]fluoromisonidazole: A pretherapy study of 37 patients. *Int. J. Radiat. Oncol. Biol. Phys.* 1996; 36(2):417–428.

22. Aboagye EO, Kelson AB, Tracy M, Workman P. Preclinical development and current status of the fluorinated 2-nitroimidazole hypoxia probe N-(2-hydroxy-3,3,3-trifluoropropyl)-2-(2-nitro-1-imidazolyl) acetamide (SR 4554, CRC 94/17): A non-invasive diagnostic probe for the measurement of tumor hypoxia by magnetic resonance spectroscopy and imaging, and by positron emission tomography. *Anticancer Drug Des.* 1998; 13(6):703–730.

23. Lewis JS, McCarthy DW, McCarthy TJ, Fujibayashi Y, Welch MJ. Evaluation of 64Cu-ATSM in vitro and in vivo in a hypoxic tumor model. *J. Nucl. Med.* 1999; 40:177–183.

24. Pinedo HM, Peters GF. Fluorouracil: Biochemistry and pharmacology. *J. Clin. Oncol.* 1988; 6(10):1653–1664.

25. Saleem A, Yap J, Osman S et al. Modulation of fluorouracil tissue pharmacokinetics by enil-uracil: In-vivo imaging of drug action. *Lancet* 2000; 355(9221):2125–2131.

26. Anderson H, Yap JT, Price P. Measurement of tumor and normal tissue (NT) perfusion by positron emission tomography (PET) in the evaluation of antivascular therapy: Results in the phase I study of combretastatin A4 phosphate (CA4P). *Proc. Am. Soc. Clin. Oncol.* 2000; 19:179a.

27. Yap JT, Rhodes CG, Cunningham VJ, Jones T, Anderson H, Price PM. Measurement of cardiac output during PET tumor blood flow studies. *Proc. Soc. Nucl. Med.* 2000.

28. Tozer GM, Prise VE, Wilson J et al. Combretastatin A-4 phosphate as a tumor vascular-targeting agent: Early effects in tumors and normal tissues. *Cancer Res.* 1999; 59:1626–1634.

29. Weissleder R. Molecular imaging: Exploring the next frontier. *Radiology* 1999; 212:609–614.

30. Yu Y, Annala AJ, Barrio JR et al. Quantification of target gene expression by imaging reporter gene expression in living animals. *Nat. Med.* 2000; 6:933–937.

31. Gibbs JB. Anticancer drug targets: growth factors and growth factor signalling. *J. Clin. Invest.* 2000; 9–13.

32. Gibbs JB. Mechanism-based target identification and drug discovery in cancer research. *Science* 2000; 287:1969–1973.

33. Bakir MA, Eccles S, Babich JW et al. c-erbB2 protein overexpression in breast cancer as a target for PET using iodine-124-labeled monoclonal antibodies. *J. Nucl. Med.* 1992; 33:2154–2160.

34. Hamil TG, Burns HD, Eng WS, Francis BE, Gibson RE, Fioravanti C. Radioiodinated farnesyl transferase inhibitors. *J. Label Compd. Radiopharm.* 1999; 42:S30–32.

35. Touroutoglou N, Pazdur R. Thymidylate synthase inhibitors. *Clin. Cancer Res.* 1996; 2:227–243.

36. Matthews DA, Villafranca JE, Janson CA, Smith WW, Welsh K, Freer S. Stereochemical mechanism of action for thymidylate synthase based on the X-ray structure of the covalent inhibitory ternary complex with 5-fluoro-2′-deoxyuridylate and 5,10-mehylenetetrahydrofolate. *J. Mol. Biol.* 1990; 214:937–948.

37. Hardy LW, Finer-Moore JS, Montford WR, Jones MO, Santi DV, Stroud RM. Atomic structure of thymidylate synthase: target for rational drug design. *Science* 1987; 235: 448–455.

38. Wells P, Gunn RN, Hughes A, Taylor GA, Price P, Newell DR. Thymidine salvage demonstrated in vivo: A specific pharmacodynamic endpoint of thymidylate synthase (TS) inhibition. *Proc. Am. Assoc. Cancer Res.* 1997.

39. Collins JM, Klecker RW, Katki AG. Suicide prodrug activated by thymidylate synthase: rationale for treatment and noninvasive imaging of tumors with deoxyuridine analogues. *Clin. Cancer Res.* 1999; 5:1976–1981.

40. Mankoff DA, Shields AF, Graham MM, Link JM, Eary JF, Krohn KA. Kinetic analysis of 2-[carbon-11]thymidine PET imaging studies: Compartmental model and mathematical analysis. *J. Nucl. Med.* 1998; 39:1043–1055.

41. Eary JF, Mankoff DA, Spence AM et al. 2-[C-11]thymidine imaging of malignant brain tumors. *Cancer Res.* 1999; 59:615–621.

42. Gunn RN, Yap JT, Wells P et al. A general method to correct PET data for tissue metabolites using a dual-scan approach. *J. Nucl. Med.* 2000; 41(4):706–11.

43. Wells P, Gunn R, Steel C, Alison M, Jones T, Price P. Measurement of cell proliferation in vivo using [2–11C]thymidine. *Proc. Am. Soc. Clin. Oncol.* 1997; 16:548a.

44. Shields AF, Mankoff DA, Link JM et al. Carbon-11-thymidine and FDG to measure therapy response. *J. Nucl. Med.* 1998; 39:1757–1762.

45. Blasberg RG, Roelcke U, Weinreich R et al. Imaging brain tumor proliferative activity with [124I]iododeoxyuridine. *Cancer Res.* 2000; 60:624–635.

46. Shields AF, Grierson JR, Dohmen BM et al. Imaging proliferation in vivo with [F-18]FLT and positron emission tomography. *Nat. Med.* 1998; 4:1334–1336.

47. Weber G. Carbohydrate metabolism in cancer cells and the molecular correlation concept. *Naturwissenschaften* 1968; 9:418–429.

48. Weber G. Enzymology of cancer cells (first of two parts). *N. Engl. J. Med.* 1977; 296(9):486–492.

49. Weber G. Biochemical strategy of cancer cells and the design of chemotherapy: G. H. A. Clowes memorial lecture. *Cancer Res.* 1983; 43:3466–3492.

50. Aloj L, Carac'o C, Jagoda E, Eckelman WC, Neumann RD. Glut-1 and hexokinase expression: relationship with 2-fluoro-2-deoxy-D-glucose uptake in A431 and T47D cells in culture. *Cancer Res.* 1999; 59:4709–4714.

51. Chung JK, Lee YJ, Kim C et al. Mechanisms related to [18F]fluorodeoxyglucose uptake of human colon cancers transplanted in nude mice. *J. Nucl. Med.* 1999; 40:339–346.

52. Brock CS, Meikle SR, Price P. Does fluorine-18 fluorodeoxyglucose metabolic imaging of tumours benefit oncology? [see comments]. *Eur. J. Nucl. Med.* 1997; 24(6):691–705.

53. Brock CS, Young H, O'Reilly SM et al. Early evaluation of tumour metabolic response using [18F]fluorodeoxyglucose and positron emission tomography: A pilot study following the phase II chemotherapy schedule for temozolomide in recurrent high-grade gliomas. *Br. J. Cancer* 2000; 82:608–615.

54. Wahl RL, Zasadny K, Helvie M, Hutchins GD, Weber B, Cody R. Metabolic monitoring of breast cancer chemohormonotherapy using positron emission tomography: Initial evaluation. *J. Clin. Oncol.* 1993; 11:2101–2111.

55. Maisey NR, Webb A, Flux GD, Padhani A, Cunningham DC, Ott RJ. FDG-PET in the prediction of survival of patients with cancer of the pancreas: A pilot study. *Br. J. Cancer* 2000; 83:287–293.

56. Findlay M, Young H, Cunningham D et al. Noninvasive monitoring of tumor metabolism using fluorodeoxyglucose and positron emission tomography in colorectal cancer liver metastases: correlation with tumor response to fluorouracil [see comments]. *J. Clin. Oncol.* 1996; 14(3):700–708.

57. Ogawa T, Uemura K, Shishido F et al. Changes of cerebral blood flow, and oxygen and glucose metabolism following radiochemotherapy of gliomas: A PET study. *J. Comput. Assist. Tomogr.* 1988; 12(2):290–297.

58. Young H, Baum R, Cremerius U et al. Measurement of clinical and subclinical tumour response using [^{18}F]-fluorodeoxyglucose and positron emission tomography: Review and 1999 EORTC recommendations. *Eur. J. Cancer* 1999; 35:1773–1782.

59. Blakenberg FG, Tait J, Ohtsuki K, Strauss HW. Apoptosis: The importance of nuclear medicine. *Nucl. Med. Commun.* 2000; 21:241–250.

60. Neeman M, Provenzale JM, Dewhirst MW. Magnetic resonance imaging applications in the evaluation of tumor angiogenesis. *Semin. Radiat. Oncol.* 2001; 1:70–82.

61. Brasch RC, Li KC, Husband JE et al. In vivo monitoring of tumor angiogenesis with MR imaging. *Acad. Radiol.* 2000; 7:812–823.

62. Blankenberg FG, Eckelman WC, Strauss HW et al. Role of radionuclide imaging in trials of antiangiogenic therapy. *Acad. Radiol.* 2000; 7:851–867.

63. Miles KA, Charnsangavej C, Lee FT, Fishman EK, Horton K, Lee TY. Application of CT in the investigation of angiogenesis in oncology. *Acad. Radiol.* 2000; 7:840–850.

64. Ferrara KW, Merritt CR, Burns PN, Foster FS, Mattrey RF, Wickline SA. Evaluation of tumor angiogenesis with US: Imaging, Doppler, and contrast agents. *Acad. Radiol.* 2000; 7:824–839.

65. Yuh WT. An exciting and challenging role for the advanced contrast MR imaging. *J. Magn. Reson. Imaging* 1999; 10:221–222.

66. Taylor JS, Tofts PS, Port R et al. MR imaging of tumor microcirculation: Promise for the new millennium. *J. Magn. Reson. Imaging* 1999; 10:903–907.

67. Matsubayashi R, Matsuo Y, Edakuni G, Satoh T, Tokunaga O, Kudo S. Breast Masses with peripheral rim enhancement on dynamic contrast-enhanced MR images: Correlation of MR findings with histologic features and expression of growth factors. *Radiology* 2000; 217:841–848.

68. Zierler KL. Theory of use of indicators to measure blood flow and extracellular volume and calculation of trans capillary movement of tracers. *Circulation Res.* 1963; 12:464–471.

69. Crone C. The permeability of capillaries in various organs as determined by the use of 'indicator diffusion' method. *Acta Physiol. Scand.* 1963; 58:292–305.

70. Kety SS. The theory and applications of the exchange of inert gas at the lungs and tissues. *Pharmacol. Rev.* 1951; 3:1–41.

71. Rosen BR, Belliveau JW, Aronen HJ et al. Susceptibility contrast imaging of cerebral blood volume: human experience. *Magn. Reson. Med.* 1991; 22:293–299.

72. Edelman RR, Mattle HP, Atkinson DJ et al. Cerebral blood flow: Assessment with dynamic contrast-enhanced T2*-weighted MR imaging at 1.5 T. *Radiology* 1990; 176:211–220.

73. Dennie J, Mandeville JB, Boxerman JL, Packard SD, Rosen BR, Weisskoff RM. NMR imaging of changes in vascular morphology due to tumor angiogenesis. *Magn. Reson. Med.* 1998; 40:793–799.

74. Bruening R, Berchtenbreiter C, Holzknecht N et al. Effects of three different doses of a bolus injection of gadodiamide: Assessment of regional cerebral blood volume maps in a blinded reader study. *Am. J. Neuroradiol.* 2000; 21:1603–1610.

75. Sorensen AG, Tievsky AL, Ostergaard L, Weisskoff RM, Rosen BR. Contrast agents in functional MR imaging. *J. Magn. Reson. Imaging* 1997; 7:47–55.

76. Rempp KA, Brix G, Wenz F, Becker CR, Guckel F, Lorenz WJ. Quantification of regional cerebral blood flow and volume with dynamic susceptibility contrast-enhanced MR imaging. *Radiology* 1994; 193:637–641.

77. Wenz F, Rempp K, Hess T et al. Effect of radiation on blood volume in low-grade astrocytomas and normal brain tissue: quantification with dynamic susceptibility contrast MR imaging. *Am. J. Roentgenol.* 1996; 166:187–193.

78. Moseley ME, Vexler Z, Asgari HS et al. Comparison of Gd- and Dy-chelates for T2 contrast-enhanced imaging. *Magn. Reson. Med.* 1991; 22:259–264.

79. Lev MH, Kulke SF, Sorensen AG et al. Contrast-to-noise ratio in functional MRI of relative cerebral blood volume with sprodiamide injection. *J. Magn. Reson. Imaging* 1997; 7:523–527.

80. Ichikawa T, Haradome H, Hachiya J, Nitatori T, Araki T. Characterisation of hepatic lesions by perfusion-weighted MR imaging with an echoplanar sequence. *Am. J. Roentgenol.* 1998; 170:1029–1034.

81. Kuhl CK, Bieling H, Gieseke J et al. Breast neoplasms: T2* susceptibility-contrast, first-pass perfusion MR imaging. *Radiology* 1997; 202:87–95.

82. Kvistad KA, Lundgren S, Fjosne HE, Smenes E, Smethurst HB, Haraldseth O. Differentiating benign and malignant breast lesions with T2*-weighted first pass perfusion imaging. *Acta Radiol.* 1999; 40:45–51.

83. Aronen HJ, Gazit IE, Louis DN et al. Cerebral blood volume maps of gliomas: Comparison with tumour grade and histologic findings. *Radiology* 1994; 191:41–51.

84. Sugahara T, Korogi Y, Kochi M et al. Correlation of MR imaging-determined cerebral blood volume maps with histologic and angiographic determination of vascularity of gliomas. *Am. J. Roentgenol.* 1998; 171:1479–1486.

85. Aronen HJ, Glass J, Pardo FS et al. Echo-planar MR cerebral blood volume mapping of gliomas. Clinical utility. *Acta Radiol.* 1995; 36:520–528.

86. Knopp EA, Cha S, Johnson G et al. Glial neoplasms: dynamic contrast-enhanced T2*-weighted MR imaging. *Radiology* 1999; 211:791–798.

87. Bagley LJ, Grossman RI, Judy KD et al. Gliomas: Correlation of magnetic susceptibility artifact with histologic grade. *Radiology* 1997; 202:511–516.

88. Roberts TP. Physiologic measurements by contrast-enhanced MR imaging: Expectations and limitations. *J. Magn. Reson. Imaging* 1997; 7:82–90.

89. Evelhoch JL. Key factors in the acquisition of contrast kinetic data for oncology. *J. Magn. Reson. Imaging* 1999; 10:254–259.

90. Parker GJM, Suckling J, Tanner SF et al. Probing tumor microvessel density by measurement, analysis and display of contrast agent uptake kinetics. *J. Magn. Reson. Imaging* 1997; 7:564–574.

91. Flickinger FW, Allison JD, Sherry RM, Wright JC. Differentiation of benign from malignant breast masses by time-intensity evaluation of contrast enhanced MRI. *Magn. Reson. Imaging* 1993; 11:617–620.

92. Kaiser WA, Zeitler E. MR imaging of the breast: fast imaging sequences with and without Gd-DTPA — preliminary observations. *Radiology* 1989; 170:681–686.

93. Gribbestad IS, Nilsen G, Fjosne HE, Kvinnsland S, Haugen OA, Rinck PA. Comparative signal intensity measurements in dynamic gadolinium-enhanced MR mammography. *J. Magn. Reson. Imaging* 1994; 4:477–480.

94. Kuhl CK, Mielcareck P, Klaschik S et al. Dynamic breast MR imaging: Are signal intensity time course data useful for differential diagnosis of enhancing lesions? *Radiology* 1999; 211:101–110.

95. Hoffmann U, Brix G, Knopp MV, Hess T, Lorenz WJ. Pharmacokinetic mapping of the breast: a new method for dynamic MR mammography. *Magn. Reson. Med.* 1995; 33:506–514.

96. Parker GM, Baustert I, Tanner SF, Leach MO. Improving image quality and T1 measurements using saturation recovery TurboFLASH with approximate K-space normalisation filter. *Magn. Reson. Imaging* 2000; 18:157–167.

97. Tofts PS. Modelling tracer kinetics in dynamic Gd-DTPA MR imaging. *J. Magn. Reson. Imaging* 1997; 7:91–101.

98. Tofts PS, Brix G, Buckley DL et al. Estimating kinetic parameters from dynamic contrast-enhanced T(1)-weighted MRI of a diffusible tracer: Standardized quantities and symbols. *J. Magn. Reson. Imaging* 1999; 10:223–232.

99. Tofts PS, Berkowitz B, Schnall MD. Quantitative analysis of dynamic Gd-DTPA enhancement in breast tumors using a permeability model. *Magn. Reson. Med.* 1995; 33:564–568.

100. Weind KL, Maier CF, Rutt BK, Moussa M. Invasive carcinomas and fibroadenomas of the breast: comparison of microvessel distributions — implications for imaging modalities. *Radiology* 1998; 208:477–483.

101. Jitsuiki Y, Hasebe T, Tsuda H et al. Optimizing microvessel counts according to tumor zone in invasive ductal carcinoma of the breast. *Mod. Pathol.* 1999; 12:492–498.

102. Buadu LD, Murakami J, Murayama S et al. Breast lesions: Correlation of contrast medium enhancement patterns on MR images with histopathologic findings and tumor angiogenesis. *Radiology* 1996; 200:639–649.

103. Yamashita Y, Baba T, Baba Y et al. Dynamic contrast-enhanced MR imaging of uterine cervical cancer: pharmacokinetic analysis with histopathologic correlation and its importance in predicting the outcome of radiation therapy. *Radiology* 2000; 216:803–809.

104. Liney GP, Gibbs P, Hayes C, Leach MO, Turnbull LW. Dynamic contrast-enhanced MRI in the differentiation of breast tumors: user-defined versus semi-automated region-of-interest analysis. *J. Magn. Reson. Imaging* 1999; 10:945–949.

105. Parker GJ, Suckling J, Tanner SF, Padhani AR, Husband JE, Leach MO. MRIW: Parametric analysis software for contrast-enhanced dynamic MR imaging in cancer. *Radiographics* 1998; 18:497–506.

106. Mayr NA, Yuh WT, Arnholt JC et al. Pixel analysis of MR perfusion imaging in predicting radiation therapy outcome in cervical cancer. *J. Magn. Reson. Imaging* 2000; 12:1027–1033.

107. Hayes C, Padhani AR, Leach MO. Assessing tumor response to treatment: Histogram analysis of parametric maps of tumor vascular function derived from dynamic contrast enhanced MR images. International Society for Magnetic Resonance in Medicine, 8th Scientific Meeting, Colorado 2000.

108. Weidner N. Intratumoral microvessel density as a prognostic factor in cancer (comment). *Am. J. Pathol.* 1995; 147:9–19.

109. Stomper PC, Winston JS, Herman S, Klippenstein DL, Arredondo MA, Blumenson LE. Angiogenesis and dynamic MR imaging gadolinium enhancement of malignant and benign breast lesions. *Breast Cancer Res. Treat.* 1997; 45:39–46.

110. Hawighorst H, Knapstein PG, Weikel W et al. Angiogenesis of uterine cervical carcinoma: Characterization by pharmacokinetic magnetic resonance parameters and histological microvessel density with correlation to lymphatic involvement. *Cancer Res.* 1997; 57:4777–4786.

111. Tynninen O, Aronen HJ, Ruhala M et al. MRI enhancement and microvascular density in gliomas. Correlation with tumor cell proliferation. *Invest. Radiol.* 1999; 34:427–434.

112. Buckley DL, Drew PJ, Mussurakis S, Monson JR, Horsman A. Microvessel density of invasive breast cancer assessed by dynamic Gd-DTPA enhanced MRI. *J. Magn. Reson. Imaging* 1997; 7:461–464.

113. Hulka CA, Edmister WB, Smith BL et al. Dynamic echo-planar imaging of the breast: Experience in diagnosing breast carcinoma and correlation with tumor angiogenesis. *Radiology* 1997; 205:837–842.

114. Cooper RA, Carrington BM, Loncaster JA et al. Tumor oxygenation levels correlate with dynamic contrast-enhanced magnetic resonance imaging parameters in carcinoma of the cervix. *Rad. Oncol.* 2000; 57:53–59.

115. Knopp MV, Weiss E, Sinn HP et al. Pathophysiologic basis of contrast enhancement in breast tumors. *J. Magn. Reson. Imaging* 1999; 10:260–266.

116. Furman-Haran E, Margalit R, Grobgeld D, Degani H. Dynamic contrast-enhanced magnetic resonance imaging reveals stress-induced angiogenesis in MCF7 human breast tumors. *Proc. Natl. Acad. Sci. U. S. A.* 1996; 93:6247–6251.

117. Bhujwalla ZM, Artemov D, Solaiyappan M, Mao D, Backer JP. Comparison of vascular volume and permeability for tumors derived from metastatic human breast cancer cell with and without metastasis supressor gene nm23. International Society for Magnetic Resonance in Medicine, 7th Scientific Meeting. Philadelphia 1999; 146.

118. Dzik-Jurasz ASK, George M, Padhani AR, Swift RI, Leach MO, Rowland IJ. Is there an association between systemic VEGF and permeability in locally advanced rectal adenocarcinoma? Initial observations. Proceedings of the International Society of Magnetic Resonance Imaging 2000; 1055.

119. Pham CD, Roberts TP, van Bruggen N et al. Magnetic resonance imaging detects suppression of tumor vascular permeability after administration of antibody to vascular endothelial growth factor. *Cancer Invest.* 1998; 16:225–230.

120. Padhani AR, O'Donell A, Hayes C. Dynamic contrast enhanced MR imaging in the evaluation of antiangiogenesis therapy. *Clin. Cancer Res.* 1999; 5:3828S.

121. Verstraete KL, De Deene Y, Roels H, Dierick A, Uyttendaele D, Kunnen M. Benign and malignant musculoskeletal lesions: dynamic contrast-enhanced MR imaging-parametric "first-pass" images depict tissue vascularization and perfusion. *Radiology* 1994; 192:835–843.

122. Boetes C, Barentsz JO, Mus RD et al. MR characterisation of suspicious breast lesions with a gadolinium-enhanced TurboFLASH subtraction technique. *Radiology* 1994; 193:777–781.

123. Gilles R, Guinebretiere JM, Shapeero LG et al. Assessment of breast cancer recurrence with contrast-enhanced subtraction MR imaging: Preliminary results in 26 patients. *Radiology* 1993; 188:473–478.

124. Heywang SH, Wolf A, Pruss E, Hilbertz T, Eiermann W, Permanetter W. MR imaging of the breast with Gd-DTPA: Use and limitations. *Radiology* 1989; 171:95–103.

125. Stomper PC, Herman S, Klippenstein DL et al. Suspect breast lesions: findings at dynamic gadolinium-enhanced MR imaging correlated with mammographic and pathologic features. *Radiology* 1995; 197:387–395.

126. Fobben ES, Rubin CZ, Kalisher L, Dembner AG, Seltzer MH, Santoro EJ. Breast MR imaging with commercially available techniques: radiologic-pathologic correlation. *Radiology* 1995; 196:143–152.

127. Brinck U, Fischer U, Korabiowska M, Jutrowski M, Schauer A, Grabbe E. The variability of fibroadenoma in contrast-enhanced dynamic MR mammography. *Am. J. Roentgenol.* 1997; 168:1331–1334.

128. Padhani AR, Gapinski CJ, James F et al. Dynamic MR enhancement in prostate cancer: Correlation with morphology and MRI stage, histological grade and serum PSA. *Clin. Radiol.* 2000; 55:99–109.

129. Barentsz JO, Engelbrecht M, Jager GJ et al. Fast dynamic gadolinium-enhanced MR imaging of urinary bladder and prostate cancer. *J. Magn. Reson. Imaging* 1999; 10:295–304.

130. Liu PF, Krestin GP, Huch RA et al. MRI of the uterus, uterine cervix, and vagina: Diagnostic performance of dynamic contrast-enhanced fast multiplanar gradient-echo imaging in comparison with fast spin-echo T2-weighted pulse imaging. *Eur. Radiol.* 1998; 8:1433–1440.

131. Barentsz JO, Jager GJ, van Vierzen PB et al. Staging urinary bladder cancer after transurethral biopsy: value of fast dynamic contrast-enhanced MR imaging. *Radiology* 1996; 201:185–193.

132. Jager GJ, Ruijter ET, van de Kaa CA et al. Dynamic turboFLASH subtraction technique for contrast-enhanced MR imaging of the prostate: Correlation with histopathologic results. *Radiology* 1997; 203:645–652.

133. Barentsz JO, Berger-Hartog O, Witjes JA et al. Evaluation of chemotherapy in advanced urinary bladder cancer with fast dynamic contrast-enhanced MR imaging. *Radiology* 1998; 207:791–797.

134. Reddick WE, Taylor JS, Fletcher BD. Dynamic MR imaging (DEMRI) of microcirculation in bone sarcoma. *J. Magn. Reson. Imaging* 1999; 10:277–285.

135. van der Woude HJ, Bloem JL, Verstraete KL, Taminiau AH, Nooy MA, Hogendoorn PC. Osteosarcoma and Ewing's sarcoma after neoadjuvant chemotherapy: Value of dynamic MR imaging in detecting viable tumor before surgery. *Am. J. Roentgenol.* 1995; 165:593–598.

136. Knopp MV, Brix G, Junkermann HJ, Sinn HP. MR mammography with pharmacokinetic mapping for monitoring of breast cancer treatment during neoadjuvant therapy. *Magn. Reson. Imaging Clin. N. Am.* 1994; 2:633–658.

137. Padhani AR, Hayes C, Assersohn L, Powles T, Leach MO, Husband JE. Response of Breast carcinoma to Chemotherapy — MR Permeability changes using Histogram Analysis. Proceedings of the International Society for Magnetic Resonance in Medicine, 8th Scientific Meeting, Colorado 2000.

138. de Vries A, Griebel J, Kremser C et al. Monitoring of tumor microcirculation during fractionated radiation therapy in patients with rectal carcinoma: Preliminary results and implications for therapy. *Radiology* 2000; 217:385–391.

139. Padhani AR, MacVicar AD, Gapinski CJ et al. Effects of androgen deprivation on prostatic morphology and vascular permeability evaluated with MR imaging. *Radiology* 2001; 218:365–374.

140. Burn PR, McCall JM, Chinn RJ et al. Uterine fibroleiomyoma: MR imaging appearances before and after embolization of uterine arteries. *Radiology* 2000; 214:729–734.

141. Jha RC, Ascher SM, Imaoka I et al. Symptomatic fibroleiomyomata: MR imaging of the uterus before and after uterine arterial embolization. *Radiology* 2000; 217:228–235.

142. Li W, Brophy DP, Chen Q et al. Semiquantitative assessment of uterine perfusion using first pass dynamic contrast-enhanced MR imaging for patients treated with uterine fibroid embolization. *J. Magn. Reson. Imaging* 2000; 12:1004–1008.

143. Hawighorst H, Weikel W, Knapstein PG et al. Angiogenic activity of cervical carcinoma: Assessment by functional magnetic resonance imaging-based parameters and a histomorphological approach in correlation with disease outcome. *Clin. Cancer Res.* 1998; 4:2305–2312.

144. Mayr NA, Yuh WT, Magnotta VA et al. Tumor perfusion studies using fast magnetic resonance imaging technique in advanced cervical cancer: A new noninvasive predictive assay. *Int. J. Radiat. Oncol. Biol. Phys.* 1996; 36:623–633.

145. Dao TH, Rahmouni A, Campana F, Laurent M, Asselain B, Fourquet A. Tumor recurrence versus fibrosis in the irradiated breast: Differentiation with dynamic gadolinium-enhanced MR imaging. *Radiology* 1993; 187:751–755.

146. Heywang-Kobrunner SH, Schlegel A, Beck R et al. Contrast-enhanced MRI of the breast after limited surgery and radiation therapy. *J. Comput. Assist. Tomogr.* 1993; 17:891–900.

147. Kerslake RW, Fox JN, Carleton PJ et al. Dynamic contrast-enhanced and fat suppressed magnetic resonance imaging in suspected recurrent carcinoma of the breast: Preliminary experience. *Br. J. Radiol.* 1994; 67:1158–1168.

148. Mussurakis S, Buckley DL, Bowsley SJ et al. Dynamic contrast-enhanced magnetic resonance imaging of the breast combined with pharmacokinetic analysis of gadolinium-DTPA uptake in the diagnosis of local recurrence of early stage breast carcinoma. *Invest. Radiol.* 1995; 30: 650–662.

149. Kinkel K, Tardivon AA, Soyer P et al. Dynamic contrast-enhanced subtraction versus T2-weighted spin-echo MR imaging in the follow-up of colorectal neoplasm. A prospective study of 41 patients. *Radiology* 1996; 200:453–458.

150. Hawnaur JM, Zhu XP, Hutchinson CE. Quantitative dynamic contrast enhanced MRI of recurrent pelvic masses in patients treated for cancer. *Br. J. Radiol.* 1998; 71:1136–1142.

151. Blomqvist L, Fransson P, Hindmarsh T. The pelvis after surgery and radio-chemotherapy for rectal cancer studied with Gd-DTPA-enhanced fast dynamic MR imaging. *Eur. Radiol.* 1998; 8:781–787.

152. Vajkoczy P, Menger MD, Vollmar B et al. Inhibition of tumor growth, angiogenesis, and microcirculation by the novel Flk-1 inhibitor SU5416 as assessed by intravital multi-fluorescencevideomicroscopy. *Neoplasia.* 1999; 1:31–41.

153. Mendel DB, Laird AD, Smolich BD et al. Development of SU5416, a selective small molecule inhibitor of VEGF receptor tyrosine kinase activity, as an anti-angiogenesis agent. *Anticancer Drug Des.* 2000; 15:29–41.

154. Shaheen RM, Davis DW, Liu W et al. Antiangiogenic therapy targeting the tyrosine kinase receptor for vascular endothelial growth factor receptor inhibits the growth of colon cancer liver metastasis and induces tumor and endothelial cell apoptosis. *Cancer Res.* 1999; 59:5412–5416.

155. Kanthou C, Prise VE, Milson J, Tozer GM. The vascular targeting agent combretastatin A4 phosphate alters the endothelial cell actin cytoskeleton and mediates changes in vascular permeability in vitro and in vivo. American Association for Cancer Research Meeting, New Orleans 2001.

156. Galbraith SM, Chaplin D, Lee F et al. Effects of combretastatin A4 phosphate on endothelial cell shape in vitro and relation to vascular targeting effects in vivo. *Anticancer Res.* 2001, in press.

157. Lodge MA, Galbraith SM, Taylor NJ et al. Reproducibility of quantitative permeability measurements in dynamic contrast-enhanced MRI studies. Proceedings of the International Society of Magnetic Resonance in Medicine, 9th Scientific Meeting, Glasgow 2001.

158. Padhani AR, O'Donell A, Hayes C et al. Dynamic contrast enhanced MR imaging in the evaluation of antiangiogenesis therapy. Molecular Targets and Cancer Therapeutics:

Discovery, Development and Cancer Therapeutics. The Joint AACR-NCI-EORTC Meeting. Washington 1999. *Clin. Cancer Res.* 1999; 5:3828S.

159. Galbraith SM, Lodge M, Taylor NJ et al. Combretastatin reduces blood flow in animal and human tumours, demonstrated by dynamic MRI. Proceedings of the International Society of Magnetic Resonance in Medicine, 9th Scientific Meeting, Glasgow 2001.

160. den Boer JA, Hoenderop RK, Smink J et al. Pharmacokinetic analysis of Gd-DTPA enhancement in dynamic three-dimensional MRI of breast lesions. *J. Magn. Reson. Imaging* 1997; 7:702–715.

161. Degani H, Gusis V, Weinstein D, Fields S, Strano S. Mapping pathophysiological features of breast tumors by MRI at high spatial resolution. *Nat. Med.* 1997; 3:780–782.

162. Port RE, Knopp MV, Hoffmann U, Milker-Zabel S, Brix G. Multicompartment analysis of gadolinium chelate kinetics: blood-tissue exchange in mammary tumors as monitored by dynamic MR imaging. *J. Magn. Reson. Imaging* 1999; 10:233–241.

163. Barbier EL, den Boer JA, Peters AR, Rozeboom AR, Sau J, Bonmartin A. A model of the dual effect of gadopentetate dimeglumine on dynamic brain MR images. J Magn Reson Imaging 1999; 10:242–253.

164. Baustert IC, Padhani AR, Brada M, Leach MO. Assessing the progressive development of the angiogenic phenotype with simultaneous permeability and perfusion MRI measurements. Cancer workshop on MR in experimental and clinical cancer research International society for magnetic resonance in medicine. St Louis 1998.

165. d'Arcy JA, Collins DJ, Rowland IJ, Padhani AR, Leach MO. A rapid acquisition dual gradient echo sequence for combined perfusion and permeability studies. British Chapter of the International Society of Magnetic Resonance in Medicine, Liverpool June 2000.

166. Brasch R, Pham C, Shames D et al. Assessing tumor angiogenesis using macromolecular MR imaging contrast media. *J. Magn. Reson. Imaging* 1997; 7:68–74.

167. Gerlowski LE, Jain RK. Microvascular permeability of normal and neoplastic tissues. *Microvasc. Res.* 1986; 31:288–305.

168. Jain R. Transport of molecules across tumor vasculature. *Cancer Metast. Rev.* 1987; 6:559–593.

169. van Dijke C, Brasch R, Roberts T et al. Mammary carcinoma model: Correlation of macromolecular contrast enhanced MR imaging characterizations of tumor microvasculature and histologic capillary density. *Radiology* 1996; 198:813–818.

170. Turetschek K, Huber S, Floyd E et al. MR Imaging Characterization of microvessels in experimental breast tumors by using a particulate contrast agent with histopathologic correlation. *Radiology* 2001; 218:562–569.

171. Ogawa S, Menon RS, Kim SG et al. On the characteristics of functional magnetic resonance imaging of the brain. *Annu. Rev. Biophys. Biomol. Struct.* 1998; 27:447–474.

172. Abramovitch R, Frenkiel D, Neeman M. Analysis of subcutaneous angiogenesis by gradient echo magnetic resonance imaging. *Magn. Reson. Med.* 1998; 39:813–824.

173. van Zijl PC, Eleff SM, Ulatowski JA et al. Quantitative assessment of blood flow, blood volume and blood oxygenation effects in functional magnetic resonance imaging. *Nat. Med.* 1998; 4:159–167.

174. Robinson SP, Collingridge DR, Howe FA, Rodrigues LM, Chaplin DJ, Griffiths JR. Tumour response to hypercapnia and hyperoxia monitored by FLOOD magnetic resonance imaging. *NMR Biomed.* 1999; 12:98–106.

175. Griffiths JR, Taylor NJ, Howe FA et al. The response of human tumors to carbogen breathing, monitored by Gradient-Recalled Echo Magnetic Resonance Imaging. *Int. J. Radiat. Oncol. Biol. Phys.* 1997; 39:697–701.

176. Taylor NJ, Baddeley H, Goodchild H et al. BOLD MR imaging of human tumour oxygenation during carbogen breathing. *J. Magn. Reson. Imaging* 2001 (accepted).

177. Tatum JL, Hoffman JM. Role of imaging in clinical trials of antiangiogenesis therapy in oncology. *Acad. Radiol.* 2000; 7:798–799.

14

DEVISING PROOF-OF-CONCEPT STRATEGIES IN ONCOLOGY CLINICAL TRIALS

PAUL S. WISSEL

Group Director, Clinical Development
GlaxoSmithKline
Collegeville, Pennsylvania

Adjunct Associate Professor
University of Pennsylvania
Philadelphia, Pennsylvania

I. INTRODUCTION
II. PROOF-OF-CONCEPT
III. ELEMENTS OF "THE CONCEPT"
IV. APPLICATION OF SURROGATE END POINTS IN PROOF-OF-CONCEPT DECISION MAKING
V. SELECTED STATISTICAL CONSIDERATIONS IN PROOF-OF-CONCEPT STUDIES
VI. PHARMACODYNAMIC PROOF-OF-CONCEPT END POINTS
VII. PHARMACOKINETIC PROOF-OF-CONCEPT END POINTS
VIII. PROCEEDING FROM PROOF-OF-CONCEPT DIRECTLY TO PHASE II
IX. GUIDELINES AND SUMMARY

I. INTRODUCTION

Novel therapies that effect the biology of human cancer have typically been investigated in four general phases of drug development. Phase I includes dose-escalation studies which assess the safety, tolerability, and pharmacokinetics of the new chemical entity (NCE) and may define dose-limiting toxicities. Phase I, as part of the standard clinical pharmacology evaluation, can also include any drug-drug interaction studies in which the NCE is co-administered with a standard agent(s). At the conclusion of phase I, a dose for phase II trials should have been determined. Phase II trials are designed to assess the early clinical activity of the NCE in patients with a specific tumor type and setting. Phase III trials assess the efficacy of the NCE compared to that of currently available standard therapy. In addition, phase III trials are designed to provide prescribing information to oncologists and a description of the expected clinical benefit using an end point that physicians, patients, and regulatory authorities would deem as important. Safety and tolerability data are collected from all patients in all phases of clinical development as well as post-approval [1]. Phase IV studies evaluate a novel compound after registration and marketing approval, and can be used to demonstrate activity or efficacy in new clinical settings or with alternative dose regimens in the same setting.

Efforts to incorporate drug development decision analysis into this sequential drug development schema has been the basis of the traditional development milestone method of drug evaluation. The planned results from a clinical study can lead an investigator or sponsor to decide on the future development (PoC) of a drug: continue as planned, end development, or change the clinical development plan. Proof-of-concept uses this well-established system of trial-based milestones and attempts to add more formality to decision making which often links the results from more than one trial together, thus, improving characterization of activity and safety. In comparison, single or multiple phase II studies, performed sequentially and with post hoc decision making (milestones), have been used (currently and in the past) to determine early clinical activity [2, 3] and have effectively screened anti-tumor agents in drug development for several decades.

The establishment of proof-of-concept decision points in clinical development has increased in importance over time. Clinical research resources for large, adequately powered phase III trials (principal investigator's time, institutional commitment, and funding) are limited and patient's commitment to the research process must be matched with the best opportunities for clinical benefit. Creating a method that allows initiation of phase III studies with trial designs and treatment arms more likely to succeed in testing an important experimental hypothesis will better utilize these commitments and resources.

II. PROOF-OF-CONCEPT

A suitable definition of *proof-of-concept* may be different for each program and drug. In general, it should conform to a standard and demonstrate, in a clinical trial setting, that a measurement reflective of efficacy has been improved by drug administration. The term *proof-of-mechanism* can be used if the end point studied has minimal correlation to an efficacy end point, but replicates the early preclinical pharmacology findings (e.g., the targeted enzyme is inhibited, the receptor is blocked, etc.) instead. Efforts made to characterize proof-of-concept prior to human dosing can be rewarding, because it requires the investigator or sponsor to acknowledge that certain questions must be addressed, such as:

1. What level of efficacy is the NCE capable of achieving?
2. Is there a surrogate end point that is well correlated to the efficacy end point?
3. What clinical strategy can assess efficacy in an expedited manner?

III. ELEMENTS OF "THE CONCEPT"

The concept in the early stages of a drug development program is that the tested therapeutic intervention will lead to a salutary effect in a specific setting and in a predictable manner. This concept is then formally confirmed in adequately powered phase III trials; often requiring two well-controlled randomized studies in the same patient setting. Generating an early framework for the phase III study design is important in planning the early drug development milestones and proof-of-concept. When the proof-of-concept is determined for an NCE, the planning is initiated prior to the first time in human dosing. This planning process may involve the 18 to 36 months prior to the start of phase III trials. When the NCE does not operate by a novel mechanism, but is perhaps an analog of an approved agent, the planning process is greatly assisted by reviewing the development program of an established drug. When the NCE is an analog of a well-described chemical series, review of the literature and attendance at public regulatory advisory committees can provide important background of the established agent's drug development path.

Finalization of these phase III designs is dependent upon selecting an appropriate control arm. Typically a recognized standard of care — as defined in the literature, by oncology societies, or by regulatory authorities — is utilized. For some clinical trial control arms, a novel regimen may be selected when it appears likely to become established as the new standard of care during the conduct of the trial. Similarly, an ideal proof-of-concept program will end with a characterization of the influence of the experimental therapy on the surrogate end point which is related to the final efficacy end point; an end point viewed as important to patients, practicing physicians, and regulatory agencies. If a surrogate marker is identified that correlates with the primary efficacy end point, then the trial design may be simplified and timelines shortened. If a proof-of-concept program with this level of clarity is not possible (which commonly occurs), grouping less compelling early end points from more than one clinical study may suffice as a useful PoC. This occurs when a surrogate marker for a true efficacy end point is not available or does not have sufficient predictive value. These include a variety of proof-of-mechanism end points, pharmacokinetic measurements and well-defined safety end points. Taken together, these early end points may be combined to determine if an NCE should be developed further. Thus, proof-of-concept may not be determined during the initial phase of clinical trials, but after more than one phase II study has been completed.

A. Phase III End Point — Clinical Benefit, Selecting the End Point for PoC

Because the purpose of a proof-of-concept trial is to enhance the confidence that future phase III trials will be positive, agreeing on the proposed phase III primary end point is a key element in planning. The phase III primary end point (when positively influenced by the novel therapy) should represent a clinical benefit that will convince physicians their patients will feel better, delay the onset of tumor-related symptoms, or live longer. If another purpose of the phase III program is to seek regulatory approval, then the primary efficacy end point (as well as the entire phase III study design) needs to be acceptable to the appropriate agencies. Clinical end points that may be suitable for phase III primary end points of efficacy include [4]:

1. **Overall survival (OS):** This is viewed as the gold standard for efficacy in an oncology trial and addresses a common goal of oncology patients — to live longer. An overall survival end point is frequently used in phase III where registration for marketing is sought throughout the world. Additionally, demonstration of a survival benefit beyond the standard control arm is a frequent end point in non-registration directed trials. These trials, when positive, can rapidly change the standard of care in the studied setting. Although the end point clarity and avoidance of site-based interpretation adds merit to this end point, study timeline considerations reduce its utility in proof-of-concept trials.

2. **Time to disease progression (TTP):** This end point is a frequently recorded secondary end point in phase III trials in which overall survival is the primary end point. TTP may provide a good assessment of treatment effect, but its correlation to overall survival varies by disease setting. When TTP is considered as a surrogate for an overall survival end point, an in-depth validation of this correlation in the specific study setting is advised. TTP, or 1-year progression-free survival, may be particularly useful for cytostatic agents, where few or no objective responses are expected [3, 5, 6]. Although this end point is not subject to cross-over treatment effects, it is dependent on disease assessment timings; typically needs a concurrent, blinded control arm to assure accurate interpretation; and requires substantial time for follow-up, data collection, and expense. When a compound provides anti-tumor activity by providing longer periods of stable disease, this end point warrants consideration for use in proof-of-concept trials.

3. **Reduction of tumor volume (response):** Measurement of this end point is well accepted as a treatment effect, is easily measurable, and can be monitored and reviewed by independent panels. Similarly, there are clear standards for classification of tumor volume reductions that are well accepted [7, 8]. Overall response rate (ORR) is defined as the number of complete and partial responses. Of note, the absence of cytotoxic drug-related tumor reduction in phase I, even at the anecdotal level, has been associated with disappointing results in later clinical development. This has also been called the Von Hoff rule [9].

4. **Reduction of pain:** With the availability of validated pain scales as a clinical research tool, this end point can be reflective of true clinical benefit. When pain scales are used to support the phase III primary end point, a detailed clinical protocol must be included and ancillary staff must be familiar with the administration of this assessment.

5. **Improving a specific quality-of-life measurement** (e.g., fatigue, hot flashes, mucositis, preservation of rectal sphincter function and laryngeal function): Symptoms that substantially impact a patient's perception of well-being can be measured by a validated instrument and have potential to become primary phase III end points [10]. If a symptom-based

drug-related change in a measurable symptom or quality-of-life (QOL) assessment is the only end point in a proof-of-concept (or phase III), suitable attention to study design and validation of the instrument is recommended [4]. If a quality-of-life endpoint can be more objectively measured (preservation of rectal sphincter function or preservation of laryngeal function), then it would be suitable as a proof-of-concept endpoint. Given the cautions associated with this approach, using an additional endpoint to complement a general QOL assessment would be prudent.

6. **Stable disease:** This end point has generally been defined as measurable disease, over time, which does not qualify as formal tumor response or progressive disease; <50% reduction or <25% increase tumor volume. In one setting, patients with tumors showing stable disease while on therapy experienced a similar increase in survival as those with tumors showing a partial response [8, 11]. This end point can be influenced by various factors other than the tested therapy (such as frequency of evaluation), but collection of the data can be useful, particularly if the trial includes a concurrent control. No standard definition of duration of stable disease that is clinically meaningful is widely accepted, which substantially limits the utility of this end point in proof-of-concept studies.

7. **Intraepithelial neoplasia (IEN):** Several examples of good correlations between IEN and later development of invasive cancer permits this end point to be considered in a variety of proof-of-concept settings (and perhaps be used in phase III treatment and prevention). These settings are well described by a recent AACR task force [12]. Further support for the use of drug-related reduction for IEN as a marker in a proof-of-concept study is seen by the FDA approval of celecoxib for the reduction in the number of adenomatous colorectal polyps in familial adenomatous polyposis (FAP), as adjunct to usual care [13].

B. Drug-Like Qualities as PoC

Defining safety and efficacy are the primary elements of a phase III program. If these objectives are not met, it is very unlikely that a NCE will be used clinically or meet regulatory requirements for approval. Beyond the assessment of safety or activity, proof-of-concept can be based on other considerations needed for a successful compound. The term "drug-like qualities" is important to any NCE with a goal of becoming a global therapeutic. Drug-like qualities are those features that would make a compound easy to use and prescribe by health professionals and include clinical pharmacologic characteristics that could be extended to a broader demographic population. When the NCE becomes widely available (post approval), administration will be under the direction of pharmacists, physicians, and nurses; a group of prescribers somewhat different from the principal investigators in phase III trials. Similarly, as a marketed drug, the strict entry criteria of phase III is no longer a requirement for patient access to the NCE and the type of patients receiving the agent may vary from the more specific phase III population. Among the properties that can be assessed as drug-like qualities are characteristics that allow or enhance an agent's ability to be viewed as a reliable and predictable therapeutic, which is compatible with optimal patient compliance. These characteristics include:

- Bioavailability (average and variability)
- Conditions limiting bioavailability (fasting, antacids, gastrointestinal surgery, etc.)
- Significant drug-drug interactions with therapeutics commonly prescribed to the target population (e.g., P450 inhibition or induction, alteration of drug clearance, protein binding, etc.)
- Size of tablets, number of tablets needed per day, duration of the infusion, frequency of dosing — issues which directly affect patient compliance
- Conditions needed to maintain drug shelf-life (e.g., photosensitivity, decomposition, etc.)
- Comparison of the above qualities with other "competing" therapies
- Substantial change in systemic exposure after chronic dosing (induction or suppression of drug metabolism)
- Known common functional polymorphisms of drug metabolic pathways

C. Safety Profile of the Novel Therapy as PoC

An important component of early-phase clinical studies is the determination of the adverse event profile of the NCE. Assessment of the novel therapeutic's safety profile is an important element in a proof-of-concept decision analysis and, in some settings, the primary element. When a safety end point is the primary component of PoC, estimating the number of patients to adequately characterize the safety profile at the phase III dose level, or dose regimen, is needed prior to the start of these studies. A key component of any study design is the sample size estimation. For example, if the significant adverse event is infrequent, the number of patients needed to successfully evaluate safety as a PoC end point may be larger than that needed for a more common safety end point. Recruiting a patient population that includes the necessary demographics is central to the planning of the proof-of-concept program. The consideration of patient demographics includes both adequate representation of the disease setting and population diversity. Will the proof-of-concept includes a balance of gender, race, age, and metabolic or genetic diversity to predict the safety experience that will occur in phase III trials? Similarly, recruiting patients with a similar tumor setting in the proof-of-concept trial and the later phase III trials strengthens the predictability. The early phase trials typically recruit patients who have therapy-refractory tumors and meet rigid performance status and organ function criteria. When these criteria are applied, the majority of patients recruited to early phase trials includes those with non-small cell lung cancer and colon cancer with minimal consideration for gender, age, and race. For example, if a drug is targeted for a patient population defined by a specific tumor setting (e.g., ovarian cancer refractory to first line therapy or hormone refractory prostate cancer), then the it would be prudent for the proof-of-concept trial to recruit a suitable cohort of these patients. Factors that should be considered in this process include class of drug (is it completely novel or an analog of an established class); information suggesting a potential for rare, serious adverse events [14]; and variability of drug exposure within a given dose level. Statistical estimation of the incidence of unacceptable adverse events may be applied in the proof-of-concept strategy. For example, if the degree of grade 3 and 4 neutropenia produced by an NCE (or regimen) must not exceed a predetermined incidence, then the early phase trials can be designed to detect this event within estimation of a confidence interval. Thus, exceeding a predetermined level of severe neutropenia would lead to a negative proof-of-concept (or that element of a multi-component proof-of-concept).

IV. APPLICATION OF SURROGATE END POINTS IN PROOF-OF-CONCEPT DECISION MAKING

The decision-making element of proof-of-concept studies can be underscored by the assessment of a surrogate end point during the dosing period of the NCE. When considering biomarker or surrogate end points (one or several) as a basis for enhancing confidence that a phase III end point can be achieved, several criteria need to be considered [15].

Preclinical studies provide one basis for selecting a proof-of-concept end point. Laboratory-based pharmacology studies have advantages of a carefully controlled environment, assurance of an adequate number of homogenous study models (*in vivo* or *in vitro*), opportunities to characterize the dose-effect curve, and the use of positive and negative controls. Potential disadvantages in relying on preclinical studies for the only proof-of-concept end point include poor interspecies correlation of the agent's pharmacokinetics, variability of the pharmacodynamic correlate surrogate end point, and divergence of dose-effect between the preclinical species and patients with cancer. When approached systematically with an understanding of the rigor of the model, important supportive information can be gained. An example underscoring the complete understanding of the preclinical model, along with the human disease to be studied, is described by Houghton [16]. It is shown that wider testing of dose-effect, schedule dependence, and understanding of variation in target cell vulnerability can correctly extend preclinical learning to the clinic. In this example, longer systemic exposure of the drug is essential for effect (Figure 14.1) and was not so identified in prior studies.

A. Assessment of Mechanism: The Type I EGFR Receptor Kinase Inhibitor

ZD1839 (geFitinib) provides an example of preclinical models that can be validated in the clinic. Initial preclinical reports described a variety of human tumor cell lines that overexpressed the EGF receptor and demonstrated kinase inhibition when exposed to low concentrations of the experimental agent [17]. These studies also demonstrated drug-related inhibition of tumor growth *in vivo*. This preliminary finding was expanded to link the drug-related inhibition of the kinase with *in vivo* tumor reduction by producing the important dose-effect correlation [18] (Figures 14.2 and 14.3). More important, demonstration that this salutary effect was also seen and enhanced when ZD1839 was co-administered with standard chemotherapy agents provided support for use of the new agent in a wider variety of patient settings

(a)

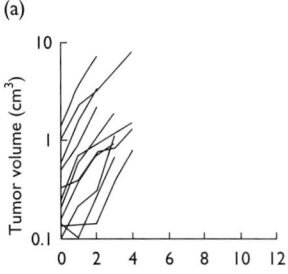

(b)

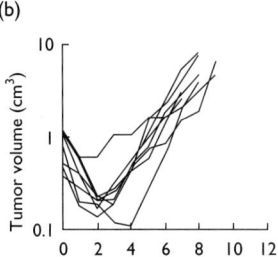

(c)

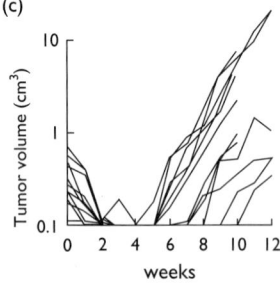

FIGURE 14.1 Schedule-dependent efficacy of irinotecan. (a) Growth of NB-1691 childhood neuroblastoma xenografts after irinotecan treatment in mice treated with a drug vehicle; (b) irinotecan, administered at a dose of 40 mg/kg for 5 days [(dx5)1] schedule]; (c) or irinotecan, given at 10 mg/kg for 5 days on 2 consecutive weeks [(dx5)2]. Note that mice in group B received a total of 200 mg/kg of irniotecan, whereas those in group C received only 100 mg/kg [16].

(Figure 14.4). An important correlation in patients has been shown between drug-related reduction of the target kinase and tumor reduction [19, 20].

B. Scanning Assessments

Scanning techniques offer a non-invasive method for monitoring the size, and occasionally the function, of a tumor. Traditional X-rays and tomography offer reproducible, standardized universally available methods of quantifying tumor size. These techniques allow changes in tumor size, which is used to determine the response to therapy, to be assessed during the time of dosing. In addition, the results may later be viewed by an independent review panel. Because response rate, in some settings, can be a useful component of proof-of-concept, this should be assessed whenever preclinical studies suggest that tumor volume reduction is a potential drug-effect in a patient with cancer.

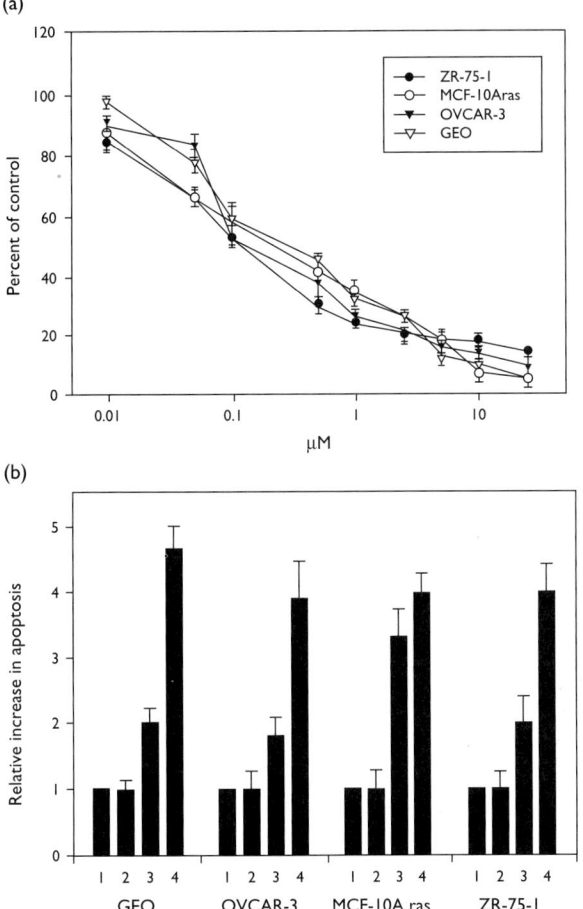

FIGURE 14.2   (a) dose-dependent growth-inhibitory effects of ZD-1839 on the soft agar growth of human ZR 75-1, MCF-10A ras, OVCAR-3, and GEO cell lines. Cells were treated with the indicated concentrations of ZD-1839 each day of 5 consecutive days. Colonies were counted after 10–14 days. Data represent the averages of three different experiments, each performed in triplicate; *bars*, SD. (b) Dose-dependent induction of programmed cell death by treatment with ZD-1839 in human ZR-75-1, MCF-10A ras, OVCAR-3, and GEO cell lines. Cells were treated each day of 3 days with the following doses of ZD-1839: columns 1, untreated controls; columns 2, 0.05 μM; columns 3, 0.01 μM and columns 4, 1 μM. Analysis of apoptosis was performed 4 days after the beginning of treatment. Data represent the averages of quadruplicate determinations; *bars*, SD [18].

Newer methodology, such as positron emission tomography (PET) offers an opportunity to assess selected functional characteristics of a tumor and, with multiple assessments over time, a drug-effect. Several examples have recently been highlighted [21], which include a trend toward increased uptake of the active agent temozolomide as [^{11}C] temozolomide in those patients who have longer response duration. Another example demonstrating the utility of PET scanning to determine a functional end point can be demonstrated in patients with colorectal cancer co-administrated [^{18}F] 5-fluorouracil and eniluracil (a potent inactivator of dihydropyrimidine dehydrogenase, the rate-limiting enzyme for 5-FU catabolism) [22]. PET scans have shown increased uptake of

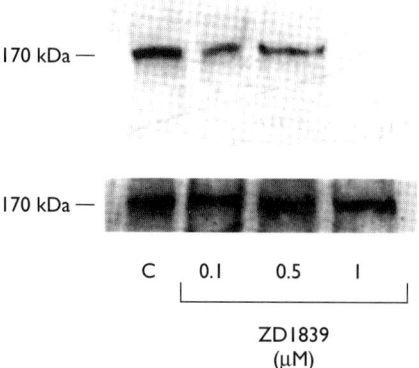

FIGURE 14.3   Dose-dependent inhibition of EGF-induced EGFR autophosphorylation by ZD-1839 in human MCF-10A ras cells. Serum-starved MCF-10A Ha-ras cells were treated for 3 h with the indicated concentration of ZD-1839, followed by addition of complete medium containing EGF (50 ng/ml) for 15 min. Protein extracts were then immunoprecipitated with the MAb C225 anti-EGFR monoclonal antibody, resolved by a 7.5% SDS-PAGE and probed with either the PY20 anti-P-tyr monoclonal antibody (top) or an antihuman EGFR monoclonal antibody (bottom). Immunoreactive proteins were visualized by enhanced chemiluminescence [18].

[^{18}F] 5-fluorouracil when co-administered with eniluracil, which suggests that there is added exposure of the active therapy (5-FU) within the tumor when the catabolic enzyme is inhibited. A third example demonstrating the importance of functional has been shown in breast cancer patients who are administered a tracer dose of glucose or methionine before and after polychemotherapy [23]. Results showed that some patients who showed tumor reduction by conventional techniques at 9–12 weeks demonstrated an earlier indication of response by PET at 6–13 days. Also, the methionine tracer may have provided better tumor definition than the glucose tracer. These three examples of PET scan capabilities suggest this modality can provide proof-of-mechanism data and, possibly in the future, provide an early correlate for efficacy.

C. Serum Biomarkers

The use of serum markers as surrogate end points in proof-of-concept studies has been tested in several settings. Advantages of this strategy include the general availability of many assays for testing in clinical chemistry labs, clinical acceptance of the marker as an indicator of disease recurrence, and a large body of literature validating its use in selected settings. Careful evaluation of the correlation of the serum marker to a therapy-induced clinical benefit is essential if it is to be considered as a surrogate end point in a proof-of-concept trial. The use of serum prostate-specific antigen (PSA) to monitor disease recurrence in prostate cancer is well accepted as a surrogate of disease recurrence [24]. Its use to monitor drug-effect in patients with hormone-refractory prostate cancer in specific settings has acceptance as changes in PSA levels correlated with patient benefit, and some agreement has been reached in defining response and progression criteria. Furthermore, clinical studies suggest a good correlation for therapy-related decreases in serum PSA and patient survival, in particular, substantial decreases in serum PSA (>50% from baseline) [25]. This concept was applied in two prospective randomized studies that led to the marketing approval of mitoxantrone by the Food and Drug Administration (FDA). One study suggested [26] a "palliative response correlated with a decrease in serum PSA level, but the decrease was a poor discriminant between patients who did and did not achieve a palliative response." The second study showed an improved PSA response in the experimental arm, but no survival or palliative advantage [27]. When these two trials were presented in a public forum as a new drug application, the experimental arm showed improved palliative responses, TTP, and serum PSA (decrease >75% from baseline) in study 1, but no effect on survival. The second study showed that the experimental therapy led to an improved PSA response and TTP, but had no influence on survival [28]. In this study, the decrease in PSA did correlate to a clinically meaningful benefit as measured by palliative measurements and TTP, but not to improved survival. In this example, selection of two primary end points was prudent and led to marketing approval of mitoxantrone. It has been demonstrated that PSA levels can rise following administration of certain differentiating agents, thus, the usefulness of a PSA response must be validated in each clinical setting. Analysis of serum PSA as prostate-specific antigen doubling time (PSA-DT) has added additional refinement to the correlation of this surrogate to a true disease end point [29]. The clinical end points that are better estimated by PSA-DT, compared to PSA, include survival after primary treatment (surgery or RT), treatment failure. and TTP.

An example of limitations of using a serum marker as a surrogate for a traditional trial end point was demonstrated in the initial trials investigating marimastat in patients with ovarian cancer. The initial phase II study recruited 415 patients with advanced ovarian, prostate, pancreatic, and colorectal cancer who had a documented 25% rise in CA-125, PSA, CA19-9, or CEA, respectively, during the run-in screening period. Of the 415 patients, 132 had advanced ovarian cancer. These data were presented by combining the patient data from all four tumor types and classifying the response of the specific serum tumor markers as a combined analysis of biologic end point [30]. The conclusion showed a salutary drug-effect on tumor markers. However, when the phase III trial was conducted, no benefit on overall survival was seen in patients with ovarian cancer receiving marimastat with standard chemotherapy compared to standard chemotherapy alone [31]. In this setting, the use of serum CA-125, in addition to other serum makers, as a proof-of-concept did not predict the phase III outcome.

Since the time of clinical testing marimastat using a serum CA-125 biomarker, refinement on the definition and utility of applying changes in serum CA-125 to characterize response and progression occurred [32, 33]. Among these important efforts, which raise the predictability of serum CA-125 as a clinically related end point, includes the comparison of CA-125 response to the standard response evaluation criteria in solid tumors (RECIST) [34]. These authors suggest that newer approaches to analysis of this biomarker ". . . indicates that CA-125 response criteria are a better prognostic tool than RECIST in the second line treatment of ovarian carcinoma . . . ." In addition, a scholarly, multidisciplinary review of this topic [35] has concluded that "CA-125 should be used routinely in phase II clinical trials to support go/no go decisions for

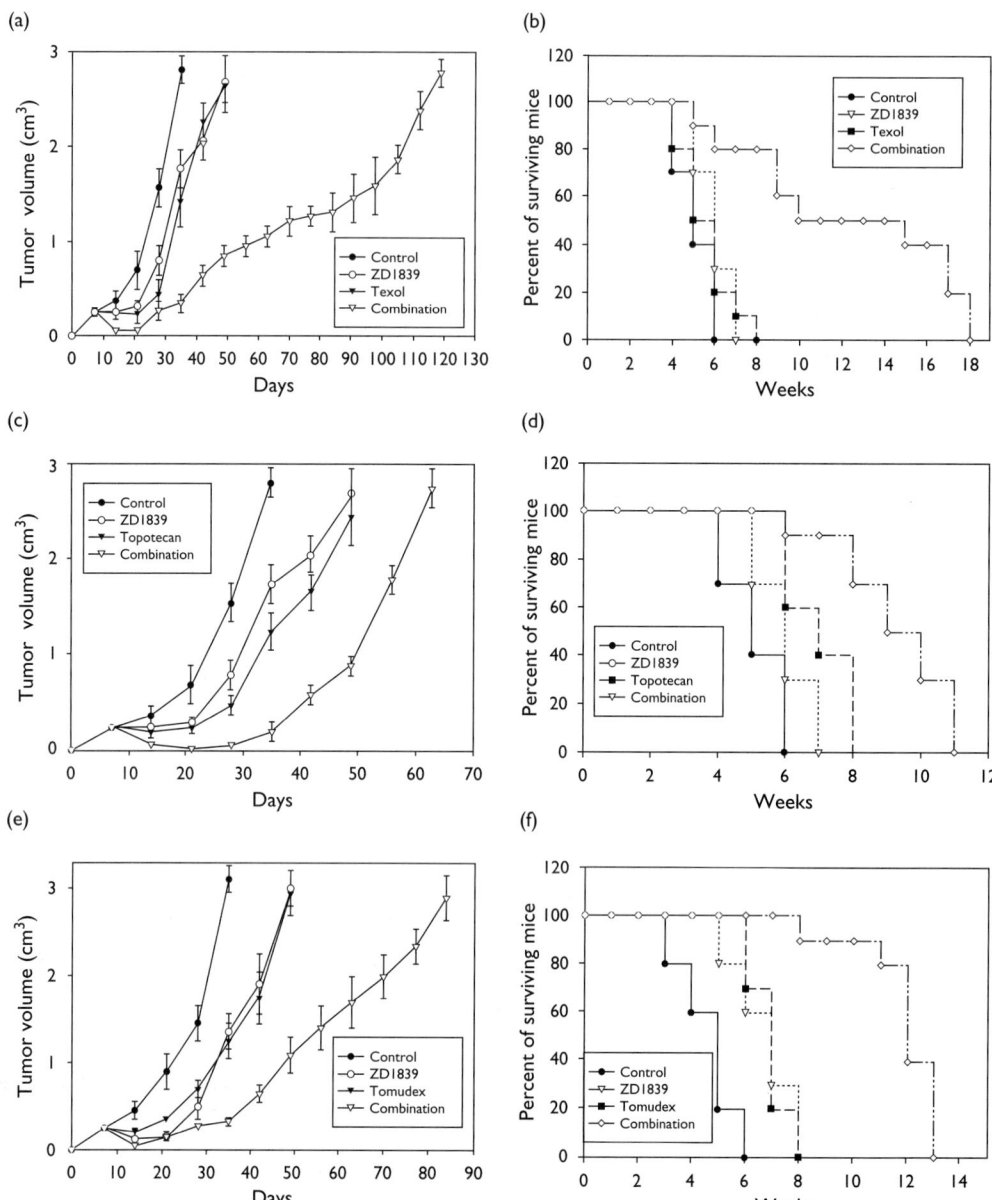

FIGURE 14.4 Antitumor activity of ZD-1839 treatment in combination with cytotoxic drugs on established GEO human colon carcinoma xenografts. Mice were injected s.c. in the dorsal flank with 10^7 GEO cells. Three different experiments with a total of 40 mice for each experiment were performed. In each experiment, each group consisted of 10 mice. Data represented the averages, *bars*, DS. In each experiment, after 7 days (average tumor size, 0.2–0.2 cm³), the mice were treated i.p. on days 1–5 of each week for 4 weeks with ZD-1839, 2.5 mg/dose, alone or in combination with paclitaxel (Taxol:A), 20 mg/kg/dose, on day 1 of each week for 4 weeks: with topotecan. (c) 2 mg/kg/dose on day 1 of each week for 4 weeks: or with raltitrexed (Tomudex:E) 12.5 mg/kg/dose, on day 1 of each week for 4 weeks. For each experiment, the Student's *t*-test was used to compare tumor sizes among different treatment groups at day 35 after GEO cell injection.

further development." The establishment of serum CA-125 as a useful biomarker in the proof-of-concept decision process has progressed over time to allow this biomarker to be considered as a go/no end point in a specific patient population.

V. SELECTED STATISTICAL CONSIDERATIONS IN PROOF-OF-CONCEPT STUDIES

A. Evaluation of Surrogate to Primary End Point Correlations

Determining the degree of correlation of the surrogate end point to the clinical benefit end point is essential in assigning a value to its inclusion in a proof-of-concept study in drug development. An important focus in planning a proof-of-concept program can be the identification of a surrogate end point(s), which is predictive of the primary phase III end point. It is assumed that the surrogate is not the primary end point, otherwise it would be readily acceptable by the clinical and regulatory community as clear evidence of clinical benefit on its own. Thus, assigning a predictability factor to the surrogate used in the proof-of-concept study is an essential step in determining the ultimate utility.

The application of statistical planning and analysis is a central element for a proof-of-concept program. Statistical planning includes sample size estimates to assure that an adequate number of patients are enrolled for purposes of assessing safety and pharmacodynamics, pharmacokinetics, and assigning a predictability for the surrogate marker to the primary end point. Although the application of statistics in early drug development will be addressed in greater depth in another chapter, it is important to briefly review how statistical considerations can help establish a link between a correlate or surrogate marker to the traditional primary trial end point.

Using response rate (fraction of patients who achieve a defined tumor volume reduction) as a surrogate for overall survival is a frequently used proof-of-concept end point and has produced thoughtful publications evaluating this

FIGURE 14.4 (*Continued*) Tumor size were significantly different between: ZD-1839 and control (two-sided P = 0.01): paclitaxel (Taxol) and control (two-sided P = 0.01: topotecan and control (two-sided P = 0.01): raltitrexed (Tomudex) control (two-sided P = 0.01: ZD-1839 plus paclitaxel (Taxol) and control (two-sided P < 0.001): ZD1839 plus paclitaxel (Taxol) and paclitaxel (Taxol) alone (two-sided P = 0.01: ZD-1839 plus paclitaxel (Taxol) and ZD-1839 alone (two-sided P = 0.01): ZD-1839 plus topotecan and control (two-sided P < 0.001): ZD-1839 plus topotecan and topotecan alone (two-sided P = 0.01): ZD-1839 plus topotecan and ZD-1839 alone (two-sided P = 0.01): ZD-1839 plus raltitrexed (Tomudex) and control (two-sided P = 0.01). The effects of ZD-1839 treatment in combination with paclitaxel (Taxol B), with topotecan (D), or with raltitrexed (Tomudex: F) on the survival of GEO tumor-bearing mice were also determined. Differences in animal survival among groups were evaluated using Mantel-Cox log-rank test. The survival of mice was significantly different between ZD-1839 plus Taxol and control (two-sided P < 0.001); ZD-1839 plus paclitaxel (Taxol) and paclitaxel (Taxol) alone (two-sided P < 0.001): ZD-1839 plus paclitaxel (Taxol) and ZD-1839 alone (two-sided P < 0.001): ZD-1839 plus topotecan and control (two-sided P < 0.001): ZD-1839 plus topotecan and topotecan alone (two-sided P = 0.05): ZD-1839 plus topotecan and control (two-sided P < 0.001): ZD-1839 plus raltitrexed (Tomudex) and control (two-sided P < 0.001): ZD-1839 plus raltitrexed (Tomudex) and raltitrexed (Tomudex) alone (two-sided P + 0.01): and ZD-1839 plus raltitrexed (Tomudex) and ZD-1839 and ZD alone (two-sided P = 0.01) [18].

relationship. Buyse and Piedbois [36] correctly identified the central questions to address when considering this link.

1. Is response to treatment a prognostic factor for survival?
2. Is response to treatment an independent prognostic factor for survival, that is, does a response to treatment add any prognostic information to other known prognostic factors?
3. Do the patients in who a response is achieved benefit from treatment in terms of their survival expectancy (or is response merely a marker of some underlying favorable characteristic)?
4. Can the efficacy of an investigational treatment be evaluated through its effect upon response rather than through its effect upon survival? [36].

These authors provide a clear example demonstrating a correlation of response rate to survival that was significantly influenced by performance status (Figure 14.5, Table 14.1). In addition, they offer insight into confounding factors that can influence this link. Advice on criteria for validating this link is also provided [37].

In general, caution must be applied when using response rate as a marker for clinical benefit and it needs to be validated in each clinical setting. Two examples using meta-analysis in specific clinical settings offer insight into the validation of response rate with clinical benefit. When data on 3791 patients with previously untreated advanced colorectal cancer were collected from 25 studies and evaluated by meta-analysis [38], it was determined that an increase in tumor response rate correlates with an increase in overall survival. Subgroup analysis based on performance status also correlated best response with survival. In an analysis of data from 26 randomized studies that included a total of 4914 women with advanced ovarian cancer, the conclusions were similar but more specific (and potentially more useful for proof-of-concept planning). Patients with ovarian cancer who experienced a substantial drug-related improvement in clinical response (with confirmatory surgical re-staging) seemed

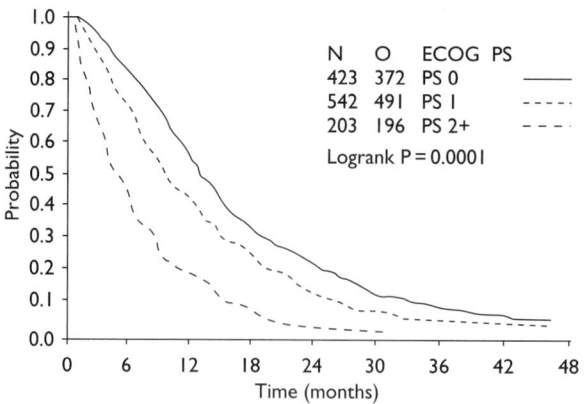

FIGURE 14.5 Kaplan Meier estimates of survival by performance status (PS) measured on WHO, ECOG scale in a meta-analysis of eight trials on 1178 patients with advanced colorectal cancer (3 patients had an unknown PS and no follow-up was available on 7 further patients) [36].

TABLE 14.1 Response versus Performance Status (PS) in a Meta-Analysis of Eight Trials on 1178 Patients with Advanced Colorectal Cancer

WHO/ECOG PS	PS 0	PS 1	PS 2+
Complete response	18 4.2%	13 2.4%	1 0.5%
Partial response	59 13.9%	63 11.5%	19 9.4%
Stable disease	209 49.2%	200 36.6%	59 29.0%
Progressive disease	139 32.7%	271 49.5%	124 61.1%

Note: 3 patients had an unknown PS, 28 patients had a PS of 3, and 1 patient had a PS of 4. From Ref. 3b.

to have improved survival [39]. Of note, the accompanying editorial [40] found the meta-analysis to be insightful but added a note of caution regarding generalization of a correlation of tumor volume reduction to improved survival:

> When studying reports of the relationship between response and survival, investigators must distinguish sharply between different units of analysis, patient versus study, and interpret the results accordingly.

Because response rate can be determined well before a survival end point is finalized, a statistical correlation can have regulatory implications for drug approval. In an editorial, Dr. Richard Pazdur (Director, Division of Oncology Drug Products, FDA) suggested that this link can provide regulatory guidance when specific criteria are met, which include pre-study discussion with the appropriate regulatory agency. A conclusion is put forward that: "In making clinical and regulatory decisions, the use of response rates and their probability in predicting clinical benefit relies not only on the response rate number but also on the duration of response, the number of complete responses, the magnitude of increase in this surrogate, and the location of the responses (e.g., hepatic versus cutaneous). Response rate, a piece for the clinical decision-making puzzle, is a puzzle in itself [41].

B. Clinical Trial Designs Leading to Proof-of-Concept Testing

A suitable proof-of-concept clinical design for a given NCE will be dependent on the class of compound and the subsequent phase III program objective. Proof-of-concept clinical trials that assess a surrogate end point should be done with a dose range that includes the phase III dose. The proof-of-concept study can have a dose-ranging objective that will help refine the phase III dose. Actual studies used to assess the surrogate end point should be carefully designed to optimize patient safety evaluation as well as to minimize time and costs. These considerations have been addressed in a number of publications [3, 5, 51–53] as well as in other chapters of this book.

C. Randomized Phase II Trials as Proof-of-Concept

Phase III trial design strengths include the use of a control arm, which is frequently the standard of care, the selection of clinically relevant end points, and the application of comparative statistics to the results. The randomized phase II study is a modification that seeks to include the strength of a concurrent control arm and the application of comparative statistical analysis. The "compromise" of this design typically involves the recruitment of fewer patients than would be required for an adequately powered, pivotal phase III study. Additionally, the randomized phase II design requires less resource and, at times, uses different clinical end points. Randomized phase II studies have been published that determine the activity of an experimental arm compared to a concurrent control [42–46]. When summarized, the balance of the pros and cons of this design can be appreciated. As fewer patients are used in a randomized phase II, compared to a phase III trial, less resources are needed, reduced time lines, and an earlier determination of proof-of-concept. However, the cons of this approach frequently include an inflated estimation of the clinical benefit expected from the experimental arm when compared to the control arm. A priori expectations of experimental arm enhancement of clinical benefit of up to 100% in response rate, 100% in TTP, and 50% in overall survival are routinely described in the statistical sections. One alternative to this practice, which is discussed within academics and industry, is the examination of all clinical end points in a trial for consistency of trend (experimental arm to control). This cross end point observation would formalize the "clinical eye," which typically reviews all end points when forming an opinion on treatment-effect. Formalizing this process could allow enhanced confidence in go/no go decisions without an increase in sample size.

VI. PHARMACODYNAMIC PROOF-OF-CONCEPT END POINTS

Some end points will have a high level of correlation, and some will correlate poorly to the targeted clinical benefit. Understanding this relationship is a key element in weighing the importance of the trial results. Perhaps the best example of early proof-of-concept in oncology was seen in the development of endocrine-modulating agents for breast cancer. The initial observation of Beatson that oophorectomy led to regression of breast cancer has been replicated several times with small-molecule drug therapy. Thus, an important correlation between hormonal suppression and effect was established. A high level of confidence can be attached to early dose-related changes, as was shown in the clinical development of letrozole. The initial clinical pharmacology studies in healthy, postmenopausal women showed that a dose-related suppression of estrone and estradiol was present (Figure 14.6) and well-tolerated while other important hormonal pathways were unaltered [54]. A follow-up pilot study demonstrated that tumor regression was seen at the predicted dose-level in postmenopausal women with progressive breast cancer [55]. The confidence from these findings led to registration-directed, randomized trials that clearly documented clinical benefit [56]. In this example, proof-of-concept could be

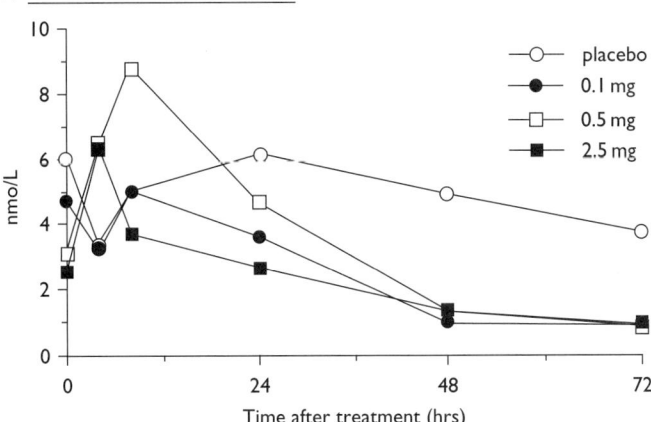

(a) Urinary oestrone concentration

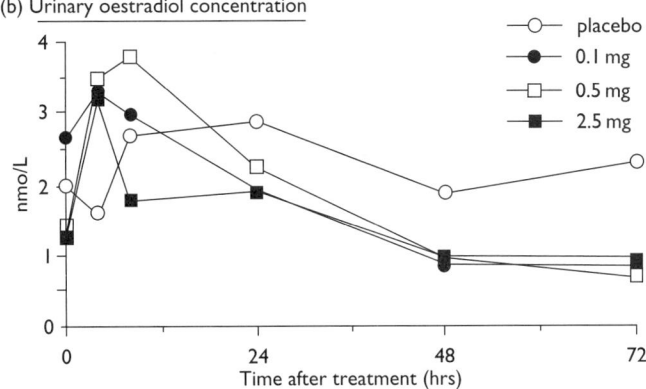

(b) Urinary oestradiol concentration

FIGURE 14.6 (a) Urinary estrone concentrations (geometric mean) after a single dose of CGS 20267 (0.1, 0.5, or 2.5 mg) or placebo. (b) Urinary estradiol concentrations (geometric mean) after a single dose of CGS 20267 (0.1, 0.5, or 2.5 mg) or placebo [54].

appropriately applied to the first study, which showed the predicted dose-effect on estrogenic hormones, or the second study in which responses were demonstrated. The number of established, effective hormonal agents for breast cancer, including a proof-of-concept pilot study in an NCE development program, will add confidence to continue development by showing that the response rate is in the range of that seen with established drugs.

When proof-of-concept is based on newly established end points, a greater understanding of the correlation to the mechanism of action and putative links to clinical benefit must be considered. In this setting, a multidisciplinary group is a useful way to debate the strengths and weaknesses of these correlations. Group consensus on the relative importance of a selected end points signal is an important step toward proof-of-concept. An example of developing a new end point as a surrogate for a traditional trial outcome was demonstrated in the early trials of a novel monoclonal antibody for the treatment of breast cancer. Treatment with this antibody resulted in a reduction in the number of micrometastatic deposits in the bone marrow of patients with breast cancer.

This model has been developed by a group with an interest in demonstrating that cytokeratin staining of bone marrow identifies tumor cells, and that their presence signifies an independent prognostic factor. Through retrospective studies, the group showed that the presence of cytokeratin positive cells in the bone marrow of stage I, II, or III patients with breast cancer was an independent negative prognostic finding [57].

Two pharmacologic trials performed by this group, using this model, are good examples of a novel approach to proof-of-concept. In one study, an experimental monoclonal antibody with an antigen target on these cells was administered to patients with positive bone marrows. In a two-week window-of-opportunity study, when monoclonal alone therapy was administered, a substantial reduction in cytokeratin positive cells was seen (Figure 14.7) [58]. In the companion study, when standard chemotherapy was applied, only minimal reduction of cytokeratin cells was seen [59]. As a proof-of-concept finding, this could imply that the monoclonal antibody has some activity and may not be cross-resistant with standard chemotherapy. The same monoclonal antibody was subsequently shown to provide a survival benefit in a randomized pilot study in patients with stage III colon cancer [60]. However, when the monoclonal antibody was tested in a phase III setting, an improvement in survival was not seen [61] and the clinical benefits of adding the antibody to standard chemotherapy was statistically demonstrated in only one of the two pivotal trials conducted. An important point for proof-of-concept planning is that a gold standard end point alone (e.g., survival) in a pilot study may not be sufficient to predict outcome of an adequately powered phase III study. Another observation to consider is that the proof-of-concept study testing the effect of

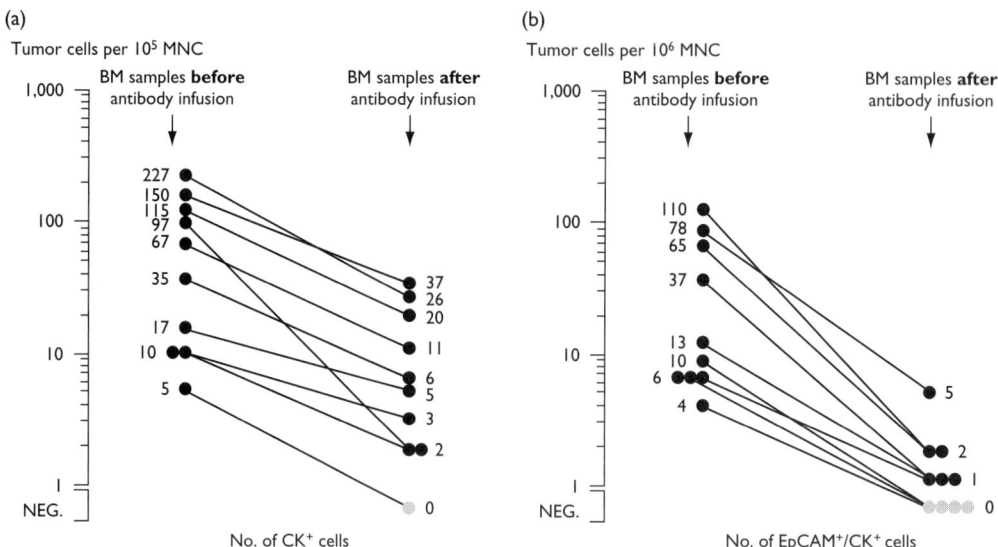

FIGURE 14.7 Direct immunocytochemical monitoring of therapeutic efficacy by repeated bone marrow analysis during passive antibody therapy with a single dose of 500 mg of Panorex. (a) CK^+ tumor cells detected in single APAAP labeling. (b) $EpCAM^+/CK^+$ tumor cells detected in double-labeling before and after Edrecolomab treatment. Closed symbols represent the absolute number (%) of cells in individual patients; corresponding bone marrow samples are connected by lines, MNC, mononuclear cells: BM, bone marrow [58].

the monoclonal antibody in the bone marrow of patients with breast cancer has yet to be validated in a phase III trial with the same population. A negative phase III study in one patient population may not predict a similar outcome in a patient with a different tumor type.

A third example, a proof-of-mechanism, is the demonstration that a targeted inhibitor effects its target. Inhibitors of the multidrug efflux pump, P-glycoprotein (also called multidrug resistance) provide an example of the need for a novel clinical end point. Multidrug resistance to xenobiotics and similar drugs is produced by an ATP-dependent P-glycoprotein that is able to actively pump chemotherapy out of a tumor cell faster than the passive diffusion gradient generates the intracellular concentration. A program of small-molecule inhibitors targeting P-glycoprotein would be expected to have a final phase III end point of increased tumor cytotoxicity by standard chemotherapy when the inhibitor is co-administered. GF120918 was a product of this drug discovery program. Identification of an early readout of drug-effect would provide added confidence to such a program. When the human natural killer lymphocyte surface protein CD56+ was shown to have a P-glycoprotein-like function, an *in vivo* surrogate was identified for a drug-effect study. In a human volunteer study [62] in which 1 in 4 received placebo, CD56+ lymphocytes were isolated before and after dosing of GF120918 and tested for rhodamine (also a substrate for the efflux pump) fluorescence by flow cytometry. Standard curves were generated by *ex vivo* studies prior to human dosing (Figure 14.8). This pre-study effort lead to a useful generation of concentration-effect results in the

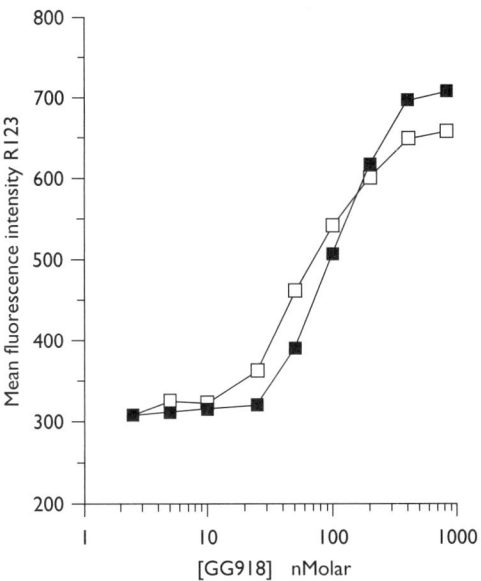

FIGURE 14.8 Effect of GG918 dose on R123 uptake in CD56 + PBLs. The Pgp antagonist was added to heparin-treated whole blood samples at concentrations ranging from 2.5–800 nM and incubated at 37 °C for 1 h prior to the addition of R123 to a final concentration of 150 ng/ml. Incubation was continued for 1 h before termination by dilution in ice-cold PBS and the gradient-purification of PBLs for antibody staining and cytometric analysis. The data shown were collected from two individuals in separate experiments. The R123 intensity values for volunteer 2 were normalized to those of volunteer 1 based on vehicle control values ■ volunteer 1: □ volunteer 2 [62].

clinical phase I human studies, which demonstrated that a GF120918-related rhodamine efflux from CD56+ lymphocytes was inhibited. Thus, the human *in vivo* data was similar to the human *ex vivo* data and provided an important proof-of-mechanism. In this example, the GF120918 proof-of-concept predicted that the P-glycoprotein pump would be inhibited in later clinical trials. However, it was not able to provide assurance that inhibiting the P-glycoprotein pump with co-administered anti-neoplastic chemotherapy reduced drug resistance in patients with cancer. Thus, if the program's goal was to inhibit P-glycoprotein function, this study would be considered as proof-of-concept. If the program's goal was to provide evidence that clinical benefit to patients with drug-resistant tumors was likely, then this study would be proof-of-mechanism.

VII. PHARMACOKINETIC PROOF-OF-CONCEPT END POINTS

The pharmacokinetic characterization of an NCE and its metabolites is a key goal in a drug development program. Basic data such as determination of clearance, volume of distribution, and routes of elimination are needed to understand the clinical pharmacology of a compound. If limited variability and predictable dose-effect are considered essential for a successful compound, such basic data can also become a proof-of-concept characteristic. The drug assay for GI147211, lurtotecan, (described later) was used in the phase I trial to generate drug assay data as each cohort was completed [63]. Because the expected dose-limiting toxicity was myelosuppression, it served as a useful marker of drug-effect. Although the demonstration of lowered neutrophil count is not a useful surrogate for drug-effect, when graphed by dose and concentration, it provides a measure of comparison between dose-levels (Figure 14.9) and patient populations (Figure 14.10). A drug development program can assign a level of variability that is acceptable for further development. Thus, quantifying a level of unacceptable variability in phase I would become a component of proof-of-concept if it were seen to impact on safety in the phase III population.

A. Assay/Measurement Validation

A reliable method of measuring any pharmacokinetic or pharmacodynamic end point used in phase I or proof-of-concept studies is essential to proper interpretation of the results. Some measurable end points, such as the complete blood count and clinical chemistry, are performed in laboratories that undergo regular inspection and certification and adhere to high standards of validation. Because these pharmacodynamic end points are also part of diagnosis and patient care, the designers of a proof-of-concept trial benefit from prior validation work. In addition, these markers are generally available in most clinical centers and sample handling specifications have already been determined. When planning proof-of-concept studies, utilization of these assays is advised whenever appropriate.

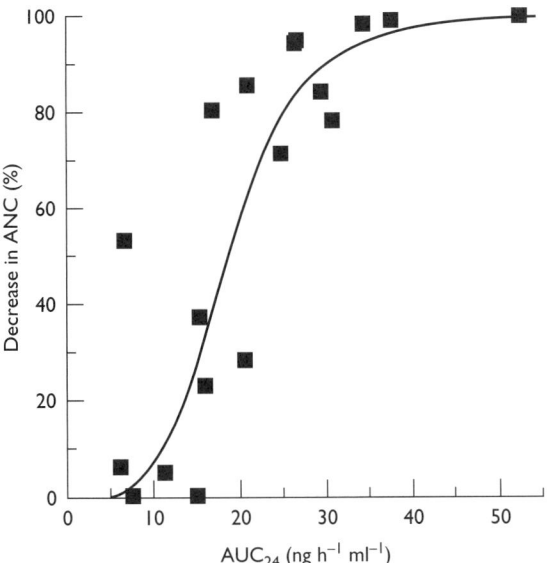

FIGURE 14.9 Relationship between the AUC of GI147211 determined on day 4 of the first course and the percent decrease in ANC. The sigmoid E_{max} model was applied [63].

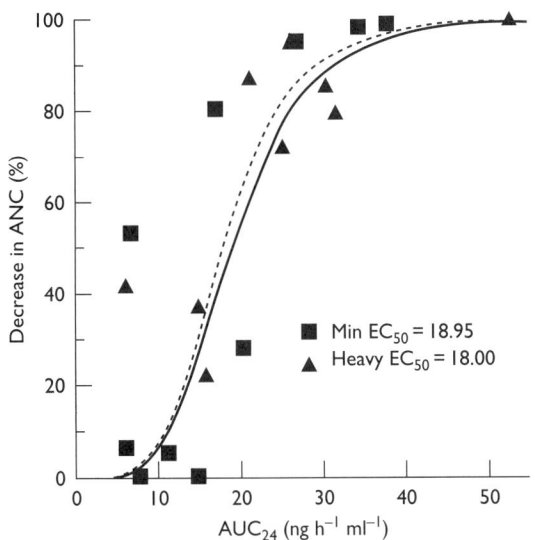

FIGURE 14.10 Relationship between AUC of GI147211 on day 4 of the first course and the percent decrease in ANC, in minimally and heavily pretreated patients. EC_{50} value in minimally pretreated patients, 18.95 (-■-) EC_{50} value in heavily pretreated patients, 18.00 (-▲-) [63].

Measurement of the parent compound, or an active metabolite, is an essential part of a phase I trial and can also become a useful component of a proof-of-concept program. Assay methodology generally includes specific validation steps and sample handling techniques. The sensitivity and specificity of the assay needs to be assessed prior to using a specific test in clinical trials, unless the results will be considered exploratory in nature. In most drug development programs, preclinical GLP toxicology studies will have started the process of laboratory validation for the analytes in human matrix. Human assay validation steps have been formalized by clear guidelines [47]. This workshop outlines principles and recommendations for full assay methodology which include:

- Generation of a standard curve with minimum standard points done in replicate and use of quality control samples
- Statistical application to this curve
- Identification of a lower and upper limit of quantitation and coefficient of variation
- Stability of analyte by matrix
- Specificity of assay methodology
- Rules for accepting and rejection of data points

An example of the usefulness of a validated pharmacokinetic assay, and pharmacodynamic end point, was demonstrated in the proof-of-concept study for the water-soluble camptothecin analog GI147211. The active parent compound has a lactone ring that forms relatively inactive carboxylate when exposed to a pH greater than 4.0. When a blood sample is obtained for pharmacokinetic measurement, exposure to physiologic pH (7.4) during sample handling could provide a misleading ratio of lactone to carboxylate. Studies performed pre-phase I addressed the sampling handling and assay issues permitting a reliable, validated assay for the first time in human studies [48]. The methods were developed to determine the true concentrations of the lactone and carboxylate fractions at the time of phlebotomy. In this example, using a validated assay as part of the proof-of-concept study resulted in meaningful correlations between the dose, plasma concentration, and selected adverse events.

Measurement of end points used in proof-of-concept studies that are not used for patient care or characterization of drug disposition also need to adhere to standards that assure an acceptable level of specificity and sensitivity. This level may be less than needed for use in a clinical care setting, but may still be acceptable for drug development purposes. For example, the measurement of phosphorylated tyrosine (pTyr) is useful when determining the drug-effect of a type 1 membrane tyrosine kinase inhibitor. It would be expected that as the drug exposure increases, the quantity of pTyr diminishes. Important considerations that increase the chance to obtain reproducible data include: optimization of tissue handling conditions, determination of a range of concentrations that fall within the expected clinical trial experience, and confirmation of the reproducibility with positive and negative controls [49]. An example of this was demonstrated in a proof-of-concept study with a monoclonal antibody that measured the effect of therapy on pTyr levels in tissue samples obtained from patient biopsies. Pre-study efforts led to an assay that was available at the time of the clinical trial [50]. The pharmacodynamic results from this clinical study confirmed that the tumor was exposed to the NCE, and the exposure was sufficient to produce enzyme inhibition. This observation is a proof-of-mechanism and could be a component of an integrated proof of concept plan.

VIII. PROCEEDING FROM PROOF-OF-CONCEPT DIRECTLY TO PHASE III

The decision to proceed into phase III registration trials considers the questions of level of support provided by the proof-of-concept program and the risk/benefit of assuming the larger cost of a phase III program (relative to phase II). The question of "skipping" phase II trials has been discussed in a clinical setting [5, 52] as well as in a clinical-regulatory setting [51, 64] with excellent points made for including or excluding a phase II program in proof-of-concept. The question of risk/benefit of conducting a phase II trial prior to conducting phase III, or directly initiating phase III studies after proof-of-concept, can be simplified by outlining the pragmatic elements of conducting both types of development plans. Attaching cost and timeline estimates to this assessment can assist in making the decision of using phase II in sequence to phase III or in parallel.

- Number of protocols and patients needed in a phase II program that would substantially enhance the original proof-of-concept
- Time from first patient recruited to final analysis of phase II
- Number of patients recruited in the phase II program
- Number of staff (or full-time equivalents) needed for the entire phase II program
- Include salary, benefits, and years of participation on the phase II trial
- Include all departments that contribute to the effective and legal conduct of a study: clinical research, biometrics, regulatory affairs, clinical supply management, compliance, data management, clinical monitoring at sites, travel costs; commonly, the costs of staff and drug supply will exceed the clinical grants to the sites
- Shift in dates for submission to regulatory agencies for marketing approval
- Change in the competitive landscape and standard of care during the time of the phase II trial (e.g., will the phase III standard therapy arm change during phase II development)

The details of this resource and timeline model is beyond the scope of this chapter. However, in assessing the utility of including a phase II program as a sequential component in clinical development — the commitment of patients, investigators, and their site staff, along with the other substantial costs commonly assigned to the sponsor — need to be considered. Similarly, reviewing literature examples of phase II results that clearly influenced the phase III trial design is critical in any decision to reduce or eliminate phase II testing. The putative advantages of "skipping" phase II needs to be balanced by the important information obtained during this stage of development; clinical activity within the targeted population, confirmation of (or final dose adjustment to) the phase III dose and a more robust understanding of the NCEs safety profile in the targeted patient population.

IX. GUIDELINES AND SUMMARY

A proof-of-concept program can offer efficiency in the drug development process through pre-phase I planning and identification of important safety, activity, and competitive landscape criteria that must be met. Similarly, the pre-planning discussion of these important elements of proof-of-concept will naturally bring together a multidisciplinary group that can make better decisions. In summary, elements of the pre-phase I planning and resources needed include:

Clinical study aspect	Description	Resources needed and background work
Surrogate end point	Measurable parameter over time that can be correlated to drug-effect and primary efficacy end point	Literature review Clinical and statistical assessment of the end point correlation For a novel surrogate, exploratory laboratory investigation capabilities are needed If surrogate involves specialty areas (e.g., surgical biopsy, radiologic imaging, pathologic tissue staining), this expertise needs to be involved
Safety assessment	A sufficient number of patients are exposed to the novel compound to assess the adverse event profile	Clinical protocols with safety assessment which, when combined, provide an adequate number of patients to predict phase III safety Data collection methodology in place (case report forms, adverse event reporting structure, medical review)
Parent drug and metabolite assay	Clinical pharmacokinetic characterization of the novel compound	Drug metabolism support for animal- and human-validated assay of the compound and selected metabolites in relevant matrices Sample handling techniques verified Bioanalyst and pharmacokineticist support
Budget and staff	Estimation of cost and timing of expenditures of study grant costs and specialties of staff needed to conduct the program and associated compensation	Management tools to predict expenditures for grants and staff over several years

If a proof-of-concept program contains a surrogate end point that is correlated to the primary efficacy end point, then the main decision point for the program may be based on a single trial, which adequately tests this question. If proof-of-concept cannot be addressed by a single end point in a single study, then a composite of important end points from more than one study can be joined to form a proof-of-concept program. These could include:

Study end point	Decision-making criteria	Resources needed
Safety of drug regimen	Acceptable tolerability relative to benefit Comparison to standard therapy or competitors safety profile Clinical and statistical estimation of acceptable adverse event profile	Investigators and sites Integrated safety database with clinical reviewers Literature review of safety and efficacy of similar, existing agents Clinical and statistical staff
Pharmacokinetics	Variability, needed frequency of dosing	Above Drug metabolism lab with validated assay Pharmacokineticist
Drug-like qualities	Pharmacokinetics, patient convenience, stability qualities	Protocols designed to capture the data and patient queries Clinical and pharmacokinetic staff
Proof-of-mechanism study	Patient-based information showing that the expected pharmacologic effect is seen	Pharmacodynamic laboratory capability.
Secondary clinical end point	Identification of clinical end point with a moderate correlation to clinical benefit	Clinical and statistical estimation of surrogate correlation to primary clinical benefit
		Utility of surrogate if strongly positive compared to minimally positive

ACKNOWLEDGMENTS

The author appreciates the review and comments of Jeremey Levin, M.D. Ph.D, Lance Leopold, MD, and Deborah Mulready Wissel, M.S.

REFERENCES

1. Simon R. Clinical trials in Cancer. In *Cancer: Principles and Practice of Oncology, 5th* edition, Chap. 20, p. 2.
2. Marsoni S, Hoth D, Simon R, Leyland-Jones B, DeRosa M, Wittes R et al. Clinical drug development: An analysis of phase II trials, 1970–1985. *Cancer Treat. Rep.* 1987; 71:71–80
3. Eisenhauer E. Phase I and II trials of novel anti-cancer agents: Endpoints, efficacy and existentialism. *Ann. Oncol.* 1998; 9:1047–1052.

 4. Schilsky R. End points in clinical trials and the drug approval process. *Clin. Cancer Res.* 2002; 8:935–938.

 5. Korn E, Arbuck S, Pluda J et al. Clinical trial designs for cytostatic agents: Are new approaches needed? *J. Clin. Oncol.* 2001; 19:265–272.

 6. Sekine I, Tamure T, Kunitoh H. Progressive disease rate as a surrogate endpoint of phase II trials for non-small-cell lung cancer. *Ann. Oncol.* 199; 10:731–733.

 7. Green S, Weiss G. Southwest Oncology Group standard response criteria, endpoint definitions and toxicity criteria. *Invest. New Drugs* 1992; 10:239–253.

 8. Therasse P, Arbuck S, Eisenhauer E et al. New guidelines to evaluate the response to treatment in solid tumors. *J. Natl. Cancer Inst.* 2000; 92:205–216/

 9. Von Hoff D, Turner J. Response rates, duration of response and dose response effects in phase I studies of antineoplastics. *Invest. New Drugs* 1991; 9:115–122.

10. Loprinzi C, Kugler J, Sloan J et al. Venlafaxine alleviates hot flashes: An NCCTG trial, pg. 2a. *Proc. ASCO* 2000.

11. Murray N, Coppin C, Coldman A et al. Drug delivery analysis of Canadian multicenter trial in non-small cell lung cancer. *J. Clin. Oncol.* 1994; 12:2333–2339.

12. O'Shaughnessy J. Treatment and Prevention of intraepithelial neoplasia: An important target for accelerated new drug approval. *Clin. Cancer Res.* 2002; 8:314–346.

13. Steinbach G, Lynch PM, Phillips RK, Wallace MH, Hawk E. Gordon GB, Wakabayashi N, Saunders B, Shen Y, Fujimura T, Su LK, Levin B. The effect of celecoxib, a cyclooxygenase-2 inhibitor, in familial adenomatous polyposis. *N. Engl. J. Med.* 2000; 342:1946–1952.

14. Feldman A, Lorell B, Reis S. Trastuzumab in the treatment of metastatic breast cancer: Anticancer therapy versus cardiotoxicity. *Circulation* 2000; 102:272–275.

15. Park JW, Kerbel RS, Kelloff GJ et al. Rationale for biomarker and surrogate endpoints in mechanism-driven oncology drug development. *Clin. Cancer Res.* 2004; 10;3885–3896.

16. Houghton PJ, Stewart C, Thompson J, Santana V, Furman W, Friedman H et al. Extending principles learned in model systems to clinical trial designs. *Oncology* 1998; 12:84–93.

17. Woodburn J, Barker A, Gibson K et al. ZD1839, an epidermal growth factor tyrosine kinase inhibitor selected for clinical development, pg. 633. *Proc. AACR* 1997; 38.

18. Ciardiello F, Caputo R, Bianco R et al. Antitumor effect and potentiation of cytotoxic drugs activity in human cancer cells by ZD-1839 (Iressa), an epidermal growth factor receptor-selective tyrosine kinase inhibitor. *Clin. Cancer Res.* 2000; 6:2053–2063.

19. Kusaba H, Tamura T, Nakagawa K et al. A phase I intermittent dose-escalation trial of ZD1839 (Iressa) in Japanese patients with solid malignant tumors. Proceedings of 11th NCI-EORTC-AACR symposium on new drugs in cancer therapy (poster and abstract). *Clin. Cancer Res.* 2000; 6:4543.

20. Goss G, Lorimer I, Miller W et al. A phase I dose-escalation, pharmacokinetic (PK) and pharmacodynamic (PD) stud of ZD1839 ('Iressa"): NCIC-CTG IND,122. Proceedings of 11th NCI-EORTC-AACR symposium on new drugs in cancer therapy (poster and abstract). *Clin. Cancer Res.* 2000; 6:4543.

21. Aboagye E. Cancer Research Campaign (CRC) program of in vivo pharmacokinetics and pharmacodynamics in drug development using positron emission tomography, Pg. 143. Proceedings of 1999 AACR*NCI*EORTC international conference.

22. Saleem A, Yap J, Osman S et al. Modulation of fluorouracil tissue pharmacokinetics by eniluracil: in-vivo imaging of drug action. *Lancet* 2000; 355:2125–2131.

23. Bubley GJ, Carducci M, Dahut W et al. Eligibility and response guidelines for phase II clinical trials in androgen-independent prostate cancer: Recommendations from the prostate-specific antigen working group *J. Clin. Oncol.* 1999; 10:3461–3467.

24. Jansson T, Westlin JE, Ahlstrom H, Lilja A, Langstrom B, Bergh J. Positron emission tomography studies in patients with locally advanced and/or metastatic breast cancer: A method for early therapy evaluation? *J. Clin. Oncol.* 1995; 13:1470–1477.

25. Kelly W, Scher H, Mazumdar M et al. Prostate-specific antigen as a measure of disease outcome in metastatic hormone-refractory prostate cancer. *J. Clin. Oncol.* 1993; 11:607–615.

26. Tannock I, Osoba D, Stockley M et al. Chemotherapy with mitoxantrone plus prednisone or prednisone alone for symptomatic hormone-resistant prostate cancer: A Canadian randomized trial with palliative end points. *J. Clin. Oncol.* 1996; 14:1756–1764.

27. Kantoff P, Halabi S, Conaway M et al. Hydrocortisone with or without mitoxantrone in me with hormone refractory prostate cancer: results of the cancer and leukemia group B 9182 study. *J. Clin. Oncol.* 1999; 17:2506–2513.

28. Public distribution of Novantrone (mitoxantrone for injection concentrate) NDA #19–297, Supplement S0014 ODAC Questions: September 11, 1996.

29. Kelloff GJ, Coffey DS, Chabner BA et al. Prostate-specific antigen doubling time as a surrogate marker for evaluation of oncology drugs to treat prostate cancer. *Clin. Cancer Res.* 2004; 10:3927–3933.

30. Nemunaitis J, Poole C, Primrose J et al. Combined analysis of studies of the effects of the matrix metalloproteinase inhibitor marimastat on serum tumor markers in advanced cancer: Selection of a biologically active and tolerable dose of longer term studies. *Clin. Cancer Res.* 1998; 4:1101–1109.

31. *Dow Jones International News*, 09/26.2000 British Biotech: Marimastat ovarian study sees no benefit.

32. Rustin GJS. Use of CA-125 to assess response to new agents in ovarian cancer trials. *J. Clin. Oncol.* 2003; 10:187s–193s.

33. Rustin GJS. Can we now agree to use the same definition to measure response according to CA-115. *J. Clin. Oncol.* 2004; 20:4035–4036.

34. Gronlund B, Hogdall C, Hilden J et al. Should CA-125 response criteria be preferred to response evaluation criteria in solid tumors (RECIST) for prognostication during second-line chemotherapy of ovarian cancer. *J. Clin. Oncol.* 2004; 20:4051–4058.

35. Rustin GJS, Bast RC, Kelloff GJ et al. Use of CA-125 in clinical trial evaluation of new therapeutic drugs for ovarian cancer. *Clin. Cancer Res.* 2004; 3919–3926.

36. Buyse M, Piedbois P. On the relationship between response to treatment and survival time. *Stat. Med.* 1996; 15:2797–2812.

37. Buyse M, Molenberghs' G. Criteria for the validation of surrogate endpoints in randomized experiments. *Biometrics* 1998; 54:1014–1029.

38. Buyse M, Thirion P, Carlson RW, Burzykowski, Molenberghs G, Piedbois P. Relationship between tumor response to first-line chemotherapy and survival in advanced colorectal cancer: A meta-analysis. *Lancet* 2000; 356:373–378.

39. Torri V, Simon R, Russek-Cohen E, Midthune D, Friedman M. Statistical Model to determine the relationship of response and survival in patients with advanced ovarian cancer treated with chemotherapy. *J. Natl. Cancer Inst.* 1992; 84:407–414.

40. Piantadosi S, McGuire W. Assessing the effect of response on survival in ovarian cancer. *J. Natl. Cancer Inst.* 1992; 84:376–380.

41. Pazdur R. Response rates, survival and chemotherapy trials. *J. Natl. Cancer Inst.* 2000; 2:1552–1553.

42. Stiff PJ, Shpall EJ, Liu PY et al. Randomized phase II trial of two high-dose chemotherapy regimens with stem cell transplantation for the treatment of advanced ovarian cancer in first remission for the treatment of advanced ovarian cancer in first remission or chemosensitive relapse" a southwest oncology group study. *Gynecol. Oncol.* 2004; 94:98–106.

43. Stadler WM, Cao D, Vogelzang NJ et al. A randomized phase II trial of the antiangiogenic agent SU5416 in hormone-refractory prostate cancer. *Clin. Cancer Res.* 2004; 10;3365–3370.

44. Edelman MJ, Clark JI, Chansky K et al. Randomized phase II trial of sequential chemotherapy in advanced non-small cell lung cancer (SWOG 9806): carboplatin/gemcitabine followed by paclitaxel or cisplatin/vinorelbine followed by docetaxel. *Clin. Cancer Res.* 2004; 10:5022–5026.

45. Oh WK, Kantoff PW, Weinberg V et al. Prospective, multicenter, randomized phase II trial of the herbal supplement, PC-SPES, and diethylstilbestrol in patients wit androgen-independent prostate cancer. *J. Clin. Oncol.* 2004; 22:3705–3712.

46. Gatzemeier U, Groth G, Butts , C et al. Randomized phase II trial of gemcitabine-cisplatin with or without trastuzumab in HER2-positive non-small-cell lung cancer. *Ann. Oncol.* 2004; 15:19–27.

47. Shah V, Midua K, Findlay J et al. Workshop/conference report: Bioanalytical method validation — a revisit with a decade of progress, July 25, 2000.

48. Selinger K, Smith G, Depee S, Aureche C. Determination of GW147211 in human blood by HPLC fluorescence detection. *J. Pharm. Biomed. Anal.* 1995; 13:1521–1530.

49. Dowlati A. Sequential tumor biopsies in early phase I clinical trials of anticancer agents for pharmacodynamic evaluations *Clin. Cancer Res.* 2001; 7:2971–2976.

50. Perez-Soler R, Donato N, Shin D et al. Tumor epidermal growth factor receptor studies in patients with non-small cell lung cancer or head and neck cancer treated with monoclonal antibody RG83852. *J. Clin. Oncol.* 1994; 12:730–739.

51. Collier M, Shepherd F, Ahmann F et al. A novel approach to studying the efficacy of AG3340, a selective inhibitor of matrix metalloproteases (MMPs), 482a. *Proc. ASCO* 1999.

52. Fazzari M, Heller G, Scher H. The phase II/III transition: Toward the proof of efficacy in cancer clinical trials. *Control. Clin. Trials* 2000; 21:360–368.

53. Bellissant E, Benichou J, Chastang C. The group sequential triangular test for phase II cancer trials. *Am. J. Clin. Oncol. (CCT)* 1996; 1:422–430.

54. Iveson T, Smith I, Ahern J, Smithers D, Trunet P, Dowsett M. Phase I study of the oral nonsteroidal aromatase inhibitor CGS20267 in healthy postmenopausal women. *J. Clin. Endo. Metab.* 1993; 77:324–331.

55. Bisagni G, Cocconi G, Scaglione G. Letrozole, a new oral non-steroidal aromatase inhibitor in treating postmenopausal patients with advanced breast cancer: A pilot study. *Ann. Oncol.* 1996; 7:99–102.

56. Dombernowsky P, Smith I, Falkson G et al. Letrozole, a new oral aromatase inhibitor for advanced breast cancer: double-blind randomized trial showing a dose effect and improved efficacy and tolerability compared with megestrol acetate. *J. Clin. Oncol.* 1998; 16:453–461.

57. Braun S, Pantel K, Muller P et al. Cytokeratin-positive cells in the bone marrow and survival of patients with stage I, II, III breast cancer. *N. Engl. J. Med.* 2000; 342:525–533.

58. Braun S, Hepp F, Kentenich C et al. Monoclonal antibody therapy with Edrecolomab in breast cancer patients: monitoring of elimination of disseminated cytokeratin positive tumor cells in bone marrow. *Clin. Cancer Res.* 1999; 5:3999–4004.

59. Braun S, Kentenich C, Janni W et al. Lack of effect of adjuvant chemotherapy on elimination of single dormant tumor cells in bone marrow of high-risk breast cancer patients. *J. Clin. Oncol.* 2000; 18:80–86.

60. Riethmuller G, Schneider-Gadicke E, Schimok G et al. Randomized trial of monoclonal antibody for adjuvant therapy of resected Dukes' C colon carcinoma. *Lancet* 1994; 343:1177–1183.

61. Punt C, Nagy A, Douillard J et al. Edrecolomab 17–1A antibody) alone or in combination with 5-fluorouracil based chemotherapy in the adjuvant treatment of stage III colon cancer: results of a phase III study. *Proc. ASCO* V 20, 2001.

62. Witherspoon S, Emerson D, Kerr B et al. Flow cytometric assay of modulation of P-glycoprotein function in whole blood by the multidrug resistance inhibitor, GG918. *Clin. Cancer Res.* 1996; 2:7–12.

63. Gerritis C, Creemers G, Schellens J et al. Phase I and pharmacological study of the new topoisomerase I inhibitor GI147211, using a daily X 5 intravenous administration. *Br. J. Cancer* 1996; 73:744–750.

64. Carter S. Clinical strategy for the development of angiogenesis inhibitors. *Oncologist* 2000; 5(Suppl 1):51–54.

15

CLINICAL TRIAL DESIGNS FOR CYTOSTATIC AGENTS AND AGENTS DIRECTED AT NOVEL MOLECULAR TARGETS

EDWARD L. KORN
LARRY V. RUBINSTEIN
SALLY A. HUNSBERGER

Biometric Research Branch
National Cancer Institute
Bethesda, Maryland

JAMES M. PLUDA

Investigational Drug Branch
Cancer Therapy Evaluation Program
National Cancer Institute
Bethesda, Maryland

ELIZABETH EISENHAUER

National Cancer Institute of Canada
Clinical Trials Group
Kingston, Ontario, Canada

SUSAN G. ARBUCK

Aventis Pharmaceuticals
Bridgewater, New Jersey
Current affiliation: Schering Plough Research Institute
Kenilworth, New Jersey

I. INTRODUCTION
II. PHASE I DOSE-FINDING TRIALS
III. PRELIMINARY EFFICACY TRIALS
IV. DEFINITIVE RANDOMIZED EFFICACY TRIALS
V. CONCLUSIONS

I. INTRODUCTION

The usual clinical development of chemotherapeutic agents proceeds through three phases of human testing. Phase I trials are designed to find the dose to be recommended for further testing by finding the highest dose that has acceptable toxicity (recommended phase II dose). Phase II trials are designed to see if the recommended dose leads to tumor shrinkage in patients with certain types of cancer; various schedules (with their corresponding recommended doses) can be tested in these trials. Phase III trials are designed to test in a randomized controlled manner whether agents (or regimens) showing promise in phase II trials lead to improved survival or quality of life as compared to standard treatment regimens. This developmental pathway is predicated on some general assumptions that are typically considered appropriate for cytotoxic agents:

1. The agent will shrink tumors at doses that have acceptable toxicity
2. Increased dosage of the agent will cause increased tumor shrinkage
3. Tumor shrinkage will lead to clinical benefit in terms of increased survival and/or quality of life, with increased tumor shrinkage leading to more clinical benefit.

Some cytostatic agents and agents directed at novel molecular targets have properties that raise questions about whether this standard developmental pathway is appropriate or optimal. First, the agent may not be expected to shrink tumors, but merely to halt progression. Secondly, there may be a plateau on the dose-efficacy curve for the agent such that higher doses may not offer more clinical benefit. Thirdly, it may be possible to identify patients before treatment who have molecular target levels in their tumors that indicate that they are particularly likely (or unlikely) to receive clinical benefit from the agent. Finally, it may be possible to monitor patients during treatment to see how well the agent is working at the molecular level. In this chapter some options for clinical trial designs for cytostatic agents and agents directed at novel molecular targets that take into account these considerations are examined. This examination is not meant to be an exhaustive listing of all possible approaches nor a definitive recommendation for certain trial designs. Other related discussions are given elsewhere [1–6].

II. PHASE I DOSE-FINDING TRIALS

If the goal of a trial is to find the maximum tolerated dose to be used for further testing, then a standard design using cohorts of 3–6 patients treated at escalating dose levels can be used, or preferably a design that escalates more quickly through non-toxic dose levels can be used [7, 8]. Even with this standard goal and design there can be challenges for non-cytotoxic agents. For example, it may be necessary for maximum benefit to treat patients with some cytostatic agents for long periods of time, making first-course toxicity (the determinant of dose levels in a typical phase I trial) inappropriate for choosing a recommended dose. The focus of this section, however, is not on finding the maximum tolerated dose. Instead, it is a discussion of other possible goals when additional information is available, specifically, a desired blood concentration level of the agent (see Section II.A) or a targeted biologic response associated with the mechanism of action of the agent that can be measured in patients (see Section II.B). To accomplish these goals sometimes requires larger numbers of patients per dose level than would be accrued in a standard phase I trial. This is of concern, because it is questionable whether it is appropriate to treat larger numbers of patients with an agent that has not yet shown any clinical activity. In addition, using these other sources of information is not without difficulties (see Section II.C).

A. Agents for which a Minimum Effective Blood Concentration Level is known

In this section it is assumed that based on preclinical evidence there is a minimum blood concentration of the agent (or its active metabolite) that is thought to be sufficient for the agent to be effective. One would like to identify a dose level of the agent that reliably yields at least this blood concentration. Although this sounds like it is a well-defined goal, there is actually some ambiguity. For example, suppose the minimum concentration desired is 100 (in some appropriate units), and at a given dose level, 5 patients have been treated with observed concentrations 95, 103, 112, 120, and 120. The observed mean of the concentrations is 110 and 80% (= 4/5) of the observations are above 100. The lower 90% confidence limit for the true mean concentration is approximately 102.5, which appears promising. However, although the observed proportion above 100 is 80%, we can be confident, at the 90% level, only that the true proportion above 100 is at least 49%, which might be considered unsatisfactory. Larger numbers of patients treated at a dose would be required to ensure that the true percentage of patients achieving a specified concentration is high, although this may be too ambitious a goal for a phase I trial. It may also be possible to incorporate the blood concentrations into a dose escalation using statistical models [9, 10].

B. Agents for which a Targeted Biologic Response can be Measured

In this section it is assumed that there is a binary (positive/negative) response measured in each patient, after treatment with the agent, which indicates whether or not the agent has had the desired effect on the target. Such a response might involve the level of a molecular target, or the change in the level of a molecular target that suggests clinical promise. The ability to measure biologic responses makes possible different criteria for designating the dose to use for further testing. Some of these criteria are discussed in Sections II.B.1–II.B.4. Note that the dose recommended based on a targeted biologic response may have little or no toxicity associated with it. In this situation, unless one is sure that the mechanism of action of the agent is understood, escalating the dose levels further might be considered [11]. On the other hand, one may encounter dose-limiting toxicity before reaching a dose that has sufficient biologic activity. In this case, the definition of sufficient activity may need to be reassessed: consider reformulating the delivery of the agent to yield less toxicity or discontinue development of the agent.

1. Finding a Dose that Guarantees a Specified Minimum Biologic Response

One may adapt the approach to assure a sufficient blood level outlined in Section II.A using binary responses of a targeted biologic effect rather than continuous concentration levels. For example, one might want to ensure with high probability that the true biologic response rate was greater than 80% at a given dose level. After patients have been treated at that dose level, one can use confidence intervals to address this issue. For example, Friedman et al. [12] observed 11 of 11 patients treated at 100 mg/m^2 of O6-benzylguanine had biologic responses defined as tumor AGT levels of less than 10 fmol/mg protein. It can be stated that with this observed response rate of 100% with 11 patients, the lower 90% confidence bound for the true response rate is 81.1%. However, if they had observed only 10 responses out of the 11 patients, then the observed response rate would be 91% and the lower 90% confidence bound for the true response rate would be 69.0%, less than 80%. With a larger sample size it is possible to have some non-responses and still have 90% confidence that the true response rate is greater than 80%; for example, the lower 90% confidence bound is 80.1% if 17 out of 18 responses are seen.

Is it possible to design a study with enough patients at a dose level to ensure with high probability that after observing the responses one can be 90% confident that the true response rate is greater than some specified level, like 80%? The answer is yes, but unless one hypothesizes that the true response rate is very close to 100% (e.g., >95%), the sample size can be prohibitively large [13].

2. Finding a Biologically Efficacious Dose

Suppose rather than trying to ensure that the true biologic response rate is 80% at a given dose level, a less ambitious goal is set. For example, suppose the goal is to ensure (in the context of a dose escalation) that if the true response rate is low or unchanging from previous doses then there will be a high probability of escalating further, whereas if the true response rate is high or increasing from previous doses then there will be a low probability of escalating further. There are many ways a trial to address this goal could be designed. Hunsberger et al. [14] consider two escalation designs based on these goals and show that cohorts of 1–6 patients can be used to find the biologically efficacious dose.

3. Is there a Dose-Response Relationship?

In this section the important scientific question of whether the biologic response is the same over a range of different doses or whether the response increases with increasing dose is addressed. Strictly speaking, answering this question does not identify a dose for further testing and trials, and answering this question might not be considered "dose finding." However, a negative trial of this type definitely has implications for the recommended dose, therefore, a brief discussion of this question is included here.

With only two dose levels, the response at each dose level could be estimated and a statistical hypothesis test to ascertain the statistical significance of the difference in biologic responses performed. With more than two dose levels, some type of linear relationship between the dose levels and the responses could be typically assumed, and a statistical test that the slope associated with the linear relationship is zero would be performed. (If the toxicity associated with the dose levels is known to be acceptable, then a randomization among the dose levels is advisable.) The sample sizes for doing these types of analyses are larger than those required for finding a biologically efficacious dose as described previously. For example, to reliably detect a dose-response relationship corresponding to true biologic response rates of 50% versus 90% would require 20 patients treated at each dose level (power = .90 for one-sided alpha = .10), with larger sample sizes required to detect smaller differences. Using more than two dose levels allows one to treat fewer patients at each dose level, but the total number of patients required to detect a dose-response relationship will actually be larger than if only two dose levels are tested. The advantage of using more than two dose levels is that it gives the ability to assess the shape of the dose-response curve, as discussed next.

4. Assessing the Shape of the Dose-Response Relationship: Finding the Optimum Biologic Dose

Trying to assess the shape of the dose-response relationship or find the "optimum biologic dose" will require larger sample sizes than those required to show that there is a positive association between dose and response. To demonstrate this, consider a trial with 10 patients treated at each of 5 doses. The proportions plotted in Figure 15.1 were based on data generated randomly by computer with this type of design with a true linear relationship of dose and response, with the true response going from 50 to 90%. With these sample sizes, it is easy to be misled about the shape of the dose-response relationship. For example, in Figure 15.1C it appears that the response has reached a plateau at dose level 4, and in Figure 15.1B there is a suggestion of a plateau starting at dose level 3. To lessen the possibility of getting misled, one can include confidence intervals around the plotted response proportions

(a)

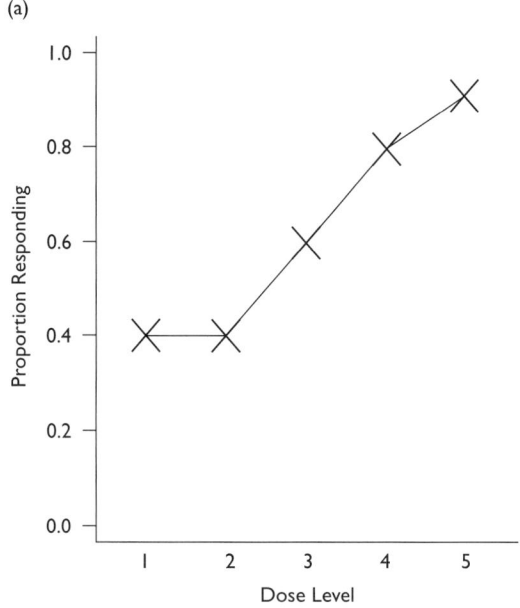

FIGURE 15.1 Hypothetical biologic response data for three trials (A, B, and C) generated randomly by the computer with 10 patients treated at each dose level. The true response proportions are 0.5, 0.6, 0.7, 0.8, and 0.9 for dose levels 1, 2, 3, 4, and 5, respectively.

(b)

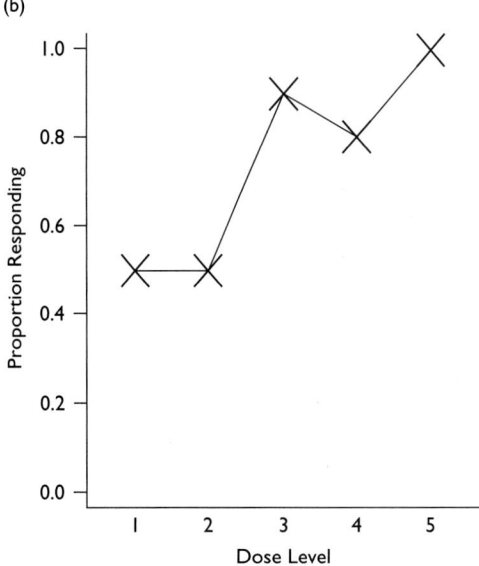

(c)

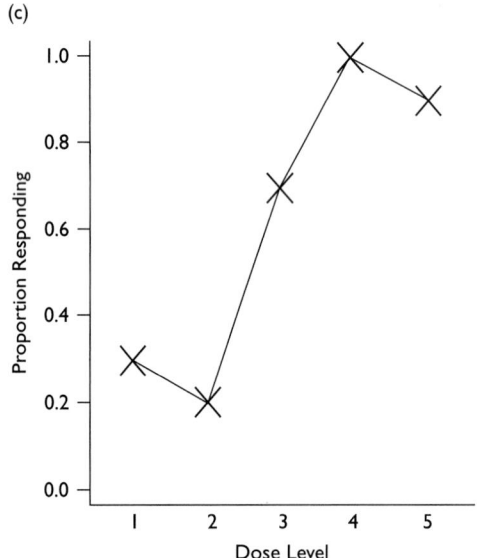

FIGURE 15.1 (*Continued*)

to display how variable the proportions are. For example, Figure 15.2 is a re-plot of Figure 15.1C with 90% confidence intervals for the proportions. It is now clear that because of the wide confidence intervals that there is no consequential evidence that there is a plateau. To assess whether or not there is a plateau in this type of data would require much larger sample sizes treated at each dose level. (The data in Figure 15.1 are sufficient to demonstrate a positive dose-response relationship, with the *p* values less than .005 for Figures 15.1A and B, and less than .001 for Figure 15.1C.)

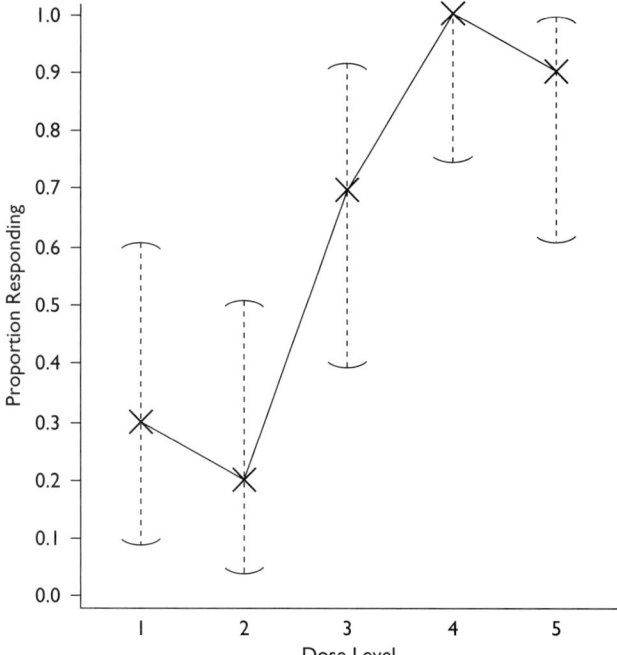

FIGURE 15.2 Re-plot of Figure 15.1C with 90% confidence intervals for each proportion.

C. Caveats and Feasibility Issues

Much of the above sections focus on how measures other than toxicity might be used to rationally determine the recommended dose of cytostatic agents and agents directed at novel molecular targets. However, there are some important factors to consider before employing these alternative endpoints into phase I trials.

First, there needs to be data from laboratory models that validate the choice of endpoint. For example, if a biologic measure of target effect in normal or tumor tissues was used as a means of defining "effective" doses in patients, there must be some evidence from *in vivo* animal studies that doses effective in producing growth delay or improved survival are also able to induce the biologic change in target tissues.

Secondly, although it is generally agreed upon that the most relevant tissue in which such effects are to be measured is tumor itself, there are substantial problems in obtaining serial biopsies suitable for laboratory evaluation from patients. Not only are there limitations on which tumor sites may be accessed for repeat assessment, there are issues of optimal timing of biopsies and minimum size that it may not be possible to address prior to the study. In addition, many samples from tumor turn out to be unacceptable for evaluation due to admixing of viable malignant cells with normal cellular populations or with necrotic tissue. For these reasons, as well as ethical concerns about invasive procedures undertaken primarily for research purposes, many investigators have chosen instead to examine easily accessible normal tissues (e.g., peripheral blood cells, skin, buccal mucosa) for evidence of molecular changes on treatment. This is reasonable when tumor tissues are not available, but results from these assays are subject to the criticism of relevance because changes in normal tissues may not be reflective of tumor tissue.

Finally, an important consideration is the reproducibility and reliability of the assay used to assess biological effects. By definition, assays conducted early in the investigation of a new agent are themselves investigational, so measurements made on the basis of the assay may be misleading. The confusion surrounding the assays for HER2 (or even the estrogen receptor in past years) serves to underscore the fact that standardization of assay methodology requires attention early in drug development. At the very least, it should be demonstrated that the assay of target effect proposed for use in dose-seeking trials shows little intra-patient variability (as evidenced by similar results on more than one occasion before drug administration) and is able to detect the level of change that is associated with anti-tumor efficacy in animal models.

Perhaps because of these factors, not many dose-finding trials have used non-toxicity endpoints [15].

III. PRELIMINARY EFFICACY TRIALS

For cytotoxic agents, a standard two-stage phase II trial enrolling up to 35–40 patients might target 5% versus 20% response rates in a patient population where response is a partial or complete tumor response [16]. These trials allow (1) the screening of agents to select (if any) the most promising to bring forward into randomized trials, (2) the treatment of fewer patients with agents that turn out to be inactive than if randomized trials were used to test all agents, and (3) the modification of the recommended dose from phase I trials based on a larger experience of treating patients. For cytostatic agents and agents directed at novel molecular targets, there are two considerations that might lead one to modify the standard approach that is used for cytotoxic agents. The first is that one may be able to measure for each patient the likelihood that the agent will be effective for them, e.g., by measuring the magnitude of the presence of the molecular target in their tumor. As discussed in the next section, this would suggest the possibility of restricting eligibility with a standard design targeting tumor response. The second consideration is that the mechanism of action of the agent may indicate that the agent is unlikely to cause rapid or any tumor shrinkage even if it did offer delay in tumor growth or prolonged survival, e.g., with cytostatic agents. Because one cannot target tumor response in this situation, different types of trial designs will be necessary as discussed in Section III.B.

A. Selecting the Patient Population to Study

If it is possible to identify which patients are more likely to respond to a molecular-targeted agent, e.g., based on the level of expression of the molecular target, then a natural strategy is to test the agent first only in patients who have tumors with high expression levels and are more likely to respond. If the agent shows sufficient activity in these patients, then it can be tested in a separate cohort of patients who are less likely to respond. One could argue about whether it is appropriate to test the agent on patients without the target expression even after it has shown activity in patients with expression, but this is usually reasonable because investigators may not be completely sure that they understand the mechanism of action of the agent. There are three complications with this strategy that will be discussed next.

The first complication is that it may not be obvious who is likely to respond, as the target may be measured on a continuous scale and with considerable measurement error. To test the agents in separate cohorts will require the identification of a "target positive" group and "target negative" group based on whatever measurements are available. However, the definitions of these groups may only be possible after a trial is complete and it is known which levels of expression are associated with greater or lesser probabilities of response. As an example, the definition of estrogen or progesterone positivity as a predictor of response to hormone therapy in breast cancer was only determined after large numbers of patients were treated, their receptor levels quantified, and a cut-off created that was clinically useful in predicting response.

The second complication is that the number of patients who are target positive may be considerably smaller than the number who are target negative. Performing trials for the target-negative patients only after trials for target-positive patients have been completed could considerably slow down the development of interesting agents. One approach to avoid delay is to have a menu of agents available for study so that patients who have a molecular target specific for an agent could be given that agent in a first trial of that agent, and patients who have none of the targets associated with the agents tested could participate in the second trial of one of the agents that showed sufficient activity in its first trial. Although we believe this approach is ideal, it may be logistically difficult because it involves sites and investigators dealing with multiple investigational agents. A compromise approach (involving only one agent) is to perform the first trial with the target-positive patients and start the second trial as soon as the first trial demonstrates a minimum level of activity, rather than waiting for the first trial to be completed. Of course, there is also the approach of starting trials for the target-positive and -negative patients at the same time, which may be reasonable if the agent has very little toxicity or there are no other promising agents available to be tested for the patient population under consideration.

The third complication is that there may not be a real-time method for assessing whether patients are target positive or target negative. (Presumably, the lack of a real-time assessment method is temporary, otherwise it is not clear how this information would be used in further clinical development of the agent.) A phase II trial could be performed on all patients to examine the target status retrospectively after the completion of the trial. Depending upon the number of patients who are in the target-positive and -negative groups, and the proportions of responders in these groups, one could accrue after the trial more patients to one or both of the groups (assuming real-time assessment is available at that time).

Even it if is not possible at present to identify which patients are more likely to respond to a molecularly targeted agent, it can be worthwhile to collect tumor specimens for future analyses. For example, retrospective analyses identified a mutation in the epidermal growth factor receptor (EGFR) gene in lung cancer that was associated with responsiveness to the EGFR kinase inhibitor gefitinib (Iressa) [17, 18].

B. Possible Trial Designs when Tumor Shrinkage is not Expected

The designs discussed in this section attempt to offer a preliminary test of the efficacy of an agent that is not expected to shrink tumors. The situation in which there is a targeted biologic endpoint that can be monitored for drug efficacy is considered separately (Section III.B.1) from the situation in which there is no endpoint of that type available and a clinical endpoint must be used (Section III.B.2).

1. Designs Using a Targeted Biologic Endpoint

A single-arm trial can be performed to estimate the proportion of patients whose endpoint is affected by the agent, as well as the magnitude of the effects on the endpoint. A small sample size (e.g., 30 patients) may be sufficient, although the endpoint must be measurable in all patients (e.g., in some situations tumor must be accessible for serial biopsy). One problem with this approach is that frequently the precise mechanism of action of a new agent is not known and/or the agent may have additional mechanisms of action to the one identified. Therefore, there is the danger of a negative trial for an agent that actually offers benefits to the patients (e.g., improvement in time to progression). On the other hand, even in the case in which targeted biologic activity is seen, this may not be considered sufficient evidence to proceed to a large randomized trial in the absence of evidence of benefit to the patients or in the absence of convincing data from other trials that the biologic measure is a surrogate for such benefit. It is suspected that because of these problems this type of design will be infrequently used as the sole preliminary efficacy trial. It is, of course, important for proof-of-principle to measure targeted biologic endpoints in trials that are using clinical outcomes as the primary determinant of activity.

2. Designs Using Clinical Outcomes Other Than Tumor Shrinkage

These trial designs naturally fall into two categories: those that use historical experience (either formally or informally) and those that do not. As the designs using historical experience have some advantages (when there are good historical databases available for comparisons), it might be reasonable for institutions without such databases to collect prospectively the required data for future studies.

a. Designs Using Historical Experience

A single-arm trial can be performed with a clinical endpoint that is expected to be affected by the agent, e.g., progression-free survival. One would compare the endpoint results to historical experience with a patient population treated with inactive agents or untreated. A 30–50 patient trial would typically be sufficient. The difficulty with this approach is ensuring that the patient population associated with the historical data is similar to the presently treated patients in terms of stage of disease and amount of prior therapy, organ function and performance status, and monitoring procedures for disease progression. Preferably the historical experience would come from patients treated at the same institutions as the presently treated patients. This approach can be used with the new agent combined with standard agents provided that the historical experience with the standard agents is known. This would be the correct approach in situations where it would be inappropriate to withhold standard therapy, or where the agent is expected only to potentiate the efficacy of a standard agent.

Rather than using progression-free survival or overall survival, one can also use this approach with a quality-of-life type endpoint, such as symptom reduction. Provided symptomatic treatment is already optimized, an observed benefit could reasonably be attributed to the new agent and could be sufficient evidence for proceeding to a phase III trial.

One can perform a single-arm trial comparing each patient's experience (e.g., tumor growth rate or time to progression) when given the new agent to his or her experience when previously given standard therapy [2]. The new agent would be viewed as a success for each patient with sufficient improvement in experience (e.g., time to progression increased by 33%). A relatively small sample size would be required, e.g., 50 patients. Some statistical issues in using this type of design with time to progression are discussed in reference 19. This type of design makes implicit use of historical experience in that it is assumed that treatment with no or inactive agents would lead to no or very few successes. The practical difficulties in using this type of design are formidable:

1. Patients must be enrolled prior to the time of treatment with the new agent so that they can be treated with the standard therapy. If they are enrolled after they have received the standard treatment, the possibilities of selection biases would be too large.
2. It might be difficult to identify suitable patients (e.g., with sufficient tumor growth on standard treatment who are still able to receive the new agent).
3. Precise rules will need to be formulated to define success in terms of improvement and to handle drop outs.
4. Because the investigators know the patients on first-line therapy will be receiving the new agent after progression, there may be bias in declaring progression early for the first-line therapy.

b. Designs Not Using Historical Experience

One can perform a "screening" randomized trial comparing the new agent to a placebo, or the new agent plus standard therapy to standard therapy alone. A standard clinical endpoint such as progression-free survival is used. By setting the alpha level to 0.20, rather than the usual 0.05, the sample sizes required will be about half of the usual required for a definitive randomized trial [6, 20]. However, with this type of trial, if the result is positive, the agent can be viewed as only promising and testing is pursued. Whether to use a screening trial or go directly to a larger definitive trial will depend on the strength of the preclinical evidence and any phase I evidence that the agent is effective (more evidence favors a definitive trial), the number of agents available for testing (more agents favors a screening trial), and the number of patients available to participate (fewer patients in a limited number of institutions favors a screening trial).

One can perform a multi-arm randomized selection design in which multiple new agents are compared to each other with the agent showing the best clinical effects chosen to be tested further. (If none of the agents demonstrate some minimal clinical effect, then an argument can be made for testing none of the agents further. However, defining an appropriate minimal clinical effect based on historical data may not be easy, see Section III.B.2.a) The sample sizes for each agent can be relatively small, e.g., 30–50 patients. However, this design will only ensure that an inferior agent will not be chosen if it is sufficiently inferior to the best agent [21]. Because most investigators and sponsors will not want to drop the study of their new agent just because it is not sufficiently superior to other new agents, this may not be a popular design.

IV. DEFINITIVE RANDOMIZED EFFICACY TRIALS

The designs for definitive randomized efficacy trials with cytostatic agents and agents directed at novel molecular targets will be similar to those used for cytotoxic agents. In particular, the agent could be compared to placebo (in settings where a treatment arm with only supportive care is acceptable), or a standard therapy could be compared to the new agent combined with the standard therapy (for situations where a negative interaction is unlikely). The sample sizes required will not be small. In situations where the new agent has not previously shown clinical activity, it is important that the definitive trial have early stopping guidelines for when the experimental arm does not appear better than the standard arm (i.e., stopping for "futility"); this could involve temporarily halting accrual after a first cohort of patients have been randomized to obtain sufficient follow-up information for assessment.

An additional consideration for targeted agents is whether to restrict eligibility to patients whose tumors express sufficient target; if the target is necessary for effect then lack of restriction can lead to a trial with insufficient power [22]. Ideally, the decision as to whether to restrict eligibility will be made based on data from the earlier development of the agent. Even if the trial does not restrict eligibility, it will typically be useful to collect information on the tumor target levels on patients for whom this information can be easily obtained. An additional consideration for cytostatic agents is that they may need to be given for a longer period of time than is usual for cytotoxic agents. This makes certain settings where time to progression is expected to be long (or some patients might be cured) less attractive for initially testing these agents.

V. CONCLUSIONS

Before abandoning standard clinical trial development for an agent, one should carefully examine the preclinical evidence that the agent is cytostatic or directed at a novel molecular target. For a putative cytostatic agent, if the evidence is not strong then the rationale can be questioned for further development of an agent that does not demonstrate tumor regressions given the large number of agents waiting to be tested. If the evidence for a cytostatic effect is strong, then some of the trial designs discussed in this chapter may be useful. For an agent directed at a novel molecular target, ideally the preclinical evidence should indicate that the agent affects the target, that affecting the target in this way has a negative effect on the tumor (cells), and that there are reliable assays for measuring the presence of the target in the tumor or the effect of the agent on the target. Frequently, this ideal will not be met as the assay development may be proceeding at the same time the agent is to be developed clinically. In this situation, the standard trial development can be used until reliable assays have been developed. At that point, the trial designs discussed in this chapter may be useful.

REFERENCES

1. Eisenhauer EA. Phase I and II trials of novel anti-cancer agents: Endpoints, efficacy and existentialism. *Ann. Oncol.* 1998; 9:1047–1052.
2. Von Hoff DD. There are no bad anticancer agents, only bad clinical trial designs — twenty first Richard and Hinda Rosenthal Foundation Award Lecture. *Clin. Cancer Res.* 1998; 4:1079–1086.
3. Gelman KA, Eisenhauer EA, Harris AL, Ratain MJ, Workman P. Anticancer agents targeting signaling molecules and cancer cell environment: Challenges for drug development? *J. Natl. Cancer Inst.* 1999; 91:1281–1287.
4. Stadler WM, Ratain MJ. Development of target-based antineoplastic agents. *Invest. New Drugs* 2000; 18:7–16.
5. Rowinsky EK. The pursuit of optimal outcomes in cancer therapy in a new age of rationally designed target-based anticancer agents. *Drugs* 2000; 60(Suppl 1):1–14.
6. Korn EL, Arbuck SG, Pluda JM, Simon R, Kaplan RS, Christian MC. Clinical trial designs for cytostatic agents: Are new approaches needed? *J. Clin. Oncol.* 2001; 19:265–272.
7. Goodman SN, Zahurak ML, Piantadosi S. Some practical improvements in the continual reassessment method for phase I studies. *Stat. Med.* 1995; 4:1149–1161.
8. Simon R, Freidlin B, Rubinstein L et al. Accelerated titration designs for phase I clinical trials in oncology. *J. Natl. Cancer Inst.* 1997; 89:1138–1147.
9. Mick R, Ratain MJ. Model-guided determination of maximum tolerated dose in phase I clinical trials: Evidence for increased precision. *J. Natl. Cancer Inst.* 1993; 85: 217–223.
10. Piantadosi S, Liu G. Improved designs for dose escalation studies using pharmacokinetic measurements. *Stat. Med.* 1996; 15:1605–1618.
11. Korn EL. Nontoxicity endpoints in phase I trial designs for targeted, non-cytotoxic agents. *J. Natl. Cancer Inst.* 2004; 96:977–978.
12. Friedman HS, Kokkinakis DM, Pluda J et al: Phase I trial of O^6-benzylguanine for patients undergoing surgery for malignant glioma. *J. Clin. Oncol.* 1998; 16:3570–3575.
13. Korn EL. Sample size tables for bounding small proportions. *Biometrics* 1986; 42:213–216 (Corr v 42, p 691).
14. Hunsberger S, Rubinstein LV, Dancey J, Korn EL. Dose escalation trial designs based on a molecularly targeted endpoint. *Stat. Med.* 2005 (in press).
15. Parulekar WR, Eisenhauer EA. Phase I trial design for solid tumor studies of targeted, non-cytotoxic agents: theory and practice. *J. Natl. Cancer Inst.* 2004; 96:990–997.

16. Simon R. Optimal two-stage designs for phase II clinical trials. *Control. Clin. Trials* 1989; 10:1–10.

17. Lynch TJ, Bell DW, Sordella R, Gurubhagavatula S, Okimoto RA, Branigan BW et al. Activating mutations in the epidermal growth factor receptor underlying responsiveness on non-small-cell lung cancer to gefitinib. *N. Eng. J. Med.* 2004; 350:2129–2139.

18. Paez JG, Janne PA, Lee JC, Tracy S, Greulich H, Gabriel S et al. EGFR mutations in lung cancer: correlation with clinical response to gefitinib therapy. *Science* 304:1497–1500.

19. Mick R, Crowley JJ, Carroll RJ. Phase II clinical trial design for noncytotoxic anticancer agents for which time to disease progression is the primary endpoint. *Control. Clin. Trials* 2000; 21:343–359.

20. Rubinstein LV, Korn EL, Freidlin B, Hunsberger SA, Ivy SP, Smith MA. Randomized phase 2 design issues and a proposal for phase 2 screening trials, *J. Clin. Oncol.* in press.

21. Simon R, Wittes RE, Ellenberg SS. Randomized phase II clinical trials. *Cancer Treat. Rep.* 1986; 69:1375–1381.

22. Betensky RA, Louis DN, Cairncross JG. Influence of unrecognized molecular heterogeneity on randomized clinical trials. *J. Clin. Oncol.* 2002; 20:2495–2499.

16

CANCER GENE THERAPY CLINICAL TRIALS: FROM THE BENCH TO THE CLINIC

EVANTHIA GALANIS

Division of Medical Oncology
Mayo Clinic and Foundation
Rochester, Minnesota

   I. REGULATORY REQUIREMENTS AND GOOD
     MANUFACTURING PRACTICES FOR GENE TRANSFER
     PRODUCTS
  II. PRECLINICAL DEVELOPMENT OF GENE THERAPY
     VECTORS/TOXICOLOGY TESTING
 III. FEDERAL AND INSTITUTIONAL APPROVAL PROCESSES
     FOR CLINICAL GENE THERAPY TRIALS
 IV. GENE THERAPY CLINICAL TRIAL DESIGN
  V. CORRELATIVE END POINTS

Gene therapy is a medical intervention based on the introduction of genetic material in human cells *in vivo* or *in vitro*. The genetic manipulation may be intended to have therapeutic or prophylactic effects or may provide a way of marking cells for later identification.

The concept of gene therapy evolved from the initial observation that certain diseases are caused by the inheritance of a single malfunctioning gene. Following early gene therapy efforts targeting inherited diseases, such as adenosine deaminase deficiency and cystic fibrosis, it became obvious that the limited efficiency of the gene transfer that could be accomplished with the existing gene transfer vehicles (vectors) could make treatment of monogenic hereditary diseases extremely challenging. As a result, the evolution of clinical gene transfer efforts has taken a different course than originally predicted, mainly focusing on cancer. To date, almost two-thirds of the gene therapy clinical trials, more than 400 trials worldwide, are focusing on cancer. One important motivation that underlies the shift has been the evolution of cancer gene therapy approaches that are less affected by the technical limitations complicating treatment of inherited genetic diseases. These approaches attempt to increase tumor cell immunogenicity and/or enhance killing via gene replacement or suicide gene transfer, and, in contrast to the manipulations directed toward overcoming metabolic diseases, do not require sustained gene expression. Although the field of clinical trials in cancer gene therapy is relatively new, over the last ten years a significant amount of information has emerged that should guide the design of future cancer gene therapy clinical trials. As with all clinical trials, conducting gene therapy clinical trials in human subjects should be viewed as a privilege, not a right, and every effort should be made to assure the safety of the patients.

The use of gene transfer for treatment of malignancies has had an excellent safety record thus far [1]. The tragic death, however, of a patient participating in a human gene therapy trial for treatment of an inherited disease focused national attention on the nature and conduct of human gene therapy trials, which significantly affected the field of cancer gene therapy. The clinical trial in question included intrahepatic artery infusion of a replication-deficient adenoviral vector encoding the ornithine transcarbamylase gene into a patient with partial ornithine transcarbamylase deficiency [2]. The second patient in the last (highest) dose cohort was treated with 2×10^{13} vector particles. After 24 hours the patient showed clinical deterioration and acute elevation in cytokine levels. What followed next was evidence of systemic inflammatory response syndrome, lack of tissue oxygenation due to adult respiratory distress syndrome (ARDS), subsequent multi-organ failure, and the first death of a human gene therapy trial subject [3]. The etiology of this lethal toxicity is most likely multifactorial. Although the injection of high doses of the adenoviral vector certainly played a role in the fatal outcome, other contributing factors possibly influencing the outcome must also be considered. The underlying ornithine transcarbamylase deficiency, the effect of mechanical ventilation on developing ARDS, as well as the presence of bone marrow aplasia in the subject's post-mortem exam may have also played a role in the sequence of events [4]. Although this event did not occur in a cancer gene therapy trial, and similar doses of other non-replicating adenoviral vectors (such p53 encoding adenovirus) administered via the hepatic artery to patients with metastatic cancer were well tolerated [5], it did have a significant impact on the field of cancer gene therapy. It emphasized some critical lessons in the conduct of all clinical trials; rules and guidelines for conducting clinical experiments should be adhered to, and quality assurance testing of materials including gene delivery vectors should be reinforced. In addition, as the field of gene therapy evolves, there is a major need to collect data regarding efficiency of gene delivery, safety and toxicity in accessible databases so that this already accumulated information can be translated into useful knowledge for all investigators.

More recently two significant adverse events occurred in a European pediatric trial of retroviral gene transfer for X-linked combined immunodeficiency, also known as gamma chain deficiency. In this trial pediatric patients with no alternative treatment options underwent bone marrow transplant with autologous CD34 bone marrow cells, stably transduced with a retrovirus expressing the gamma-c gene. Nine out of ten patients were cured with this approach. However, almost three years after gene therapy, uncontrolled exponential clonal proliferation of mature T cells occurred in the two youngest patients. Both patients' clones showed retrovirus vector integration and proximity to the LMO2 proto-oncogene promoter leading to abnormal transcription of expression of LMO2. This side effect, although not having significant implications in the conduct of cancer gene therapy trials employing retroviral vectors to destroy cancer cells, since in this setting the risk of incorporation to normal cells and secondary malignancy is extremely low, it will definitely impact the design of clinical trials employing retrovirus transduced hematopoietic stem cells [6].

This chapter will focus on some of the most important considerations in the design of gene therapy trials. The American Society of Gene Therapy, recognizing the importance of proper training in the evolution of the field, has been organizing Clinical Gene Transfer Training Course, in association with its annual meetings.

I. REGULATORY REQUIREMENTS AND GOOD MANUFACTURING PRACTICES FOR GENE TRANSFER PRODUCTS

All gene therapy products and most somatic cell therapy products in the United States are regulated by the Food and Drug Administration (FDA). As of 2005, there are no FDA-approved gene transfer products in the USA. Therefore, all gene transfer clinical trials need to have an Investigational New Drug (IND) application approved prior to enrolling patients. The process for manufacture and quality control of gene transfer vectors used for direct administration to clinical trial subjects or for *ex vivo* modification of cells must be documented in an IND submission to the FDA. There are multiple components used during the production of gene transfer vectors including cell banks, viral banks, and molecular constructs. In order to ensure production of a consistent and high-quality vector product, each component used during production must be controlled through testing and characterization. Poor control of production processes can lead to the introduction of adventitious agents or other contaminants or to inadvertent changes in the proper stability of the biological product that may not be detectable in final product testing. For this reason the methods and the agents involved in the production process should be clearly defined. The division of cell and gene therapy, Center for Biologics Evaluation and Research (CBER), applies a stepwise approach to the requirements for testing and characterization of components, which allows greater flexibility at early phases and requires strict compliance with regulations by phase III.

Good manufacturing practice (GMP) should be applied in the production of clinical grade gene transfer products. GMP is the part of quality assurance which ensures that medicinal products are consistently produced and controlled to the quality standards appropriate to their intended use and as required by the marketing or product specification. There are two main components of GMP: production control and quality control. Production control is focused on manufacturing, including suitability of the facility and staff for manufacturing, development of standard operating procedures, and record keeping. Quality control is concerned with sampling specification and testing and with recommendation and review of procedures ensuring satisfactory quality. Important steps pertaining to quality assurance of the gene transfer products include:

1. Characterization of the plasmids that have been used for preparation of the vector (such as plasmids used for preparation of the retroviral producer lines, adenoviral shuttle vectors, or the plasmid used for transient transfections for the production of adeno-associated viruses (AAV) or retroviral vectors); the description and derivation of plasmid is important including the backbone, gene insert, regulatory elements, selection markers; a diagram of the construct; and the confirmation of identity, frequently performed with restriction analysis. Additional requirements for plasmids include sterility; characterization of endotoxin levels; purity; activity, i.e., gene expression; concentration; and sequence analysis.

2. Cell banks, established for cell lines used in production such as packaging cells, producer cells, and feeder cells, should be characterized regarding derivation; culture conditions and reagents used; cryopreservation and storage conditions; and stability including genetics, phenotypic stability, and viability. In addition, safety testing including mycoplasma, adventitious viruses, species specific pathogens, bacteria, and fungi is required.

3. Characterization of free agents used in the production projects include characterization of cytokines, growth factors, antibiotics, cell selection devices, monoclonal antibodies, and plasmids. Final concentration of the reagents, source, vendors, certificates of analysis for critical reagents, and the clinical grade of licensed products needs to be available.

4. The final product should be tested for purity. This includes testing for total DNA cell content, testing for homogeneity of size and structure, excluding contamination with RNA or host DNA, testing for proteins if present as contaminants, testing for replication competent viruses resulting from recombination or complementation, testing for toxic materials involved in production, and testing for the presence of endotoxins. In addition, the final product should be free of adventitious agents including viruses, bacteria, fungi, and mycoplasma and should be tested for sterility, identity, and activity. Consistency in purity should be confirmed from lot to lot.

II. PRECLINICAL DEVELOPMENT OF GENE THERAPY VECTORS/TOXICOLOGY TESTING

In the development of new vector systems for gene transfer, clinical pharmacology and toxicology studies are frequently conducted in conjunction with the development of product manufacturing. The overall goal of preclinical animal and *in vitro* studies is to support the safety and the rationale for use of the product in human subjects. There are several goals to be achieved by preclinical testing that contribute to the design and conduct of the initial clinical trial. These include:

1. Identification of doses that confirm the desired biologic effect
2. Definition of the safe starting dose in escalation scheme

3. Identification of pharmacodynamic measures of biological activity
4. Identification of safety and toxicity parameters to monitor in the clinical trial
5. Definition of inclusion and/or exclusion criteria based on observed toxicities
6. Designating stopping rules for the clinical trial based on the toxicity of the profile observed in animals

Traditional drug development programs evaluating the safety of small molecule or protein therapeutics typically conduct toxicology testing in normal animals using a well-defined paradigm to establish the acute, subacute, and cumulative toxicities of an agent prior to its first use in humans. The advantages of this approach are that a wide range of doses may be investigated to give high multiples of the expected human exposure. In addition, metabolism and pharmacokinetics in different species may be established as a basis for comparison for clinical dosing. However, there are limitations to this approach when applied to toxicity testing of gene transfer agents. Species specificity of the transgene product, limitations in the doses that are feasible to administer, and the interaction of the agent with a specific receptor should be taken into consideration when designing toxicology studies. In gene transfer research, demonstration of safety must also take into account toxicities due to both expression of the transgene, as well as any specific adverse effects associated with a vector, and mode of delivery used to introduce the foreign gene. Additionally, any underlying pathology associated with the disease investigated may either exacerbate or confound toxicity related to the gene transfer system. These points must be considered when designing a preclinical protocol to evaluate the safety and efficacy of a gene transfer agent.

Preclinical studies in support of use of gene transfer vector in clinical studies should be conducted in compliance with the regulations for good laboratory practice (GLP, 21CFR part 58). Although preclinical pharmacology and efficacy studies in animals as well as *in vitro* pharmacology studies are not always expected to be conducted in full compliance with GLP, toxicology studies including *in vitro* toxicity studying, single and repeat dose toxicity testing in animals, *in vivo* reproductive toxicity and carcinogenicity studies, as well as biodistribution studies for gene transfer research are expected to follow the guidelines set forth by the regulations.

III. FEDERAL AND INSTITUTIONAL APPROVAL PROCESSES FOR CLINICAL GENE THERAPY TRIALS

There are both institutional and federal levels of oversight for clinical gene transfer trials. Two important institutional committees include the Institutional Review Board (IRB) and the Institutional Biosafety Committee (IBC). The IRB's role is to protect the rights of research participants by conducting a risk-benefit assessment and assuring that the informed consent document accurately reflects this balance. This includes assessment of risk for physical, psychological, and social harm in the context of anticipated benefit.

The IRB has the authority to approve or disapprove gene transfer protocols independent of the other regulatory bodies involved at the regular or federal level. The IBC reviews trial design, biosafety, and containment as well as compliance with National Institutes of Health (NIH) U.S. guidelines. The aim of this review is to minimize risks to close contacts and to the community as well as to the individual research participants.

At the federal level, the FDA oversees gene therapy trials at all institutions, reviews safety and efficacy data, and represents the regulatory authority. The FDA is ultimately responsible in authorizing clinical trials to proceed, and can also put clinical trials on hold or close clinical trials as necessary in light of new information. NIH guidelines apply to investigators conducting gene transfer research that is founded by the NIH or performed at an institution that receives NIH support for any type of recombinant DNA research. The NIH Recombinant DNA Advisory Committee (RAC) is a federal advisory committee providing advice and recommendations to the NIH director regarding recombinant DNA research. It conducts public review and discussions of the science, safety, and ethics of human gene transfer research. The oversight function of RAC includes reviewing gene transfer protocols, safety information, and issues both relevant to specific protocols and of general importance to the field. NIH guidelines define the roles and responsibilities of the institutions, investigators, and the institutional biosafety committee. Gene transfer protocols subjected to NIH guidelines should be registered with the NIH Office of Biotechnology Activities (OBA) and undergo initial RAC triaging regarding the need for an in-depth review. In addition to the clinical protocol, the initial submissions include responses to Appendix M Points to Consider in the Design and Submission of Protocols for the Transfer of Recombinant DNA into Human Subjects (http://www.4od.nih.gov/oba/rac/documents1.htm). Approximately 20–30% of protocols are selected for in-depth review by RAC. The recommendations of RAC subsequently are sent to the principal investigator and the institutional IRB, IBC, and FDA. IRB review and approval can occur before or after RAC review. The same applies for FDA review and authorization of IND application. During the review process, early RAC input is encouraged by the NIH and FDA. The final IBC approval cannot occur until RAC review is completed and no research participant may be enrolled prior to completion of the RAC review process. In addition, within 20 days of enrollment of the first participant, the principal investigator must submit to the NIH Office of Biotechnology Activities a response to RAC recommendations, a copy of the final protocol if applicable, a copy of final informed consent, and a copy of IRB and IBC approval.

IV. GENE THERAPY CLINICAL TRIAL DESIGN

Most of the gene therapy trials are currently stage I/II studies with the minority of them being phase III trials. The classic phase I design with three patients per dose level has been employed for most of the gene therapy trials. Several clinical trials during the last decade have proven the safety of intratumoral administration of a variety of vectors both replicating and non-replicating for different therapeutic transgenes. Among them are retroviral, adenoviral vectors, vaccinia virus, and DNA/liposome complexes. Sites of administration include skin and subcutaneous tumor deposits, lymph nodes [7], the central nervous system, [8–10], prostate gland [11–12], and a variety of other intra-abdominal and thoracic visceral organs such as liver and lungs [13–14]. As it pertains to systemic administration of viral vectors, clinical trials have been performed mainly with adenoviruses, both selectively replicating and non-replicating and the paranyxovirus PV701 can oncolytic strain of Newcastle disease virus) [30–31]. Hepatic artery administration of a non-replicating adenovirus encoding the tumor-suppressor gene p53 showed that very high adenoviral doses of 7.5×10^{13} particles could be associated with hypotension [15]. In contrast, lower doses of both a non-replicating p53 adenovirus (2.5×10^{13} particles) and 2×10^{12} particles of the replicating adenovirus ONYX-015 administered through the hepatic artery were well tolerated [16]. The most common side effects associated with the administration of the ONYX virus include mild constitutional symptoms and reversible LFT elevation. Intravenous administration of ONYX-015 in doses up to 2×10^{12} viral particles was also well tolerated except for mild to moderate constitutional symptoms [17].

Tolerance of intravenous administration of PV702 improved significantly with the use of initial lower desensitizing doses, allowing a 5-1 to 10-fold increase in the maximum tolerated dose [30, 31].

From the above, it becomes obvious that for vector systems previously used in the clinic through a specific route of administration, that have a proven safety record, alternative phase I designs such as the accelerated titration design, i.e., treating one patient per dose level with conversion to the standard cohort of three design, should grade 2 or higher toxicity occur, may be appropriate [18]. It appears that for both adenoviruses and retroviruses the maximum number of infectious particles delivered intratumorally is only limited by the titers that can be produced. Different rules apply, however, when intra-arterial or intravenous vector administration is contemplated or when novel replicating viral vectors are introduced to the clinic. In this setting, safety has to be convincingly demonstrated and more conservative study designs should be applied.

When determining a phase II dose during a phase I gene therapy study, the aim should be to identify the dose that can achieve the maximum biologic effect, which can occasionally reach a plateau at doses below the maximum tolerated dose. This emphasizes the need for convincing correlative end points that should be incorporated in all phase I/II clinical gene therapy trials.

Initially gene transfer had been envisioned by many as being able to eradicate cancer as a single modality, but a principle has recently emerged investigating the value of combining gene transfer with traditional anticancer modalities such as chemotherapy and radiation therapy. For example, preclinical cytotoxic synergy has been demonstrated between the conditionally replicating adenoviruses (oviruses) and different chemotherapy agents [19]. These results have been confirmed in a clinical trial in head and neck patients where viral monotherapy led to objective responses in only 15% of the patients as compared to 60% of the patients when this treatment was combined with 5-FU/cisplatin chemotherapy [20]. Similarly, intratumoral administration of replication deficient p53 adenovirus along with cisplatin appears to be synergistic in a variety of tumor cell lines [21], including lung cancer cells. Two of the 24 patients with non-small cell lung cancer refractory to platinum agents exhibited partial responses and stable disease was seen in 17 patients in a clinical trial [22]. Furthermore, combination of gene transfer with radiation therapy is a subject of ongoing evaluation. Based on encouraging preclinical work, a phase I/II trial of radiation therapy in combination with 3 biweekly intratumoral injections of Ad p53 in patients with locoregionally advanced non-small cell lung cancer achieved a one-year progression-free survival of 45.5%, which is superior to historic controls [23]. Although the potential of combining gene transfer agents with conventional treatment modalities such as chemotherapy and radiation therapy has become more obvious, the design of combination studies needs to be carefully considered. When limited experience exists with the gene transfer agent alone, an appropriate design may include administration of the gene transfer agent for one of two treatment cycles followed by the combined modality approach. If there is adequate prior experience with the gene transfer agent, up front administration of the conventional chemotherapy agent or radiation therapy in combination with the gene transfer agent is appropriate. In this setting the investigators need to be particularly aware and sensitive to unexpected side effects, with severity, specificity or frequency that exceeds the expected, based on the prior experience with the gene transfer agent alone or the conventional therapeutic modality as single agent. Possibly interim assessment of observed toxicity should be required and appropriate early stopping rules/safeguards should be applied.

V. CORRELATIVE END POINTS

In gene transfer trials, it is essential that meaningful correlative endpoints are employed in order to correlate the employed doses with biological effect and select the most appropriate dose for phase II setting. This usually requires repeat tumor biopsies, a task not always easy when performed in a multi-center setting or for deep-seated tumors. Significant parameters to examine include transfer of DNA to the target tissue, usually by employing PCR-based methodology, and even more important, expression of the transgene as indicated by the presence of mRNA by RT-PCR or at the protein level usually employing immunohistochemistry or FACS analysis. In case of replicating vectors, one additional element is the demonstration of replication. Although assessment of replication by *in situ* hybridization is appealing, since it allows assessment of the nature and distribution of the infected cells, it is limited by sampling variations and small amount of tissue assessed, which can lead in false negative results. Depending on the vector type, the presence of viral genomes in the peripheral blood is not always an adequate demonstration of viral replication. For example, non-replicating adenoviral vectors can be detected in the peripheral blood using sensitive PCR technology. Therefore, decrease of adenoviral titers in the peripheral blood with a subsequent increase during the second round of viral replication is necessary in order to convincingly demonstrate replication of replicating adenoviral vectors.

Another important consideration pertains to the use of provisionally replicating viruses that exploit specific molecular alterations. Examples include

ONYX-015 (replicates in cells with malfunctioning p53) [24] and reovirus (replicates in cells with activated ras pathway) [25]. Collection of information prospectively as part of clinical trials that would subsequently allow the correlation of clinical efficacy with the molecular alteration thought to be responsible for the selective replication of the virus should be encouraged. In later stages of development this may prove crucial in tailoring molecular therapies to the appropriate patient population. For example, there was a lack of correlation between the p53 mutation status and response to ONYX-015 in a trial of hepatic artery administration of the virus [16].

Another issue to be addressed is viral kinetics, i.e., distribution of virus after administration to humans via a specific route. For example, a phase I/II trial of intratumoral administration of p53 encoding adenovirus (Ad p53) in patients with recurrent head and neck cancer [26] showed that Ad p53 DNA was detected in the blood by PCR 30 minutes after Ad p53 injection and gradually eliminated over the next 48 hours. Cytotoxicity assays (CPE) performed in patients treated at 3×10^{10} and 10^{11} pfu (the highest two-dose levels) showed that viable Ad p53 was present in blood at the highest level 30 minutes after intratumoral injections, decreased at a rate of 2 to 4 orders of magnitude by 90 minutes, and further decreased to very low or undetectable titers by 24 hours to be completely eliminated by 48 hours after injection. Ad p53 was detected in the urine from some patients who received doses of 3×10^9 pfu or greater, and was present in urine from all patients who received doses of 3×10^{10} pfu or greater at 3–17 days from the last viral administration. These data demonstrated a relationship between dose and secretion of the viral vector in the urine. Ad p53 was also detected in the sputum and/or saliva samples of 6 high-dose patients tested; the virus was detected within one day of injection and was cleared to background levels within 7 days. Similarly, the HSV-tk adenovirus was detected in a dose-dependent manner in the urine of all patients after intraprostatic administration [11]. Studies such as these are important in order to not only elucidate what happens to a specific viral agent after administration and determine the optimal frequency of repeat dosing, but also in order to address public safety issues, especially when replicating agents that have potential for transmission are employed. Although a significant public health issue relates to the exposure of health-care providers and family members to potentially harmful viral vectors, only limited information is available. In one study of intratumoral administration of adenoviral vectors, two health providers with the greatest risk of exposure were tested. No elevation of neutralizing antibodies was observed in their serum, and neither serum nor urine contained infectious p53 particles or Ad p53 DNA [26]. This issue has unfortunately been only minimally or inadequately addressed in most clinical trials. A conscious effort should be made to address this theoretical risk in future trials, especially when novel replicating viral agents are employed.

In addition, it is important to characterize the immune response against the vector and/or transgene if applicable, which certainly can affect the effectiveness of treatment, especially after systemic administration of the viral agent. For example, a significant concern since the early days of adenoviral gene transfer has been the presence of anti-adenoviral neutralizing antibodies.

Indeed, in all of the adenoviral trials the level of neutralizing antibodies appeared to increase significantly within three to four weeks after administration of the virus. Antibody titers, however, did not appear to correlate with adenoviral dose or course of treatment and did not prevent the expression of therapeutic levels of the transgene after intratumoral administration or viral replication after intra-arterial administration [16, 26].

Despite systematic efforts in most gene therapy trials to assess the distribution of viral vectors/transgenes by performing repeat tissue biopsies, the results are often suboptimal. Biopsies are invasive procedures that can only be performed to a limited extent and are subject to sampling errors. There is therefore an emerging need for assessment of viral dissemination by using non-invasive monitoring procedures. This information in turn can prove very useful in order to judge the adequacy of delivery, possibly predict toxicity, and determine optimal dosing. Examples of novel technology that hopefully will be incorporated in clinical trials in the near future include use of positron emission tomography (PET scanning) employing [^{124}I]-5-iodo-2′-fluoro-1-β-D-arabinofuranosyl-uracil (FIAU) in order to image cells infected with viruses of the herpes simplex group (HSV). FIAU is a substrate for the phosphorylation catalyzed by viral thymidine kinase (TK). These phosphorylated nucleoside analogs are trapped within the tumor cells and accumulate to levels that are measurable by current imaging techniques. Using PET, as few as 1×10^7 viral particles injected into 0.5-cm colorectal xenografts could be detected by [^{124}I] FIAU PET imaging. The PET signal in this particular study was significantly greater at 48 hours compared to 8 hours after viral injection, indicating that the PET scan can detect changes in TK activity resulting from local viral proliferation. In addition, FIAU PET scanning was able to detect differences in viral inactivity at 0.5 log increments. Thus, PET may prove a useful modality for the localization of provisionally replication-competent HSV-1 viruses [27]. Similarly, PET or SPECT can also be used to follow the expression of the herpes simplex virus thymidine kinase gene when used as therapeutic transgene [28]. Another novel approach in this direction is the construction of trackable viral vectors expressing inert (non-immunogenic, non-functional, and accurately measurable) soluble marker peptides such as CEA and β-HCG. Oncolytic vaccine strain measles viruses were generated expressing CEA or β-HCG. A correlation was observed between expression of the marker peptide and viral gene expression, and *in vivo* kinetics of this trackable virus could be easily followed by measuring the concentration of the marker peptides in culture supernatants or in the serum. Measuring peptide levels in the serum could serve as a real-time indicator of viral gene expression; therefore facilitating the rational development of effective and individually tailored cancer virotherapy [29]. The first clinical trial of intraperitoneal administration of a measles virus derivative expressing CEA (MV-CEA) in patients with recurrent ovarian cancer is ongoing.

In summary, correlative endpoints including evaluation of expression of the transgene, immunological response to transgene or vector (when appropriate), vector kinetics, and assessment of viral replication if replicating vectors are important in order to validate the clinical utility and optimize gene transfer and virotherapy approaches. More traditional endpoints such as assessment of safety and efficacy, and their association with laboratory correlates are also key elements, when evaluating a new gene transfer based approach. There is gradually increasing hope that new developments in the field of gene transfer, including vector targeting, new vector systems, replicating vectors, and novel transgenes, along with constructive use of lessons learned in the recent past will allow the safe and efficient incorporation of gene transfer and virotherapy approaches in the treatment of cancer.

REFERENCES

1. Galanis E, Russell S. Cancer gene therapy clinical trials: Lessons for the future. *Br. J. Cancer* 2001; 85(10):1432–1436.
2. Batshaw ML, Wilson JM, Raper S, Yudkoff M, Robinson MB. Recombinant adenovirus gene transfer in adults with partial ornithine transcarbamylase deficiency (OTCD). *Hum. Gene Ther.* 1999; 10:2419–2437.
3. Department of Health and Human Services: Recombinant DNA Advisory Committee National Institutes of Health. *Hum. Gene Ther.* 2000; 11(11):1591–1621.
4. Schnell MA, Zhang Y, Tazelaar J et al. Activation of innate immunity in nonhuman primates following intraportal administration of adenoviral vectors *Mol. Ther.* 2001; 3;708–722.
5. Hacein-Bey-Abina S, Von Kalle C, Schmidt M et al. LMO2-associated clonal T cell proliferation in two patients after gene therapy for SCID-X1 *Science.* 2003; 302(5644):415–419.
6. Atencio I, Warren R, Venook AP et al. A phase I clinical trial of intra-arterial adenovirus p53 (SCH 58500) gene therapy for colorectal tumors metastatic to the liver. American Society of Gene Therapy 4th Annual Meeting 2001 (Abstract #871).
7. Stopeck At, Hersh EM, Akporiaye ET et al. Phase I study of direct gene transfer of an allogeneic histocompatibility antigen, HLA-B7, in patients with metastatic melanoma. *J. Clin. Oncol.* 1997; 15:341–349.
8. Ram Z, Culver KW, Oshiro EM et al. Therapy of malignant brain tumors by intratumoral implantation of retroviral vector-producing cells. *Nat. Med.* 1997; 3:1354–1361.
9. Klatzman D, Valery CA, Bensimon G et al. A phase I/II study of herpes simplex virus type I thymidine kinase "suicide" gene therapy for recurrent glioblastoma. *Hum. Gene Ther.* 1998; 9:2595–2604.
10. Rainov NG. A phase III clinical evaluation of herpes simplex virus type 1 thymidine kinase and ganciclovir gene therapy as an adjuvant to surgical resection and radiation in adults with previously untreated glioblastoma multiforme. *Hum. Gene Ther.* 2000; 11:2389–2401.
11. Herman JR, Adler HL, Aguilar-Cordova E et al. In situ gene therapy for adenocarcinoma of the prostate: A phase I clinical trial. *Hum. Gene Ther.* 1999; 10:1239–1249.
12. Sweeney P, Pisters LL. Ad5CMVp53 gene therapy for locally advanced prostate cancer – where do we stand? *World J. Urol.* 2000; 18:121–124.
13. Rubin J, Galanis E, Pitot HC et al. Phase I study of immunotherapy of hepatic metastases of colorectal carcinoma by direct gene transfer of all allogeneic histocompatibility antigen, HLA-B7B7. *Gene Ther.* 1997; 4:419–425.
14. Galanis E, Hersh EM, Stopeck AT et al. Immunotherapy of advanced malignancy by direct gene transfer of an interleukin-2 DNA/DMRIE/DOPE lipid complex: Phase I/II experience. *J. Clin. Oncol.* 1999; 17(10):3313–3323.
15. Venook AP, Bergsland EK, Ring E et al. Gene therapy of colorectal liver metastases using a recombinant adenovirus encoding WT p53 (SCH 58500) via hepatic artery infusion: a phase I study. *Proc. Am. Soc. Clin. Oncol.* 1998; 1661(17):431a.
16. Reid T, Galanis E, Abbruzzese J et al. Intra-arterial administration of a replication-selective adenovirus (d11520) in patients with colorectal carcinoma metastatic to the liver. a phase I trial. *Gene Ther.* 2001; 8(21):1618–1626.
17. Nemunaitis J, Swisher SG, Timmons T et al. Adenovirus mediated p53 gene transfer in sequence with cisplatin to tumors of patients with non-small cell lung cancer. *J. Clin. Oncol.* 2000; 18:609–622.

18. Simon RM, Friedlin B, Rubinstein LV, Arbuck S, Collins J, Christian M. Accelerated titration designs for phase I clinical trials in oncology. *JNCI* 1997; 89:1138–1147.

19. Heise C, Sampson-Johannes A, Williams A, McCormick F, Von Hoff DD, Kirn DH. OXYX-015, an E1B gene-attenuated adenovirus, causes tumor-specific cytolysis and anti-tumoral efficacy that can be augmented by standard chemotherapeutic agents. *Nat. Med.* 1997; 3:639–645.

20. Khuri FR, Nemunaitis J, Ganly I et al. A controlled trial of intratumoral ONYX-015, a selectively-replicating adenovirus, in combination with cisplatin and r-fluorouracil in patients with recurrent head and neck cancer. *Nat. Med.* 2000; 6(8):879–885.

21. Nielsen LL, Lipari P, Dell J, Gurnani M, Hajian G. Adenovirus-mediated p53 gene therapy and paclitaxel have synergistic efficacy in models of human head and neck, ovarian, prostate, and breast cancer. *Clin. Cancer Res.* 1998; 4:835–846.

22. Nemunaitis J, Cunningham C, Buchanan A et al. Intravenous infusion of a replication-selective adenovirus (ONYX-015) in cancer patients: Safety, feasibility and biological activity. *Gene Ther.* 2001; 8:746–759.

23. Swisher SG, Roth JA, Komaki R et al. A phase II trial of adenoviral mediated p53 gene transfer (RPR/INGN 201) in conjunction with radiation therapy in patients with localized non-small cell lung cancer (NSCLC). *Proc. Am. Soc. Oncol.* 2000; 19:461a.

24. Bischoff JR, Kirn DH, Williams A et al. An adenovirus mutant that replicates selectively in p53-deficient human tumor cells. *Science* 1996; 274:373–376.

25. Coffey MC, Strong JE, Forsyth PA, Lee PW. Reovirus therapy of tumors with activated Ras pathway. *Science* 1998; 282:1332–1334.

26. Clayman GL, El-Nagger AK, Lippman SM et al. Adenovirus-mediated p53 gene transfer in patients with advanced recurrent head and neck squamous cell carcinoma. *J. Clin. Oncol.* 1998; 16(6):2221–2232.

27. Bennett JJ, Tjuvajev J, Johnson P et al. Positron emission tomography imaging for herpes virus infection: implications for oncolytic viral treatments of cancer. *Nat. Med.* 2001; 7(7):859–863.

28. Tjuvajev JG, Finn R, Watanabe K et al. Noninvasive imaging of herpes virus thymidine kinase gene transfer and expression: A potential method for monitoring clinical gene therapy. *Cancer Res.* 1996; 56:4087–4095.

29. Peng KW, Facteau S, Wegman T, O'Kane D, Russell SJ. Non-invasive *in vivo* monitoring of trackable viruses expressing soluble marker peptides. *Nat. Med.* 2002; 8(6):527–531.

30. Pecora AL, Rizvi N, Cohen GI et al. Phase I trial of intravenous administration of PV701, an oncolyticvirus, in patients with advanced solid cancers. *J. Clin. Oncol.* 2002; 20(9):2220–2222.

31. Lorence RM, Pecora AL, Major PP et al. Overview of phase I studies of intravenous administration of PV701, an oncolytic virus. *Curr. Opin. Mol. Ther.* 2003; 5(6):618–624.

17

MOLECULAR TARGETS FOR RADIOSENSITIZATION

ROGER OVE

JAMES A. BONNER

Department of Radiation Oncology
University of Alabama at Birmingham
Birmingham, Alabama

I. INTRODUCTION
II. GROWTH FACTOR RECEPTORS
III. RAS
IV. MODULATION OF P53
V. DNA DAMAGE RECOGNITION AND REPAIR
VI. OTHER PROMISING APPROACHES
VII. CONCLUSIONS
VIII. ADDENDUM

I. INTRODUCTION

Modulation of radiation sensitivity has been a topic of both laboratory and clinical investigation for many years [1]. Recently, the scientific community has gained a better understanding of molecular cell biology including such topics as DNA repair, cell cycle control, internal signal transduction, and apoptosis. This improved understanding of radiation-induced effects at the molecular level coupled with historical efforts to enhance radiation effects has placed the radiation oncology scientific community in a position to capitalize on many potential avenues of radiosensitization.

Historically, the first efforts at radiosensitization involved the combination of radiation with conventional chemotherapy agents as well as hypoxic cell sensitizers. The use of cytotoxic chemotherapy agents can be curative in many hematological malignancies; however, cures with chemotherapy alone are uncommon in patients with epithelial or other types of solid tumors. This dichotomy of effects stems from the fact that it is not possible to obtain the several logs of cell kill required for eradication of gross solid tumors [2]. Cytotoxic chemotherapy agents can contribute to radiosensitization in the treatment of solid tumors. However, the challenge for investigators in this area is to develop methods of utilizing cytotoxic agents in a manner to radiosensitize tumor cells and not normal cells (enhance the therapeutic ratio). Hypoxic radiosensitizers, in particular tirapazamine (TPZ), have been utilized in an effort to take advantage of the distinction between normal cells and tumor cells in terms of their oxygen tension levels. These agents have shown the most promise in clinical trials when used in conjunction with cisplatin [3], and when used concurrently with radiotherapy for advanced head and neck cancer [4, 5]. While these classical agents continue to hold promise and are actively pursued in clinical trials, this review will focus on radiosensitization approaches that are developing to capitalize on the increasing ability to target molecular events in the tumor cells. As these areas of research progress, it will be important to integrate our new understanding of tumor control at the molecular level with our past understanding of classical radiosensitization parameters.

The DNA double-strand break has long been accepted as an important event in cellular injury due to radiotherapy. Therefore, mechanisms for DNA damage recognition and repair may be targets for therapeutic intervention [6]. However, such approaches have not yet come to clinical trial, although laboratory work has shown potential [7–12]. Other approaches to addressing biological radiosensitization targets include targeting growth factors and signal transduction pathways. This area of research has not been fully realized in the form of multiple clinical trials, but initial trials are under way with agents targeting cell surface growth factor receptors including their enzymatically active domains and downstream signal transduction cascades. The most widely studied current receptor is epidermal growth factor receptor (EGFr). Several anti-EGFr antibodies have been synthesized. In addition to anti-EGFr antibodies, such as cetuximab (C225) [13], agents have been developed that interact with the active tyrosine kinase intracellular portion of the receptor [14]. These agents have been explored in several clinical trials. However, there is a paucity of trials that have explored the combination of these agents with radiotherapy in an effort to examine radiosensitization. Indeed, it is not immediately obvious why interaction with EGFr or similar growth factor receptors would lead to synergy with radiation therapy. However, such synergy may occur through several mechanisms, as will be discussed later in this chapter.

This chapter will focus on four current approaches to radiosensitization; primarily addressing new molecular targets for radiosensitization that have reached clinical trial, or that are likely to form the basis of clinical trials in the near future. These selected areas provide examples of various cellular mechanisms that can be altered to affect radiosensitivity. This chapter will also highlight studies of the epithelial growth factor receptors, which include Her1, Her2, Her3, and Her4. The focus will be primarily on EGFr (Her1), which is the most commonly exploited receptor. It will also address interactions with the downstream signal transduction cascade, which includes Ras inhibition and subsequent inhibition of the mitogen-activated protein (MAP) kinase pathway. Much of the work taking place in clinical trials with and without radiation involves inhibition of farnesylation, which disrupts the ability of Ras to localize to the cell membrane. As Ras activation acts immediately downstream of the EGFr tyrosine kinase, this approach is closely related to that of EGFr modulation (Figure 17.1). A third molecular target for radiosensitization is related to the exploitation of cell cycle control, and involves such gene targets as p16, p21, and p53. The final topic to be reviewed is the potential

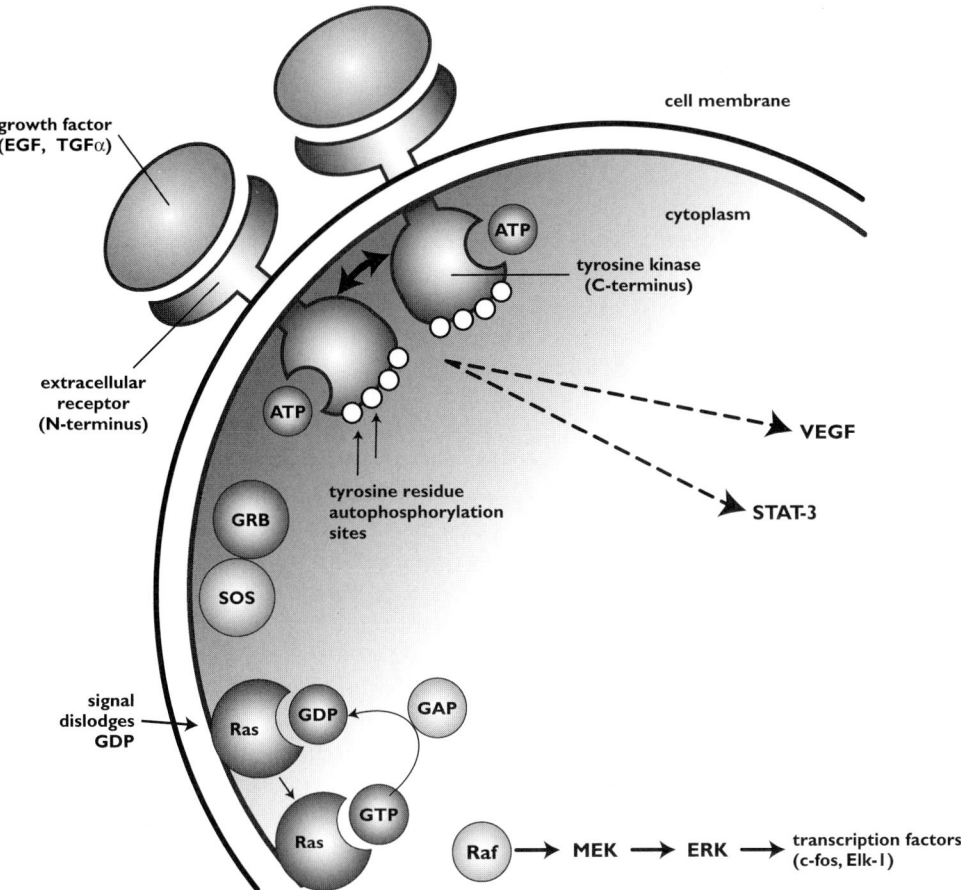

FIGURE 17.1 Schematic of EGFr signal transduction. EGFr is a class I transmembrane tyrosine kinase receptor with each receptor interacting with a separate ligand (EGF). Interaction induces dimerization and autophosphorylation of the intracellular C terminus portion, which leads to conformational changes enhancing tyrosine kinase activity and allowing interaction with substrates. The growth stimulus is transmitted via the growth factor receptor binding protein (GRB) and son of sevenless (SOS), which leads to dissociation of GDP from membrane bound Ras. Ras then binds with GTP, which is more prevalent than GDP in the cytoplasm. This leads to interaction with Raf and stimulation of the MAP kinase pathway. Ras is returned to the rest state by GAP, which dephosphorylates GTP. EGFr also leads to increased VEGF production, and in addition has anti-apoptotic effects by decreasing levels of phophorylated STAT-3. See Color Plate 23.

exploitation of DNA damage recognition and repair, as our understanding of these processes continues to improve. Although these potential modalities have been investigated for several years, they have yet to come to clinical trials. In part, this may be due to the fact that DNA repair takes place within the nucleus, which makes these targets somewhat more difficult to access than surface receptors or processes that take place in the cytoplasm. However, it is becoming increasingly possible to target intranuclear targets, and it is likely that targeting the recognition and repair pathways of DNA damage will reach clinical application within the next few years.

II. GROWTH FACTOR RECEPTORS

EGFr has been studied for roughly twenty years. It was originally identified through the study of a mutant tyrosine kinase that induced tumors in animals [15]. EGFr is a 170-kDa transmembrane glycoprotein that interacts with external ligands to activate its tyrosine kinase activity. Ligand interaction with the extracellular receptor portion activates the intracellular tyrosine kinase component of EGFr (Figure 17.1). EGFr is closely related to other tyrosine kinase growth factor receptors such as the Her2/neu and insulin receptors. EGFr is present in many cell types, with hematopoietic cells as a notable exception. The N terminus of EGFr is located in the extracellular domain, while the C terminus resides inside the cell. A hydrophobic transmembrane region separates the two. Unlike the oncogenic mutant tyrosine kinase to which its discovery is linked, EGFr requires a ligand for activation. Ligands that activate EGFr include epidermal growth factor (EGF) as well as transforming growth factor alpha (TGFα).

Interest in EGFr has been stimulated by the discovery that it is overexpressed in multiple tumor types including melanomas, cancers of the head and neck, gastrointestinal malignancies, lung cancer, and prostate cancer. Depending on the tumor cell type, the percentage of tumors found to have EGFr overexpression ranges between 50–90%. Head and neck cancers tend to overexpress EGFr in nearly 100% of cases. Although the discovery of EGFr overexpression in multiple malignancies has been exciting, it is even more important to note that EGFr overexpression in tumors is frequently associated with much lower expression of EGFr in surrounding normal tissue [16]. This latter finding suggests that EGFr can be used as a selective target for cancer cells while sparing normal tissue. The number of EGFr receptors per epithelial cell is typically 10^4 to 10^5 per cell, dependent on cell type, with numbers exceeding 10^6 in some cell lines such as A431 (human gynecologic squamous cell cancer).

EGFr is the only known receptor for epidermal growth factor. It is also one of the few known receptors for TGFα. However, it is known that TGFα can stimulate the MAP kinase pathway even while EGFr is blocked with a monoclonal antibody. This suggests that there is an alternative receptor for TGFα [17]. Several other ligands can activate EGFr. Interaction of the ligand with the extracellular domain causes ATP-induced phosphorylation of various intracellular components. These phosphorylations lead to activation of signal transduction cascades, which include the Ras/Raf MAP kinase cascade that has activity in regulating apoptosis and cell cycle control.

Binding with ligands promotes the formation of EGFr dimers, which is associated with increased tyrosine kinase activity, autophosphorylation of EGFr, and interaction with substrates. EGFr is a subclass I transmembrane tyrosine kinase, which exists as monomers on the cell surface, each of which independently interacts with ligands. Ligand interaction induces dimerization, and the proximity of the intracellular domains of the receptor induces phosphorylation. Autophosphorylation of the intracellular tyrosine kinase portion induces conformational changes that allow interaction with various intracellular substrates [18].

Both TGFα and EGF are capable of inducing angiogenesis [14]. Angiogenesis has been shown to be inhibited *in vivo* by cetuximab-induced blockade of EGFr in a mouse pancreatic cancer xenograft model [19, 20]. Intracellular targets activated by EGFr tyrosine kinase include phospholipase C-γ (PLCγ), phosphatidylinositol-3′-kinase (PI3K), G proteins, Ras, GTPase activating protein (GAP), growth factor receptor binding protein 2 (Grb2), and Src kinases. The best known and most completely elucidated activated pathway is the Ras/Raf MAP kinase pathway. PI3K is a component of multiple signal transduction pathways and is associated with lipid metabolism [21].

Several approaches have been explored in an attempt to create radiosensitization through various interactions with EGFr. The receptor can be blocked by a specific antibody, such as cetuximab in the case of EGFr or trastuzumab in the case of Her2. Another approach is to interfere with the tyrosine kinase cytoplasmic component of EGFr, as is currently being explored with the small molecule gefitinib (ZD1839). Such disruption of the receptor can lead to radiosensitization via several potential mechanisms, which will be discussed below. Mechanisms for radiosensitization include direct effects on tumor cell molecular biology, as well as indirect effects such as immune system interaction and angiogenesis inhibition. Direct effects in principle should be measurable with *in vitro* methods, but paradoxically clonogenic survival analysis does not consistently demonstrate cetuximab radiosensitization [22]. Recent results support this view, and suggest that radiosensitization arises from complex processes involving the surrounding tissue matrix [23].

It has long been known that activation of Ras and its subsequent downstream events can lead to radiation resistance [24]. A high percentage of tumors have a Ras mutation, which leads to sustained activation of Ras, and this activation is associated with poor prognosis and radiation resistance [25–27]. Blockage of EGFr or interference with its tyrosine kinase can lead to an increase in radiation sensitivity that is similar to the radiosensitization created by interference with Ras function and the subsequent disruption of downstream events [28, 29].

One of the downstream events stemming from irradiation under conditions of EGFr blockade, which may be transmitted by the MAP kinase pathway, is alteration of radiation-induced redistribution of the cell cycle. It has been shown in prostate cancer cell lines that inhibition of the EGFr leads to an increase in the percentage of cells in G2-M phase, the most radiation-sensitive portion of the cell cycle. A decreased proportion of cells in the radioresistant S-phase was also observed [29]. These results have been confirmed recently and in addition, it has been shown that the cetuximab/EGFr interaction may lead to an increase in cell populations in the G1 phase [30, 31]. Irradiation in the presence of cetuximab blockade has been shown to result in a shift in the percentage of cells in G2-M as well as G1, with decreased populations in the radioresistant S-phase, and the overall effect is potentially favorable for radiosensitization.

Anti-EGFr-induced radiosensitization may also be intimately involved with DNA double-strand break repair. Administration of cetuximab has been shown to lead to a redistribution of DNA-PK in the cell [30]. Blockade of the EGFr with cetuximab leads to a decrease in DNA-PK in the nucleus of the cell and increased levels in the cytosol. DNA-PK is the primary enzyme involved in double-strand break repair, and the cetuximab effects on DNA-PK localization may play a role in cetuximab-induced radiosensitization. Detection of DNA damage and signaling of this event may also be altered by EGFr blockade. ATM (protein mutated in ataxia-telangiectasia) is rapidly phosphorylated after irradiation, and it phosphorylates other targets involved in cell cycle control and DNA repair, such as p53 and members of the hMre11/hrad50/nibrin complex. ATM levels are upregulated by irradiation and downregulated by EGF [32]. The impact of cetuximab on ATM levels and activity is unclear, and may depend on cell type. Further investigation of this relationship is warranted.

Apoptosis, and the multiple cellular processes associated with apoptosis, may also play a crucial role in increased radiosensitivity with EGFr blockade. EGF/EGFr interaction leads to an increase in mitosis and inhibition of apoptosis. It has been shown by several laboratories that blockade of EGFr with cetuximab leads to an increase in apoptosis [31, 33]. It is believed that irradiation can activate the downstream events of the EGFr/Ras/MAP kinase pathway independently of epidermal growth factor [34]. This concept has been further supported in prostate cancer cell lines [29] and squamous cancer cell lines as well as breast cancer cell lines [17]. Activation of the MAP kinase pathway can lead to both cell cycle arrest and apoptosis as well as proliferation. Following irradiation alone, it has been suggested that MAP kinase activation is involved in the proliferative status of the tumor cell. This activation can be disrupted by an EGFr blockade with cetuximab, which leads to another possible mechanism of radiosensitivity. However, increased levels of activated MAP kinase were not detected in several cell lines after irradiation and cetuximab exposure [31]. In some cell lines, EGFr appears to influence apoptosis through the signal transducers and activators of transcription (STAT) protein family, in particular via the STAT-3 pathway [33, 35]. Both concurrent cetuximab with radiation or cetuximab alone have been shown to induce markedly decreased levels of phosphorylated STAT-3, which is associated with an anti-apoptotic effect [31].

Cetuximab has also been shown to lead to a decrease in angiogenesis. Decreased levels of vascular endothelial growth factor (VEGF) have been detected after cetuximab administration [19]. The mechanism of this decrease is currently unknown. Decreased angiogenesis has been seen *in vivo* following cetuximab administration [23]. Histological evaluation of tissue following irradiation and cetuximab administration also shows decreased angiogenesis, in addition to granulocytic infiltration. Additionally, radiosensitization due to cetuximab is more reliably measurable *in vivo* than *in vitro* [22, 23, 31]. Although this decrease in angiogenesis and VEGF expression is not measurable *in vitro*, it may be one of the more important implications of cetuximab blockade *in vivo* and clinically.

Her2/neu blockade may also lead to an increase in radiosensitivity. This concept has been observed in breast cancer cell lines overexpressing Her2 [36]. Blockade of the Her2 receptor has been associated with downregulation of VEGF [37]. This finding is analogous to similar findings observed with EGFr blockade. Gefitinib inhibits the tyrosine kinase activity of Her2/neu in addition to EGFr [38]. The study of radiotherapy in combination with blockade of the Her2 receptor will be the subject of future works.

A. EGFr and Clinical Trials of Radiosensitization

The preceding section reviewed the multiple interactions that may occur between radiation and EGFr inhibition. These interactions may lead to radiosensitization. It is possible that these interactions will vary in importance depending on the tumor type. Therefore, the study of radiotherapy and anti-EGFr treatment is being taken to the clinic to determine whether these theoretical arguments and laboratory findings translate into clinically meaningful radiosensitization.

Both EGFr blockade with cetuximab and disruption of the tyrosine kinase portion of EGFr via the small molecule gefitinib have been explored recently in clinical trials. Cetuximab has been studied concurrently with radiotherapy. The first of these trials was a phase I trial for head and neck cancer preformed at the University of Alabama at Birmingham (UAB) [39, 40]. In this phase I trial 12 of 15 patients had long-term disease-free survival (greater than 18 months), in excess of the 50% expected disease-free survival for these high-risk inoperable patients. Many patients had a dramatic clinical response (one of these cases is illustrated with pre- and post-treatment tomography in Figure 17.2). Morbidity was essentially equivalent to radiation therapy alone. Currently a phase III trial of radiotherapy with and without cetuximab is under way internationally with an accrual goal of 410 patients. Gefitinib has shown promise in the laboratory. There are several protocols under way utilizing gefitinib to determine dose escalation and pharmacokinetics. There are also phase II and phase III trials targeting lung cancer utilizing gefitinib currently with chemotherapy [41].

B. Connection with VEGF and Specific Inhibitors of VEGF

Modulation of angiogenesis may also hold potential for synergy with radiotherapy. As noted above, EGFr inhibition has been shown to downregulate angiogenesis via decreased production of VEGF [19, 20, 23]. Although a decrease in tumor angiogenesis would be clearly beneficial, it is unclear how this would lead to synergy with radiotherapy. However, recent results shed some light on the mechanism.

Exposure to radiation has been shown to lead to an increase in production of VEGF, presumably due to the generalized proliferative effect of the growth stimulus [42]. Thus, the administration of antibody to VEGF or angiostatin (an anti-VEGF compound) may counter this proliferative effect on the vascular endothelium. Experiments assessing the efficacy of concomitant administration of anti-VEGF antibody with radiation have shown this combination to be effective and synergistic *in vivo* [42, 43]. The same combination was shown to be no more effective than radiation alone on tumor cell lines *in vitro*. The combination was also effective when acting upon vascular endothelial cells *in vitro*. Greater than additive effects with radiation were seen with *in vivo* tumors and *in vitro* endothelial cells, which suggests that the mechanism of synergy is due to the effect on tumor vasculature rather than a direct effect on tumor cells.

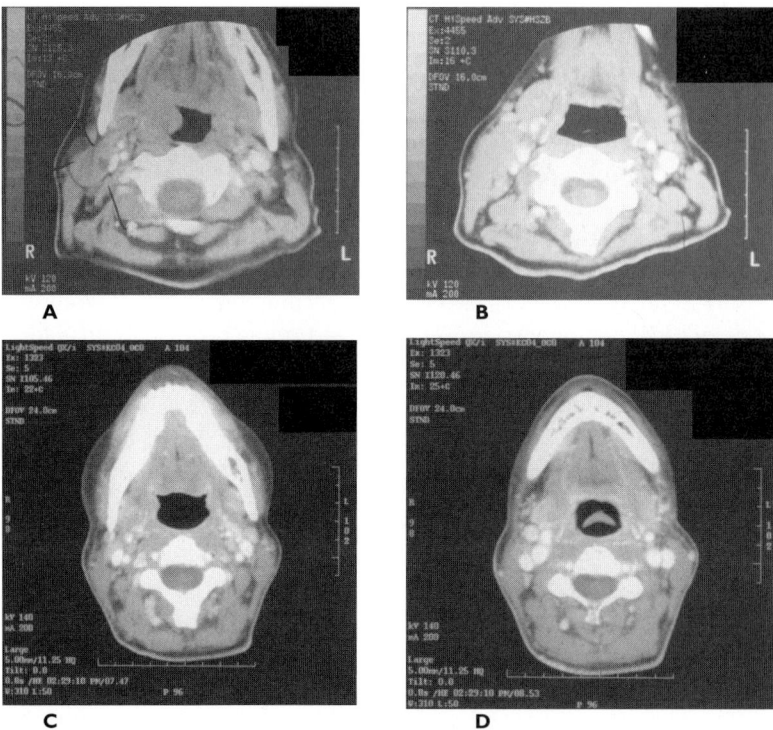

FIGURE 17.2 Pre- and post-treatment CTs from a 43-year-old female with T2 N2C squamous cell carcinoma of the right tonsil treated with concurrent cetuximab and RT (76.8 Gy at 1.2 Gy b.i.d.) on the phase I UAB protocol. The patient had bulky right-sided adenopathy (5 × 4.5 cm clinically) at the level of the primary (A) and right-sided adenopathy seen best on a cut immediately above the hyoid bone. Follow-up CT one month after completion of therapy shows a dramatic clinical response at these levels (C corresponds to A and D corresponds to B) with minimal residual adenopathy and restoration of symmetry in the oropharynx. Right-sided planned neck dissection shortly after the follow-up scan removed 23 nodes with no residual carcinoma found. The patient is currently NED at 1.5 years.

Similarly, angiostatin has been studied *in vivo* with concomitant radiotherapy [43]. These experiments were performed on a Lewis lung cancer mouse xenograft. Angiostatin is a proteolytic fragment of plasminogen, which has been shown to inhibit tumor growth by suppressing angiogenesis. In these *in vivo* experiments (from the University of Chicago), synergy with radiation was demonstrated in much the same way as it was shown with anti-VEGF antibodies.

It is not immediately obvious that reduction in tumor vasculature would lead to an improved tumor response, in view of the negative impact of hypoxia on radiosensitivity. Somewhat surprisingly, administration of anti-angiogenesis factors were demonstrated to lead to an increase in tumor oxygenation despite a decrease in vascular density [44, 45]. This is attributed to a decrease in the amount of oxygen consumption, or possibly a difference in the quality of the microvasculature [45].

Angiogenesis inhibitors show considerable promise as possible synergistic agents for use with radiotherapy, which complements their potential systemic activity. Cetuximab and other agents targeting the EGFr appear to act in part via the anti-angiogenesis pathway, which may contribute to synergy with radiation. Although angiogenesis inhibitors have been explored in numerous recent trials, the use of these inhibitors in combination with radiotherapy will be the subject of future trials.

III. RAS

For many years the Ras family has been considered a promising set of onco-genes for exploitation in the radiosensitization context. In 1988, Sklar demonstrated that transfection of NIH 3T3 mouse cells with mutant Ras (several Ras alleles with missense mutations) resulted in radioresistance [24]. After many years of study, the concept of Ras inhibition as a method of radiosensitization has reached the clinic. These clinical trials have involved the farnesyl transferase inhibitors (FTI), which interfere with the ability of mutated Ras to bind to the inner surface of the cell membrane [46]. Ras is the most commonly mutated oncogene in human cancers. There are several known human alleles, denoted K-Ras, H-Ras, N-Ras, and R-Ras. K-Ras is found to be mutated in 30% of cancers overall and in 50% of colon cancers and 90% of pancreatic cancers. Another important human variant is H-Ras, so named due to its association with the Harvey rat sarcoma virus. It was the first to be discovered, but it is less commonly mutated in human cancers than K-Ras. The alleles N-Ras and R-Ras are less commonly associated with human cancers, although both can transform cells [47]. Ras forms one of the initial components of a signal transduction cascade in human cells (Figure 17.1). It is a membrane-bound protein with intrinsic GTPase activity, and the transformation of GTP to GDP is involved in Ras inactivation fol-lowing triggering of the downstream cascade. The structure of Ras contains a binding domain for GDP or GTP, and binding to GDP represents the stable off state. When Ras is activated by a tyrosine kinase, such as EGFr, the wild-type Ras is dissociated from GDP. Binding with GTP then occurs (GTP is more prevalent in the cytosol than GDP), and Ras-GTP represents the active form. Activity is transient due to rapid inactivation with the assistance of GAP with GTP being transformed to GDP.

Common mutations of Ras, typically at codon 12, lead to a sustained sig-nal in the absence of stimuli. Sustained signaling along the MAP kinase path-way promotes proliferation and inhibits apoptosis. The primary signaling cascade consists of the elements Ras/Raf/MEK/ERK/Elk-1/c-fos. This sequence forms a cascade of activating phosphorylations, the final elements of which produce an anti-apoptotic signal that leads to an increase in DNA synthesis and eventual mitosis. Ras also interacts with other signaling cas-cades including stress activated protein kinase (SAPK), which have an oppo-site pro-apoptotic influence.

Ras and Raf interact when Ras is in the bound state with GTP [48]. In many cases of human cancer, Ras is found to be mutated such that its GTPase activity is lost, yet it retains its kinase activity. This prevents the Ras oncogene from becoming inactivated by transformation of GTP to GDP, yet it allows Ras to continue activating the MAP kinase pathway. This failure to reverse the normally transient active state leads to persistent proliferation.

Ras is normally found as a membrane-bound protein on the inner surface of the cell membrane (Figure 17.1). This location allows it to remain in close proximity to tyrosine kinases such as EGFr, which it requires for activation. Posttranscriptional modification of Ras is required via the process of prenylation, which modifies the C terminal end of Ras. In the case of K-Ras this process takes place via the enzyme farnesyl transferase and involves the attachment of a 15 carbon compound. A similar process takes place in case of H-Ras with a different lipid residue added. It has been shown by several investigators that interfering with the ability of Ras to bind to the membrane by blocking farnesylation disrupts its function [49].

Various cell lines with Ras mutations have been shown to exhibit radioresistance [24, 50]. Several attempts have been made to exploit a developing understanding of the molecular biology of Ras to reverse radioresistance. One of the earlier attempts involved inactivating Ras mRNA via antisense technology [51]. A more elaborate scheme involved single chain antibodies targeting K-Ras transfected by an adenoviral vector [52]. The intracellular single chain was able to restore radiosensitivity in cells with mutant K-Ras. In general, radiosensitization via Ras disruption targets only cells with mutant Ras. This strategy potentially allows specificity to tumor cells. The first attempt to induce enhanced radiosensitivity via interference with the membrane binding of Ras was undertaken with lovastatin, a drug which non-specifically interferes with lipid metabolism. Lovastatin was shown to induce radiosensitivity, and this was attributed to disruption of farnesylation [53, 54]. These results have since been improved upon via the use of more specific FTIs such as FTI-277 [55]. These results were shown to be effective in inducing increased radiosensitivity in human tumor cell lines with a known Ras mutation. Failure to modify the radiosensitivity of cells without a Ras mutation offers the potential for selectively targeting tumor cells without relying on tumor specific vectors.

Similar to the case with anti-EGFr agents, the FTIs appear to have multiple effects that may contribute to radiosensitization. Growth inhibition induced by FTIs may not be entirely due to inhibition of activated Ras. Induction of p21 (WAF/CIP), a cyclin-dependent kinase inhibitor activated by p53, is seen after transfection with prenylation inhibitors, which leads to cell cycle arrest in G1 and G2 [56–58]. These events occur for cells with wild-type Ras as well as mutant cells.

A. Ras and Clinical Trials of Radiosensitization

Specific FTIs have been explored in clinical trials including a clinical trial with concurrent radiotherapy [46]. This trial involved a total of 13 patients with pancreatic cancer, head and neck cancer, and lung cancer treated to doses between 59.4 and 70 Gy with the radiation dose dependent on the tumor site. The peptide FTI-778123 was administered on weeks 1, 2, 4, 5, and 7 of radiotherapy with an escalating dose schedule. No grade 3 or 4 toxicities have been observed to date with two complete responses seen (head and neck) and two partial responses, all in the second dose-escalation ($280 \text{ mg/m}^2\text{/day}$). Escalation to $560 \text{ mg/m}^2\text{/day}$ is currently being evaluated.

IV. MODULATION OF p53

The transcription factor p53 is the most commonly mutated gene in human cancers. Its normal function relates to cell cycle control via CDK inhibitors (primarily p21), stimulation of DNA repair via GADD45, and induction of apoptosis. Levels are affected by a feedback mechanism involving MDM2, and loss of this feedback in the mutant p53 case leads to increased levels of dysfunctional p53 protein. Upregulation of wild-type p53 can occur through multiple cellular insults including DNA damage and viral infection. Failure of damage to the genetic material to induce a checkpoint, stimulate DNA repair, and conditionally promote apoptosis could lead to propagation of mutations. For this reason p53 is known as the "guardian of the genome." Resistance to chemotherapy and radiotherapy in mutant p53 cells arises largely from failure of apoptosis.

Transfection of p53 into cells has been shown to lead to increased radiosensitivity in several cases of mutant cell lines. Results have been inconsistent, with some wild-type cells showing a response and some mutant lines becoming resistant. The adenoviral vector has been the most commonly used transfection vehicle, and Ad-p53 has been shown to increase radiosensitivity in mutant p53 colon and ovarian cancer cell lines [59, 60]. Ad-p53 with concurrent irradiation has been shown to be synergistic *in vivo*, using a mutant p53 head and neck cancer mouse model xenograft [61]. Restoration of the G1-S checkpoint and apoptosis was observed as well as radiosensitization. Additionally, pro-apoptotic regulators of apoptosis (bax and bak) have been shown to be upregulated after transfection of wild-type p53 [62]. Transfection of Ad-53 (RPR/INGN 201) has been shown to radiosensitize non-small cell lung cancer (NSCLC) cells and not to sensitize normal lung fibroblasts [63].

Retroviral vectors have also been used to transfect p53. Radiosensitivity was induced in a line of p53 mutant breast cancer cells, but was not observed in wild-type breast cancer cells [64]. An increase in sensitivity to chemotherapy agents was not seen for these lines.

Effectiveness of p53 transfection appears to be dependent on the particular target cancer cells [65]. Ad-p53 was effective in both wild-type and mutant prostate cancer cells [66]. Ad-53 also induced increased radiosensitivity in p53 normal glioma cells [67]. The transfection led to increased levels of active p53 and increased apoptosis. Failure of p53 transfection to radiosensitize some p53 mutants may stem from the presence of other mechanisms of resistance on an individual basis.

Wortmannin, an inhibitor of PI3K, leads to an inhibition of radiation-induced upregulation of p53/p21 in wild-type cells [68]. However, in this study little change in p53 and p21 levels were seen in mutant cells, while radiosensitization was seen in both wild-type and mutant cells. Overall levels of p53 are an unreliable indicator of the potential effects of wortmannin, as mutant p53 is typically overexpressed. The presence of radiosensitization in the mutant case suggests that wortmannin sensitizes via a mechanism unrelated to p53, but the mechanism remains unclear at present. Increased activity of PI3K has been shown to lead to radioresistance in melanoma cell lines, resistance which was reduced by administration of wortmannin [21]. Wortmannin is an inhibitor of many protein kinases, in particular DNA-PK, the primary kinase involved in the repair of DNA double-strand breaks. Wortmannin causes radiosensitization in ATM mutant cells, but not in DNA-PK deficient cells, which suggests that radiosensitization occurs via disruption of DNA-PK and that this is independent of ATM [69].

Potential problems with clinical implementation of these p53 altering treatments are complex. Resistance to p53 gene therapy can occur from p53 inactivation via MDM2 feedback inhibition, the presence of inactivating proteins of viral origin (HPV E6 or adenoviral E1b), or the failure of adenoviral infection. Multiple phase I trials of p53 gene therapy are under way with concurrent radiotherapy and p53 gene therapy currently being investigated by ECOG in the setting of NSCLC [70, 71]. Phase II NSCLC data of Ad-p53 gene therapy (RPR/INGN 201) with concurrent radiotherapy has recently been reported [72]. Tumors were directly injected during bronchoscopy or under CT guidance. Eight of eleven patients undergoing biopsy after treatment were pathologically negative.

V. DNA DAMAGE RECOGNITION AND REPAIR

Repair mechanisms for DNA damage remain under investigation, and to some extent have been elucidated in recent years. Nucleotide excision repair, the removal and replacement of chemically altered nucleotides, is controlled by a series of genes denoted ERCC1 through 5 (excision repair cross-complementing) [73]. Cross-complementing genes are those human genes that reverse a defect upon transfection into a mutant cell line. Nucleotide damage is frequently caused by UV radiation and some chemicals. Defects in this repair mechanism are found in xeroderma pigmentosum and Cockayne's syndrome, which renders such patients sensitive to UV radiation. However, the lethal events caused by higher LET ionizing radiation more typically involve DNA breaks, and the ERCC genes are less relevant.

Similar methods of cross-complementation have uncovered the family of human genes denoted XRCC1 through 7, which reverse the sensitivity to ionizing radiation exhibited by certain mutant rodent cell lines [6]. XRCC1 is known to be involved in the repair of single-strand DNA damage [74]. Other XRCC complementation groups are related to double-strand break repair. This double-strand break repair tends to take place via non-homologous end-joining (repair without use of the sister chromatid) in eukaryotic cells, and is related to the V(D)J recombination that plays a central role in generating random immunoglobulins and receptors during development. Several of the XRCC genes have been identified. XRCC4 is mutated in the Chinese hamster mutant XR-1 [75]. The protein product of XRCC4 is now known to form a dimer with DNA ligase IV, and XRCC4 has been shown to be phosphorylated by DNA-PK [76]. Both DNA-PK and DNA ligase IV are components of non-homologous end-joining, along with ku70, ku80, and XRCC4. Ku70 and ku80, along with the catalytic subunit of DNA-PK (DNA-PKcs), bind to the free ends of the DNA breaks and protect them from degradation [77]. The XRCC4 DNA ligase IV dimer is then recruited and repair takes place and the details of the repair process remain a topic of investigation. The genes XRCC5 and XRCC6 have been found to code for the proteins ku70 and ku80, respectively. XRCC7 codes for DNA-PKcs. The precise roles of XRCC2 and XRCC3 are presently under investigation and evidence suggests involvement in DNA break repair as well as contributing to centromere stability and chromosome segregation [78–80]. XRCC2 and XRCC3 are part of the hRad51 family of proteins, which are human analogs of homologous recombination proteins in yeast [78, 80].

It may be possible to induce radiosensitization by directly modulating DNA damage recognition and repair mechanisms. Dysfunctional DNA repair has been shown to lead to an increase in radiosensitivity [81–83]. In view of the complexity of the DNA repair process, there are many possible approaches that could potentially lead to clinical translation. Guidance in selecting appropriate molecular targets stems from known human mutations that give rise to alterations in clinical radiation sensitivity. Promising targets include NBS1, ATM, and hMre11, which are the genes mutated in Nijmegen breakage syndrome (NBS) ataxia-telangiectasia (AT), and ataxia-telangiectasia-like disorder (ATLD), respectively. The nature of these syndromes is described below. The gene products of ATM, NBS1, and hMre11 may be targeted by several means, either by interfering with synthesis or interacting with the protein products. The V(D)J related double-stranded DNA-PK repair mechanism is also a potential target.

NBS is closely related to the better known AT syndrome with both characterized by chromosomal instability, immune deficiency, and high incidence of malignancy. Both populations present in childhood. Malignancies tend to be hematopoietic in both cases, and chromosomal instability predominantly affects chromosomes 7 and 14. The clinical presentation of the syndromes is somewhat different. AT patients present with severe neuromotor dysfunction with cerebellar degeneration, dilation of facial blood vessels, and immune deficiency related to humoral (primarily IgA) and cell-mediated immunity. NBS patients present with microcephaly, mental retardation, facial erythema, café-au-lait spots, and IgA deficiency. NBS is less common than AT, with only 50 patients known world-wide. NBS patients are considered to have a greater predisposition to cancer and genomic instability, which may account for the low incidence of homozygotes in the population, despite an incidence of heterozygotes of 1–4% in the general population [84].

NBS1 is a gene that codes for the protein nibrin, which has been implicated as part of a double-stranded DNA repair complex. Nibrin has recently been found to be equivalent to p95, a component of a five protein complex including hMre11 and hRad50, which rapidly localizes to the areas of DNA damage [85]. p95 has been shown to be an essential component in the association of hMre11 and hRad50, without which these proteins do not colocalize in response to radiation. It is believed that these proteins form a complex immediately upon synthesis (the independent proteins are detected only at very low levels). There is evidence that this complex acts similarly to ATM in that it appears to be involved as a sensor of DNA damage. Unlike ATM, NBS1 mutations do not interfere with the G2-M checkpoint, although there is evidence indicating G1-S is disrupted [86].

Recently an additional related syndrome has been described in a handful of patients, denoted as ATLD, in which other elements of the nibrin/hRad50/hMre11 complex are mutated. Gene expression experiments for these mutants as well as for NBS cells and AT cells show a six-fold under-expression of Jun Kinase activity relative to normal cells following exposure to radiation [87]. This finding suggests the possibility that apoptosis may play a role in increased radiosensitivity of these mutant lines. An additional relationship between ATM and NBS has recently been uncovered, in which nibrin is phosphorylated by ATM in response to ionizing radiation leading to transient S-phase arrest [88–90].

The breast cancer associated gene BRCA1 may be related to the nibrin/hRad50/hMre11 mechanism and have effects relating to DNA repair. BRCA1 is intimately involved with Rad51, colocalizing with it, phosphorylating it, and altering its cellular localization in response to DNA damage [91, 92]. These results establish a potential role for BRCA1 with homologous DNA repair [91]. BRCA1 mutant cells are radiosensitive with transfection of wild-type BRCA1 restoring radioresistance [93, 94]. BRCA1 has recently been shown to colocalize with the hMre11-hRad50-p95 complex after exposure to ionizing radiation [94]. Cells with mutated BRCA1 did not show similar colocalization. It has been suggested that BRCA1 is part of a larger complex including ATM, nibrin, hMre11, hRad50, and components of transcription-coupled repair, and that this complex may be involved in detection of DNA damage and maintenance of genomic stability [95]. However, localization of the nibrin/hRad50/hMre11 complex to sites of DNA damage occurs in the absence of functional BRCA1 [96]. Although both BRCA1 and the nibrin complex play roles in DNA damage recognition and repair, the degree to which these proteins are co-dependent is unclear.

AT, NBS, and ATLD patients are known to be extremely sensitive to radiation — two to three times more sensitive compared to normal cells [87, 97, 98]. In the case of AT, heterozygotes are also more radiosensitive than normals [99]. This finding has not been clearly established for NBS or ATLD. NBS is a rare disorder, and ATLD (hMre11 mutants) is even less common, with only a handful of known patients. The functions of ATM and the hMre11-hRad50-nibrin complex have recently been better elucidated. The hMre11-hRad50-nibrin complex has been implicated as part of a DNA double-strand break recognition complex [85]. Nibrin is phosphorylated by ATM at a known site, and this phosphorylation is essential for the function of the complex [88–90]. This phosphorylation takes place in response to double-strand breaks (ionizing radiation), and leads to a transient S-phase arrest. Nibrin is expressed in extremely small quantities, expression is not upregulated by ionizing radiation, and it represents an attractive target for radiosensitization. The protein hMre11 is also phosphorylated after irradiation, and it is phosphorylated *in vitro* by ATM. It is not known if these actions are essential for the function of the complex.

Competitive inhibition of nibrin has been evaluated on human cancer cell lines demonstrating modest radiosensitization [100]. The competitive inhibitor was formed by synthesizing a truncated version of nibrin intracellularly, such that the mutant protein would bind to the complex but be unable to interact with DNA breaks. Methods that do not require degradation and recycling of the wild-type complex may offer improved radiosensitization.

Disruption of DNA-PK double-strand break repair has been explored to a limited extent. Wortmannin is a non-specific protein kinase inhibitor that disrupts intracellular signal transduction and inhibits DNA-PK. It is argued that this is the mechanism of wortmannin-induced radiosensitization [69]. Adenoviral transfection of a single chain intracellular antibody to ku protein (a component of DNA-PK), directed with a nuclear localization sequence, failed to lead to detectable radiosensitization [101]. The single chain antibody was designed to bind with the full ku protein and conceivably may not have interacted with a relevant epitope. Further work is necessary to determine whether DNA-PK double-strand break repair can be targeted to enhance the effects of radiation.

ATM has shown potential as a target for radiosensitization. Some preliminary reports have indicated radiosensitization via antisense targeting of ATM in glioma and prostate cell lines [11, 12]. In these *in vitro* studies, cDNAs coding for multiple RNA antisense chains were transfected, which disabled ATM synthesis at multiple sites. According to current models, ATM is involved in DNA damage recognition and checkpoint control. ATM is also implicated in maintaining the accuracy of DNA repair [102]. In the presence of normal ATM, cells with intact p53 tend to induce p53 expression and activate the G1-S checkpoint in response to radiation damage. In the case of mutant ATM, cells are radiosensitive, which may in part be due to p53 mediated apoptosis. Therefore use of ATM as a target may conflict with eventual adenoviral targeting schemes that take advantage of p53 dysfunction in cancer cells [103]. However, it is currently unclear if ATM-related radiosensitivity is truly dependent on apoptosis [104]. ATM is involved in both the G1-S and G2-M checkpoints, the latter of which is independent of p53 and may be more important in conferring radiosensitivity. It may also be involved in the S checkpoint and spindle checkpoint [105, 106].

VI. OTHER PROMISING APPROACHES

Based on favorable results in the context of photodynamic therapy, the redox agent motexafin gadolinium (MGd) has been evaluated recently with concurrent radiotherapy and chemotherapy [107, 108]. MGd is a metalloporphyrin that tends to localize in tumors and has been shown to be a radiosensitizer *in vitro* and *in vivo*. It catalyzes the production of superoxide anion and hydrogen peroxide. *In vivo* animal models have also demonstrated an improved mean time to regrowth when used with concurrent chemotherapy consisting of carboplatin, bleomycin, and doxorubicin [109]. MGd has the additional property of allowing MRI imaging of the redox agent distribution. A phase I dose-escalation trial has been carried out on a small series of biliary and pancreatic cancer patients. No response data is available at present [110]. Concurrent radiotherapy was delivered up to 50.4 Gy in 28 fractions. MGd was evaluated on 61 patients with brain metastases with radiotherapy (30 Gy in 10 fractions) [107]. Survival was similar to historical results with whole brain radiotherapy alone, although a 72% radiological response rate was seen. Hepatic toxicity was the dose-limiting toxicity.

Prostaglandin inhibitors, in particular inhibitors of cyclooxygenase 2 (Cox2), have shown promise as radiosensitizers. Cox2 is an important enzyme that has recently been shown to have potential as a cancer prevention agent. Both Cox1 and Cox2 are associated with prostaglandin synthesis. Cox1 is considered a housekeeping gene and Cox2 is an inducible counterpart that tends to be overexpressed under situations of cell stress. Cox2 is overexpressed in several types of cancer [111, 112]. Cox2 inhibitors have demonstrated promise in cancer prevention, in particular for colon cancer [111]. Cox2 has also been shown to be overexpressed in vascular endothelium and is believed to be associated with the angiogenesis of prostate cancer [111]. Irradiation can transiently increase Cox2 expression. In a series of experiments employing Western blots, Cox2 protein expression was evaluated at doses of 5, 10, and 15 Gy [113]. A 100% increase in Cox2 protein expression was observed at 15 Gy.

Demonstrating the fact that many of these new agents have some common effects, angiogenesis and apoptosis may be important mechanisms by which Cox2 inhibitors sensitize cells to irradiation. Cox2 increases levels of VEGF, induces production of factors stimulating endothelial cell migration, and inhibits endothelial cell apoptosis [114]. *In vivo* experiments utilizing a sarcoma/mouse xenograft demonstrated radiosensitization with the Cox2 inhibitor SC-236 [115]. There was no increase in normal tissue effect. Cox2 does not appear to be involved in repair of radiation injury, unlike Cox1 [116]. SC-236 has also been shown to be a radiosensitizer in the setting of a glioma xenograft, and radiosensitization was also seen *in vitro* with the clonogenic survival assay [117]. This *in vitro* response indicates that the mechanism of synergy with radiation involves more than angiogenesis. The nature of the mechanism is unclear, as changes in cell cycle distribution and differences in apoptosis were not seen following SC-236 administration. In addition to affects associated with angiogenesis and apoptosis, Cox2 may play a role in the cancer physiology by modulating immune surveillance via prostaglandin E2 [118, 119]. These agents appear to require further mechanistic studies, but show promise as future clinically applicable agents in the effort to enhance the radiation response.

Promising preclinical data have lead to several ongoing clinical oncology trials. A head and neck cancer prevention trial utilizing celecoxib is currently under way at MD Anderson for patients with premalignant lesions. NSCLC trials incorporating celecoxib with and without radiotherapy and chemotherapy are currently under way at MD Anderson, Vanderbilt University, and the Hoosier Oncology Group (HOG). Esophagus cancer phase I/II trials are being initiated by HOG using celecoxib for cancer prevention and also for treatment with concurrent cisplatin/5-FU and radiotherapy. Celecoxib is also being explored clinically in phase I/II trials with concurrent chemoradiation for pancreatic cancer and rectal cancer (MD Anderson), with the rectal cancer trial involving concurrent celecoxib, radiotherapy, and CPT-11.

VII. CONCLUSIONS

Multiple new agents are showing promise as radiosensitizers in the laboratory, and several of these are coming to clinical trial. Agents that interfere with growth factor receptors or their downstream signaling cascades are currently receiving a great deal of attention. For example, one of these agents (cetuximab) is under investigation in a phase III trial with radiotherapy for head and neck cancer. The mechanism of radiosensitization for the new approaches is multifocal. Modulation of VEGF and alteration of angiogenesis seems to play a role in several cases including cetuximab, FTI, and Cox2 inhibition. The importance of angiogenesis suggests that the standard measure of radiosensitization, the clonogenic assay, may be inadequate and more clinically relevant *in vivo* assays are required.

Basic research into the underlying molecular biology of cancer is leading to an increasing understanding of the complex mechanisms controlling cell growth, signal transduction, DNA repair, and cell death. Methods for selectively targeting tumor cells remain underdeveloped. With recent important advances in the geometric targeting of radiotherapy, it is likely that radiotherapy will remain a mainstay of cancer therapy in the future. Research on the complex interplay between irradiation and the molecular biology of the cell promises to increase tumor control and decrease morbidity of treatment.

VIII. ADDENDUM

Due to delays between preparation of the manuscript for this chapter and final publication, some of the material in the chapter does not reflect advances in the field over the intervening period. It was not feasible to rewrite the chapter to reflect the current status of the field. Since the chapter was written, several clinical trials involving radiosensitizers have completed, and several are currently underway.

The most significant advances in the clinical use of nonchemotherapy radiosensitization have taken place in the area of EGFr inhibition, particularly monoclonal antibody inhibition of EGFr. The international phase III trial of radiotherapy with or without cetuximab accrued 424 patients and was reported at ASCO 2004, with a minimum follow-up of 24 months [1, 2]. The addition of cetuximab resulted in statistically significant improvements in local control and survival, both with a p value of 0.02, without an increase in toxicity. The degree of survival improvement was comparable to that seen with the addition of radiosensitizing concurrent chemotherapy, based on the recent MACH-NC meta-analysis of nearly 17,000 patients enrolled in 87 randomized trials [3]. In both cases there is an absolute survival improvement of approximately 8%. At this point it is unclear if the survival improvement seen with hyperfractionated radiotherapy will be additive to this, when hyperfractionated therapy is combined with cetuximab or chemotherapy. This issue is being addressed in current trials. The RTOG is currently conducting a randomized phase II postoperative head and neck cancer trial, using cetuximab with different chemotherapy agents concurrently with radiotherapy. There is also an ongoing RTOG lung cancer trial with concurrent cetuximab and radiotherapy.

Cetuximab is a chimeric antibody, which may contribute the typical follicular rash seen in many patients. There are now several humanized anti-EGFr antibodies being evaluated in preliminary clinical trials. Other inhibitors of EGFr continue to be promising. In particular the tyrosine kinase inhibitor ZD1839 has engendered considerable interest, and is currently being evaluated as a radiosensitizer in head and neck and lung cancer trials, and the CALGB is evaluating it with chemoradiation for NSCLC [4].

Farnesyl transferase and combination farnesyl geranylgeranyltransferase inhibitors have been evaluated in phase I trials with radiotherapy for lung cancer, cancer of the head and neck, and pancreatic cancer [5]. Promising responses have been observed, with acceptable toxicity. While clinical results on the use of these agents as a single-modality treatment have been negative, the potential benefit with concurrent radiotherapy remains.

Tirapazamine has been evaluated in multiple preliminary trials with various chemotherapy agents, and in addition there have been several recent radiotherapy trials for lung cancer and cancer of the head and neck. SWOG performed a pilot study with the agent in the setting of small cell lung cancer, with concurrent cisplatin, etoposide, and radiotherapy [6]. Promising results have been observed in the setting of head and neck cancer, both definitive and recurrent, with better results seen in those patients with hypoxia evident on misonidazole-PET imaging [7, 8]. Phase III data should be available in the near future.

Cox-2 inhibitors have been explored in numerous clinical trials, with the majority of these being cancer prevention trials in patients at high risk for malignancy. These trials have been disrupted, and in many cases discontinued, by increased cardiac risk reported after preliminary analyses in a few prevention studies. A smaller number of clinical trials continue to explore the use of Cox-2 inhibition as a radiation sensitizer, a role in which the drug is not taken over a prolonged period of years and the potential benefit outweighs the risk. This approach continues to hold promise, and clinical trials continue, with a locally advanced head and neck cancer trial at the University of Alabama at Birmingham [9], and a lung cancer trial at MD Anderson Cancer Center [10]. The RTOG is currently conducting a study of concurrent celecoxib with radiotherapy for lung cancer, and recently closed a similar study for cervical cancer. Results for these studies are not yet available.

Radiation therapy remains a mainstay of cancer therapy for many potentially curable malignancies. Biological sensitizers remain an active topic of research and there remains considerable activity on the clinical trial front. In the case of the most successful biologic radiosensitizer to date (cetuximab), there is little activity in the absence of radiation, yet as an enhancer of radiotherapy a survival benefit was seen. This is an important lesson to keep in mind, as many promising agents are abandoned after failing to show cytotoxic activity on their own.

ADDENDUM REFERENCES

1. Bonner J, Giralt J, Harari PM et al. Cetuximab prolongs survival in patients with locoregionally advanced squamous cell carcinoma of head and neck: A phase III study of high dose radiation therapy with or without cetuximab. *J. Clin. Oncol.* 2004; 22(14S):5507.
2. Bonner JA, Raisch KP, Buchsbaum DJ et al. Combination radiation and epidermal growth factor receptor blockade in head and neck cancer. *Cancer Invest.* 2004; 23.
3. Bourhis J, Amand C, and Pignon J -P, Update of MACH-NC (meta-analysis of chemotherapy in head and neck cancer) database focused on concomitant chemoradiotherapy. *J. Clin. Oncol.* 2004; 22(14S): 5505.
4. Ready N, Herndon J, Vokes EE et al. Initial cohort toxicity evaluation for chemoradiotherapy (CRT) and ZD1839 in stage III non-small cell lung cancer (NSCLC): A CALGB stratified phase II trial. *J. Clin. Oncol.* 2004; 22(14S): 7078.
5. Martin NE, Brunner TB, Bernhard EJ et al. A phase I trial of the farnesyltransferase and geranylgeranyltransferase-I inhibitor L-778,123 (L-778) and radiotherapy for locally advanced pancreatic cancer. *J. Clin. Oncol.*, 2004; 22(14S): 4098.
6. Le Q, Chansky K, Williamson SK et al. SWOG 0004 – pilot study of tirapazamine (TPZ) plus cisplatin/etoposide (PE) and concurrent thoracic radiotherapy (RT) in limited small cell lung cancer (LSCLC). in *ASCO Proceedings, 2002.*
7. Rischin D, Peters L, Smith J et al. Preliminary results of TROG 98.02 – a randomized phase II study of 5-fluorouracil, cisplatin and radiation versus tirapazamine, cisplatin and radiation for advanced squamous cell carcinoma of the head and neck. in *ASCO Proceedings*, 2003.
8. Cohen EEW, Rosine D, Loh E, Haraf DJ, Vokes EE, and Bourhis J, A phase I study of cisplatin, tirapazamine and accelerated re-irradiation in unresectable recurrent head and neck cancer. *J. Clin. Oncol.*, 2004; 22(14S): 5511.
9. George J, Peters G, Carroll W, Nabell L, and Ove R, Radiosensitization with a Cox-2 inhibitor, with chemoradiation for cancer of the head and neck. *J. Clin. Oncol.*, 2004; 22(14S): 5542.
10. Liao ZX, Chen Y, Komaki R, Cox JD, and Milas L, A phase I study combining thoracic radiation (RT) with celecoxib in patients with non-small cell lung cancer (NSCLC). *Proc. Am. Soc. Clin. Oncol.*, 2003; 22: 216.

REFERENCES

1. Adams GE. Chemical radiosensitization of hypoxic cells. *Br. Med. Bull.* 1973; 29(1):48–53.
2. Rowinsky EK. The pursuit of optimal outcomes in cancer therapy in a new age of rationally designed target-based anticancer agents. *Drugs* 2000; 60(Suppl 1):1–14; discussion 41–42.
3. Dorie MJ, Brown, JM. Tumor-specific, schedule-dependent interaction between tirapazamine (SR 4233) and cisplatin. *Cancer Res.* 1993: 53(19):4633–4636.
4. Rischin D et al. Phase I trial of concurrent tirapazamine, cisplatin, and radiotherapy in patients with advanced head and neck cancer. *J. Clin. Oncol.* 2001; 19(2):535–542.
5. Brown JM. Therapeutic targets in radiotherapy. *Int. J. Radiat. Oncol. Biol. Phys.* 2001; 49(2):319–326.
6. Maity A et al. Potential molecular targets for manipulating the radiation response. *Int. J. Radiat. Oncol. Biol. Phys.* 1997; 37(3):639–653.
7. Buchsbaum DJ et al. Approaches to enhance cancer radiotherapy employing gene transfer methods. *Gene Ther.* 1996; 3(12):1042–1068.
8. Rosenzweig KE et al. Radiosensitization of human tumor cells by the phosphatidylinositol3-kinase inhibitors wortmannin and LY294002 correlates with inhibition of DNA-dependent protein kinase and prolonged G2-M delay. *Clin. Cancer Res.* 1997; 3(7):1149–1156.

9. Zhang W et al. Radiosensitization and inhibition of deoxyribonucleic acid repair in rat glioma cells by long-term treatment with 12-O-tetradecanoylphorbol 13-acetate. *Neurosurgery* 1993; 32(3):432–437; discussion 437.

10. Zhang N et al. Isolation of full-length ATM cDNA and correction of the ataxia-telangiectasia cellular phenotype. *Proc. Natl. Acad. Sci. U. S. A.* 1997; 94(15):8021–8026.

11. Fan Z et al. Adenovirus-mediated antisense ATM gene transfer sensitizes prostate cancer cells to radiation [in process citation]. *Cancer Gene Ther.* 2000; 7(10):1307–1314.

12. Guha C et al. Antisense ATM gene therapy: A strategy to increase the radiosensitivity of human tumors. *Gene Ther.* 2000; 7(10):852–858.

13. Prewett M et al. The biologic effects of C225, a chimeric monoclonal antibody to the EGFR, on human prostate carcinoma. *J. Immunother. Emphasis Tumor Immunol.* 1996; 19(6):419–427.

14. Raymond E, Faivre S, Armand JP. Epidermal growth factor receptor tyrosine kinase as a target for anticancer therapy. *Drugs* 2000; 60(Suppl 1):15–23; discussion 41–42.

15. Gamett DC, Tracy SE, Robinson HL. Differences in sequences encoding the carboxyl-terminal domain of the epidermal growth factor receptor correlate with differences in the disease potential of viral erbB genes. *Proc. Natl. Acad. Sci. U. S. A.* 1986; 83(16):6053–6057.

16. Dassonville O et al. Expression of epidermal growth factor receptor and survival in upper aerodigestive tract cancer. *J. Clin. Oncol.* 1993; 11(10):1873–1878.

17. Dent P et al. Radiation-induced release of transforming growth factor alpha activates the epidermal growth factor receptor and mitogen-activated protein kinase pathway in carcinoma cells, leading to increased proliferation and protection from radiation-induced cell death. *Mol. Biol. Cell.* 1999; 10(8):2493–2506.

18. Ullrich A, Schlessinger J. Signal transduction by receptors with tyrosine kinase activity. *Cell* 1990; 61(2):203–212.

19. Bruns CJ et al. Epidermal growth factor receptor blockade with C225 plus gemcitabine results in regression of human pancreatic carcinoma growing orthotopically in nude mice by antiangiogenic mechanisms. *Clin. Cancer Res.* 2000; 6(5):1936–1948.

20. Buchsbaum DJ et al. Treatment of Mia-PaCa-2 pancreatic cancer with IMC-C225 Anti-EGFr antibody, gemcitabine, and radiation. *Proc. Rad. Res. Soc.* 2001; Abstract P22–278.

21. Krasilnikov M et al. Contribution of phosphatidylinositol 3-kinase to radiation resistance in human melanoma cells. *Mol. Carcinogen.* 1999; 24(1):64–69.

22. Saleh MN et al. Combined modality therapy of A431 human epidermoid cancer using anti-EGFr antibody C225 and radiation. *Cancer Biother. Radiopharm.* 1999; 14(6):451–463.

23. Milas L et al. In vivo enhancement of tumor radioresponse by C225 antiepidermal growth factor receptor antibody. *Clin. Cancer Res.* 2000; 6(2):701–708.

24. Sklar MD. The ras oncogenes increase the intrinsic resistance of NIH 3T3 cells to ionizing radiation. *Science* 1988; 239(4840):645–647.

25. Neubauer A et al. Prognostic importance of mutations in the ras proto-oncogenes in de novo acute myeloid leukemia. *Blood* 1994; 83(6):1603–1611.

26. Slebos RJ et al. K-ras oncogene activation as a prognostic marker in adenocarcinoma of the lung. *N. Engl. J. Med.* 1990; 323(9):561–565.

27. Cohen-Jonathan E et al. Farnesyltransferase inhibitors potentiate the antitumor effect of radiation on a human tumor xenograft expressing activated HRAS. *Radiat. Res.* 2000; 154(2):125–132.

28. Sartor CI. Biological modifiers as potential radiosensitizers: Targeting the epidermal growth factor receptor family. *Semin. Oncol.* 2000; 27(6 Suppl 11):15–20; discussion 92–100.

29. Hagan M et al. Ionizing radiation-induced mitogen-activated protein (MAP) kinase activation in DU145 prostate carcinoma cells: MAP kinase inhibition enhances radiation-induced cell killing and G2/M-phase arrest. *Radiat. Res.* 2000; 153(4):371–383.

30. Huang SM, Harari PM. Modulation of radiation response after epidermal growth factor receptor blockade in squamous cell carcinomas: Inhibition of damage repair, cell cycle kinetics, and tumor angiogenesis. *Clin. Cancer Res.* 2000; 6(6):2166–2174.

31. Bonner JA et al. Enhanced apoptosis with combination C225/radiation treatment serves as the impetus for clinical investigation in head and neck cancers. *J. Clin. Oncol.* 2000; 18(21 Suppl):47S–53S.

32. Gueven N et al. Epidermal growth factor sensitizes cells to ionizing radiation by down-regulating protein mutated in ataxia-telangiectasia. *J. Biol. Chem.* 2001; 276(12):8884–8891.

33. Grandis JR, Zeng Q, Drenning SD. Epidermal growth factor receptor-mediated stat3 signaling blocks apoptosis in head and neck cancer. *Laryngoscope*, 2000; 110(5 Pt 1):868–874.

34. Bonner JA et al. Ionizing radiation-induced MEK and Erk activation does not enhance survival of irradiated human squamous carcinoma cells. *Int. J. Radiat. Oncol. Biol. Phys.* 1998; 42(4):921–925.

35. Grandis JR et al. Requirement of Stat3 but not Stat1 activation for epidermal growth factor receptor-mediated cell growth in vitro. *J. Clin. Invest.* 1998; 102(7):1385–1392.

36. Pietras RJ et al. Monoclonal antibody to HER-2/neureceptor modulates repair of radiation-induced DNA damage and enhances radiosensitivity of human breast cancer cells overexpressing this oncogene. *Cancer Res.* 1999; 59(6):1347–1355.

37. Petit AM et al. Neutralizing antibodies against epidermal growth factor and ErbB-2/neu receptor tyrosine kinases down-regulate vascular endothelial growth factor production by tumor cells in vitro and in vivo: Angiogenic implications for signal transduction therapy of solid tumors. *Am. J. Pathol.* 1997; 151(6):1523–1530.

38. Moulder SL et al. Small molecule EGF receptor tyrosine kinase inhibitor ZD1839 (IRESSA) inhibits HER2/Neu (erb-2) overexpressing breast cancer cells. *Proc. Am. Soc. Clin. Oncol.* 2001; Abstract 8.

39. Ezekiel MP, Robert F, Meredith RF. Phase I study of anti-epidermal growth factor receptor (EGFr) antibody (C225) in combination with irradiation in patients with advanced squamous cell carcinoma of the head and neck (SCCHN). *Proc. Am. Soc. Clin. Oncol.* 2000; Abstract 1522(17):395.

40. Bonner JA et al. Continued response following treatment with IMC-C225, and EGFr MoAb, combined with RT in advanced head and neck malignancies. *Proc. Am. Soc. Clin. Oncol.* 2000; Abstract 5F.

41. Baselga J, Averbuch SD. ZD1839 ("Iressa") as an anticancer agent. *Drugs* 2000; 60(Suppl 1):33–40; discussion 41–42.

42. Gorski DH et al. Blockage of the vascular endothelial growth factor stress response increases the antitumor effects of ionizing radiation. *Cancer Res.* 1999; 59(14):3374–3378.

43. Mauceri HJ et al. Combined effects of angiostatin and ionizing radiation in antitumour therapy. *Nature* 1998; 394(6690):287–291.

44. Teicher BA. Angiogenesis and cancer metastases: therapeutic approaches. *Crit. Rev. Oncol. Hematol.* 1995; 20(1–2):9–39.

45. Lee CG et al. Anti-Vascular endothelial growth factor treatment augments tumor radiation response under normoxic or hypoxic conditions. *Cancer Res.* 2000; 60(19):5565–5570.

46. Hahn SM et al. Phase I trial of the farnesyl protein transferase (FPTase) inhibitor L-78123 in combination with radiotherapy. *Proc. Am. Soc. Clin. Oncol.* 2000; Abstract 906.

47. Graham SM et al. Aberrant function of the Ras-related protein TC21/R-Ras2 triggers malignant transformation. *Mol. Cell Biol.* 1994; 14(6):4108–4115.

48. Marais R et al. Differential regulation of Raf-1, A-Raf, and B-Raf by oncogenic ras and tyrosine kinases. *J. Biol. Chem.* 1997; 272(7):4378–4383.

49. Bernhard EJ et al. The farnesyltransferase inhibitor FTI-277 radiosensitizes H-ras-transformed rat embryo fibroblasts. *Cancer Res.* 1996; 56(8):1727–1730.

50. Bernhard EJ et al. Direct evidence for the contribution of activated N-ras and K-ras oncogenes to increased intrinsic radiation resistance in human tumor cell lines. *Cancer Res.* 2000; 60(23):6597–6600.

51. Pirollo KF et al. Evidence supporting a signal transduction pathway leading to the radiation-resistant phenotype in human tumor cells. *Biochem. Biophys. Res. Commun.* 1997; 230(1):196–201.

52. Russell JS et al. Radiosensitization of human tumor cell lines induced by the adenovirus-mediated expression of an anti-Ras single-chain antibody fragment. *Cancer Res.* 1999; 59(20):5239–5244.

53. Miller AC et al. Differences in radiation-induced micronuclei yields of human cells: Influence of ras gene expression and protein localization. *Int. J. Radiat. Biol.* 1993; 64(5):547–554.

54. Miller AC et al. Increased radioresistance of EJras-transformed human osteosarcoma cells and its modulation by lovastatin, an inhibitor of p21ras isoprenylation. *Int. J. Cancer* 1993; 53(2):302–307.

55. Bernhard EJ et al. Inhibiting Ras prenylation increases the radiosensitivity of human tumor cell lines with activating mutations of ras oncogenes. *Cancer Res.* 1998; 58(8):1754–1761.

56. Sepp-Lorenzino L, Rosen N. A farnesyl-protein transferase inhibitor induces p21 expression and G1 block in p53 wild type tumor cells. *J. Biol. Chem.* 1998; 273(32): 20243–20251.

57. Vogt A et al. The geranylgeranyltransferase-I inhibitor GGTI-298 arrests human tumor cells in G0/G1 and induces p21(WAF1/CIP1/SDI1) in a p53-independent manner. *J. Biol. Chem.* 1997; 272(43):27224–27229.

58. Miquel K et al. GGTI-298 induces G0-G1 block and apoptosis whereas FTI-277 causes G2-M enrichment in A549 cells. *Cancer Res.* 1997; 57(10):1846–1850.

59. Gallardo D, Drazan KE, McBride WH. Adenovirus-based transfer of wild-type p53 gene increases ovarian tumor radiosensitivity. *Cancer Res.* 1996; 56(21):4891–4893.

60. Spitz FR et al. Adenoviral-mediated wild-type p53 gene expression sensitizes colorectal cancer cells to ionizing radiation. *Clin. Cancer Res.* 1996; 2(10):1665–1671.

61. Chang EH et al. Restoration of the G1 checkpoint and the apoptotic pathway mediated by wild-type p53 sensitizes squamous cell carcinoma of the head and neck to radiotherapy. *Arch. Otolaryngol. Head Neck Surg.* 1997; 123(5):507–512.

62. Pearson AS et al. Up-regulation of the proapoptotic mediators Bax and Bak after adenovirus-mediated p53 gene transfer in lung cancer cells. *Clin. Cancer Res.* 2000; 6(3):887–890.

63. Kawabe S et al. Adenovirus-mediated wild-type p53 gene expression radiosensitizes non-small cell lung cancer cells but not normal lung fibroblasts. *Int. J. Radiat. Biol.* 2001; 77(2):185–194.

64. Maeda T et al. Radiosensitivity of human breast cancer cells transduced with wild-type p53 gene is influenced by the p53 status of parental cells. *Anticancer Res.* 2000; 20(2A):869–874.

65. Wu GS, El-Deiry WS. Apoptotic death of tumor cells correlates with chemosensitivity, independent of p53 or bcl-2. *Clin Cancer Res.* 1996; 2(4):623–633.

66. Colletier PJ et al. Adenoviral-mediated p53 transgene expression sensitizes both wild-type and null p53 prostate cancer cells in vitro to radiation. *Int. J. Radiat. Oncol. Biol. Phys.* 2000; 48(5):1507–1512.

67. Lang FF et al. Enhancement of radiosensitivity of wild-type p53 human glioma cells by adenovirus-mediated delivery of the p53 gene. *J. Neurosurg.* 1998; 89(1):125–132.

68. Kubota N et al. Wortmannin sensitizes human glioblastoma cell lines carrying mutant and wild type TP53 gene to radiation. *Cancer Lett.* 2000; 161(2):141–147.

69. Chernikova SB, Wells RL, Elkind MM. Wortmannin sensitizes mammalian cells to radiation by inhibiting the DNA-dependent protein kinase-mediated rejoining of double-strand breaks. *Radiat. Res.* 1999; 151(2):159–166.

70. Weill D et al. Adenoviral-mediated p53 gene transfer to non-small cell lung cancer through endobronchial injection. *Chest* 2000; 118(4):966–970.

71. Roth JA et al. Gene replacement strategies for treating non-small cell lung cancer. *Semin. Radiat. Oncol.* 2000; 10(4):333–342.

72. Swisher SG, Roth JA, Komaki R. A phase II trial of adenoviral mediated p53 gene transfer (RPR/INGN 201) in conjunction with radiation therapy in patients with localized non-small cell lung cancer (NSCLC). *Proc. Am. Soc. Clin. Oncol.* 2000; 19:461a.

73. Sancar A. Mechanisms of DNA excision repair. *Science,* 1994; 266(5193):1954–1956.

74. Thompson LH et al. Molecular cloning of the human XRCC1 gene, which corrects defective DNA strand break repair and sister chromatid exchange. *Mol. Cell Biol.* 1990; 10(12):6160–6171.

75. Li Z et al. The XRCC4 gene encodes a novel protein involved in DNA double-strand break repair and V(D)J recombination. *Cell* 1995; 83(7):1079–1089.

76. Critchlow SE, Bowater RP, Jackson SP. Mammalian DNA double-strand break repair protein XRCC4 interacts with DNA ligase IV. *Curr. Biol.* 1997; 7(8)588–598.

77. Hanakahi LA et al. Binding of inositol phosphate to DNA-PK and stimulation of double-strand break repair. *Cell* 2000; 102(6):721–729.

78. Liu N et al. XRCC2 and XRCC3, new human Rad51-family members, promote chromosome stability and protect against DNA cross-links and other damages. *Mol. Cell* 1998; 1(6):783–793.

79. Pierce AJ et al. XRCC3 promotes homology-directed repair of DNA damage in mammalian cells. *Gene Dev.* 1999; 13(20):2633–2638.

80. Griffin CS et al. Mammalian recombination-repair genes XRCC2 and XRCC3 promote correct chromosome segregation. *Nat. Cell Biol.* 2000; 2(10):757–761.

81. Kelland LR, Edwards SM, Steel GG. Induction and rejoining of DNA double-strand breaks in human cervix carcinoma cell lines of differing radiosensitivity. *Radiat Res.* 1988; 116(3):526–538.

82. Schwartz JL et al. Faster repair of DNA double-strand breaks in radioresistant human tumor cells. *Int. J. Radiat. Oncol. Biol. Phys.* 1988; 15(4):907–912.

83. Wlodek D, Hittelman WN. The repair of double-strand DNA breaks correlates with radiosensitivity of L5178Y-S and L5178Y-R cells. *Radiat. Res.* 1987; 112(1):146–155.

84. Shiloh Y. Ataxia-telangiectasia and the Nijmegen breakage syndrome: Related disorders but genes apart. *Annu. Rev. Genet.* 1997; 31:635–662.

85. Carney JP et al. The hMre11/hRad50 protein complex and Nijmegen breakage syndrome: Linkage of double-strand break repair to the cellular DNA damage response. *Cell* 1998; 93(3):477–486.

86. Sullivan KE et al. Cell cycle checkpoints and DNA repair in Nijmegen breakage syndrome. *Clin. Immunol. Immunopathol.* 1997; 82(1): 43–48.

87. Stewart GS et al. The DNA double-strand break repair gene hMRE11 is mutated in individuals with an ataxia-telangiectasia-like disorder. *Cell* 1999; 99(6): 577–587.

88. Zhao S et al. Functional link between ataxia-telangiectasia and Nijmegen breakage syndrome gene products [see comments]. *Nature* 2000; 405(6785):473–477.

89. Gatei M et al. ATM-dependent phosphorylation of nibrin in response to radiation exposure. *Nat. Genet.* 2000; 25(1):115–119.

90. Lim DS et al. ATM phosphorylates p95/nbs1 in an S-phase checkpoint pathway. *Nature* 2000; 404(6778):613–617.

91. Scully R et al. Association of BRCA1 with Rad51 in mitotic and meiotic cells. *Cell* 1997; 88(2):265–275.

92. Gowen LC et al. BRCA1 required for transcription-coupled repair of oxidative DNA damage. *Science* 1998; 281(5379):1009–1012.

93. Scully R et al. Genetic analysis of BRCA1 function in a defined tumor cell line. *Mol. Cell* 1999; 4(6):1093–1099.

94. Zhong Q et al. Association of BRCA1 with the hRad50-hMre11-p95 complex and the DNA damage response [in process citation]. *Science* 1999; 285(5428):747–750.

95. Wang Y et al. BASC, a super complex of BRCA1-associated proteins involved in the recognition and repair of aberrant DNA structures. *Gene Dev.* 2000; 14(8):927–939.

96. Wu X et al. Independence of R/M/N focus formation and the presence of intact BRCA1. *Science* 2000; 289(5476):11.

97. Chan DW et al. Lack of correlation between ATM protein expression and tumour cell radiosensitivity. *Int. J. Radiat. Biol.* 1998; 74(2):217–224.

98. Taylor AM, Metcalfe JA, McConville C. Increased radiosensitivity and the basic defect in ataxia telangiectasia. *Int. J. Radiat. Biol.* 1989; 56(5):677–684.

99. Arlett CF, Priestley A. An assessment of the radiosensitivity of ataxia-telangiectasia heterozygotes. *Kroc. Found. Ser.* 1985; 19:101–109.

100. Carney JP. 2001; personal communication.

101. Stackhouse MA. 2001; personal communication.

102. Debenham PG et al. Molecular studies on the nature of the repair defect in ataxia- telangiectasia and their implications for cellular radiobiology. *J. Cell Sci.* 1987; (Suppl 6): 177–189.

103. Bischoff JR et al. An adenovirus mutant that replicates selectively in p53-deficient human tumor cells [see comments]. *Science* 1996; 274(5286):373–376.

104. Enns L et al. Radiosensitivity in ataxia telangiectasia fibroblasts is not associated with deregulated apoptosis. *Radiat. Res.* 1998; 150(1):11–16.

105. Takagi M et al. Defective control of apoptosis, radiosensitivity, and spindle checkpoint in ataxia telangiectasia. *Cancer Res.* 1998; 58(21):4923–49299.

106. Morgan SE, Kastan MB. p53 and ATM: Cell cycle, cell death, and cancer. *Adv. Cancer Res.* 1997; 71:1–25.

107. Carde, P et al. Multicenter phase ib/ii trial of the radiation enhancer motexafin gadolinium in patients with brain metastases. *J. Clin. Oncol.* 2001; 19(7):2074–2083.

108. Xu S et al. Effects of Motexafin gadolinium on tumor metabolism and radiation sensitivity. Int. *J. Radiat. Oncol. Biol. Phys.* 2001; 49(5):1381–1390.

109. Miller RA et al. Motexafin Gadolinium (MGd): A REDOX active drug that enhances tumor response to chemotherapy. *Proc. Am. Soc. Clin. Oncol.* 2001; Abstract 453.

110. Fakih M et al. Phase I and pharmacokinetic trial of thrice weekly Motexafin Gadolinium (MGd) with daily radiotherapy (RT) in advanced biliary tree and pancreatic cancers. *Proc. Am. Soc. Clin. Oncol.* 2001; Abstract 454.

111. Yoshimura R et al. Expression of cyclooxygenase-2 in prostate carcinoma. *Cancer* 2000; 89(3):589–596.

112. Gupta S et al. Over-expression of cyclooxygenase-2 in human prostate adenocarcinoma. *Prostate* 2000; 42(1):73–78.

113. Steinauer KK et al. Radiation induces upregulation of cyclooxygenase-2 (COX-2) protein in PC-3 cells. *Int. J. Radiat. Oncol. Biol. Phys.* 2000; 48(2):325–328.

114. Gately S. The contributions of cyclooxygenase-2 to tumor angiogenesis. *Cancer Metast. Rev.* 2000; 19(1–2):19–27.

115. Kishi K et al. Preferential enhancement of tumor radioresponse by a cyclooxygenase-2 inhibitor. *Cancer Res.* 2000; 60(5):1326–1331.

116. Houchen CW, Stenson WF, Cohn SM. Disruption of cyclooxygenase-1 gene results in an impaired response to radiation injury. *Am. J. Physiol. Gastrointest. Liver Physiol.* 2000; 279(5):G858–865.

117. Petersen C et al. Enhancement of intrinsic tumor cell radiosensitivity induced by a selective cyclooxygenase-2 inhibitor. *Clin. Cancer Res.* 2000; 6(6):2513–2520.

118. Soslow RA et al. COX-2 is expressed in human pulmonary, colonic, and mammary tumors. *Cancer* 2000; 89(12):2637–2645.

119. Buttar NS, Wang KK. The "aspirin" of the new millennium: Cyclooxygenase-2 inhibitors. *Mayo Clin. Proc.* 2000; 75(10):1027–1038.

18

PATIENT ACCRUAL TO CLINICAL TRIALS

SUSAN QUELLA

Mayo Clinic
Mayo Alliance for Clinical Trials (Mayo ACT)
Rochester, Minnesota

I. INTRODUCTION
II. SETTING UP THE ENVIRONMENT

I. INTRODUCTION

It has been estimated that in the United States, only 3% of the eligible oncology patient population enrolls in clinical trials [1]. It would be relatively easy to improve on these numbers if there were defined steps for accruing patients to clinical trials. Unfortunately, there are no defined steps, and techniques for accruing patients are as diverse as the research professionals themselves. There are several practical rules that one must remember, however. These rules will be discussed below.

II. SETTING UP THE ENVIRONMENT

A. Rule 1: Be Committed to the Research

Before a healthcare professional can sit down with a patient in need of treatment options for a critical and perhaps life-threatening cancer, they need to be committed to all the options they offer [1]. If the patient senses any ambivalence concerning research and clinical trials, the chances of having that patient enter a trial are low. Studies have shown that patients can be influenced by the media, friends, family, and healthcare professionals, but ultimately they want the information from their physician in a patient-centered, supportive, and reflective manner [2, 3]. If their physician presents the clinical trial information positively, the patient is more likely to enroll [1, 4].

B. Rule 2: Educate the Team

Due to the complex nature of modern health care, no single individual can accrue all patients to a clinical trial. It must be a team effort led by physicians and assisted by nurses and clinical research assistants. It is critical that this entire healthcare team be committed to conducting the study. If one member of the team is ambivalent or negative about the trial, that will become apparent to the patient. This may discourage a patient who was initially open to the possibility of enrolling in a clinical trial. If an uninformed staff member is the patient's initial contact, it could be extremely frustrating for the patient if they want information about particular clinical trials.

To develop a positive cohesive team, communication between members is essential. Regular meetings assist the team in becoming familiar with the clinical trial and regulatory issues. It also develops a team mechanism to accrue patients and conduct the study successfully.

C. Rule 3: Educate the Public

It takes a new drug approximately 14 years to move from the development stage in a laboratory to the consumer for use [5]. The single largest impediment to a speedy process is the slow patient accrual into the clinical trials needed to test that new drug. According to the Harris Interactive Survey [6], the three most common barriers to patient recruitment are the patient, the healthcare provider, and the clinical trial. This survey found that 85% of cancer patients polled were unaware of clinical trials as a treatment option or unaware that a clinical trial could be an option for them.

Clinical trials are a vital step in the research process because they move the science from the laboratory to the patient. The impact of cancer on our population is devastating. Approximately 554,000 people die of cancer in the United States each year [7]. This translates to more than 1500 people dying each day of a disease that is only controlled and will finally be cured through research. Yet, only 3% of cancer patients enter a clinical trial [1, 8]. There are many reasons for this disparity. After subtracting the 85% of cancer patients that are unaware of clinical trials, those persons who may have heard of clinical trials but do not have any knowledge of what they are, how they are conducted, or how to access them, are left [1]. Many people know what clinical trials are, but are suspicious or fearful of them after hearing frightening media reports concerning past trial improprieties by unethical practitioners [1, 8]. Often, patients think that clinical trials are a "last resort" treatment option and do not wish to discuss them. They may also think that they may be "used" as "guinea pigs." Some patients have the misconception that clinical trials are less effective than the standard care [8]. They also are suspicious of the randomization process and believe all clinical trials employ placebos as one study arm. They are afraid of being randomized to the placebo arm and not receiving treatment at all. Finally, many people believe their third-party payers will not cover their costs, which, they think, may be higher than standard care. Only 1.5% of Medicare patients enroll in clinical trials [9]. Often patients will be told by Medicare employees that Medicare will not cover "experimental treatments," even though Medicare covers all items and services used to diagnose and treat patients in a qualifying clinical trial and all reasonable costs associated with treatment of side effects occurring from the clinical trial treatment [10, 11]. Moreover, three recent major studies presented at the American Society of Clinical Oncology (ASCO) Annual Meeting (May 2000) proved that costs were comparable between clinical trials and standard therapy [12, 13].

Many practitioners are unaware of the process in accessing clinical trials, or they may know how to do so, but do not have the time or the resources to dedicate to research. Most practitioners are too busy to take time out of their schedules to inform and enroll patients. Moreover, the cost of data management and staff resources is prohibitive. The cost of enrolling one patient into a phase III National Cancer Institute (NCI) or industry-sponsored clinical trial is estimated to be $2000, according to an ASCO survey (1999) [13]. The survey also found that conducting the trial required 1800 nurse hours and 1500 data manager hours. Oncologists stated that if they participated in a clinical trial, they had to subsidize the cost significantly and the pressure to seek reimbursement was increasing. An additional cost of the research budget must be dedicated to support the Internal Review Board (IRB) activities. Institutional costs are increasing to provide compliance with increasingly complex regulations that govern human subject research. Also, there is an enormous paperwork burden, which can only increase as cancer patients are surviving longer and being followed longer [1].

An additional barrier to physician participation is the unwillingness to turn the patient over to another practitioner for treatment. Many physicians feel that once they have referred their patient to someone for the purpose of getting them into a trial, they lose control of that patient's medical course or they may not see that patient again.

The third most common barrier to patient recruitment is the protocol itself. In an effort to ensure patient safety and keep the research as "pure" as possible, the eligibility criteria have become exceedingly stringent. Many physicians feel that it is almost impossible to find patients to fit the criteria. Patients who are searching for a protocol become frustrated when they cannot find a protocol for which they qualify. In addition, there are not enough protocols to cover all the disease sites and specific disease stages for all patients.

Interventions aimed at enhancing public knowledge and understanding of clinical trials promote increased trial participation. For medical professionals to present the most advanced treatments to the public and forward research at a more reasonable speed, thereby translating new drugs or treatments into standard care, it is important to encourage and assist in public education. With increasing positive public education, more patients will be willing to participate and clinical trials will move through the process more quickly. The patient needs to know the facts about clinical trials and be aware that the hospital/clinic they are coming to is making research a top priority and will be presenting clinical trials to them if warranted. They need to be taught the difference between misconception and reality. They need to know that the costs are not higher, placebo arms are used infrequently, and that cancer clinical trials are the state-of-the-art cancer treatment.

One successful recruitment technique is the use of posters and informational pamphlets in the lobby, in the examination rooms, and near patients' seating areas. Posters in the lobby may state that a particular hospital or clinic is a member of a research group or a cooperative cancer research group and is committed to offering state-of-the-art cancer clinical trials to their patients. Some posters and pamphlets may inform patients about the phases of clinical trials, participant protection regulated by federal agencies, or the reasons why clinical trials are so important. Posters and pamphlets in the examination rooms may state that cancer clinical trials may be the patient's chance of receiving the most advanced treatment, and when the treatment is successful, they are the first to benefit. Also, the posters may state that when patients take part in a cancer clinical trial, they may be helping themselves and future patients. To show patients that the healthcare team is interested in discussing clinical trials with them, the posters could state: "Ask your doctor or nurse about current clinical trials."

D. Rule 4: Develop an Outreach Program

Increasing community awareness of an institution's participation in research is important to increase patient accrual to clinical trials. An outreach program is simply a plan to go into the community and educate the public about clinical trials. Large posters and pamphlets work well. Health fairs, church organizations, local county fairs, local mass media, and student activities are a few of the many opportunities that have proven effective. Creating awareness may be as generic as just wanting to educate the public about research, or it may be as specific as looking for people to recruit to a trial that is currently open. Using the media is effective. If a specific trial needs to be advertised, an IRB-approved script performed on local TV or radio can be used.

Names of possible participants can be found in an institution's tumor registry, and IRB-approved letters describing the trial and asking for their interest can be sent to them. Educating other departments in the hospital/clinic about specific trials and asking for referrals is an additional option.

Local presentations in the clinic or the community can be helpful. One powerful technique is a first-hand presentation from a patient who has had a positive experience in a clinical trial. The Harris Interactive Survey [6] reported that of the cancer clinical trial patients polled, most experiences were very positive. Of past clinical trial participants, 97% stated that they were treated with respect and dignity. Also, 97% rated their quality of care as "excellent" or "good." Positive experiences were reported by 93% of participants and 82% did not feel they were treated as guinea pigs. Of the participants, 81% believed they were not subjected to more tests and procedures than they would have undergone with standard care, and 76% would definitely recommend a clinical trial to someone else.

E. Rule 5: Know the Community

Assess the community in which the potential participants reside. This can include racial and ethnic background, socioeconomic status, education and literacy levels, community and cultural norms, health beliefs and practices, and needs and values in addition to an assessment of their understanding of clinical trials. Once the lines of communication are open, maintain them with periodic information concerning the research, final trial results, implications to that population, and plans for future research. Something as simple as thank you notes or postcards with trial updates are effective. Continued communication promotes cooperation, awareness of the research processes, and trust in the medical establishment and in research. It will also show the participants that they are valued partners in the research process.

Due to the massive acculturation of America, significant heterogeneity can exist in a single community. Not only can socioeconomic, educational, and literacy levels differ, but health practices and beliefs can be very different. Recruitment strategies must be developed with those beliefs and practices in mind. Other factors that need to be taken into account may be transportation abilities, child care, ability to access the medical facility, ability to leave work, and in some cultures, the ability to gain permission from their leaders.

F. Rule 6: Designate a Liaison

To facilitate a mutually beneficial community and clinic/hospital collaboration and cooperation, it is important to designate one or two representatives from the research staff to act as liaisons between the community, the staff, and the researchers. These representatives should involve the clinic or hospital staff, community leaders, local organizations, and school leaders frequently. They should become known in the community as research representatives and eventually be looked upon as trusted community members. They may offer to set up a booth at health fairs, church gatherings, festivals, block parties, or school activities. These representatives may hold informational meetings to other staff members in the clinic or hospital. They can facilitate the identification of potential trial participants and encourage them to consider a particular trial. They may also be able to identify any possible early trial problems in either the community or the medical setting. If the community involved is comprised mainly of minority populations — a readily identifiable subset of the U.S. population distinguished by racial, ethnic and/or cultural differences, or mixed racial and/or ethnic parentage [14] — consider having a minority representative who can explain the healthcare practices and beliefs of that particular community to the staff and carry information concerning the trial back to the community.

G. Rule 7: Know and Respect the Ethical Principals Regarding Research

When any research is planned, whether on animals or on humans, ethical issues must be considered. When research is performed on humans, the ethical principles established by the National Commission in 1978 (The Belmont Report) must be respected and followed [15–17]. All researchers and their staff must follow these three basic principles:

1. *Respect for persons.* This principal involves two ethical considerations: (1) individuals are to be treated as autonomous agents and

(2) persons with diminished autonomy are entitled to protection. When researchers conduct research involving humans, respect for the rights of the individual requires that the participant enter into the research voluntarily and with adequate information.

2. *Beneficence.* This principal stipulates that persons are treated in an ethical manner not only by respecting their decisions and protecting them from harm, but also by making efforts to secure their well-being. Two complementary expressions of beneficent actions have been formulated: (1) do no harm and (2) maximize possible benefits while minimizing possible harm.

3. *Justice.* This principal stipulates that injustice occurs when some benefit to which a person is entitled is denied without good reason, or when some burden is imposed unduly. When researchers recruit subjects for research, they should not systematically include some individuals or groups because of their easy availability, their compromised position, or their malleability. Rather, subjects should be recruited based on their relation to the problem being studied.

Researchers must commit to recruiting participants who will provide the most useful, valid, and most general knowledge concerning the question that is being tested. They must not recruit participants only because they are readily available, malleable, or compromised in some way. On the other hand, participants must not be denied access to a trial for reasons not related to their health status or to the goals of the trial.

H. Rule 8: Develop a System

Before offering clinical trials to patients, develop a smooth, working system that benefits both patients and medical professionals. Fit this system into the established routine of the clinic. One staff member may determine eligibility and suitability for a specific trial. Another staff member may approach the patient initially and discuss the clinical trial, the reason it is offered, the objectives and goals of the study, and what to expect while on that study. A consent form should be presented to the patient and all questions answered before turning the patient over to the physician to witness the patient's signature and sign the document. There are many possibilities that are dependent upon the size of the staff and workload. The system will flow more efficiently if a system is developed before research is initiated.

I. Rule 9: Invite the Person to Participate

Far too often, research personnel forget to invite the patient to participate in the study. It is assumed that if the trial is presented, the patient will understand that they are wanted or needed on the trial and go along with the plan. Potential participants must be offered all the treatment options available to them for their disease, symptoms, or treatment side effects [17]. The clinical trial should be offered as a part of the available treatment armamentarium.

Information regarding why the trial is being run, what its objectives and the goals are. A basic design of the trial should also be incorporated. After this, invite the patient to become a participant. Offer the consent form to read, go over the consent form with the patient, answer questions truthfully, discuss any concerns, and clarify any conflicting information. Then leave the room and give the participants plenty of time to think about their options without feeling rushed. A trusting relationship with the research team is important in the decision-making process. By educating the participants, including their significant family members, and following up with supplemental written material when possible, the research team can help the participants arrive at an informed decision. This can make participants more compliant and enhance symptom management. If the potential participant agrees to go into the trial, go back to the trial design and follow up with more complex information — the treatment schedule, what will be expected of the participant, and what side effect management is planned. Reiterate what is on the consent form. Because the patient is in a situation that is very stressful and retention is a distinct problem, continue to refer back to the consent form information periodically throughout the patient's clinical trial process.

J. Rule 10: Tailor your Approach

An effective approach for accruing patients into phase III trials may be different from the approach for phase I trials. Phase I trials are often the first human trial when the drug or device leaves the laboratory and are described in Chapter 11.

Potential participants in phase I trials must be approached in a compassionate, but honest manner. It must be emphasized that phase I trials are not curative or life-prolonging in many cases [5, 18]. It should also be emphasized that there may be unexpected side effects with unclear management. For example, skin rash, which is sometimes severe, has emerged as a common side effect in a number of phase I trials. Management of this side effect is still unclear. Patients must be assured they will be very closely monitored and if serious adverse events occur, they will be taken off the trial.

When accruing patients to phase II trials, it must be understood by the participants that only a small number of patients have been tested with the drug or combination of drugs or a new schedule of administration in the phase I trial, and there is little information concerning safety and effectiveness in larger numbers of people with different types of cancers or co-morbid conditions. Patients should also be told that they will be closely monitored for unexpected side effects and if serious adverse events occur, they will be taken off the trial.

Phase III trials are usually much larger and much longer than phase II trials. Normally, there are greater than 100 participants accrued at several community sites to get a better picture of the effectiveness of the treatment. The goals of phase III trials are to determine if the new drug/combination or new schedule is more effective and if it is safe or safer than the standard treatment [5, 18]. Often, phase III trials will also look at survival time and quality of life. The results of phase III trials could determine a new standard treatment for specific cancers. Phase III trials incorporate randomization to test a group of participants on the standard treatment against the new treatment. In certain cases, phase III trials are designed with more than two arms to test more than one question. Eligibility criteria will address a specific cancer, stage of cancer, past treatments, range of lab values, co-morbid conditions, age, and gender as well as other factors.

Potential participants in phase III trials must understand that if they are randomized to the newer treatment, and it is more effective than the standard treatment, they are the first to benefit. If they are randomized to the standard treatment, they may not benefit as much as those randomized to the new treatment. However, there is ongoing analysis so the study may be stopped early if one treatment is clearly superior. If this is the case, then all patients will have the chance to receive the most effective treatment. Patients must also be told that despite the phase I and II trials, the new treatment may not have been tested on large numbers of patients and unexpected side effects can occur. Patients will be closely monitored and taken off the trial if serious adverse effects occur.

K. Rule 11: Know the Regulations Governing the Informed Consent Process

The Civil Rights Movement in the 1960s triggered a conscious effort by the government to change the belief that society's need for scientific knowledge placed the individual's rights second. The prevailing attitude had been that the end justified the means. At times, trials went a little far to prove their hypothesis. In 1966, the U. S. Office of the Surgeon General issued the first regulation requiring internal review for all clinical research proposals [18]. This began a shift toward placing the individual's rights over society's needs. In response to the Tuskegee debacle of the 1940s, the Department of Health, Education, and Welfare (now Department of Health and Human Services) published the first regulations on the protection of human research subjects [18, 19]. In 1974, Congress passed the National Research Act, which required each institution conducting human research to submit the research proposal to an IRB for evaluation of safety and efficacy [20]. The National Research Act Commission required that each research design must offer a high probability of generating useful knowledge, the probable benefits must outweigh the risks, the selection of patients must be just, the subjects must give their informed consent, and the subject's right to privacy and confidentiality must be protected [9, 18, 19, 21].

In keeping with the National Research Act, rules were established that required *written* informed consent for patients participating in federally supported research studies. The language of the federal regulations directing this process stipulated that the prospective research subject be given "sufficient opportunity to consider whether or not to participate, that there be no coercion or undue influence, and that the subject is provided information that is in a language that is *understandable* to him/her" [19, 21–23].

L. Rule 12: Ensure that Consent Forms are Readable and Understandable

The consent document was thus created to serve a major role in providing the patient with the information necessary to make a truly *informed* decision. However, it quickly became evident that some healthcare providers relied heavily on a document that most patients could not understand, which left it impossible for patients to reach true informed consent by the use of the document alone. Patients need a role in the decision-making process and they need information to make that decision, but they need a collaborative relationship with their physician and healthcare team with more than a written document to assist in making an *informed* decision.

It is important to understand that the consent document was also created for the protection of the patient, not the physician or institution presenting it. Although, according to Cassileth et al., that has not always been understood by some patients or physicians [4]. In their 1980 study of 200 cancer patients undergoing surgery, only 40% had read the document carefully and the majority of the patients felt that the purpose of the document was to protect the physician's rights in case something went wrong. They may have believed correctly. An article by Williams et al. [13] stated that informed consent documents are frequently designed "less to inform the patient than to list all the possible adverse occurrences — irrespective of their probability — to cover the provider in any eventuality."

Although the IRB system was developed to act as a safety net for the review of protocols and consent documents, studies have demonstrated that the educational level of patients is often not considered when consent documents are written and not taken into account when determining what is appropriate for patients [6, 9, 14]. First, IRB members tend to be college educated and/or professional. Second, after just a few months of reviewing consent documents, IRB members become acclimated to the language and its meaning. Meade et al. [20] proved that out of the consent documents taken from 46 NCI studies in 1990, 96% of them were computer analyzed (SMOG formula) as written at a grade 12.0 to 17.5, with a mean grade level of 14.3, i.e., a college/scientific level. These documents were slightly less difficult to read and understand than medical journals, but substantially more difficult than material from the popular press. They were all passed by the IRB without difficulty.

Are we providing consent information in "language that is understandable to him/her"? The Governmental Statistical Abstract of the United States [25] estimated that 23% (44 million) adult Americans were Level One illiterate (functionally illiterate) in 1997 and did not have enough reading and writing skills to function effectively in our society. Fifty million (28%) adult Americans were Level Two (marginally illiterate) and reading at a sixth to seventh grade level [25]. To further define the problem, 44 million adult Americans do not understand verbal descriptions, written instructions, audiovisuals, or audiotapes. They may have any level of education, although reading levels have often been found to be three to four grade levels below the stated years of schooling [20, 26, 27]. High school graduates can actually get through high school without advancing beyond a seventh or eighth grade reading level. Despite the rising levels of education and training, the average reading skills of the American adult continue to remain at an eighth to ninth grade level. Also, 28% of Americans are only marginally competent in language skills. They may not be able to order from a catalog, follow an instruction sheet, read a thermometer, read the information on an aspirin bottle (which requires a tenth grade reading level), order from a menu, or find their way on a map. They may have difficulty reading the instructions on a frozen food package (which usually requires an eighth grade reading level), or addressing an envelope [20, 22, 28]. They are of every race, age, nationality, cultural background, and occupation. They are rich and poor and everything in between [26]. Healthcare providers must be aware of these issues and adjust accordingly.

It has also been found that many consent documents contain sentences with greater than 50 words, and many contain sentences with 70 or 80 words [26]. The use of too many adverbs and adjectives can make the document too wordy and difficult to understand. Medicolegal jargon is the norm, and long sentences, small type, tiny margins, lack of pictures and graphics, and document length further reduce reader comprehension.

Controversy exists concerning the importance in lowering the readability levels of consent forms to enhance comprehension. Whereas Young et al. [24] demonstrated a significantly higher patient understanding of the simplified language consent form (6th grade level), as compared to the standard form (16th grade level), Davis et al. [29] argued that lowering the readability level alone appeared to have little impact on patient comprehension. What did appear to have more impact was document length; improved presentation using instructional graphics, pictures, headers, and questions; as well as colors and bold type. Coyne et al. [30] demonstrated that simplifying the language did little to enhance understanding, but did reduce anxiety and apprehension and promoted trust in the medical providers and in the research itself.

M. Rule 13: Train the Team in the Consent Process

Informed consent is one tool that can help give the patient autonomy in a situation when patients are already very close to losing their independence. To do this, healthcare professionals need to re-think the process of obtaining informed consent. Rather than view it as a paper-signing event, informed consent should be viewed as a process that evolves over time by incorporating formal and informal teaching practices, and is presented to the patient in language that imparts large volumes of information that is understandable [31].

From the beginning of their dialogue with patients, the informed consent process needs to be a priority. One of the most important aspects of this process is the interaction between the patient and the healthcare team. No written form can be a substitute for the dialogue between the patient and the healthcare professional who needs to creatively communicate complex information. Patients want and need a provider-patient relationship built on trust in which the provider's counsel is predominant in the decision-making process. According to Doak [26], patients must know enough about their condition to understand the nature and the continuity of the treatment. To obtain *informed* consent, information needs to be presented to the patient in meaningful dialogue by persons fluent in lay language and familiar with the details of the procedures being explained and with the elements of informed consent.

There is not just one strategy to obtaining informed consent. Printed information must be accompanied by pictures, repetitious dialogue, question and answer sessions, videos, and demonstrations. In addition, it is important to understand that the process is ongoing and should continue throughout the course of treatment, after treatment, and to include discharge planning and follow-up care.

Why is it so important that trial patients understand their treatment? Society has become increasingly technological with new products, ideas, and more complicated functions. In a 1990 publication of *Megatrends 2000*, John Naisbitt stated "we are poised on the threshold of a great era in biotechnologic advancement that cannot be ignored" [8]. Medical care is becoming intensely complex as technology, genetic therapy, and medical knowledge advances. Although these advances greatly aid in the treatment of disease, explaining these treatments has become increasingly difficult and time intensive. Patients fear the immersion into, what can be for them, a foreign culture with its intimidating centers, technology, and the complicated medical language that defies comprehension. Fear and mistrust result. Exacerbating this problem, less time is spent in the hospital and in dialogue with the healthcare team. The resulting division between the patient and the healthcare team makes it even more difficult for patients to ask questions, express concerns, and receive adequate information. Many research centers have hired clinical research assistants to counter this problem by contacting the patient periodically to anticipate problems, answer questions, and stay connected to the patients, thereby facilitating comprehension, compliance, autonomy, and retention.

In summary, a minority of cancer patients participate in clinical trials. Unless this situation is addressed, the pace of introducing new, more effective agents into cancer therapy will be slowed. Specific efforts by healthcare workers to make the process of clinical trial enrollment user-friendly following some of the ideas outlined above is one approach to enhancing clinical trial participation.

REFERENCES

1. Cohen GI. Clinical research by community oncologists. *CA Cancer J. Clin.* 2003; 53:73–81.
2. AMA Council on Ethical and Judicial Affairs. Ethical use of placebo controls in clinical trials. CEJA Report 2-A, 1996.
3. Barrett R. A nurse's primer on recruiting participants for clinical trials. *Oncol. Nurs. Forum* 2002; 29:7.
4. Cassileth BR. Informed consent- why are its goals imperfectly realized? *N. Engl. J. Med.* 1980; 302:896–900.
5. Jenkins J, Hubbard S. History of clinical trials. *Sem. Oncol. Nurs.* 1991; 7(4):228–234.
6. Harris Survey: A Quantitative Survey of Public Attitudes Toward Cancer Clinical Trials. 1999, in press.
7. American Cancer Society Fact Sheet, 2002.
8. Engelking C. Facilitating clinical trials: The expanding role of the nurse. *Cancer* 1991; 67:1793–1797.
9. Meier E. Politically Speaking: Groups support insurance coverage for clinical trials. *ONS News* 2000; 15(4):9.
10. Russo F. The clinical-trials bottleneck. Medicine. *The Atlantic Monthly* May 1999; 30–36.
11. Scott J, Cooper M, Larson T. Making clinical trials financially viable. *Oncol. Issues* 2000; 15(1):14–16.
12. Blayney DW. Clinical trials in the spotlight. *Oncologist* (commentary) 1999; 4:348–351.

13. Williams MV, Parker RM, Baker DW et al. Inadequate functional health literacy among participants at two public hospitals. *JAMA* 1995; 274:1677–1682.

14. NIH guidelines on the inclusion of women and minorities as subjects in clinical research. *NIH Guide* 1994; 23(10):3.

15. OPRR. Protecting Human Research Subjects. Institutional Review Board Guidebook, 1993.

16. OPRR. Protection of Human Subjects. Title 45, Code of Federal Regulations, 1991; Part 46, Revised.

17. National Commission for the Protection of Human Subjects of Biomedical and Behavioral Research. The Belmont Report, 1979.

18. Hubbard S. Principles of clinical research. *Handbook of Oncology Nursing* 1985; 67–90.

19. Kiev AA. A history of informed consent doctrine. Applied Clinical Trials 1993; 2(5):56–69.

20. Meade C, Howser D. Consent forms: How to determine and improve their readability. *Oncol. Nurs. Forum* 1992; 19(10):1523–1528.

21. Tarnowski K, Allen D, Mayhall C, Kelly P. Readability of pediatric biomedical research informed consent forms. *Pediatrics* 1990; 85(1): 58–62.

22. Hammerschmidt D, Keane M. Institutional review board (IRB) review lacks impact on the readability of consent forms for research. *Am. J. Med. Sci.* 1992; 304(6):348–351.

23. Hopper K, Lambe H, Shirk S. Readability of informed consent forms for use with iodinated contrast media. *Radiology* 1993; 187(1):279–283.

24. Young DR, Hooker DT, Freeberg FE. Informed consent documents: Increasing comprehension by reducing reading level. *IRB* 1990; 12:1–6.

25. Wagner JL, Alberst SR, Sloan JA et al. Incremental costs of enrolling cancer patients in clinical trials: A population-based study. *J. Natl. Cancer Inst.* 1999; 19:847–853.

26. Doak CC, Doak LG, Root JH. *Teaching Patients with Low Literacy Skills.* Lippincott and Company, Philadelphia, Pennsylvania, 1985.

27. Murgatroyd R, Cooper R. Readability of informed consent forms. *Am. J. Hosp. Pharm.* 1991; 48:2651–2652.

28. Duffy MM. Selecting educational materials for patients with limited reading abilities. *ANNA J.* 1988; 15(2):114–117.

29. Davis TC, Holcombe RF, Berkel HJ, Pramanik S, Divers SG. Informed consent for clinical trials: A comparative study of standard versus simplified forms. *JNCI* 1998; 90(9):668–675.

30. Coyne CA, Ronghui X, Raich P et al. A randomized controlled trial of an easy-to-read informed consent statement for clinical trial participation. *J. Clin. Oncol.* 2003; 21(5):836–842.

31. Berry DL, Dood MJ, Hinds PS, Ferrell BR. Informed consent: Process and clinical issues. *Oncol. Nurs. Forum* 1996; 23(3)507–508.

INDEX

A

ABC transporters, pharmacogenetics, 291–292

Active control trials
non-inferiority design, 281–282
superiority design, 281

Acute lymphocytic leukemia, microarray research, 59

Acute myeloid leukemia, microarray research, 59

Adapter proteins, as drug targets, 12

Adenovirus ONYX-015, and gene therapy, 385

ADEPT, see Antibody-directed enzyme prodrug technique

Ad p53, see p53 encoding adenovirus

Adult respiratory distress syndrome, and gene therapy, 380

Affymetrix, high-density oligonucleotide chips, 47–48

ALEXA dyes, for spotted arrays, 49

Algorithms
for agent validation, 238–240
for microarray data analysis, overview, 39–40
pharmacokinetic modeling, 316–317

ALL, see Acute lymphocytic leukemia

AML, see Acute myeloid leukemia

Angiogenesis, as drug target, 17–19

Angiogenesis inhibitors, and radiotherapy, 399

Angiostatin, and radiotherapy, 398

Animal models, in anticancer agent validation, 243–244

Anti-angiogenesis studies, microvessels, 320–321

Anti-angiogenic therapy, PET studies, 305–307

Antibodies
anti-tumor therapeutics, 209
bispecific antibodies, 210
conjugated anticancer drug studies, 146–151
immunotherapies, see Anti-tumor antibody immunotherapeutics

Antibody-directed enzyme prodrug technique, for tumor targeting, 84

Antigen-loaded autologous dendritic cells, as cancer vaccines, 217–218

Antisense oligonucleotides
delivery, 198–199
design chemistry, 196–197
design overview, 193–194
design principles, 194–196
evaluation, 200–202
overview, 191–193

pharmacological evaluation, 199–200
safety evaluation, 202
target validation and optimization, 197–198

Anti-tumor antibody immunotherapeutics
applications, 209
bispecific antibodies, 210
categories, 208
developments, 208
early work, 207–208
immunoconjugates, 210–212
immunotoxins, 210
radio-immunoconjugates, 211

Anti-vascular therapy
microvessels, 320–321
PET studies, 305–307

Apollon, 224, 228

Apoptosis
in cancer therapeutic evaluation, 311
and drug targeting, 15–16
and radiosensitization, 396

Approval processes
drugs, see Drug approval
gene therapy, 383–384

ARDS, see Adult respiratory distress syndrome

AT, see Ataxia-telangiectasia

Ataxia-telangiectasia, and radiosensitization, 403

427

Ataxia-telangiectasia-like disorder, and radiosensitization, 403
ATLD, *see* Ataxia-telangiectasia-like disorder
Aurora-2, as drug target, 11
Aurora-2 kinase, as drug target, 11

B
Baculoviral inhibitor of apoptosiis repeat domains, in IAPs, 224
Bcl-2 protein, and drug targeting, 16
Bcl-xL, and drug targeting, 16
Biomarkers
    definition, 250–251
    and drug effect *in vivo*, 252
    evaluation in tumor tissue, 258–260
    future work, 261
    ideal type, 251–252
    as predictive factors, 252–253
    as prognostic factors, 253–254
    in proof-of-concept assessments, 347–348
    tissue choice, 255–258
Biopsy, tumor tissues, 258–259
BIR domains, *see* Baculoviral inhibitor of apoptosiis repeat domains
Bispecific antibodies, as therapeutics, 210
Bladder cancer, microarray research, 60–61
Blood concentration, phase I dose-finding trials, 367
Blood oxygenation level dependent contrast, in vascular imaging, 326, 328
BOLD contrast, *see* blood oxygenation level dependent contrast
Bortezomib, for proteasome targeting, 19
Breast cancer
    microarray research, 61
    proof-of-concept of agents, 351–352
Buccal mucosa cells, in biomarker assays, 256–257

C
CA4P, *see* Combretastatin phosphate
CAMs, *see* Cell adhesion molecules

Cancer detection, mass spectrometry techniques, 155–158
Cancer Genome Anatomy Project, microarray data mining, 52
Cancer therapeutics, PET evaluation
    anti-angiogenic therapy, 305–307
    anti-vascular therapy, 305–307
    apoptosis, 311
    cellular proliferation evaluation, 308–310
    dihydropyrimidine dehydrogenase modulation, 304–305
    gene expression, 307
    mitogenic signal transduction, 308
    multidrug resistance, 303–304
    overview, 302–303
    receptor occupancy, 303
    thymidylate synthase inhibition, 308
    tumor energy metabolism, 310
    tumor hypoxia, 304
Cancer vaccines
    basic elements, 213–214
    cell-based vaccines, 215–217
    early experiments, 213
    gangliosides, 215
    immune adjuvants, 217–218
    overview, 212–213
    peptide vaccines, 214–215
CancerVax, characteristics, 216
CARD motif, *see* Caspase recruitment domain motif
Caspase recruitment domain motif, in IAPs, 224
Caspases, and IAPs, 225–226
Cassette-dosing, in anticancer agent validation, 240–241
Catalyst analysis
    for FPT hypothesis, 101
    Sch 44342, 95
Cathepsin B-activated prodrugs, for tumor targeting, 89
CBER, *see* Center for Biologics Evaluation and Research
CDER, cancer agent review, 266
CDKs, *see* Cyclin-dependent kinases
Cell adhesion molecules, as drug targets, 18–19
Cell-based cancer vacccines, characteristics, 215–217
Cell line models, *in vitro,* for agent validation, 238–240

Cell surface molecules, and tumor targeting, 85
Cellular proliferation, in cancer therapeutic evaluation, 308–310
Center for Biologics Evaluation and Research, cancer agent review, 266
Cetuximab
    development, 5
    and radiosensitization, 396
CGAP, *see* Cancer Genome Anatomy Project
CGP 57148
    drug targets for, 8
    mass spectrometry studies, 155
Chaperones, as drug targets, 19
Chemotherapeutics, for tumor targeting
    ADEPT, 84
    background, 83–84
    cathepsin B-activated prodrugs, 89
    and cell surface molecules, 85
    enzyme-activated targeting, 85
    enzymes for prodrugs, 89–90
    fibroblast activation protein alpha activated prodrugs, 89
    future research, 90
    glucuronidase-activated doxorubicin, 86–87
    N-l-leucyl-doxorubicin, 85–86
    matrix-metalloprotease activated prodrugs, 88
    passive targeting, 84–85
    plasmin-activated doxorubicin, 88
    prostate-specific antigen activated doxorubicin, 87
    super-Leu-doxorubicin, 87–88
Chemotherapy protectants, trial designs, 282
Chk1, as drug target, 11
Chromatin remodeling factors, as drug targets, 19–20
Chromatographically prepared components, ESI-mass screening, 161
CI-1033, development, 5
Cisplatin, mass spectrometry studies, 144–146
c-kit, as drug target, 6
Clinical end points, tumor markers as, 280
Clinical trial design
    for approval, 280–282
    gene therapy, 384–386

overview, 365–366
phase I dose-finding trials,
366–372
phase I trials, 268–269
phase II trial, 269–270
Clinical trials
CDER and CBER reviews, 266
early, *see* Early clinical trials
FDA regulatory approach,
266–267
IND process, 265
IND regulations, 264–265
IND submission support,
267–268
NDA process, 265–266
overview, 263–264
patient population
approach development,
419–420
community assessment,
416–417
consent forms, 420–421
consent process team,
422–423
ethical principals, 417–418
governing regulations, 420
liason designation, 417
outreach program, 416
participant invitation,
418–419
public education, 414–416
research committment, 413
system development, 418
team education, 414
and proof-of-concept
testing, 350
for protectants, 282
radiosensitization and EGFr, 397
Ras radiotherapy, 400–401
Colorectal cancer, microarray
research, 59–60
Combretastatin phosphate,
clinical study, 320–321
COMPARE, for anticancer agent
validation, 239
Composite end points, in drug
approval, 276–277
Condensed phase systems, mass
spectrometry screening,
160–161
Contrast agent
hemoglobin in vascular
imaging, 328
kinetics and microvessel
function, 312–313
Correlative end points, gene
therapy, 386–389

Cyclin-dependent kinases, *see also*
Serine/threonine kinases
as drug targets, 10–11
Cyclooxygenase 2 inhibitors, in
radiosensitization, 406
Cytochrome P4503A,
pharmacogenetics, 293
Cytokines
as cancer vaccines, 218
NMR studies, 127, 130
Cytoplasmic oncogenic
serine/threonine kinases, as
drug targets, 8
Cytosolic tyrosine kinases, as drug
targets, 7–8
Cytostatic agents
definitive randomized efficacy
trials, 376
overview, 365–366
phase I dose-finding trials
feasibility issues, 371–372
for minimum effective blood
concentration, 367
overview, 366–367
targeted biologic response,
367–370
preliminary efficacy trials
overview, 372
patient population selection,
372–374
and tumor shrinkage, 374–376

D
Data mining, microarray data,
39–40, 52, 73–74
DCE-MRI, *see* Dynamic
contrast-enhanced magnetic
resonance imaging
DCs, *see* Dendritic cells
DD, *see* Differential display
Definitive randomized efficacy
trials, overview, 376
Dendritic cells, as cancer vaccines,
217–218
Differential display, and DNA
microarrays, 44
Dihydropyrimidine dehydrogenase
PET studies, 304–305
pharmacogenetics, 288
5,10-Dihydropyrimidino[4,5-b]-
quinolin-4[1H]-ones, drug
target for, 8
Diseases, classification with
microarrays, 58
DNA, in circulating tumor
cells, 259

DNA damage, and
radiosensitization, 402–405
DNA double-strand break repair,
and radiosensitization,
395–396
DNA microarrays
advantages, 44–45
control choice, 66–67
detection sensitivity, 65–66
and drug action mechanisms, 57
gene function research, 63–64
gene regulation research, 64–65
high-density oligonucleotide
chips, 46–48
high-throughput proteomics,
overview, 68–69
novel technologies, 51
nylon filter arrays, 45–46
pathogenesis research, 62–63
in proteomics, 68
result validation, 67
spotted arrays, 48–50
spotted oligonucleotide arrays,
50–51
Dose-response relationship, phase I
dose-finding trials, 368–370
Dosing schedules
cassette-dosing, 240–241
cell line studies, 239–240
Doxorubicin
glucuronidase-activated, 86–87
Leu-Dox, 85–86
plasmin-activated, 88
PSA-activated, 87
super-Leu, 87–88
DPD, *see* Dihydropyrimidine
dehydrogenase
Drug actions, microarray studies,
56–57
Drug approval
accelerated, surrogate end
points, 277–278
clinical trial designs, 280–282
composite clinical benefit end
points, 276–277
efficacy end points, 272–273
and patient-reported outcomes,
275–276
and Quality of Life, 275–276
regular, surrogate end points,
278–280
requirements, 271–272
Drug development
approval requirements, 271–272
end-of-phase meetings, 271
IND submission support,
267–268

Drug development *(continued)*
  phase I trial design, 268–269
  phase II trial design, 269–270
Drug discovery
  generic cascade, 235–237
  mass spectrometry application,
    140–141
  NMR in
    1D line-broadening, 118–120
    1D STD, 120–123
    overview, 107–109
    screening overview, 110–111
    screening techniques, 126
    SHAPES method, 123
    2D screening, 111–118
  protein arrays, 71–72
Drug effects
  and biomarker assay tissue
    choice, 255–258
  biomarker indicators, 252
  in vivo technical issues, 254–255
Drug efficacy
  cellular proliferation evaluation,
    308–310
  definitive randomized efficacy
    trials, 376
  overview, 285–286
  preliminary trials, 372–376
Drug response
  cellular proliferation evaluation,
    308–310
  PET drug studies, 303–304
Drug safety, overview, 285–286
Drug screening, with mass
  spectrometry, 158–160
Drug target studies
  adapter proteins, 12
  and angiogenesis, 17–19
  and apoptosis, 15–16
  chaperones, 19
  chromatin remodeling factors,
    19–20
  discovery with microarrays,
    55–56
  growth factors, 3–4
  GTP-binding proteins, 12–13
  oncogenic transcription factors,
    13–15
  overview, 1–2
  protein degradation, 19
  protein phosphatases, 11–12
  serine/threonine kinases, 8–11
  tyrosine kinases, 4–8
Drug transporters,
  pharmacogenetics, 291–292
Dynamic contrast-enhanced
  magnetic resonance imaging,
  microvessels

contrast agent kinetics,
    312–313
  measurement precision, 325
  overview, 311–312
  protocol standardization, 321
  quantification and modeling,
    321, 323, 325
  T1-weighted imaging, 314–321
  T2*-weighted imaging, 313–314
  technique validation, 325
Dynamics analysis, by NMR,
  137–139

E
Early clinical trials
  biomarker assay tissue choice,
    255–258
  biomarker as predictive factors,
    252–253
  biomarkers, 250–251
  biomarkers and *in vivo* drug
    effect, 252
  biomarkers as prognostic
    factors, 253–254
  biomarkers in tumor tissues,
    258–260
  drug effects *in vivo* 254–255
  future work, 261
  ideal biomarkers, 251–252
  overview, 249–250
  surrogate end-point necessity,
    251
  surrogate markers, 250–251
  target agent definition, 250
ECF agents, in MR imaging, 326
EES, *see* Extravascular contrast
  agents
EGFr, *see* Epidermal growth factor
  receptors
Endocrine-modulating agents,
  proof-of-concept, 351–352
End points
  clinical end points, 280
  composite end points, 276–277
  correlation in proof-of-concept,
    348–350
  correlative end points, 386–389
  pharmacodynamic end points,
    300–302
  pharmacodynamic proof-of-
    concept, 351–355
  pharmakinetic proof-of-
    concept, 355–357
  phase III, and proof-of-concept,
    339–341
  preliminary efficacy trials, 374
  primary end point, 348–350

for regular drug approval,
    278–280
  surrogate, *see* Surrogate end
    points
  targeted biological end point,
    374
Enediyne antibiotics, mass
  spectrometry studies, 146–151
Enzyme-activated tumor targeting
  glucuronidase-activated
    doxorubicin, 86–87
  Leu-doxorubicin, 85–86
Enzymes, for tumor prodrugs,
  89–90
Epidermal growth factor receptor
  kinase inhibitor type I, 343
Epidermal growth factor receptors
  as antibody targets, 209
  as drug target, 4–5
  and radiosensitization, 392,
    394–397
ER, *see* Estrogen receptor
ERK, *see* Extracellular regulated
  kinase
Erlotimib, *see* OSI-774
ESI-mass spectrometry,
  chromatographically
  prepared components, 161
Esophogeal cancer, microarray
  research, 60
EST, *see* Expressed sequence tag
Estrogen receptor, PET occupancy
  studies, 303
expO, *see* EXpression Project for
  Oncology
Expressed sequence tag, and DNA
  microarrays, 44
EXpression Project for Oncology,
  58
Extracellular regulated kinase, in
  mitogenic signaling, 3
Extravascular contrast agents, in
  microvessel studies, 312–313

F
FAP prodrugs, *see* Fibroblast
  activation protein alpha
  activated prodrugs
Farnesyl protein transferase
  inhibitors
  discovery, 94–95
  hypothesis development, 99
  training set, 96–98
Farnesyl transferase inhibitors,
  and RAS radiotherapy,
  399–401
FBAL, *see* α-Fluoro-β-alanine

FDA, *see* Food and Drug Administration
[18]FDG, *see* [18]Fluorodeoxyglucose
FGF-2, *see* Fibroblast growth factor 2
Fibroblast activation protein alpha activated prodrugs, 89
Fibroblast growth factor 2, NMR studies, 127
Flavopiridol, targets for, 10–11
FlexJet technology, for spotted oligonucleotide arrays, 50
FLT3, as drug target, 7
Fluorescence, for spotted arrays, 49–50
α-Fluoro-β-alanine, and dihydropyrimidine dehydrogenase, 304
[18]Fluorodeoxyglucose, tumor energy metabolism evaluation, 310
Fluoropyrimidine resistance, and thymidylate synthase, 289
5-Fluorouracil, and dihydropyrimidine dehydrogenase, 288
Food and Drug Administration anticancer drug clinical trials, 263–264
  CDER and CBER reviews, 266
  end points for accelerated approval, 277–278
  gene therapy approval, 384
  IND process, 265
  IND regulations, 263–264
  NDA process, 265–266
  and Quality of Life, 275
  regulatory approach, 266–267
FPT inhibitors, *see* Farnesyl protein transferase inhibitors
FTI, *see* Farnesyl transferase inhibitors
5-FU, *see* 5-Fluorouracil

G
Gangliosides, cancer vaccine, 215
Gas-phase ESI-mass spectrometry sampling, condensed phase systems, 160–161
GDP, and RAS radiotherapy, 399–400
Gefitinib, *see* ZD1839
Geldanamycin analogs, development, 5
GEML, *see* Gene expression markup language

Gene expression, cancer therapeutic evaluation, 307
Gene expression markup language, and microarray data mining, 74
Gene expression microarrays and drug action mechanisms, 56–57
  overview, 63–65
Gene therapy
  clinical trial approval processes, 383–384
  clinical trial design, 384–386
  correlative end points, 386–389
  overview, 379–381
  and preclinical development, 382–383
  product regulations, 381–382
Genotype, TPMT, 287–288
GF120918, proof-of-concept study, 354–355
GI147211, proof-of-concept study, 357
Glass-based protein arrays, overview, 70
Gleevec
  drug targets for, 8
  mass spectrometry studies, 155
Glucuronidase-activated doxorubicin, for tumor targeting, 86–87
GM-CSF, as immune adjuvant, 218
GMP, *see* Good manufacturing practice
Good manufacturing practice, gene transfer products, 381–382
Grb2
  as drug target, 12
  in growth factor-induced mitogenic signaling, 3
Growth factor receptors, and radiosensitization, 394–397
Growth factors
  induced mitogenic signaling, 3–4
  NMR studies, 127
GTP, and RAS radiotherapy, 399–400
GTP-binding proteins, as drug targets, 12–13

H
Hairy cell leukemia, antibody therapeutics, 210
HDACs, *see* Histone deacetylases
Heat shock protein 70, 17
Heat shock protein 90, 19

Hematological toxicity, hematological, and TPMT, 287
Hemoglobin, in vascular imaging, 326, 328
Hepatocellular carcinoma, microarray research, 62
Hepatocyte growth factor, as drug target, 6
HER-2, as drug target, 4–5
Her2/neu, and radiosensitization, 396–397
HER/ErbB receptor tyrosine kinases, as drug targets, 4–5
HGF, *see* Hepatocyte growth factor
HIF-1, *see* Hypoxia-inducible factor 1
High-density oligonucleotide chips, as DNA microarrays, 46–48
High-throughput proteomics DNA microarrays, 68–69
  glass-based protein arrays, 70
  nonliving microarrays, 69–70
High-throughput screening
  cell-free screens, 237–238
  cell line studies, 239
  hollow fiber assay, 241–242
  overview, 93, 107–109
Histone deacetylases, as drug targets, 19–20
HMFG protein, *see* Human milk fat globule protein
HNCA experiment, in 3D triple-resonance NMR, 114
HN(CO)AC experiment, in 3D triple-resonance NMR, 114
HOG, *see* Hoosier Oncology Group
Hollow fiber assay, in anticancer agent validation, 241–242
Hoosier Oncology Group, radiosensitization studies, 406–407
HPV, *see* Human papillomavirus
Hsp70, *see* Heat shock protein 70
Hsp90, *see* Heat shock protein 90
2D ^{1}H-^{15}N HSQC spectroscopy in SAR by NMR, 112–116
  2D-trNOE alternative, 116–118
HTS, *see* High-throughput screening
Human milk fat globule protein, 209
Human papillomavirus, 115
Human tumor xenograft, 242–243

7-Hydroxystaurosporine, targets
    for, 11
Hypoxia, PET studies, 304
Hypoxia-inducible factor 1, 14

I
IAPs, *see* Inhibitors of apoptosis
IαB, and IAPs, 226
IBC, *see* Institutional Biosafety
    Committee
IEN, *see* Intraepithelial neoplasia
IFN, *see* Interferons
IGF-IR, *see* Insulin-like growth
    factor 1 receptor
IL-4, *see* Interleukin-4
IL-13, *see* Interleukin-13
Imaging
    DCE-MRI, *see* Dynamic
        contrast-enhanced magnetic
        resonance imaging
    microvessels, new techniques,
        326, 328
    pharmacodynamic end points,
        300–302
    T1-weighted, *see* T1-weighted
        imaging
    T2*-weighted, microvessel
        studies, 313–314
Immune adjuvants, as cancer
    vaccines, 213–214, 217–218
Immunoconjugates, as
    therapeutics, 210–212
Immunotoxins, as therapeutics,
    210
IND, *see* Investigational New
    Drug Application
Inhibitors of apoptosis
    as cancer therapy targets,
        227–229
    overview, 223
    and Smac/DIABLO, 227
    structure and function, 224–226
Institutional Biosafety Committee,
    gene therapy approval,
    383–384
Institutional Review Board, gene
    therapy approval, 383–384
Insulin-like growth factor 1
    receptor, as drug target, 6
Interferons, cDNA microarray
    studies, 57
Interleukin-4, NMR studies, 130
Interleukin-13, NMR studies, 130
International Review Board,
    clinical trial consent
    forms, 421

Intraepithelial neoplasia, phase III
    end point for proof-of-
    concept, 341
Investigational New Drug
    Application
    and FDA regulatory approach,
        266–267
    process, 265
    regulations, 264–265
    submission support, 267–268
IRB, *see* Institutional Review Board
Iressa, *see* ZD1839
Irinotecan, pharmacogenetics, 292
Isotope labeling, in 3D triple-
    resonance NMR, 113–114

J
Jaguar software package, for
    Affymetrix chips, 47–48
JNK pathway, and IAPs, 226

L
N-l-Leucyl-doxorubicin, for tumor
    targeting, 85–86
Leu-Dox, *see* N-l-Leucyl-
    doxorubicin
Leukemia, microarray research, 59
Line-broadening techniques, 1D
    NMR, 118–120
Livin, 224, 228
Living protein arrays, overview, 71
Lymphoma, microarray
    research, 59

M
Macromolecular magnetic
    resonance assays,
    microvasular function, 326
MAGE-1, peptide vaccines,
    214–215
Magnetic resonance imaging
    DCE-MRI, *see* Dynamic
        contrast-enhanced magnetic
        resonance imaging
    microvessels, new techniques,
        326, 328
MAP kinases, as drug
    targets, 10
Marker peptides, and gene
    therapy, 388
Mass spectrometry
    in cancer detection, 155–158
    condensed phase systems,
        160–161

in drug discovery, overview,
    140–141
overview, 107, 109
and protein arrays, 73
thiotepa, 142
Mass spectrometry/nuclear
    magnetic resonance screening
    assay
    flow diagram, 162–164
    MMP-1 inhibitors, 164–168
    overview, 161–162
    SEC-MS component, 164
Mass spectrometry studies
    cisplatin and analogs, 144–146
    early drug screening, 158–160
    enediyne antibiotics, 146–151
    Gleevec, 155
    methotrexate, 143
    mitoxantrone, 143–144
    photofrin, 151–153
    structure determination and
        characterization, 141
    taxanes, 153–155
    taxol, 153–155
Matrix-metalloprotease activated
    prodrugs, for tumor
    targeting, 88
Matrix-metalloproteinase 1
    inhibitors, MS/NMR
    screening assay, 164–168
Matrix-metalloproteinases
    as drug target, 18
    dynamics analysis by NMR,
        138–139
    NMR studies, 130, 132
    structure and design, 134–137
Mdm2 gene product, and drug
    targeting, 16
MDR, *see* Multidrug resistance
MEK, as drug target, 10
Melanoma, microarray
    research, 62
Methotrexate, mass spectrometry
    studies, 143
MGd, *see* Motexafin gadolinium
MGED, *see* Microarray Gene
    Expression Database Group
Microarray Gene Expression
    Database Group, data
    mining, 73
Microarray research
    bladder cancer, 60–61
    breast cancer, 61
    colorectal cancer, 59–60
    for disease classification, 58
    and drug action mechanism,
        56–57

and drug target discovery, 55–56
esophogeal cancer, 60
future research, 74–76
gene expression, 56–57, 63–65
gene function, 63–64
gene regulation, 64–65
hepatocellular carcinoma, 62
leukemia, 59
lymphoma, 59
melanoma, 62
ovarian cancer, 61
pathogenic mechanisms, 62–63
and pharmacogenetics, 57–58
prostate cancer, 61
Microarrays
  commercial hybridization
    services, 52
  commercial suppliers, 43–44
  commercial *vs.* self-made, 53
  data mining, 52
  data organization, 39–40
  DNA, *see* DNA microarrays
  glass-based protein arrays, 70
  in-house production, 53–55
  living protein arrays, 71
  nonliving protein arrays, 69–70
  overview, 38–39
  protein, *see* Protein microarrays
  related web sites, 40–42
  technological evolution, 39
Microvessel density, measurement
    validation, 318–319
Microvessels
  DCE-MRI studies
    measurement precision, 325
    protocol standardization, 321
    quantification and modeling,
      321, 323, 325
    technique validation, 325
  MRI studies
    contrast agent kinetics,
      312–313
    overview, 311–312
    T1-weighted imaging,
      314–321
    T2*-weighted imaging,
      313–314
  new MR approaches, 326, 328
Mitogenic signal transduction
  cancer therapeutic
    evaluation, 308
  growth factor induced, 3–4
Mitoxantrone, mass spectrometry
    studies, 143–144
MMP-3, *see* Stromelysin
MMPs, *see* Matrix-
    metalloproteinases

Modeling
  in anticancer agent validation,
    243–244
  cell lines for, 238–240
  chromatin remodeling
    factors, 19–20
  microvessels with DCE-MRI,
    321, 323, 325
  pharmacokinetic algorithms,
    316–317
  validation studies, 238–240,
    243–244
Monoclonal antibodies, anti-tumor
    therapeutics, 209
Motexafin gadolinium, in
    radiosensitization, 405–406
MS, *see* Mass spectrometry
MTHFR reductase,
    pharmacogenetics, 293
Multidrug resistance, PET studies,
    303–304
MVD, *see* Microvessel density
Myc, as drug target, 13

N
National Institutes of Health, gene
    therapy approval, 384
NBS, *see* Nijmegen breakage
    syndrome
NCE, *see* New chemical entity
NDA, *see* New drug application
New chemical entity
  drug-like qualities as proof-of-
    concept, 341
  overview, 337–338
  pharmacokinetic proof-of-
    concept end points,
    355–356
  safety profile as proof-of-
    concept, 342–343
New Drug Application
  and FDA regulatory approach,
    266–267
  process, 265–266
NF-κB, *see* Nuclear factor-κB
Nibrin, and radiosensitization,
    403–404
NIH, *see* National Institutes of
    Health
Nijmegen breakage syndrome, and
    radiosensitization, 403
NMR, *see* Nuclear magnetic
    resonance studies
NOESY experiments, for
    protein–ligand complexes,
    132–137

Nonliving protein arrays,
    overview, 69–70
Non-small cell lung cancer, as
    target, 209
NSCLC, *see* Non-small cell lung
    cancer
Nuclear factor-κB
  as drug target, 14
  and IAPs, 226
Nuclear magnetic resonance
    studies
  cytokines, 127, 130
  in drug discovery
    1D line-broadening, 118–120
    1D STD, 120–123
    overview, 107–109
    screening overview, 110–111
    screening techniques, 126
    SHAPES method, 123, 126
    2D screening, 111–118
  for dynamics analysis, 137–139
  growth factors, 127
  matrix-metalloproteinases,
    130, 132
  overview, 107–109
  protein–ligand complexes,
    132–137
  protein structure overview, 126
Nylon filter arrays, as DNA
    microarray, 45–46

O
OBA, *see* Office of Biotechnology
    Activities
Office of Biotechnology
    Activities, gene therapy
    approval, 384
Oil-based immune adjuvants, as
    cancer vaccines, 217
Oligonucleotides, antisense, *see*
    Antisense oligonucleotides
Oligonucleotide scanning
    arrays, 198
Olumoucine, targets for, 11
Oncogenic cell cycle
    serine/threonine kinases,
    10–11
Oncogenic transcription factors,
    as drug targets, 13–15
ORR, *see* Overall response rate
Orthotopic models, in anticancer
    agent validation, 243–244
OS, *see* Overall survival
OSI-774, development, 5
Ovarian cancer, microarray
    research, 61

Overall response rate, phase III end point for proof-of-concept, 340

Overall survival, phase III end point for proof-of-concept, 340

P

p53 encoding adenovirus, and gene therapy, 387

p53 tumor suppressor gene, and apoptosis, 15–16

p210[bcr-abl], as drug target, 8

Pain reduction, phase III end point for proof-of-concept, 340

Passive tumor targeting, chemotherapeutics for, 84–85

Pathogenesis, microarray research, 62–63

Patient population
clinical trials
approach development, 419–420
community assessment, 416–417
consent forms, 420–421
consent process team, 422–423
ethical principals, 417–418
governing regulations, 420
liason designation, 417
outreach program, 416
participant invitation, 418–419
public education, 414–416
research committment, 413
system development, 418
team education, 414
for preliminary efficacy trials, 372–374
selection for PET drug studies, 303–304

Patient-reported outcomes, and drug approval, 275–276

PBMCs, *see* Peripheral blood mononuclear cells

PCR, *see* Polymerase chain reaction

PD-153053, 5

PD-168393, 5

PDGFR, *see* Platelet-derived growth factor receptors

Peptide vaccines, 214–215

Peripheral blood mononuclear cells, in biomarker assays, 256

Peroxisome proliferator-activated receptors
as drug targets, 14–15
microarray research, 60

PET, *see* Positron emission tomography

P-glycoprotein, and proof-of-concept, 354–355

PGP protein, pharmaco-genetics, 291

Pharmacodynamic end points
overview, 300
PET, 300–301
PET acquisition and processing, 302
PET radiotracers, 300–301

Pharmacodynamics, in anticancer agent validation, 244

Pharmacogenetics
ABC transporters, 291–292
cytochrome P4503A, 293
dihydropyrimidine dehydrogenase, 288
irinotecan, 292
and microarrays, 57–58
MTHFR reductase, 293
overview, 285–286
thiopurine methyltransferase, 286–288
thymidylate synthase, 289–291
UDP-glucuronosyltransferase 1A1, 292

Pharmacology
antisense oligonucleotides, 199–200
in biomarker predictivity, 253

Pharmacophores
definition, 94–95, 99
validation, 99–104

Phase I dose-finding trials
design, 366–372
feasibility issues, 371–372
for minimum effective blood concentration, 367
overview, 366–367
targeted biologic response
dose for minimum, 367–368
dose-response relationship, 368–370
efficacious dose, 368
overview, 367

Phase I trials, design, 268–269

Phase II trials
design, 269–270
as proof-of-concept, 351

Phase III end point, and proof-of-concept, 339–341

Phase III trials
patient accrual, 419–420
proof-of-concept to, 358

Phenotype, TPMT, 287–288

3-[*N*-Phenyl]carboxamide-2–iminochromene derivatives, drug targets for, 8

Phosphorodiamidate morpholino oligomer, for c-myc target, 13

Photofrin, mass spectrometry studies, 151–153

PI-3 kinase, as drug target, 9

PKA, *see* Protein kinase A

PKB, *see* Protein kinase B

PKC, *see* Protein kinase C

Placebo control, for drug approval, 280–281

Plasmin-activated doxorubicin, for tumor targeting, 88

Platelet-derived growth factor receptors
as antibody targets, 209
as drug target, 5–6

PMO, *see* Phosphorodiamidate morpholino oligomer

PoC, *see* Proof-of-concept

Polo-like kinase, as drug target, 11

Polymerase chain reaction
and gene therapy, 386
and in-house microarray production, 53–54

Polymorphism
and thymidylate synthase, 290–291
and TPMT, 287

Positron emission tomography
cancer therapeutic evaluation
anti-angiogenic therapy, 305–307
anti-vascular therapy, 305–307
apoptosis, 311
cellular proliferation evaluation, 308–310
dihydropyrimidine dehydrogenase, 304–305
gene expression, 307
mitogenic signal transduction, 308
multidrug resistance, 303–304
overview, 302–303
receptor occupancy, 303
thymidylate synthase inhibition, 308
tumor energy metabolism evaluation, 310
tumor hypoxia, 304

and gene therapy, 388
pharmacodynamic end point
    imaging
    acquisition and processing,
        302
    overview, 300–301
    radiotracers, 301
    in proof-of-concept assessments,
        344, 346–347
PPARs, *see* Peroxisome
    proliferator-activated receptors
Preliminary efficacy trials
    overview, 372
    patient population selection,
        372–374
    and tumor shrinkage, 374–376
Primary end point, correlation to
    surrogate end point, 348–350
PRO, *see* Patient-reported
    outcomes
Prodrugs
    activating enzymes for, 89–90
    cathepsin B-activated
        prodrugs, 89
    fibroblast activation protein
        alpha activated prodrugs, 89
    matrix-metalloprotease
        activated prodrugs, 88
Programmed cell death,
    see Apoptosis
Promoters, and thymidylate
    synthase, 289
Proof-of-concept
    and clinical trial design, 350
    concept elements, 339–341
    definition, 338
    drug-like qualities as, 341–342
    guidelines, 359–360
    pharmacodynamic PoC end
        points, 351–355
    pharmacokinetic PoC end
        points, 355–357
    to phase III, 358
    randomized phase II trials as,
        351
    safety profile as, 342–343
    surrogate end points
        mechanism assessment, 343
        scanning assessments, 344,
            346–347
        serum biomarkers, 347–348
    surrogate to primary end point
        correlation, 348–350
Proof-of-principle, therapeutic
    mechanisms of action
    anti-angiogenic/anti-vascular
        therapies, 305–307

dihydropyrimidine
    dehydrogenase modulation,
        304–305
gene expression, 307
mitogenic signal transduction,
    308
thymidylate synthase inhibition,
    308
Prostaglandin inhibitors, in
    radiosensitization, 406
Prostate cancer, microarray
    research, 61
Prostate-specific antigen, proof-of-
    concept trial, 347
Prostate-specific antigen activated
    doxorubicin, 87
26S Proteasome, as drug
    target, 19
Protein arrays
    in drug discovery, 71–72
    glass-based arrays, 70
    living arrays, 71
    nonliving arrays, 69–70
ProteinChip, and mass
    spectrometry, 73
Protein degradation, as drug
    target, 19
Protein kinase A, 8–9
Protein kinase B, 8–9
Protein kinase C, 8–9
Protein kinases, 4
Protein–ligand complexes, NMR
    studies, 132–137
Protein microarrays
    for characterizations, 72–73
    and mass spectrometry, 73
Protein phosphatases, as drug
    targets, 11–12
Proteins
    conjugated anticancer drug
        studies, 146–151
    cytokine NMR studies,
        127, 130
    growth factor NMR
        studies, 127
    matrix-metalloproteinase NMR
        studies, 130, 132
    microarray characterizations,
        72–73
    NMR studies overview, 126
Proteomics
    array-based studies, 68
    high-throughput, *see* High-
        throughput proteomics
PS-341, *see* Bortezomib
PSA, *see* Prostate-specific
    antigen

Q
QOL, *see* Quality of Life
Quality of Life
    and drug approval, 275–276
    phase III end point for proof-of-
        concept, 340–341
Quantitative structure–activity
    relationships
    FPT inhibitory activity, 95
    overview, 94
Quinazoline, development, 5

R
R115777, Ras target, 13
RAC, *see* Recombinant DNA
    Advisory Committee
Rac, as drug target, 12
Radio-immunoconjugates, as
    therapeutics, 211
Radiosensitization
    and DNA damage, 402–405
    DNA double-strand break, 392
    EGFr and clinical trials, 397
    first efforts, 391–392
    overview, 394–397
    p53 modulation, 401–402
    Ras protein clinical trials,
        400–401
    Ras protein overview, 399–400
    various approaches, 405–407
    VEGF and inhibitors, 397–399
Radiotherapy protectants, trial
    designs, 282
Radiotracers, in PET
    imaging, 301
Raf-1, as drug target, 10
Randomized phase II trials, as
    proof-of-concept, 351
Ras protein
    as drug target, 12–13
    in growth factor-induced
        mitogenic signaling, 3
    radiosensitization and clinical
        trials, 400–401
    radiosensitization overview,
        395, 399–400
RDA, *see* Representational
    difference analysis
Receptor occupancy, PET studies,
    303
Receptor tyrosine kinases, in
    growth factor-induced
    mitogenic signaling, 3
Recombinant DNA Advisory
    Committee, gene therapy
    approval, 384

Representational difference
analysis, and DNA
microarrays, 44
Response rates
phase II trials, 270
in regular drug approval,
273–275
Ret, as drug target, 7
Retroviral vectors, and p53
radiotherapy, 401
Rho, as drug target, 12
RNase H digestion-based
screening, antisense
oligonucleotides, 198
Roscovitine, targets for, 11
RR, *see* Response rates
RTKs, *see* Receptor tyrosine
kinases

S

Safety, antisense oligonucleotides,
202
Safety profile, as proof-of-concept,
342–343
SAGE, *see* Serial analysis of gene
expression
SAHA, *see* Suberoylanilide
hydroxamic acid
SAR, *see* Structure-activity
relationship
Sch 44342
catalyst analysis, 95
discovery, 94–95
SCH66336, Ras target, 13
SELDI, *see* Surface-enhanced laser
desorption mass spectrometry
Sequence-walking, antisense
oligonucleotides, 197
Serial analysis of gene expression
and DNA microarrays, 44
microarray database mining, 52
Serine/threonine kinases, *see also*
Cyclin-dependent kinases
as drug targets, 8–12
Serum biomarkers, in proof-of-
concept assessments,
347–348
SHAPES method, in NMR,
123, 126
Signal transduction, cancer
therapeutic evaluation, 308
Single-arm trials, for drug
approval, 280
Single-drug regimens, in active
control trials, 281–282
Skin, in biomarker assays,
255–256

Smac/DIABLO, IAP interactions,
227
SNPs, and pharmacogenetics,
57–58
Software packages
for Affymetrix chips, 47–48
micrroarray overview, 39–40
nylon filter arrays, 46
Spotted arrays, as DNA
microarrays, 48–50
Spotted oligonucleotide arrays,
as DNA microarrays,
50–51
Src homology 2 domain, mass
spectrometry screening, 160
SSH, *see* Subtractive suppression
techniques
ST1571, *see* CGP 57148
1D STD, in NMR, 120–123
Stromelysin, SAR by NMR,
111–112
Structure–activity relationship
by NMR, 111–116
overview, 93–94
SU-5416, clinical study, 320
Suberoylanilide hydroxamic acid,
HDAC targeting, 20
Subtractive suppression
techniques, and DNA
microarrays, 44
Super-Leu-doxorubicin, for tumor
targeting, 87–88
Surface-enhanced laser desorption
mass spectrometry, 73
Surrogate end points
for accelerated drug approval,
277–278
correlation to primary end
point, 348–350
in proof-of-concept
mechanism assessment, 343
scanning assessments, 344,
346–347
serum biomarkers, 347–348
for regular drug approval,
278–280
Surrogate markers
definition, 250–251
necessity, 251
Surrogate tissues
in biomarker assays, 257–258
buccal mucosa cells as,
256–257
peripheral blood mononuclear
cells as, 256
shortcomings, 258
skin as, 255–256
Survivin, 16–17, 224, 228–229

T
T1-weighted imaging, microvessel
studies
analysis methods, 318
anti-angiogenesis/anti-vascular
studies, 320–321
clinical experience, 319–320
pathophysiological basis, 314
quantification, 315–317
validation, 318–319
T2*-weighted imaging,
microvessel studies, 313–314
Tarceva, *see* OSI-774
Targeted agents, definition, 250
Targeted biological end point,
preliminary efficacy trials, 374
Targeted biologic response, phase
I dose-finding trials
dose for minimum, 367–368
dose-response relationship,
368–370
efficacious dose, 368
overview, 367
Target negative groups, in
preliminary efficacy trials, 373
Target positive groups, in
preliminary efficacy trials, 373
Target selection, *see also* Drug
targets
antisense oligonucleotides, 198
Target validation, anticancer agent
validation, 234–235
Taxanes, mass spectrometry
studies, 153–155
Taxol, mass spectrometry studies,
153–155
Telomerase
and anticancer agent validation,
235
as drug target, 17
Thiopurine methyltransferase,
pharmacogenetics, 286–288
Thiotepa, mass spectrometry
studies, 142
[threedimensional]3D
microarrays, as DNA array
technology, 51
Thymidylate synthase
in cancer therapeutic
evaluation, 308
pharmacogenetics, 289–291
Time to disease progression
phase II trials, 270
phase III end point for proof-of-
concept, 340
in regular drug approval,
273–275
and serum biomarkers, 347

Time to treatment failure,
definition, 277
Tissues
for biomarker assays, 255–258
for phase I dose-finding trials,
371–372
Toxicity, hematological, and
TPMT, 287
Toxicology, and gene therapy
development, 382–383
TPMT, *see* Thiopurine
methyltransferase
Transfection, and p53
radiotherapy, 401
2D-Transferred NOE
as HSQC alternative, 116–118
protein-ligand complexes, 132
Transgenic models, in anticancer
agent validation, 243–244
Transporters, pharmacogenetics,
291–292
trastzumamab, development, 5
Trichostatin A, HDAC
targeting, 20
TS, *see* Thymidylate synthase
TSA, *see* Trichostatin A
TTF, *see* Time to treatment failure
TTP, *see* Time to disease
progression
Tumor cells, circulating,
collection, 259
Tumor hypoxia, PET studies, 304
Tumor markers, as clinical end
points, 280
Tumors
and biomarker predictivity, 253
energy metabolism evaluation,
310
Tumor shrinkage, and preliminary
efficacy trials, 374–376
Tumor-specific antigen, in cancer
vaccines, 213–214
Tumor suppressor proteins, and
HIF-1α, 14
Tumor targeting
chemotherapeutics

ADEPT, 84
background, 83–84
cathepsin B-activated prodrugs,
89
and cell surface molecules, 85
enzyme-activated targeting, 85
enzymes for prodrugs, 89–90
fibroblast activation protein
alpha activated
prodrugs, 89
future research, 90
glucuronidase-activated
doxorubicin, 86–87
N-l-leucyl-doxorubicin, 85–86
matrix-metalloprotease
activated prodrugs, 88
passive targeting, 84–85
plasmin-activated doxorubicin,
88
prostate-specific antigen
activated doxorubicin, 87
super-Leu-doxorubicin, 87–88
Tumor tissues, biomarker
evaluation, 258–260
TYMS, *see* Thymidylate synthase
Tyrosine kinases, as drug targets,
4–8

U
UCN-01, *see*
7-Hydroxystaurosporine
UDP-glucuronosyltransferase 1A1,
pharmacogenetics, 292
uPA, *see* Urokinase
Urokinase, as drug target, 18

V
Validation studies
animal models, 243–244
antisense oligonucleotides,
197–198
cassette-dosing, 240–241
high-throughput cell-free
screens, 237–238

hollow fiber assay, 241–242
human tumor xenograft,
242–243
overview, 233–234
pharmaceutical considerations,
241
pharmacodynamics, 244
target validation, 234–235
in vitro cell line models,
238–240
in vivo testing, 240
Vascular endothelial growth
factor
as antibody targets, 209
and radiosensitization, 397–399
Vascular endothelial growth factor
inhibitors, 397–399
Vascular endothelial growth factor
receptors
as antibody targets, 209
as drug target, 6
VEGF, *see* Vascular endothelial
growth factor
VEGFRs, *see* Vascular endothelial
growth factor receptors
Velcade, *see* Bortezomib

W
Wortmannin, and p53
radiotherapy, 401–402

X
Xenografts, human tumor,
242–243
XIAP, and apoptosis, 226
X-ray structures, MMP, 138–139

Z
ZD0473, cell line studies, 239
ZD1839
development, 5
proof-of-concept mechanism
assessment, 343